NMS Surgery

NMS *Surgery*

5th EDITION

Editors

Bruce E. Jarrell, MD, FACS
Vice Dean for Research and Academic Affairs
Professor of Surgery
Department of Surgery
University of Maryland School of Medicine
Baltimore, Maryland

R. Anthony Carabasi, III, MD
Professor of Surgery and Radiology
Director, Division of Vascular Surgery
Jefferson Medical College
Thomas Jefferson University
Philadelphia, Pennsylvania

Question Editor

Eugene Kennedy, MD
Professor of Surgery and Radiology
Jefferson Medical College
Thomas Jefferson University
Philadelphia, Pennsylvania

Wolters Kluwer | Lippincott Williams & Wilkins
Health
Philadelphia • Baltimore • New York • London
Buenos Aires • Hong Kong • Sydney • Tokyo

Acquisitions Editor: Donna M. Balado
Managing Editor: Elizabeth Stalnaker
Marketing Manager: Jennifer Kuklinski
Production Editor: Paula C. Williams
Designer: Doug Smock
Compositor: Aptara, Inc.
Printer: C&C Printing—China

Fifth Edition

Library of Congress Cataloging-in-Publication Data

Surgery / editors, Bruce E. Jarrell, R. Anthony Carabasi III ; question editor, Eugene Kennedy. — 5th ed.
    p. ; cm. — (NMS)
    Includes index.
    ISBN-13: 978-0-7817-5901-4
    ISBN-10: 0-7817-5901-3
  1. Surgery—Examinations, questions, etc. 2. Surgery—Outlines, syllabi, etc. I. Jarrell, Bruce E.
II. Carabasi, R. Anthony. III. Series: National medical series for independent study.
    [DNLM: 1. Surgical Procedures, Operative—Examination Questions. 2. Surgical Procedures,
Operative—Outlines. 3. Surgery—Examination Questions. 4. Surgery—Outlines. WO 18.2 S9601 2007]
    RD37.2.S96 2007
    617.0076—dc22

                                                                                   2007001103

DISCLAIMER

Care has been taken to confirm the accuracy of the information present and to describe generally accepted practices. However, the authors, editors, and publisher are not responsible for errors or omissions or for any consequences from application of the information in this book and make no warranty, expressed or implied, with respect to the currency, completeness, or accuracy of the contents of the publication. Application of this information in a particular situation remains the professional responsibility of the practitioner; the clinical treatments described and recommended may not be considered absolute and universal recommendations.

The authors, editors, and publisher have exerted every effort to ensure that drug selection and dosage set forth in this text are in accordance with the current recommendations and practice at the time of publication. However, in view of ongoing research, changes in government regulations, and the constant flow of information relating to drug therapy and drug reactions, the reader is urged to check the package insert for each drug for any change in indications and dosage and for added warnings and precautions. This is particularly important when the recommended agent is a new or infrequently employed drug.

Some drugs and medical devices presented in this publication have Food and Drug Administration (FDA) clearance for limited use in restricted research settings. It is the responsibility of the health care provider to ascertain the FDA status of each drug or device planned for use in their clinical practice.

To purchase additional copies of this book, call our customer service department at **(800) 638-3030** or fax orders to **(301) 223-2320**. International customers should call **(301) 223-2300**.

Visit Lippincott Williams & Wilkins on the Internet: http://www.lww.com. Lippincott Williams & Wilkins customer service representatives are available from 8:30 am to 6:00 pm, EST.

Contents

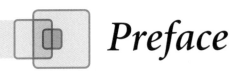

Preface

This is the fifth edition of *NMS Surgery*. Surgery is changing, and we are addressing these changes with this edition. All chapters have been updated. We have given special attention to the first chapter, Principles of Surgical Physiology, and have attempted to clarify this difficult topic. There is also the addition of an online comprehensive examination consisting of new questions and answers and explanations. In keeping with the original purpose of the *National Medical Series for Independent Study*, this book continues to present the core material of the specialty of surgery. The text is not meant to be all-inclusive and does not contain minutiae that we felt would be of little use to the reader. The authors have included not only didactic material but also facts that they find useful in clinical practice. Where controversy exists, we have attempted to present all sides fairly and to indicate factors that are essential in the decision-making process. We have also tried to stress situations in which surgeons and all others involved in patient care must work closely to make the most appropriate decisions regarding treatment.

The study questions and answers and explanations have been carefully updated and provided in both print and electronic format to be used in preparation for the United States Medical Licensing Examination Step 2.

The fifth edition of *NMS Surgery* is written primarily for students and residents in general surgery, but practicing surgeons as well as physicians in other specialties will no doubt find it a useful reference. We hope that all readers will find that the book represents a declaration of the state of surgical art in the year 2007.

Bruce E. Jarrell

R. Anthony Carabasi III

Contributors

Nasim Ahmed, MD
Clinical Assistant Professor
Robert Wood Johnson School of Medicine

William R. Alex, MD
Resident, Division of Cardiothoracic Surgery
Jefferson Medical College
Thomas Jefferson University

Vincent T. Armenti, MD, PhD
Professor of Surgery
Department of Surgery
Temple University School of Medicine
Interim Director
Department of Kidney Transplantation
Temple University Hospital

Andrew H. Borom, MD
Tallahassee Orthopedic Clinic

R. Anthony Carabasi, III, MD
Professor of Surgery and Radiology
Director, Division of Vascular Surgery
Jefferson Medical College
Thomas Jefferson University

W. Bradford Carter, MD
Assistant Professor
Department of Surgery
University of Arizona Health Sciences Center
Attending Surgeon
Department of Surgery, Section of Trauma
University Medical Center
Tucson Medical Center

Karen A. Chojnacki, MD, FACS
Assistant Professor
Department of Surgery
Thomas Jefferson University
Department of Surgery
Thomas Jefferson University Hospital

Murray J. Cohen,MD
Professor and Interim Chair
Department of Surgery
Jefferson Medical College
Thomas Jefferson University

Herbert E. Cohn, MD
Anthony E. Narducci Professor of Surgery and
Vice Chairman
Department of Surgery
Thomas Jefferson University

Bruce L. Dalkin, MD, FACS
Associate Professor of Clinical Urology
Department of Surgery
University of Arizona College of Medicine

Paul J. DiMuzio, MD
Associate Professor
Department of Surgery
Thomas Jefferson University

Richard N. Edie, MD
Professor of Surgery
Jefferson Medical College
Thomas Jefferson University
Attending Surgeon
Thomas Jefferson University Hospital

John L. Flowers, MD
Attending Surgeon
Greater Baltimore Medical Center
Baltimore, Maryland

James S. Gammie, MD
Associate Professor of Surgery
Division of Cardiac Surgery
Department of Surgery
University of Maryland School of Medicine

Diane R. Gillum, MD
General Surgery
Breast Specialty Care of South New Jersey and
    Pennsylvania

Scott D. Goldstein, MD
Associate Professor
Department of Surgery, Division of Colon and
    Rectal Surgery
Jefferson Medical College
Director, Division of Colon and
    Rectal Surgery
Thomas Jefferson University Hospital

Allan J. Hamilton, MD
Professor of Surgery
Division of Neurosurgery
Department of Surgery
University of Arizona College of Medicine

Bruce E. Jarrell, MD, FACS
Vice Dean for Research and Academic Affairs
Professor of Surgery
Department of Surgery
University of Maryland School of Medicine

Steven B. Johnson, MD, FACS
Professor of Surgery
Divisions of Trauma and Critical Care
Department of Surgery
University of Maryland School of Medicine

Mark B. Kahn, MD
Associate Professor or Surgery
Jefferson Medical College
Thomas Jefferson University

John C. Kairys, MD
Assistant Professor of Surgery, Director of
  Graduate Medical Education
Department of Surgery
Jefferson Medical College
Attending Surgeon
Department of Surgery
Thomas Jefferson University Hospital

Kris R. Kaulback, MD, FACS
Assistant Professor
Department of Surgery
Thomas Jefferson University
Assistant Professor
Department of Acute Care Surgery
Thomas Jefferson University Hospital

Robert A. Larson, MD, RVT
Assistant Professor of Surgery
Division of Vascular Surgery
Thomas Jefferson University
Attending Surgeon
Division of Vascular Surgery
Thomas Jefferson University Hospital

Matthew E. Lissauer, MD
Assistant Professor of Surgery
Divisions of Trauma and Critical Care
Department of Surgery
University of Maryland School of Medicine

Joseph V. Lombardi, MD
Assistant Professor of Surgery
Department of Surgery
Thomas Jefferson University Hospital

Paul A. Mancuso, MD, FACS, FASCES
Staff Surgeon
Colon and Rectal Surgery Chapter
Department of Colon and Rectal Surgery
Florida Hospital

David J. Maron, MD, MBA
Assistant Professor of Surgery
Division of Colon and Rectal Surgery
University of Pennsylvania
Assistant Professor of Surgery
Division of Colon and Rectal Surgery
Penn Presbyterian Medical Center

John H. Moore, Jr., MD
Clinical Associate Professor of Surgery
Division of Plastic Surgery
Jefferson Medical College
Attending Plastic Surgeon
Thomas Jefferson University
Consulting Surgeon
Magee Rehabilitation Hospital

Michael J. Moritz, MD
Chief, Transplant Services
Lehigh Valley Hospital

David D. Neal, MD, FACS
Clinical Associate Professor of Surgery
Department of Surgery
University of Arizona College of Medicine

D. Bruce Panasuk, MD
Clinical Assistant Professor of Surgery
Department of Surgery
Thomas Jefferson University
Associate Progream Director of the General
  Surgery Residency
Christiana Care Health System

Pauline K. Park, MD
Associate Director, Division of Trauma and
  Surgical Critical Care
Assistant Professor, Department of Surgery
Jefferson Medical College
Thomas Jefferson University

Vincent D. Pellegrini, Jr., MD
James L. Kernan Professor and Chair
Department of Orthopaedics
University of Maryland School of
  Medicine

Kandace Peterson, MD
Eastern Virginia School of Medicine

Benjamin Philosophe, MD, PhD
Associate Professor
Department of Surgery
Head, Division of Transplantation
University of Maryland Medical System

John S. Radomski, MD, FACS
Chairman, Department of Surgery
Our Lady of Lourdes Medical Center

Ernest L. Rosato, MD
Associate Professor of Surgery
Division Director, General Surgery
Department of Surgery
Thomas Jefferson University

Francis E. Rosato, Jr., MD
Department of Surgery
Jefferson Medical College
Thomas Jefferson University

John T. Ruth, MD
Professor of Clinical Orthopaedic Surgery
Department of Orthopaedic Surgery
University of Arizona
Active Staff
Department of Orthopaedic Surgery
University Medical Center

Robert T. Sataloff, MD, DMA, FACS
Professor and Chairman, Associate Dean for
    Clinical Academic Specialties
Department of Otolaryngology–Head and
    Neck Surgery
Drexel University College of Medicine
Clinical Service Chief
Department of Otolaryngology–Head and
    Neck Surgery
Hahnemann University Hospital

Joseph R. Spiegel, MD, FACS
Associate Professor of Otolaryngology, Head
    and Neck Surgery
Jefferson Medical College
Thomas Jefferson University
Vice Chairman, Department of Otolaryngology,
    Head and Neck Surgery
Graduate Hospital

Eric Strauch, MD
Associate Professor of Surgery
Division of Pediatric Surgery
Department of Surgery
University of Maryland School of Medicine

Nick Tarola, MD
Surgical Resident
Jefferson Medical College
Thomas Jefferson University

Jerome J. Vernick, MD
Clinical Professor of Surgery
RWJ School of Medicine
Chief of Surgery
Jersey Shore University Medical Center

Charles W. Wagner, MD
Professor of Surgery and Pediatrics
University of Arkansas for Medical
    Sciences/Arkansas Children's Hospital
Medical Director, Arkansas Regional Organ
    Recovery Agency

James A. Warneke, MD
Associate Professor
Department of Surgery, Section of Surgical
    Oncology
University of Arizona College of Medicine
General Surgery Program Director
Department of Surgery
University Medical Center

Ronald J. Weigel, MD, PhD
Professor and Vice Chairman
Department of Surgery
Jefferson Medical College
Thomas Jefferson University

Martin E. Weinand, MD, FACS
Professor of Surgery
Division of Neurosurgery, Department of
    Surgery
University of Arizona College of Medicine
Chief and Program Director
Division of Neurosurgery, Department of
    Surgery
Arizona Health Sciences Center

Michael S. Weinstein, MD, FACS
Assistant Professor
Department of Surgery
Thomas Jefferson University
Assistant Professor
Department of Surgery
Thomas Jefferson University Hospital

Howard H. Weitz, MD
Professor, Department of Medicine
Jefferson Medical College
Co-Director
Jefferson Heart Institute

Hunter Wessels, MD
Professor of Urology
Department of Urology
Harborview Hospital
University of Washington School of
    Medicine

David A. Zwillenberg, MD
Clinical Associate Professor of
    Otolaryngology
Assistant Professor of Pediatrics
Thomas Jefferson University

PART **I**

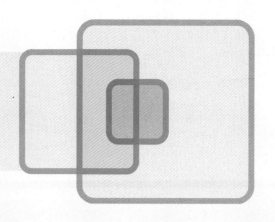

Introduction

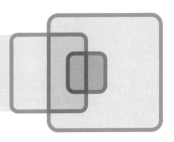

chapter 1

Principles of Surgical Physiology

STEVEN B. JOHNSON · MATTHEW LISSAUER

I   **FLUID AND ELECTROLYTES**

  A   Normal body composition

1. **Body water** accounts for 50%–70% of body weight. There is a higher percentage of water in young people, thin people, and men and a lower percentage of water in older people, obese people, and women.
   a. **Compartments**
      (1) **Intracellular.** This compartment accounts for 30%–40% of body weight (**65% of total body water**). Most of the body's intracellular water is contained in skeletal muscle cells (**lean body mass**); very little water is contained in adipose cells, which accounts for the lower percentage of water in obese and older people.
      (2) **Extracellular.** This compartment accounts for about 20%–30% of body weight (**35% of total body water**) and includes two compartments.
         (a) **Interstitial.** Accounts for 15%–20% of total body weight (**25% of total body water**).
         (b) **Intravascular.** Accounts for 5% of total body weight (**10% of total body water**). Maintenance of the intravascular compartment is essential to survival and is the primary consideration of fluid resuscitation for maintenance of homeostasis. Many regulatory mechanisms exist to supplement this compartment from the interstitial first, then intracellular compartments if the intravascular volume drops.
   b. **Two-thirds rule.** Determining the exact size of any one of the three compartments is virtually impossible because of the variation among patients (and within the same patient). The two-thirds rule is a simple method of approximating the value: Total body water comprises approximately two thirds of body weight; of this, two thirds is intracellular, and one third is extracellular (i.e., intravascular and interstitial). Of the extracellular portion, two thirds is interstitial, and one third is intravascular. This rule provides a starting point for assessment of the normal patient but must always be adjusted to the clinical presentation of the patient.
   c. **Blood volume.** Knowing how to calculate the approximate blood volume for a patient is important. Using the two-thirds rule, approximately 7% of body weight is blood volume. This calculation is based on lean body mass for a 70-kg man, and it varies depending on the patient's age, gender, and body habitus.
2. **Electrolyte composition.** Electrolytes determine the amount of water that exists in any one space at any time. Electrolyte concentrations in the intracellular space differ compared with the extracellular spaces (i.e., intravascular and interstitial). **Water follows electrolytes across cell membranes to equilibrate osmolality.**
   a. **Compartments.** (Table 1-1) Due to ion pumps (principally Na^+/K^+ ATPase), intracellular and extracellular compartments have different electrolyte compositions.
      (1) **Intracellular.** Principal osmotic cation is potassium. Has higher concentration of osmotic particles than extracellular compartment thus allowing water to flow into the cell, creating turgidity.
      (2) **Extracellular.** Interstitial and intravascular composition nearly but not quite identical. Principal osmotic cation is sodium.

TABLE 1-1   Electrolyte Composition

Intracellular Electrolytes	Interstitial Compartment	Intravascular Compartment	Compartment
Anions			
Bicarbonate (HCO_3^-)	10 mEq/L	30 mEq/L	27 mEq/L
Phosphate (PO_4^{3-})	Combined	Combined	Combined
Sulfate (SO_4^{2-})	150 mEq/L	3 mEq/L	3 mEq/L
Chloride (Cl^-)	—	114 mEq/L	103 mEq/L
Cations			
Calcium (Ca^{2+})	—	3 mEq/L	5 mEq/L
Magnesium (Mg^{2+})	40 mEq/L	2 mEq/L	3 mEq/L
Potassium (K^+)	150 mEq/L	4 mEq/L	4 mEq/L
Sodium (Na^+)	10 mEq/L	144 mEq/L	142 mEq/L
Organic acids	—	5 mEq/L	—
Various proteins	40 mEq/L	1 mEq/L	16 mEq/L
Totals*	200 mEq/L	153 mEq/L	154 mEq/L

*Total of osmotically active particles.

   b. Maintaining equilibrium. Change in osmotic pressure in one compartment causes water to redistribute from the other compartments until equilibrium is returned.

B **Maintenance**

   1. **Water.** The amount of water required by a person depends on the person's weight, age, gender, and illness.

   a. **Methods of calculating water requirements.** There are numerous methods to calculate normal water needs for maintenance.

   (1) **The amount of body water excreted can be used as an estimate.** The major water loss from the body is through urine production. Generally, 0.5 mL/kg/hour is the minimum needed to excrete the daily solute load. The next highest daily water loss is insensible loss (i.e., sweat, respiration, stool; see I D 2), which is estimated as 600–900 mL/24 hour. In a 70-kg man, minimal water maintenance would be:

   (70 kg × 0.5 mL/kg/hour × 24 hr) + 750 mL/24 hour = 1590 mL/24 hours.

   Again, this is the minimum and does not take into account any excess loss such as fever, which will increase the insensible loss.

   (2) **Body weight can be used to estimate the maintenance fluid requirement.** This method is often used for pediatric patients because their body weights vary widely. Estimations are 100 mL/kg/day or 4 mL/kg/hour for the first 10 kg of body weight, 50 mL/kg/day or 2 cc/kg/hr for the second 10 kg of body weight, and 20 mL/kg/day or 1 cc/kg/hour for each additional kilogram of body weight. An easy way to remember this is the first 20 kg of weight = 60 cc/hour (10 kg × 4 cc/kg/hour + 10 kg × 2 cc/kg/hour) and then 1 cc/kg/hour above that, so a 50-kg person = 90 cc/hour.

   (3) **A given amount of water per kilogram of body weight can be used to determine water maintenance requirements.** The value used for this method is generally 35–40 mL/kg/day, adjusted higher or lower based on age (the elderly often require only 15 mL/kg/24-hour maintenance).

   (4) **A given amount of fluid can be used, regardless of body weight.** Standard orders often include fluid rates of 100–125 mL/hour as a maintenance rate. Again, this should be adjusted for individual patients.

   b. **Evaluating maintenance rates.** Different patients not only have different maintenance needs, but replacing water or removing excess water may be of concern (see I C 1). Because water requirements vary, the most important aspect of water administration is evaluating the adequacy for the patient in question. Fever, environmental temperature, and respiratory rate can increase insensible loss and increase maintenance requirements. Simple

TABLE 1-2   Electrolyte Composition of Gastrointestinal Secretions

Organ	Volume/day	Na$^+$ mEq/L	K$^+$ mEq/L	Cl$^-$ mEq/L	HCO$_3^-$ mEq/L
Stomach	1–5 L	20–150	10–20	120–140	Nil
Duodenum	0.1–2 L	100–120	10–20	110	10–20
Ileum	1–3 L	80–140	5–10	60–90	30–50
Colon	0.1–2 L	100–120	10–30	90	30–50
Gallbladder	0.5–1 L	140	5	100	25
Pancreas	0.5–1 L	140	5	30 (higher when not stimulated)	115 (lower when not stimulated)

methods in the noncritically ill population to monitor adequacy of fluid administration include:

  (1) **Urine output variations.** If urine output is high (i.e., >1 mL/kg/hour), then less water may be required. If urine output is low, more water may be required, or further assessment may be necessary.

   (a) **Elderly.** As people age, muscle mass and the number of glomeruli decrease.

     (i) The elderly should not be expected to produce as much urine as younger people.

     (ii) Elderly patients can be pushed into congestive heart failure (CHF) by continued water administration for a low urine output. If responses to fluid bolus or increased infusion is not seen, further diagnostic workup is needed to assess fluid, renal, and circulatory status.

  (2) **Tachycardia.** Can be a sign of dehydration, low intravascular volume.

 c. **Adjusting fluid rates for individual patients.** Based on the above clinical parameters, rates can be adjusted up or down. Besides providing maintenance fluids, replacing lost fluids or removing excess fluids should alter the fluid rate and composition given to patients (Table 1-2).

  (1) **Injury, illness, and surgery.** Can result in fluid losses due to blood loss, third spacing, insensible losses from diarrhea, fever, etc. Providing more than calculated maintenance fluid to replace losses (such as 1.5 or 2 times maintenance) is necessary. Adequacy of the rate can be judged from the above criteria.

   (a) The natural response in patients stressed by injury, illness, or surgery is to retain sodium and water due to the hormonal response to stress—antidiuretic hormone (ADH) secretion—therefore, urine output may be misleading in these patients.

  (2) **Total parenteral nutrition and maintenance fluids.** Patients receiving total parenteral nutrition (TPN) generally should have their maintenance fluid calculated as part of their nutrition. A patient on TPN who does not have ongoing abnormal water losses rarely requires additional fluids.

  (3) **Diuresis.** Patients who require diuresis already are overloaded with fluid, and intravenous (IV) fluids should be held. However, there may be electrolyte or nutritional aspects of fluid administration that require water as a carrier for other substances during diuresis.

2. **Sodium.** Normally, people take 150–200 mEq of sodium daily. Much is excreted in the urine. If the body needs to conserve sodium, it can reduce renal excretion to less than 1 mEq/day. Daily homeostasis is easily maintained with 1–2 mEq/kg/day.

3. **Potassium.** The normal daily intake of potassium is approximately 40–120 mEq/day, with about 10%–15% excreted in urine. An amount of 0.5–1 mEq/kg/day is appropriate to maintain homeostasis.

4. **What is a good maintenance IV?** (Table 1-3) Using the previous estimates for a 70-kg male, the weight formula for IV fluid would equal 110 cc/hour. Minimal sodium maintenance would require 70–140 mEq/day, and minimal potassium requirements would be 35–70 mEq/day. In 0.5% normal saline (NS), there is 77 mEq/L sodium, and if one adds 20 mEq/L of potassium, then using 0.5% NS with 20 mEq/L KCL at 110 cc/hour would equal about 2.6 L of fluid, 200 mEq of sodium, and 52 mEq of potassium . . . pretty close!

TABLE 1-3 Electrolyte Concentration in Various Intravenous Fluids

Fluid	Na$^+$ mEq/L	K$^+$ mEq/L	Mg^{++} mEq/L	Ca^{++} mEq/L	Cl$^-$ mEq/L	Lactate mEq/L	Osmolarity mOsm/L
Normal saline (0.9% NaCl)	154	0	0	0	154	0	308
1/2 normal saline (0.5% NaCl)	77	0	0	0	77	0	154
Hypertonic saline (3% saline)	513	0	0	0	513	0	1027
Lactated Ringer's	130	4	0	2.7	98	28	525
Plasmalyte*	140	5	3	0	98	0	294

*Plasmalyte also contains 27 mEq/L acetate and 23 mEq/L gluconate.

C Water and electrolyte deficits and excesses

1. **Water**
   a. **Hypovolemia:**
      (1) **Signs of acute volume loss** include tachycardia, hypotension, and decreased urine output.
      (2) **Signs of gradual volume loss** include loss of skin turgor, thirst, alterations in body temperature, and changes in mental status.
      (3) **Replacing water deficits.** Acute deficits should be replaced acutely; chronic deficits should be replaced more slowly, with half of the deficit replaced over the first 8 hours and the rest in 24–48 hours. In the case of hypernatremia with hypovolemia, do not allow the sodium concentration to drop more than 0.5–1 mEq/hour.
   b. **Hypervolemia:** Well tolerated in healthy patients—they will just urinate the excess.
      (1) **Signs of acute hypervolemia:** Acute shortness of breath, tachycardia.
         (a) **Complications** of acute CHF can arise in patients with **poor cardiac function** given too much fluid acutely. Therefore, it is important to monitor these patients closely.
      (2) **Signs of chronic hypervolemia:** Peripheral edema, pulmonary edema.
         (a) Diuresis may be needed in some patients to reduce volume.

2. **Sodium: close relationship to volume status**
   a. **Hyponatremia**
      (1) **Definition and categories.** *Hyponatremia* is defined as a serum sodium level of 130 mEq/L or less. The first step in diagnosis and treatment is to assess the osmolar and volemic state.
         (a) **Hyperosmolar:** Dilutional hyponatremia from hyperglycemia, mannitol infusion, or presence of other osmotically active particles.
         (b) **Normo-osmolar: Pseudohyponatremia.** Hyperglycemia, hyperlipidemia, and hyperproteinemia interfere with the lab measurement of sodium.
         (c) **Hypo-osmolar: True hyponatremia.**
            (i) **Hypovolemic:** Most common. Normally, hypovolemia leads to ADH secretion and the inability to excrete free water. Intake of free water via thirst mechanisms or infusion of hypotonic solution leads to hyponatremia. **Total body sodium usually is low.**
            (ii) **Hypervolemic: Total body sodium usually is high.** The pathology is often related to low cardiac output (the kidneys see less blood flow, and free water is not excreted) or hypoalbuminemic (e.g., cirrhosis) or other edematous states where salt (renin-angiotensin system) and free water (ADH) cannot be excreted by the kidneys.
            (iii) **Euvolemic:** Could be either of the states above, or more frequently in the perioperative patient, **syndrome of inappropriate antidiuretic hormone (SIADH)**

secretion. ADH secretion can be stimulated by the stress response to trauma and surgery. Free water is retained.

(2) **Symptoms.** Acute hyponatremia is associated with acute cerebral edema, seizures, and coma. Chronic hyponatremia is well tolerated to Na concentrations of 110 mEq/L. Symptoms generally include confusion/decreased mental status, irritability, and decreased deep tendon reflexes.

(3) **Diagnosis and categorization.** Clinical exam and lab determination of osmolar state are often enough for diagnosis, but if in doubt, especially with hypo-osmolar hyponatremia, check urine osmolarity and sodium concentration.

    (a) **Hypovolemic, hypo-osmolar hyponatremia:** Urine osmolarity high; Na low.

    (b) **Hypervolemic, hypo-osmolar hyponatremia:** Similar picture.

    (c) **Euvolemic, hypo-osmolar hyponatremia:** Urine osmolarity high; urine Na high.

(4) **Treatment**

    (a) **Hyperosmolar:** Correct hyperglycemia or source of other actively osmotic particles.

    (b) **Normo-osmolar:** No treatment required.

    (c) **Hypo-osmolar:**

        (i) **Hypovolemic:** Treat with isotonic fluid infusion to restore fluid and sodium deficit. **If sodium deficit is severe, sodium replacement can be considered.**

       (ii) **Hypervolemic:** Treat underlying medical cause first, then usually salt and free water restriction are appropriate.

      (iii) **Euvolemic:** First determine if the true cause is one of the above states. If SIADH is the cause, free water restriction usually is enough. Do not replace salt because this can paradoxically lower serum sodium, as the kidney excretes sodium and conserves water.

b. Hypernatremia

(1) **Definition and categories.** *Hypernatremia* is defined as a serum sodium level greater than 150 mEq/L.

    (a) **Hypovolemia:** Hypernatremia almost always represents a volume deficit, with more free water being lost than sodium.

    (b) **Hypervolemia:** Iatrogenic infusion of too much sodium can lead to hypervolemic hypernatremia, but this is rare.

(2) **Symptoms** can include those of volume depletion (e.g., tachycardia, hypotension) as well as other signs of dehydration (e.g., dry mucous membranes, decreased skin turgor). Lethargy, confusion, and coma result from water shifts from the intracellular compartment in the central nervous system (CNS).

(3) **Diagnosis/etiology: Diagnosis usually simple.** High serum sodium with obvious fluid losses. In surgical patients, fluid losses may be due to:

    (a) **Extrarenal:** Insensible losses due to fever, mechanical ventilation, burns, diarrhea, or measured losses from the gastrointestinal (GI) tract.

    (b) **Renal:** Excessive free water excretion.

        (i) Osmotic diuresis from hyperglycemia or mannitol administration.

       (ii) High output dilute urine from the polyuric phase of acute tubular necrosis (ATN).

(4) **Treatment.**

    (a) **Hypovolemic:** Need to replace volume. Calculate free water deficit first:

Water deficit = 0.6 × body weight in kilograms × (pNA/140 − 1)

    Then, calculate one half the deficit to replace in the first 8 hours and the remainder in the next 16 hours. If the hypovolemic state is severe (i.e., shock), initial therapy can be isotonic fluids for resuscitation. If the deficit is less severe, or once perfusion adequate, it is permissible to switch to 0.5% NS or dextrose 5% in water (D5W).

    (b) **Hypervolemia:** If the patient's total body water is increased, first decrease the amount of sodium administered. If sodium intake (e.g., antibiotics, TPN, drips in normal saline) cannot be decreased, free water can be infused to lower the serum sodium level, but this does not decrease the total body sodium or water content. Diuretics can be used as well.

3. **Potassium**
   a. **Hypokalemia**
      (1) **Definition.** In general, K^+ <3.5 mEq/L is considered hypokalemia. *Severe hypokalemia* is defined as a serum potassium level of 3 mEq/L or less. In some patients (cardiac), it is desirable to have a K^+ >4.0.
      (2) **Symptoms** of hypokalemia include ileus and weakness. Weakness can become profound enough to cause respiratory failure. Profound depletion results in cardiac dysrhythmias. Electrocardiogram (ECG) changes can become manifest below a K^+ of 3.0 mEq/L and include, in increasing order of severity, T-wave flattening or inversion, depressed ST segments, development of U waves, prolonged QT interval, and finally ventricular tachycardia.
      (3) **Diagnosis/etiology: Diagnosis simple and based on blood chemistry.** More important is to understand the cause. Rarely found in healthy humans with a normal diet and normal kidneys. Causes can be one of four categories.
         (a) **Renal:** Diuretics, vomiting (renal excretion of K^+ to preserve Na^+), renal tubular acidosis.
         (b) **Extrarenal:** Diarrhea, burns.
         (c) **Intracellular shift:** Insulin, alkalotic state.
         (d) **Medical disease:** Hyperaldosteronism, Cushing syndrome
      (4) **Treatment.** If symptoms are severe, administer as much potassium IV as needed to reduce symptoms. If symptoms are mild or nonexistent, can infuse 20 mEq/hour maximum in the unmonitored patient and 40 mEq/hour in the monitored patient. A general rule of thumb is that every 10 mEq of K^+ should raise serum concentration by 0.1 mEq/L. Administration for more chronic conditions can be via enteral supplements. Remember, serum K^+ concentration is not an indication of total body stores of potassium. If the serum K^+ is repleted but total body stores are low (as most K^+ is intracellular), serum K^+ will drop again quickly as K^+ shifts into cells.
   b. **Hyperkalemia**
      (1) **Definition.** *Hyperkalemia* is usually defined as a serum potassium level of 6 mEq/L or greater.
      (2) **Symptoms** of hyperkalemia are rare but include diarrhea, cramping, nervousness, weakness, and flaccid paralysis. More often, cardiac dysrrhythmias are manifest before other symptoms become severe. ECG changes include **peaked T waves**, widened QRS, and can eventually degenerate into ventricular fibrillation.
      (3) **Diagnosis/etiology.** There are numerous causes, among the more common are the following:
         (a) **Renal failure:** With inappropriate consumption/administration of K^+
         (b) **Extracellular shift:**
            (i) Rhabdomyolysis
            (ii) Massive tissue necrosis
            (iii) Metabolic acidosis
            (iv) Hyperglycemia
         (c) **Medical disease:**
            (i) Addison's disease
      (4) **Treatment.** Can be divided into two phases. Acutely, the goal is to stabilize the cardiac membrane and to lower serum potassium. Once the patient is stabilized, maneuvers to remove K^+ permanently from the system should be instituted.
         (a) **Acutely symptomatic patient:**
            (i) **IV calcium** stabilizes cardiac myocyte membranes and can prevent dysrhythmias. One gram of Ca^{++} gluconate IV is a standard dose.
            (ii) **Glucose/insulin** administration can be used to shift K intracellularly acutely and quickly. One ampule of D_{50} with 10 units of regular insulin is often enough.
            (iii) **Bicarbonate** administration will also shift K^+ intracellularly.
         (b) **To remove K^+ and to lower body stores permanently:**
            (i) Ion-exchange resin: used either by mouth (PO) or rectally. Binds K^+ in the colon, facilitating excretion.

        (ii) Lasix: Only use if kidneys are able to excrete, and keep a close eye on other electrolytes and fluid balance.

        (iii) Dialysis.

4. Chloride

  a. Hypochloremia

    (1) Definition. *Hypochloremia* is defined as a chloride level less than 90 mEq/L.

    (2) Symptoms. Usually associated with dehydration or hypokalemia due to vomiting or other GI loss.

    (3) Diagnosis/etiology. Hydrochloric acid (HCl) from the stomach is lost from vomiting, leading to low chloride and a buildup of bicarbonate. This causes a metabolic alkalosis. It is often associated with paradoxic aciduria. Normally, the kidneys would excrete bicarbonate to reduce pH; however, as the dehydration becomes more severe, the kidneys drive to retain sodium predominates. The kidney excretes both K^+ and H^+ to conserve sodium.

    (4) Treatment for hypochloremia involves replacement of the chloride and volume deficit with sodium chloride solutions and replacement of K^+ as needed.

  b. Hyperchloremia

    (1) Definition. *Hyperchloremia* is defined as a plasma chloride level greater than 110 mEq/L.

    (2) Cause. The most common cause of hyperchloremia in surgical patients is the administration of large amounts of chloride in IV solutions. The chloride content in normal saline (154 mEq/L) is significantly higher than that in plasma (90–110 mEq/L).

    (3) Diagnosis/etiology. Excess chloride in relation to sodium decreases the strong ion difference, thereby causing more water to dissociate and more H^+ ions to be present.

    (4) Treatment. Decrease the amount of chloride being infused. Look for all sources (IV antibiotics) in addition to IV fluids. If isotonic saline needs to be administered for other reasons, consider sodium bicarbonate or sodium acetate to reduce chloride load. For instance, 1/2 NS with 1.5 amps $NaHCO_3$/L has 152 mEq/L Na, only 77 mEq/L chloride and 75 mEq/L bicarbonate.

5. Calcium

  a. Hypocalcemia

    (1) Definition. *Hypocalcemia* is defined as a serum calcium level less than 8 mg/dL.

    (2) Symptoms of hypocalcemia include neuromuscular irritability, with perioral and extremity numbness that may progress to carpopedal spasm and tetany. Premature ventricular contractions can be reduced with treatment of hypocalcemia as prolongation of the QT interval is noted in these patients. Classic signs include Trousseau and Chvostek's signs.

    (3) Diagnosis/etiology. There are numerous causes of hypocalcemia. In surgical patients, the suppression of normal parathyroid function from adenomatous or hyperplastic glands that have been removed is most common, followed by accidental removal of the parathyroids during thyroid surgery. In critically ill patients, lactate, citrate from blood transfusions, and numerous medicines can cause hypocalcemia.

    (4) Treatment.

      (a) Asymptomatic outpatients can be supplemented orally. An investigation into possible medical causes (vitamin D deficiency, renal failure, excess dietary phosphate, or other causes of hyperphosohatemia, etc.) should be investigated.

      (b) Symptomatic patients need to be monitored and treated. If symptoms are mild, large doses of oral calcium are often adequate (especially in the postparathyroidectomy patient). Severely symptomatic patients should be repleted with IV calcium until symptoms resolve and an appropriate oral regimen is tolerated.

  b. Hypercalcemia

    (1) Definition. *Hypercalcemia* is defined as a serum calcium level of 10.5 mg/dL or greater.

    (2) Symptoms. Fatigue, confusion, nausea, vomiting, diarrhea, dehydration, and anorexia are common. When related to hyperparathyroidism, renal calculi and ulcer disease are more common.

    (3) Diagnosis/etiology. Hypercalcemia has a multitude of causes.

(a) **Endocrine:** primary hyperparathryoidism (most common), thyrotoxicosis.
(b) **Malignancy:** Most common, up to 20%–30% of cancer patients will have hypercalcemia. Osteolytic lesions, PTHrP-secreting lesions are often the cause.
(c) **Granulomatous disease:** sarcoidosis, tuberculosis.
(d) **Medications:** excess calcium ingestion, vitamin D toxicity, thiazide diuretics.
(e) **Other causes:** renal disease, milk alkali syndrome, familial hypocalciuric hypocalcemia.

(4) **Treatment.** Severe, symptomatic hypercalcemia is a medical emergency and requires immediate treatment. The first line of therapy is aggressive isotonic resuscitation, leading to diuresis and excretion of calcium. If unsuccessful, lasix can be added, assuming that the patient is fluid resuscitated. The next line of therapy is medical. Medications to stop osteoclastic activity is the mainstream. Bisphonates, calcitonin, and steroids are all used. Mithromycin is no longer available in the United States.

II ACID–BASE DISTURBANCES

A **Regulatory systems** The human body requires a very narrow pH range of 7.35 to 7.45 to function properly. There are three main systems in the body that maintain the pH within normal parameters. CO_2, strong ions, and weak acids.

1. **Carbon dioxide:** CO_2 **production can exceed 15,000** mmol/day from metabolic processes. The lungs effectively excrete this entire amount to maintain normal CO_2. If PCO_2 increases, water dissociates and HCO_3^- and H^+ form based on the Henderson-Hasselbach equation, thus decreasing pH. The reverse happens for lower PCO_2 concentrations. Either a loss of bicarbonate or again in protons can cause acidosis.

   Henderson-Hasselbach: $pH = pK \times \log [HCO_3^-/(0.03 \times PCO_2)]$

2. **Strong ions** are defined as ions that completely dissociate in water. Na^+, Cl^-, Ca^{++}, Mg^{++}, K^+ are examples. In a pure salt solution, ion concentrations are equal, and pH is neutral. In plasma, however, there are more cations that anions. To maintain electrical neutrality, water dissociates, H^+ is excreted, and HCO_3^- concentration increases, hence a pH of 7.4 and not 7.0.

3. **Weak acids.** This includes the buffering systems of the body. Weak acids can exist as negatively charged molecules or accept H^+ and exist uncharged. They include proteins and phosphates.

B **Acidosis** The body's pH decreases when the PCO_2 increases, the concentration of HCO_3^- increases, the concentration of strong anions increases, or the concentration of weak acids increases. A pH less than 7.35 is considered pathologic, but patients can compensate from the following disorders of acid–base metabolism or have a mixed picture with a pH in the normal range.

1. **Respiratory acidosis.** Decreased ventilation relative to CO_2 production leads to increased CO_2 concentration.
   a. **Causes**
      (1) The most common cause of respiratory acidosis is **decreased alveolar ventilation.**
         (a) Respiratory depression
            (i) Drugs (narcotics)
            (ii) Alcohol
            (iii) Excess sedation/analgesia (opioids, benzodiazepines)
            (iv) Anesthetic agents
         (b) Central nervous disorders
            (i) Stroke
            (ii) Trauma
         (c) Physical
            (i) Iatrogenic (too-low minute ventilation on the ventilator)
            (ii) Intrisic lung disease (acute respiratory distress syndrome [ARDS], chronic obstructive pulmonary disease [COPD])
            (iii) Respiratory muscle weakness (myasthenia gravis, spinal cord injury)

(2) Increased CO_2 production. Excess administration of carbohydrate via enteral or parenteral administration can increase the respiratory quotient and increase production of CO_2. Most patients can compensate, but if the patient is weak or mechanically ventilated he or she may not be able to do so. Also, if the overfeeding is severe, compensation may be difficult.

  b. Treatment. The primary method of treatment for respiratory acidosis is to increase alveolar ventilation. In cases of drug overdose, this may be accomplished with appropriate reversing agents. However, most of the causes of alveolar hypoventilation require intubation with mechanical ventilation to clear CO_2 and return the pH to normal values.

2. Metabolic acidosis results either from a loss of HCO_3^-, an accumulation of strong anions, or accumulation of weak acids.

  a. Causes

    (1) Weak acid accumulation. All will have anion gap, etiology includes loss of HCO_3^- to maintain electric neutrality.

      (a) Acid accumulation can occur because of **renal failure** and the inability of the kidneys to clear the acids that are by-products of metabolism.

      (b) Lactic acidosis. A common cause of metabolic acidosis is lactic acid. Lactic acid could be considered a strong anion, however, as it nearly completely dissociates in water. It usually results from inadequate tissue perfusion, leading to anaerobic metabolism.

      (c) Diabetic ketoacidosis. Acetoacetate and β-hydroxybutarate are weak acids.

      (d) Toxins. Polyethylene glycol, methanol. Methanol is metabolized to formaldehyde and then formic acid.

    (2) Strong anion accumulation. Normal anion gap.

      (a) Hyperchloremic acidosis. Excess chloride induces water to dissociate, H to accumulate and pH to drop.

    (3) Loss of bicarbonate. Normal anion gap.

      (a) Excess renal excretion of bicarbonate.

      (b) Diarrhea.

  b. Treatment. The primary treatment for metabolic acidosis is correction of the underlying metabolic problem and proper fluid and electrolyte management. Bicarbonate administration should rarely be used unless pH is dangerously low (<7.2) and the underlying defect is in the process of being corrected. If the primary defect is excess loss of bicarbonate (diarrhea, renal tubular acidosis), bicarbonate therapy should be considered as treatment.

C **Alkalosis**

1. Respiratory alkalosis

  a. Causes

    (1) Respiratory alkalosis in the spontaneously breathing patient is caused by an increase in alveolar ventilation and subsequent reduction in CO_2 levels. This situation can be caused by any entity that causes hyperventilation, such as anxiety, pain, shock, sepsis, toxic substances (salicylate poisoning), or CNS dysfunction. Some processes causing hypoxia or intrapulmonary shunts can lead to hypocarbia and alkalosis (think of pulmonary embolus!). In the mechanically ventilated patient, iatrogenic overventillation is frequent.

  b. Treatment of respiratory alkalosis includes decreasing minute ventilation and allowing the CO_2 levels to return to normal. Turning down the ventilator and increasing sedation and analgesia will correct nearly all cases. Most cases are self-limited, however, as patients cannot keep excessive ventilatory drive for extended periods.

2. Metabolic alkalosis. pH increases to over 7.45, and the HCO_3^- level is greater than 26 mEq/L.

  a. Causes. The most common cause of metabolic alkalosis is loss of gastric contents. HCl and large volumes of water are lost. To compensate for dehydration, the kidney excretes H to conserve Na (paradoxical aciduria). The concentration of strong anions is reduced, and water is less likely to dissociate, further decreasing H and increasing pH. Other causes of metabolic alkalosis include drugs that limit renal excretion of HCO_3^-, such as steroids and diuretics. Overadministration of alkali (e.g., in ulcer therapy), acetate in TPN that is used to replace

TABLE 1-4   Acid–base Disorders

Disorder		PCO$_2$	HCO$_3^-$	pH	Expected Compensation
Respiratory acidosis	Acute	↑	Normal	<7.35	1–4 mEq/L HCO$_3^-$ for each 10 mm Hg PCO$_2$ rise
	Compensated	↑	↑	7.35–7.40	
Respiratory alkalosis	Acute	↓	Normal	>7.45	2–5 mEq/L HCO$_3^-$ for each 10 mm Hg PCO$_2$ drop
	Compensated	↓	↓	7.40–7.45	
Metabolic acidosis	Acute	Normal	↓	<7.35	Expected PCO$_2$ = 1.5(HCO$_3^-$) + 8
	Compensated	↓	↓	7.35–7.40	
Metabolic alkalosis	Acute	Normal	↑	>7.45	Expected PCO$_2$ = 0.7(HCO$_3^-$) + 20
	Compensated	↑	↑	7.40–7.45	

other anions, and citrate in transfused blood that is converted to CO_2 and water and then to HCO$_3^-$ by the kidneys can also result in metabolic alkalosis.

    b. Treatment. In almost all forms of metabolic alkalosis, a chloride and volume deficit is present. The first step is to stop the loss of chloride and to replace the water and chloride with isotonic sodium chloride and potassium supplementation.

  D **Diagnosing acid–base disorders based on the blood gas (Table 1-4)**

    1. Look at the pH.

      a. pH less than 7.35 equals acidosis.

        (1) Look at HCO$_3$. If low, metablic acidosis is indicated; if high, may have mixed disorder or compensating response to respiratory acidosis.

        (2) Look at PCO$_2$. If high, respiratory acidosis is indicated; if low, compensating for metabolic acidosis or a mixed picture is present.

      b. pH greater than 7.45 equals alkalosis.

        (1) Look at HCO$_3$. If high, metabolic alkalosis is indicated; if low, may be compensating for respiratory alkalosis or a mixed picture is present.

        (2) Look at PCO$_2$. If low, respiratory alkalosis is indicated; if high, may be compensatory for metabolic alkalosis or a mixed picture is present.

      c. pH normal. Could be a mixed disorder or compensated disorder (or no disorder!). For example, if HCO$_3^-$ is low, and PCO$_2$ is high, either mixed respiratory acidosis and metabolic alkalosis or full compensation of one for the other is indicated.

III   **COAGULATION**

  A **Mechanisms of hemostasis**   Hemostasis can be divided into three phases.

    1. Primary hemostasis

      a. Platelet adherence: The first step in controlling hemorrhage is platelet adherence to the injured vessel. Glycoprotein receptor Ib in conjunction with von Willebrand factor mediates this step.

      b. Platelet activation: Activated platelets produce thromboxane A$_2$ and other vasoconstrictors, which reduce blood flow through the injured vessel. Glycoprotein IIb/IIIa is expressed, which promotes platelet-platelet adhesion (fibrinogen required) and formation of the **platelet plug.**

    2. Clot formation. Tissue factor exposed due to vessel injury or in response to inflammation begins the clotting cascade. The cascade has traditionally been taught as having an intrinsic and extrinsic pathway; however, in vivo, both pathways act in concert. The extrinsic system usually begins the cascade with amplification by mechanisms of the intrinsic system. Components of the extrinsic system also activate the intrinsic system.

      a. Extrinsic pathway: Tissue factor binds factor VII and activates it (VIIa). VIIa subsequently activates factor X. Xa then converts prothrombin to thrombin.

    b. Intrinsic pathway: In general, factor XIIa activates XI then XIa activates IX. IX then converges with the extrinsic pathway by activating factor X. This pathway can be initiated either by exposure to a negatively charged surface (exposed collagen from a damaged vessel) or thrombin itself activates factor IX.

    c. Both pathways converge at factor X: Factor Xa then mediates activation of thombin with factor Va as a cofactor. Thrombin mediates fibronogen conversion to fibrin. Finally, factor XIIIa mediates cross linking of fibrin.

  3. Regulation and fibrinolysis. The coagulation system is a cascade, meaning that each step in the process is a point of multiplication. Each activated intermediate factor is able to activate many of the factors in subsequent steps. Additionally, thrombin itself acts as a positive feedback loop by activating factor IX. The fibrinolyic system acts to keep the coagulation cascade under control and to remove clot once healing has started to occur.

    a. Tissue factor pathway inhibitor (TFPI) may inhibit TF-VIIa complexes.

    b. Protein C and protein S degrade factors V and VIII.

    c. Antithrombin III inhibits thrombin-Xa complexes.

    d. Fibronolysis: tissue-type plasminogen activator (t-PA) and urokinase-type plasminogen activator (uPA) mediate conversion of plasminogen to plasmin, which cleaves fibrin.

  B **Coagulopathy** A good history and physical should elucidate any problems with coagulation.

Lab studies should not be routinely ordered preoperatively in a patient with a negative history. Where the history is positive, studies can then be used to confirm and specify the diagnosis.

  1. History

    a. Include any perceived coagulopathy by the patient.

      (1) Bruising

      (2) Petechia

      (3) Easy bleeding/nosebleeds

      (4) History of unexplained bleeding from other procedures (dental/surgical)

    b. Family history

    c. Risk factors

      (1) Liver disease

      (2) Renal failure

  2. Physical. Evidence of bruising, petechia, etc.

  3. Lab evidence

    a. Platelet count: Normal is 150,000–400,000/mL blood.

      (1) Keep >50,000/mL for general hemostasis.

      (2) <10,000/mL at risk for spontaneous bleeding.

      (3) >100,000 necessary if major surgery is being planned.

    b. Bleeding time: measure of platelet function. Disorders of platelet function include:

      (1) Uremia

      (2) Drugs (aspirin, clopidogrel, gp IIa/IIB inhibitors)

      (3) von Willibrand's disease

      (4) Low count

    c. Prothrombin time: measures extrinsic cascade. Since factors II (thrombin), VII, and X are produced by the liver, PT represents a good measure of vitamin K–dependent coagulation factors. It is therefore used to monitor warfarin therapy. The international normalized ratio (INR) is a normalization factor to equate lab values between labs.

    d. Activated partial thromboplastin time (aPTT): measures intrinsic cascade. Useful for following patients on IV unfractionated heparin therapy.

    e. Thrombin time: tests the conversion of fibrinogen to fibrin via thrombin. Is elevated when fibrinogen is depleted or nonfunctioning and in the presence of heparin.

  C **Specific hypocoagulopathic states**

    1. First, ensure bleeding is not a surgical complication. Do not necessarily blame postoperative bleeding on coagulopathy until surgical bleeding is ruled out.

2. **Liver disease:** In severe liver disease, hepatocytes cannot manufacture clotting factors. PT/INR is elevated. Treatment includes replacing factors with **fresh frozen plasma (FFP)** or **cryoprecipitate** and medical management of the liver disease.

3. **Renal disease:** Uremia causes platelet dysfunction. Treatment can be with ddAVP, which causes release of von Willibrand's factor or FFP.

4. **Disseminated intravascular coagulopathy (DIC):** Microvascular coagulation due to inflammation from sepsis, trauma, and other severe insults leads to a consumption of factors. Lack of factors then leads to coagulopathy. The mainstay of treatment includes treating the underlying cause. Replacement of factors may exacerbate the condition, and paradoxically, anticoagulant therapy may be beneficial.

5. **Consumption/dilution:** due to severe trauma, sepsis, major surgery, and their attendant fluid resuscitation. Treatment involves correcting the underlying cause and replacing factors with FFP. Other mechanisms include **hypothermia and acidosis** in trauma patients, both of which inhibit proper clotting mechanisms.

6. **Medically induced**
   a. **Aspirin:** permanently binds COX and prevents platelet aggregation.
   b. **Plavix:** blocks ADP-mediated platelet aggregation.
   c. **Gp IIb/IIIA inhibitors:** inhibit platelet aggregation.
   d. **Warfarin:** blocks vitamin K–dependent liver synthesis of factors II, VII, IX, and X.
   e. **Heparin and heparinoids:** augment antithrombin-III function.
   f. **Fibrinolytics:** tPA, urokinase, etc., mediate fibrinolysis.

7. **Hemophilia**
   a. **Hemophilia A:** congenital deficiency of factor VIII. Treament is factor replacement. FFP can be used in emergent situations.
   b. **Hemophilia B:** congenital deficiency of factor IX. Treatment is factor replacement. FFP can be used in emergent situations.

8. **von Willibrand disease:** The most common congenital coagulopathy (1%–2% of adults). Deficiency of von Willibrand factor. Treatment is intranasal DDAVP in mild cases, IV DDAVP prior to surgical procedures, and cryoprecipite or FFP in emergencies.

9. Others
   a. **Autoimmunity**
   b. **Cancer**
   c. **Snake venom**

10. **Recombinant activated factor VII (rfVIIa)** is approved for use in treating hemophiliacs who have developed antibodies to factors VIII and IX. While not replacing the missing factors, supraphysiologic doses of rfVIIa cause a thrombin burst and clot to form. This fact has led to it being studied for various other coagulopathies, including warfarin therapy when quick reversal is needed (i.e., intracranial bleed) and in severe traumatic coagulopathy.

D **Specific hypercoagulable states**

1. **Surgical patients.** Many surgical patients are at risk for DVT. Risk factors include major abdominal or pelvic surgery; orthopedic surgery, especially lower extremity; trauma, especially spine, pelvis, and lower extremity fractures; prolonged immobilization; cancer; smoking; obesity; central line placement; and others. Because of these risks, *always assess your patients for thromboembolic prophylaxis!* Heparin 5000 units subcutaneously q8° or low-molecular-weight heparin such as Lovenox 30 mg subcutaneously BID or 40 mg subcutaneously QD should be used. In patients who have contraindications to prophylaxis (intracranial bleed), inferior vena cava filters should be considered.

2. **Congenital risk factors.** Suspect if patients have multiple DVT or DVT without another known risk factor. Treatment is usually anticoagulation.
   a. **Protein S deficiency**
   b. **Protein C deficiency**
   c. **Factor V leiden mutation**
   d. **Antithrombin III mutations**

IV **PACKED RED BLOOD CELL TRANSFUSION THERAPY**

A **Risks of transfusion**   The longer blood is stored, the worse it performs. Over time, cells lyse, and 2,3-DPG levels fall, causing oxygen to bind more avidly.

1. **Febrile reactions/allergic:** most common immune reaction. Usually related to either cytokines or donor leukocyte or other contaminants, or a mild antibody response. Usually self-limited. Can be prevented by leukodepletion and pretransfusion antipyretics.

2. **Electrolyte disturbances**
   a. **Hyperkalemia:** Lysed cells can cause hyperkalemia.
   b. **Hypocalcemia:** Citrate in stored blood can bind calcium.

3. **Coagulapathy:** pRBC's do not contain clotting factors or platelet. Large volume transfusion without these other products can cause a coagulopathy.

4. **ABO incompatibility:** Etiology is intravascular immune reaction, leading to clumping and lysis of red cells with mismatched blood. Signs and symptoms include hemoglobinuria, fever, chills, coagulopathy, renal failure, and circulatory collapse. Prevention is key by ensuring correct patient identity and blood type to avoid these **preventable reactions.**
   a. **ABO system:** Patient's blood type is based on the ABO antigen system. Type A people make antibodies to B antigens, and type B to A. Type AB makes no ABO antibodies and hence is a universal recipient. Type O makes antibodies to A and B, and so these patients are universal donors (the cells have no ABO antigens), but they can receive only type O blood.

5. **Delayed hemolytic reaction:** Usually takes 3–7 days to manifest. Signs and symptoms include fever, malaise, hyperbilirubinemia, and decreasing hematocrit. Usually related to minor antibody systems such as the Rh system. Usually but not always preventable with recipient antibody screening. Treatment includes hydration and supportive care.
   a. **Rh system:** A system of minor antigen-antibody that can cause reactions.

6. Disease transmission: Many virsues can be transmitted by blood. Prior to screening, this was a real risk. With modern screening methods such as nucleic acid technology screening, the risk is reduced but is not negligible.
   a. **HIV:** Estimated to be 1:800,000.
   b. **Hepatitis C:** Estimated to be 1:600,000.
   c. **Hepatitis B:** Estimated to be 1:220,000.
   d. **Others:** Risks less known but have been described. HTLV 1 and 2, West Nile virus, Creutzfeld-Jacob disease.

7. **Immunosuppression:** Probably the most significant but least thought of risks of blood transfusion. Negative outcomes include:
   a. **Morbidity** in the form of increased **infectious complications,** including ventilator-associated pneumonia.
   b. Possible increases in **cancer recurrence** following potentially curative surgery.
   c. **Increased mortality** in intensive care unit (ICU) patients.

B **Indications for transfusion**   Given the negative effects of transfusions, who should be transfused?

1. **Prior transfusion triggers** of a hemoglobin of 10 mg/dL or hematocrit of 30% were artificially set. Transfusion decisions should be based on individual patient circumstances. In general, it is safe to let the Hgb drop to 7 mg/dL and even lower in healthy, young individuals.
   a. **Cardiac patients: May need higher Hgb levels, but this is debatable.**
   b. **Trauma patients:** Exsanguinating patients should be given blood as resuscitation, as their Hgb is still high acutely, but they are losing blood and its attendant oxygen-carrying capacity.
      (1) **Patients in class 3 hemorrhagic shock** (1500 cc blood loss, signs of hypotension should be transfused empirically).
   c. **ICU patients:** If needed, direct measurements of oxygen delivery and extraction can help to guide transfusion therapy.

    d. General patients: Only transfuse if symptomatic. Signs and symptoms from anemia can include tachycardia, tachypnea, and acidosis.

C **Alternatives to transfusion**

    1. **If the time of blood loss is known: elective surgery**

        a. **Autologous banked blood**

        b. **Epoetin alpha:** Can increase the hematocrit preoperatively to help avoid transfusion.

        c. **Use of auto-transfusion technology:** Recycle blood lost during surgery.

        d. **Acute normovolemic hemodilution:** Once a patient is anesthetized, blood can be removed, stored, and replaced with crystalloid or colloid to maintain euvolemia. This has two benefits. Blood lost during surgery has a lower hematocrit, and therefore fewer red cells are shed. Those that are shed can be replaced with fresh (not stored) autologous blood.

        e. **Directed donor: risk of virus transmission lower, but similar risks of immunomodulation and other reactions**

        f. **Hemostatic agents** prevent blood loss in the first place!

            (1) **FFP/cryoprecipitate** for patients with coagulopathy.

            (2) **DDAVP** for patients with platelet dysfunction.

            (3) **Aprotinin:** inhibits serine proteases, including plasmin.

            (4) **Lysine analogs:** ε-aminocaproic acid.

            (5) **Topical hemostatics:** fibrin glue.

    2. **Acute unexpected blood loss**

        a. **Autotransfusion** may still be an option, if readily available.

            (1) **Emergent aortic rupture**

            (2) **Trauma laparotomy**

        b. **Quick prevention of further blood loss is the best therapy.**

    3. **Chronic anemia**

        a. **Accept a lower Hematocrit.**

        b. **Epoetin alpha.**

V   SURGICAL WOUNDS AND WOUND HEALING

A **Classification of surgical wounds** Wounds are typically classified according to **how the wound was made, how much contamination is present,** and **the expected rate of infection.** There are four categories that determine if a wound should be closed or left opened and allowed to heal by secondary intention.

    1. **Clean wounds** are incisions made under sterile conditions for a nontraumatic procedure that does not enter the bowel, tracheobronchial tree, genitourinary system, or the oropharynx and is not infected. A wound created to repair a hernia is an example of a clean wound. The infection rate for clean wounds should be less than 2%, and all clean wounds should be closed primarily.

    2. **Clean-contaminated wounds** are similar to clean wounds, except that the bowel, tracheobronchial tree, genitourinary system, or the oropharynx was entered. There is minimal contamination of the wound, and the biliary, respiratory, and genitourinary tracts do not have any evidence of active infection. Routine cholecystectomy, colon resection, appendectomy, and bladder surgery are examples of the a clean-contaminated wound. The infection rate for clean-contaminated wounds should be 3%–4%, and these wounds are typically closed primarily unless other risk factors are present.

    3. **Contaminated wounds** are similar to the clean and clean-contaminated wounds, except that there is major contamination of the wound during the performance of the procedure (e.g., gross spillage of stool from the colon; infection in the biliary, respiratory, or genitourinary system). Fresh traumatic wounds fall into this category. Examples of this type of wound are a bowel obstruction with enterotomy and spillage of contents and acute cholecystitis with pus in the gallbladder and spillage of pus. The infection rate for contaminated wounds should be 7%–10%, and these wounds are often left open.

    4. **Dirty and infected wounds** occur when an established infection is present before a wound is made in the skin. Examples of this type of wound include an appendiceal abscess, traumatic

wound with contaminated devitalized tissue, and perforated viscus. The infection rate for dirty wounds is 30%–40%, and these wounds should be left open.

B **Normal wound-healing phases** The normal process of acute wound healing has sequential phases, eventually resulting in re-establishment of tensile strength. Depending on the extent of infection and hematoma present, this process can be delayed. Prolonged delayed healing for whatever reason can convert an acute wound into a chronic nonhealing wound.

1. **Coagulation phase.** Immediately following injury, the injured tissue and blood vessels release local mediators intended to stop bleeding and begin healing. This results in vasoconstriction and increased permeability of local blood vessels, formation of fibrin, and platelet aggregation.

2. **Inflammatory phase.** The injured tissue of the wound develops an inflammatory response comprised of cellular, vascular, and mediator changes. In the absence of infection or other factors that delay wound healing, the inflammatory phase lasts approximately 1 week.

   a. **Cellular.** The increased vascular permeability and chemokine release that occurs during the coagulation phases allows recruit and wound infiltration by polymorphonuclear cells (PMN). Activation and localization of PMN cells allows removal of necrotic tissue and debris, including invading microbes. After 24–48 hours, macrophages replace PMNs as the predominant inflammatory cells in the wound. Macrophages are necessary for remodeling of the extracellular matrix to facilate subsequent fibroblast migration and activity. Epithelial cell migration begins to occur, resulting in bridging across apposed tissue edges. Typically, by 48–72 hours, epithelial bridging and adherence across surgically closed wound edges has occurred.

   b. **Vascular.** Disruption of blood vessels makes the wound area hypoxic. Hypoxia and the wound growth factors stimulate the growth of blood vessels (angiogenesis) from existing capillaries into the hypoxic area of the wound, making healing more effective. The initial hemostatic vasoconstriction converts to inflammatory vasodilitation, promoting fluid and mediator influx into the wounded region. These changes account for the localized erythema and edema associated with the wound.

   c. **Mediators.** Injured cells, platelets, and recruited inflammatory cells release multiple mediators that promote wound remodeling and healing. Tissue growth factors such as transforming growth factor-beta and platelet-derived growth factor promote influx of fibroblasts. Chemokines and cytokines promote recruitment of additional inflammatory cells. Matrix metalloproteinases facilitate breakdown of injured tissue and remodeling of the wound.

3. **Proliferative phase.** As the inflammatory response in the wound subsides, fibroblasts that have migrated into the wound begin to form collagen, and wound strength begins to increase. Until collagen is synthesized in the wound, the strength of the wound is provided by the fibrin in the clot or scab. As myofibroblasts that have migrated into the wound multiply and begin to contract, the wound gets smaller. Wound contraction continues for several weeks or until the skin edges meet. Collagen production in the wound continues for approximately 3 weeks, then returns to the normal level.

4. **Wound remodeling.** Approximately 3 weeks after the injury occurred, the wound is essentially healed, and a scar is formed. During this period, the initial collagen that was synthesized during the proliferative phase in a haphazard way is degraded, and new collagen is synthesized and aligned along lines of stress. This newly directed collagen also has more cross links between collagen strands, which increases the strength of the scar. The scar tissue reaches approximately 90% of the original tissue strength in an average of 6 weeks; however, scar remodeling can continue for years.

C **Acute wound care of surgical and nonsurgical wounds**

1. **Hemostasis** must be obtained before wounds can be cleaned, debrided, and closed.

   a. If adequate hemostasis is not obtained, a wound hematoma will develop. The presence of a wound hematoma extends the inflammatory phase of wound healing and increases the risk of wound infection. If the hematoma becomes infected, the inflammatory phase becomes more pronounced (i.e., all of the components of the inflammatory phase are increased), and healing is delayed.

    b. Hemostasis in most wounds can be obtained by direct pressure and by careful ligation of larger bleeding vessels. If hemostasis cannot be obtained by these methods because of congenital or acquired coagulopathy, the wound should be tightly packed until the coagulopathy can be controlled.

  2. Cleansing

    a. For optimum wound healing, all **nonviable tissue, foreign bodies, and gross infection** should be removed. The inflammatory phase is shortest with a clean, viable wound, which leads to the best strength and cosmetic result.

      (1) The first step is to remove all foreign material visible to the naked eye. In some instances, foreign material may be ground into the tissue (e.g., gravel in a motorcycle accident victim), and the tissue may need to be resected. Gross material can usually be removed with forceps, scalpels, or scrub brushes.

      (2) After foreign material is removed, nonviable tissue should be resected. Sharp debridement of grossly nonviable tissue is the most common approach. If tissue viability is questionable, then additional techniques such as IV fluorescein or tissue oxygen tension measurement can be utilized. These methods are cumbersome to perform during the acute care of a wound. A common and acceptable alternative is to not immediately debride the questionable tissue and to reinspect it in 24–48 hours.

    b. After grossly visible foreign material and necrotic tissue have been removed, removal of **microscopic debris** and **bacteria** is beneficial. This is most commonly accomplished with 0.9% normal saline irrigation under pressure. Copious irrigation of the wound with nontoxic solutions reduces bacterial load without damaging underlying viable tissue. Use of betadine solutions, typically used for cleaning and disinfecting skin, should be avoided on open wounds because they can cause tissue damage and impede wound healing.

D **Methods of wound closure**

  1. Primary closure. In wounds with a low risk for infection (i.e., clean wounds, clean-contaminated wounds, and minimally contaminated wounds), closure allows for the best result. In primary closure, the skin edges are approximated shortly after the wound is incurred, using any acceptable closure method.

  2. Secondary intention. Wounds with a high risk for infection and wounds that are already infected are usually left open and allowed to heal by epithelialization and wound contraction. Epithelialization begins at the skin edges and concentrically progresses to the middle of the granulation bed. Infection and necrotic tissue will prevent granulation and wound epithelialization from occurring. Very large wounds can heal with good cosmetic results. Occasionally, wounds are too large for the epithelium to migrate over, and a skin graft is needed for final closure or to accelerate closure.

  3. Delayed primary closure. Wounds that are heavily contaminated (e.g., perforated appendicitis) are likely to develop an infection if closed primarily, and therefore the skin should be left open. After 3–5 days, the wound may be primarily closed if no residual contamination is obvious. Good wound care and the body's natural defenses decrease the bacterial count sufficiently to allow closure during this time frame. However, if the wound is closed earlier or later, bacterial counts will be higher and sufficient to cause a wound infection.

  4. Skin grafts. A skin graft is a split portion of the skin containing the epidermis and part of the dermis obtained from a normal skin donor site. Split-thickness skin grafts are used on well-granulating, noninfected, nonepithelialized superficial wounds to provide epithelial coverage for healing. Eventually, full incorporation including vascularization of the graft to the wound site occurs, allowing complete skin coverage. The thickness of these grafts is usually 15 microns but can vary from very thin (0.05 inch) to full-thickness epidermis and dermis. The thicker the graft, the more durable it is, and the less the wound contracts. However, the thicker the graft, the less frequently the donor site will heal or be able to be used again. As a result, very thick graft donor sites have more scarring and delayed healing, and there is less donor skin available for large wounds (e.g., a burn).

  5. Flaps. Some wounds have underlying tissue loss in addition to skin loss and require replacement of this tissue for adequate return of function or cosmesis. These tissues require vascularization and must be transferred with their blood supply to survive.

a. **Rotation flap.** The flap retains its normal blood supply but is mobilized to a different location to fill in a defect.

b. **Free flap.** The tissue is completely removed from its normal blood supply and is moved to another area of the body, where the blood vessels are reanastomosed to the local blood supply. This method allows tissues, such as a great toe, to be moved to the hand to replace a lost thumb.

E Wound dressings

1. **Sutured wounds.** It takes approximately 48 hours for the epithelium to migrate across a sutured wound and seal it. If there is no further drainage at that time, dressings are not needed except where necessary for patient comfort. Until the wound seals, it needs a dressing to absorb any drainage and to wick it away from the wound so that bacteria do not accumulate and multiply.

2. **Open wounds**

a. In the **open wound that has necrotic debris,** the purpose of the dressing is to help clean and debride the wound. The most common form of dressing for this type of wound is the **wet-to-dry dressing.** In this dressing, a thin piece of gauze is moistened, placed in the wound, and covered with dry dressing. The gauze is then allowed to dry. When the dry gauze is removed, it takes necrotic debris with it. The disadvantage of this type of dressing is that viable tissue is also removed, which slows wound healing.

b. A **clean open wound** or a dirty wound that has been cleaned by wet-to-dry dressings is most effectively treated with **wet-to-wet dressings,** in which the gauze is not allowed to dry. This keeps the tissues moist, does not debride healthy tissue, removes exudates, and enhances wound healing.

c. **Large, open dermal wounds** (e.g., skin graft donor sites) or large abrasions heal by epithelial migration and need a dressing that protects the underlying dermis and promotes epithelial migration. Dressings such as nonadhering petroleum-base impregnated gauze allow formation of a scab under the gauze, which facilitates epithelial migration. Nonpermeable dressings also can be applied to these wounds to keep the dermis moist and to allow epithelialization to occur faster.

F Factors that inhibit wound healing

1. **Malnutrition.** Malnutrition interferes with wound healing, and the more severe the malnutrition, the greater the deleterious impact on healing. In malnourished patients undergoing elective or urgent operation, a short course (10–14 days) of nutrition preoperatively improves wound healing. Nutritional support should be continued postoperatively in the malnourished patient. For the well-nourished patient undergoing surgery, nutritional support is not necessary for proper wound healing if normal nutrition will resume within 5–7 days. Preoperative albumin is the best guide to the risk of malnutrition-related wound healing impairment.

2. **Diabetes.** Hyperglycemia inhibits virtually all aspects of the body's inflammatory response and immune system, which leads to increased susceptibility to infection and decreased wound strength. If the patient's glucose is well controlled (80–120 mg/dL), the wound healing should be virtually normal. Therefore, aggressive control of blood glucose during the perioperative period is essential. These patients may require frequent blood glucose determinations and a constant insulin infusion.

3. **Jaundice.** Jaundice has been associated with inhibiting normal wound healing. This may be due either to the hyperbilirubinemia or the underlying liver dysfunction causing jaundice and other hepatic-related metabolic abnormalities . In jaundiced patients, an operation should be performed if the patient's liver function is good and the operation will solve the jaundice (e.g., common bile duct stone, obstructive pancreatic cancer). If the jaundice is caused by liver dysfunction (e.g., hepatitis, cirrhosis), operations should be delayed until the underlying liver dysfunction is improved.

4. **Uremia.** Like jaundice, urea has been associated with an inhibitory effect on wound healing that is related to azotemia or the renal dysfunction (e.g., malnutrition, renal toxin accumulation). The best approach in patients with renal failure who need an operation is to aggressively dialyze them if the operation is urgent or to place them on a dialysis schedule (usually three times per

week) to eliminate the toxic substances. With adequate dialysis, the inhibitory effects of uremia on wound healing can be reversed.

5. **Steroids** inhibit all phases of wound healing, and these inhibitory effects are potentiated by malnutrition. If possible, steroids should be avoided in surgical patients. Azathioprine, an immunosuppressive drug frequently used in transplantation, affects wound healing in a similar manner as steroids. Cyclosporine, another immunosuppressive drug frequently used in transplantation, does not appear to adversely affect wound healing.

6. **Chemotherapy.** All chemotherapeutic agents have been shown to have inhibitory effects on wound healing, but these effects appear to be clinically insignificant. Chemotherapeutic agents mainly inhibit the early phase of wound healing. Therefore, if chemotherapy is necessary shortly after an operation, it should be delayed for at least 7–10 days.

7. **Smoking** leads to a state of chronic hypoxia and vasoconstriction. With long-term smoking, there is also associated vascular disease. These factors combine to inhibit wound healing. To avoid wound healing compromise, patients should be encouraged to stop smoking well in advance of surgery. It is especially important for a patient to stop smoking for microvascular procedures, such as flap procedures in plastic surgery. Carboxyhemoglobin levels can be checked to ensure that the patient has stopped.

G **Factors that promote wound healing**

1. **Vitamin A.** In animal studies, vitamin A has been found to aid wound healing defects induced by steroids, chemotherapy, diabetes, and irradiation. Vitamin A promotes inflammation and the production of collagen in the wound. The dose for vitamin A can be as high as 500,000 units/day for 3 days followed by 50,000 units/day for 2 weeks.

2. **Hyperbaric oxygen** has been used in patients with nonhealing wounds, such as osteomyelitis and those induced by radiation. However, the role of hyperbaric oxygen is unclear.

VI   NUTRITION AND THE SURGICAL PATIENT

A **Sources of energy**   Humans store and utilize three sources of caloric energy: fat, glucose, and protein. Protein requires conversion to glucose via hepatic gluconeogenesis in order to be used as a caloric fuel source. Glucose can be stored as glycogen and used as a short-term reservoir of energy. The majority of energy is stored as fat and to a lesser degree as protein in the form of skeletal muscle.

B **Requirements**   The body requires protein and caloric needs to met in order for normal metabolic functions to occur. Although protein can be used as a caloric source for energy, adequate protein intake is important for muscle mass maintenance and other protein-dependent, nonenergy-producing processes.

1. **Caloric requirements.** The basal metabolic rate (BMR) is the amount of energy utilized by an unstressed, fasted individual at rest. The resting energy expenditure is the amount of energy utilized by an unstressed, nonfasted individual at rest and is 1.2 times the BMR or approximately 25 kcal/kg/day. The total energy expenditure (TEE) is the actual amount of energy that an individual utilizes and is equal to the resting energy expenditure (REE) multiplied by a stress factor that is determined by the magnitude of hypermetabolic change. The TEE can be increased significantly above the REE by hypermetabolic conditions such as surgery, trauma, sepsis, and burns. Fever increases the TEE approximately 10% for each degree centigrade over normal. Major polytrauma or large burns can increase daily energy expenditure by nearly twice the BMR. The TEE can be increased by voluntary work, such as exercise. Conversely, during starvation, the BMR decreases as the body adjusts to conserve body mass. An accurate measurement of caloric requirements can be performed by indirect calorimetry or the Fick equation.

2. **Protein requirements** are normally very low because each protein molecule has a specific purpose and is therefore not generally available as an energy source. Some protein is lost daily as shed epithelium (e.g., bowel mucosa, skin) and must be replaced, and some protein is metabolized for energy during daily periods of starvation. Generally, daily protein requirements are

only 0.8–1.0 g/kg/day, which is significantly less than the average American eats daily. The amount of protein required to meet catabolic losses is determined by measuring the nitrogen balance (Nitrogen$_{in}$ – Nitrogen$_{out}$). Typically, the nitrogen balance should be slightly positive. A negative nitrogen balance is indicative of inadequate protein intake to meet catabolic losses.

   a. During **starvation,** the body makes every attempt to conserve protein. Because glycogen stores are metabolized within the first 24 hours of starvation, another source of glucose must be found for the tissues that cannot, or usually do not, use fats (i.e., brain cells, red and white blood cells). Proteins are broken down and converted to glucose in the liver by gluconeogenesis to supply the brain and blood cells with glucose. In unstressed starvation, protein catabolism can be prevented by exogenous administration of glucose. During starvation, the brain adapts to use **ketones,** which are produced when fat is metabolized. This decreases the amount of protein that must be metabolized as a glucose source. After all of the available fat is metabolized, protein is degraded at a high rate until the total body protein stores are approximately one half of baseline, at which time death occurs.

   b. During **severe illness,** the body is not able to conserve energy and protein stores as it does during starvation.

      (1) The hormonal milieu increases the BMR, decreases the ability to utilize fats and ketones, and thereby increases the dependence on glucose as an energy source. This glucose can come only from protein that is being degraded and converted to glucose.

      (2) As the degree of illness or injury increases, the **catabolic rate increases** accordingly, leading to a rapid breakdown of protein stores and multiorgan dysfunction, if not checked. During the acute phase of severe illness or stressed starvation, protein catabolism is minimally affected by exogenous administration of glucose.

      (3) Primary treatment in these conditions is to eliminate the underlying cause of the stress response and to provide enough calories and protein to replace metabolic and catabolic losses.

   c. As the **illness begins to subside,** the hormonal milieu changes, which leads to less retention of salt and water and a **change from a catabolic protein environment to an anabolic environment.** The nitrogen balance is positive, meaning that less nitrogen is lost than is administered to the patient. This balance represents protein that is being laid down and thus improvement of the patient's health.

C Evaluation of nutritional status

   1. The **thin, cachectic** patient with hollowed cheeks, no body fat, and very little muscle is obviously in a poor nutritional state. Generally, patients who have acutely lost 10% of their body weight are considered malnourished and need nutritional support.

   2. The **obese** patient and the **well-developed** patient may need as much nutritional support as the patient in a poor nutritional state, depending on the underlying disease process.

   3. Previously well-nourished people generally are able to endure a major operation and 5–10 days of starvation without an increase in morbidity or mortality. If the period of starvation extends beyond 10 days, nutritional support is necessary.

   4. Patients with **severe illness** who will be unable to eat for more than 10 days should receive nutritional support earlier. Because it takes several days for nutritional support to take effect, it is more effective to begin such support if there is any question of nutritional deficit rather than to wait until there is a severe deficit to correct.

D Therapy

   1. Goals. The overall goal of nutritional support is to supply adequate energy in the form of calories and adequate protein for building proteins in the body. A ratio of 150 cal:1 g of protein is optimal, and most forms of nutritional support adhere closely to this ratio. Mineral and trace elements have been extensively researched and are included in most formulas in adequate amounts to prevent deficiencies or toxicities. The average hospitalized patient requires approximately 2000 cal daily and approximately 60 g of protein.

   a. Energy. An adequate amount of energy substrates (i.e., carbohydrates, fats) should be supplied to provide enough calories to allow the tissues of the body to function properly and to decrease protein catabolism. Excessive caloric provision should be avoided. There are four ways to determine caloric requirements:

    (1) Indirect calorimetry: Measures amount of oxygen inhaled minus amount of oxygen exhaled to determine amount of oxygen consumed. Since oxygen consumption (VO_2) measured in mL O_2/min is directly correlated to kcal/day (1 mL O_2/min equals approximately 7 kcal/day), measurement of the amount of O_2 consumed can determine daily caloric requirements.

    (2) Fick equation: Amount of oxygen consumed, and therefore kcal required, is determined by multiplying the cardiac output by the arterial-venous oxygen content difference.

    (3) Harris-Benedict equations: Daily caloric requirements are determined by calculating the REE from gender-based equations using gender, height, weight, and age variable and then multiplying by an estimated stress factor.

    (4) Estimated REE (25 kcal/kg/day) multiplied by an estimated stress factor.

  b. Protein. The approximate protein requirement for most adults is 0.8 g/kg/day or 56 g for the hypothetical 70-kg man. During severe illness with a high catabolic rate, this requirement may increase to 2 g/kg/day of protein or greater. Adequacy of protein nutrition can be determined by the following:

    (1) Nitrogen balance: The majority of catabolized protein is lost as urinary urea nitrogen with approximately 2–4 g of nitrogen lost in stool. Protein grams divided by 6.25 equals nitrogen grams. Amount of nitrogen intake minus nitrogen output should be positive if adequate nitrogen is being administered.

    (2) Additional assessment of adequacy of protein nutrition is the measurement of **visceral proteins** (e.g., albumin, transferrin, prealbumin). Due to the long half-life of albumin, it should only be used as an assessment of malnutrition in outpatient and elective surgery patients. Prealbumin has a shorter half-life and is more reflective of protein nutrition in hospitalized patients.

    (3) **Weight gain** in hospitalized patients is probably the **poorest method of determining adequacy of protein nutritional support.** Because most patients needing nutritional support in the hospital are stressed, they tend to retain water and become edematous. Also, because they are stressed, they will be catabolic and losing lean body weight, despite the increase of their actual body weight from fluid gain. When the acute phase of the stress is over and the patient becomes anabolic, weight gain is a useful measure of nutritional adequacy.

    (4) The **best overall method to determine adequacy of protein nutrition** is to observe the overall condition of the patient, obtain nitrogen balances (maximum of twice weekly), follow visceral proteins (prealbumin twice weekly), and increase protein administration as needed. There is no limit to the maximum amount of protein that can be administered. When more protein is administered than can be utilized, it is burned as an energy source or stored as fat, with the excess nitrogen being excreted as urea. If urea production exceeds the kidneys' ability to excrete the urea, the BUN levels will rise.

2. Enteral nutrition. The preferred route to provide nutrition is enterally. This can be performed by standard oral intake or by administration directly into the stomach or small intestine via a feeding tube. The provision of enteral nutrition maintains gut mucosal integrity and reduces complications. There is compelling evidence that the gut is important in critically ill patients; if unused for even brief periods, the mucosa begins to atrophy and lose its barrier function. This atrophy and loss of barrier function allows bacteria and toxins contained in the bowel to enter the bloodstream (bacterial translocation). Bacterial and toxin translocation has been associated with the systemic inflammatory response syndrome, sepsis, and multiorgan dysfunction. In addition to the translocation phenomenon, the atrophied mucosa is unable to digest food when food is ultimately presented, which leads to further delays in adequate nutrition and to possible infections of the GI tract (e.g., bacterial overgrowth, pseudomembranous colitis).

  a. Formula compositions. When possible, patients should be fed by mouth. However, for many reasons such as critical illness, aspiration risk, depressed mental status, or inability to take adequate calories or protein orally, the oral route may not be feasible. In these situations, the administration of enteral feeding formulas is necessary. These formulas are designed to provide adequate nutrition and may be routine formulas or ones that are highly specialized to serve the nutritional needs of unique patient populations.

(1) Standard formulas provide a balanced calorie-to-protein ratio with approximately 50%–65% of calories from carbohydrates, 10%–20% from proteins, and the remaining calories from fats. Caloric density is approximately 1.0–1.2 kcal per milliliter, and they include the essential fats, minerals, and trace elements. Most patients can be maintained on standard formulas.

(2) Elemental formulas are amino acid or small peptide–based for ease of digestion and lower residue. Patients with short gut syndrome or distal enterocutaneous fistulas benefit from these formulas.

(3) Caloric-dense formulas contain more calories per milliliter than standard formulas, typically 1.5–2.0 kcal per milliliter. Patients needing fluid restriction or very high caloric requirements may benefit from these formulas.

(4) Protein-dense formulas provide increased protein (20%–25% of calories) compared with other formulas and are used for patients with very high protein needs.

(5) Fat-based formulas provide more calories from fats rather than glucose compared with other formulas. These formulas attempt to reduce CO_2 production by altering the respiratory quotient and may be beneficial in patients with compromised minute ventilation such as severe COPD and ARDS patients.

(6) Immunomodulating formulas provide glutamine and typically omega fatty acids in an attempt to enhance immunologic function. Efficacy of these formulas appears limited, and at this time, their use should be infrequent, most commonly in major trauma patients.

  b. Route of administration. Enteral nutrition formulas can be delivered by tubes placed into the GI tract directly (gastrostomy, feeding jejunostomy) or via the nose (nasogastric, nasoduodenal, or nasojejunal). An abdominal radiograph to determine proper tube placement should be obtained prior to starting tube feedings on feeding tubes placed orally or nasally at the bedside. Postpyloric placement (jejunostomy, nasoduodenal, nasojejunal) of feeding tubes are associated with decreased risk of aspiration and earlier tolerance but are more difficult to place, leading to potential delays in initiation of enteral nutrition. Early initiation of enteral nutrition is associated with better tolerance and should be considered even in the immmediate postoperative period following abdominal surgery or trauma.

  c. Rate of administration. Enteral nutrition should be started as continuous infusion via a properly placed gastric or postpyloric tube. A reasonable starting point is full strength at 20 mL/hour and increased by 20 mL/hour every 6–12 hours until the goal rate is obtained or excessive residuals are noted. The goal rate is determined by the patient's caloric needs and the caloric density of the formula. Gastric residual volumes of tube feedings should be checked every 4 hours to determine if excessive residual volumes are present, even if feedings are postpyloric. The volume of residual that is excessive is controversial but typically is considered the greater of 200 mL or four times the rate. If residual volumes are high, the infusion should be stopped and then resumed after 4 hours.

  d. Complications of enteral feeding. Aspiration of gastric contents is the most common complication of enteral nutrition but can be reduced by monitoring residual volumes; postpyloric placement, especially jejunostomy; and maintaining the head of bed up 45 degrees. Bloating, mesenteric ischemia (rare), and diarrhea may occur with tube feedings, but adjustments in composition and rate can minimize these issues. Inadequate nutritional supplementation caused by frequent stopping of the tube feeding is not uncommon unless concerted efforts are made to avoid unnecessary cessations.

3. Parenteral (intravenous) nutrition. Total parenteral nutrition (TPN) allows the provision of adequate nutrition when the GI tract is not able to be utilized due to malabsorption, obstruction, fistulas, or anatomic changes. When possible, nutrition should be provided enterally, and combined enteral and parenteral administration is sometimes beneficial.

  a. Formula composition. TPN solutions should contain components of nutritional requirements, since other sources may not be available. The components are usually composed of various amounts of the following:

  (1) Carbohydrates, predominantly as glucose solution, providing approximately 50% of total calories and causing TPN to have a high osmolality. Partial parenteral nutrition (PPN) contains lower concentration of glucose and is not significantly hyperosmolar.

(2) Amino acid solution, providing approximately 10% of total calories but more importantly providing essential amino acids for protein metabolism, especially in hypercatabolic patients

(3) Fats, administered either continuously or intermittently as lipid emulsion, are necessary to avoid essential fatty acid deficiency. Lipid emulsions also provide the most calories in the smallest volume (fat has the highest caloric density) and produce less carbon dioxide (lowest respiratory quotient), which may be important in patients with volume restrictions or compromised ventilation. Administration of lipid emulsions can lead to hypertriglyceridemia, and levels should be routinely monitored in patients receiving lipids. The fat emulsions can be administered separately (preferred) or mixed with the other components.

(4) Electrolytes, including the monovalent cations, sodium and potassium; the divalent cations, calcium and magnesium; and the anions, chloride and acetate (converted to bicarbonate in the liver), which can be adjusted according to patient needs but must be administered in appropriate combinations to maintain ionic neutrality

(5) Vitamins and trace elements must be provided to avoid acquired deficiencies. Specifically, the exogenous administration of B vitamins, vitamin E/selenium (lipid peroxidation and free radical scavaging), zinc (wound healing, immunity), and chromium (insulin sensitivity) should be considered in patients receiving TPN.

(6) Medications may be incorported into TPN, although this is not often done routinely. Parenteral stress ulcer prophylaxis medications are the most frequently added medications, and after dosing stabilization, insulin may also be added.

b. Route of administration. The usual route of administration of TPN is via a percutaneously placed venous line with the tip located in the superior vena cava. The high osmolality of TPN causes phlebitis and sclerosis if infused into a peripheral vein; therefore, a large, high-flow central vein that quickly dilutes the TPN is necessary. Typically, a subclavian vein approach is used, but peripherally inserted central catheter (PICC) lines and the internal jugular vein approach can be used. Because PPN is less hyperosmolar and therefore does not cause phlebitis, it can be delivered via a peripheral vein.

c. Rate of administration. TPN is typically provided continuously at a rate that provides adequate calories to meet the patient's needs and is dependent of caloric density and degree of hypermetabolism. Frequently, patients are started at half the goal rate for 12 hours before advancing to full rate to avoid severe hyperglycemia. Similarly, some advocate decreasing the TPN rate by half for 6–12 hours prior to stopping to avoid hypoglycemia. Cycling of TPN to allow patients to be disconnected for periods of time during the day can be accomplished but should only be prescribed by experienced personnel and on selected patients.

d. Complications of parenteral nutrition. Complications of parenteral nutrition include those related to line placement (hemothorax, pneumothorax); infections (line sepsis, pneumonia, acalculous cholecystitis); hyperglycemia (associated with increased infection risk and death); hepatic dysfunction; and abnormalities in electrolytes, vitamins, fatty acids, and trace elements. TPN is associated with higher morbidity and mortality than enteral nutrition. In patients unable to receive adequate enteral nutrition, this increased risk is unavoidable but should not be incurred if sufficient enteral nutrition can be provided.

VII THE INTENSIVE CARE UNIT

A **Definition** An ICU is a specialized unit of the hospital that provides close monitoring and care of critically ill patients who require specific care that is not routinely available in other areas of the hospital, including the following:

1. **Airway control (intubation)** (see VII B).

2. **Ventilator support.** The need for mechanical ventilation is the most common reason to be admitted to an ICU, and except for occasional cases of chronically ventilated patients, all patients requiring mechanical ventilation will be managed in an ICU.

3. **Invasive monitoring.** While patients are monitored whenever they are in a hospital, it is only in the ICU that invasive techniques such as arterial lines, pulmonary artery catheters, and intracranial pressure monitoring take place.

4. **Vasoactive and antiarrhythmic drips.** Medications such as dopamine, dobutamine, and nitroprusside are usually only administered in the ICU. It is likely that if patients are intubated, on a ventilator, their condition will be such that they will require a vasoactive drip of some sort. In some cases, low doses of these medications will be administered in a regular hospital ward, but large doses that need to be changed frequently to keep the patient in homeostasis will have to be administered in the ICU.

5. **Intensive patient care.** The acuity of a patient's condition may require close nursing and physician observation and management, which can only be provided in an ICU setting where one nurse cares for only one or two patients at a time and physicians are present at all times in the unit. Appropriate patients for the ICU are those with acute hypoxia and respiratory failure, organ dysfunctions, active fluid and medication resuscitations, and extensive wounds.

B Airway control

1. **Intubation.** The placement of an artificial airway to prevent airway obstruction or to provide mechanical ventilation is referred to as endotracheal intubation. An artificial airway can be placed translaryngeally, either orotracheal or nasotracheal, or it can be placed directly into the trachea by an incision in the lower anterior neck, referred to as a tracheostomy. When intubation is required emergently and cannot be performed translaryngeally, then a cricothyroidotomy should be performed for airway control. The decision to intubate a patient by whichever route is a critical decision with serious consequences if performed too late. An assessment of airway control and the need for endotracheal intubation should be performed early and repeated frequently based on the acuity of the patient. There is no simple way to accurately make the decision to intubate a patient. In general, the assessment should include the following parameters. If these show a definite need for intubation, then intubation is necessary and should be performed.

   a. The **respiratory rate** is the most simple to assess. The normal respiratory rate is 12–16 breaths per minute (bpm). If a patient's respiratory rate is over 40 bpm, then there is a need to be intubated. If a patient is breathing 30–40 bpm, some therapy must be initiated to get the respiratory rate below 30 bpm or the patient will tire and go into respiratory failure (most humans cannot sustain respiratory rates of 30 bpm or greater for very long without fatigue). Respiratory rates of 20–30 bpm are usually tolerated but are definitely abnormal and must be watched closely. Respiratory rates on the low end of the spectrum are almost always caused by some neurologic disorder (e.g., alcohol, drugs, head injury), and these will determine if intubation is needed.

   b. **Respiratory effort** represents the work of breathing that the patient is performing. Patients exerting a significant effort as characterized by use of accessory respiratory muscles, difficulty speaking in full sentences, forceably exhaling, or uncomfortably inhaling should be considered to be in need of intubation. If left to progress without intervention, these patients become overly tired and somnolent with progressive hypoventilation potentially leading to respiratory arrest.

   c. **Tidal volume** is the amount of air moved in and out of the lungs with each normal breath. The normal volume is 5 mL/kg. Of this 2–3 mL/kg is dead space that does not contribute to gas exchange. Tidal volume can be measured at the bedside relatively easily but is typically estimated by observing the extent of air movement that a patient can accomplish. The tidal volume should not be much below 5 mL/kg or there will be virtually no gas exchange, and the patient should be intubated and ventilated. Failure to have an adequate tidal volume or respiratory rate can lead to hypercapnia. An acute increase in PCO_2 with respiratory acidosis due to alveolar hypoventilation is an indication for endotracheal intubation and mechanical ventilatory support.

   d. **Hypoxia** can be an indication for intubation but also can be managed by increased oxygen concentrations provided noninvasively. In addition to facilitating provision of increased FiO_2, intubation can allow for increased airway pressures to be provided that reduce intrapulmonary shunt and improve oxygenation. Patients with acute arterial oxygen saturations less than 92% should be considered for supplemental oxygen or intubation to improve their oxygenation status.

e. **Impending airway obstruction** is an indication for intubation to prevent complete obstruction and loss of the airway. Anatomical changes as a result of trauma, tumors, edema, or vocal cord abnormalities can interfere with airway patency, as can functional changes as a result of depressed neurologic status from head trauma, drugs, anesthesia, or stroke. If concern for impending airway obstruction is present, it is preferable to intubate early rather than later to allow easier passage of the endotracheal tube in a controlled manner.

C **Ventilator support**   Once the decision has been made to intubate, the next decision is how to manage the patient on the ventilator. Ventilator support should address two basic issues: ventilation and oxygenation. Ventilation determines CO_2 elimination and is dependent on alveolar minute ventilation. Alveolar minute ventilation is total minute ventilation minus dead space ventilation. Total minute ventilation is the product of respiratory rate times tidal volume and is expressed as liters per minute. To alter PCO_2, adjustments in rate and tidal volume should be made with increases in minute ventilation, resulting in decreases in PCO_2. Oxygenation or PO_2 is determined by the partial pressure of alveolar oxygen and the intrapulmonary shunt. Increasing the FiO_2 will increase alveolar oxygen while increasing mean airway pressure, such as by increasing positive end expiratory pressure (PEEP), will decrease shunt and increase PO_2. The mode of ventilation will alter how ventilation and oxygenation are achieved; however, more commonly, the mode influences patient tolerance of mechanical ventilation. For any patient receiving ventilatory support, ventilator-associated lung injury is an inherent risk to mechanical ventilation. This risk is increased with larger tidal volumes (volutrauma), higher airway pressures (barotrauma), or higher inhaled oxygen concentrations (oxygen toxicity).

1. **Modes of ventilation.** The modes of ventilation determine how the ventilator will provide a mechanical breath to the patient and are based on pressure or volume. There are more modes than are discussed here, but these will suffice in the vast majority of patients.

   a. **Synchronized intermittent mandatory ventilation (SIMV).** A preset rate and tidal volume are provided by the ventilator. Additional spontaneous breathing by the patient can occur that provides additional minute ventilation (tidal volume and rate) dependent on the patient's work of breathing capability. The work of breathing is shared between the machine's minute ventilation and the patient's spontaneous minute ventilation. This is the usual mode of ventilation when weaning a patient: By turning down the ventilator rate, the patient assumes more work of breathing until the ventilator is no longer needed. Pressure support (see below) can be added to this mode to facilitate the spontaneous breaths.

   b. **Assist or volume control (AC/VC).** A preset rate and tidal volume are provided by the ventilator, and all additional breaths by the patient are assisted by the ventilator, providing a full preset tidal volume. Minute ventilation becomes the result of the preset tidal volume times the preset ventilator's plus patient's rates. This allows the patient to receive full ventilatory support without expending extra energy on the work of breathing. Weaning cannot occur in this mode, and pressure support cannot be added to this mode.

   c. **Pressure support (PS).** Rather than providing a preset tidal volume or rate, the pressure support mode pressurizes the ventilator circuit to a preset level above the baseline pressure when the patient initiates a breath and maintains that level until the patient stops inhaling. The patient is able to initiate and terminate the respiratory cycle in this mode. Inspired tidal volume is determined by the amount of pressure support and the patient's intrinsic work of breathing capacity. Increasing the amount of pressure support reduces the work of breathing for the same tidal volume or allows a larger tidal volume for the same amount of work. The pressure support mode facilitates the patient's comfort and aids in weaning from the ventilator. The usual starting point of pressure support is 5–10 mm Hg above the baseline pressure (CPAP/PEEP) and can be used alone or in combination with SIMV.

   d. **Continuous positive airway pressure (CPAP) and PEEP.** For a basic understanding, these modes are considered similar, as both modes result in the ventilator circuit being pressurized to a specified level above atmospheric at all times, during inspiration and expiration. This increases mean airway pressure and the number of alveoli that are inflated, which increases the surface area of the lung that is available for gas exchange. This results in a decrease in intrapulmonary shunt and is considered a primary way to increase oxygenation. Usually, CPAP/PEEP of 5 mm Hg above atmospheric pressure is used and is increased as necessary to improve oxygenation. Because these modes increase intrathoracic pressure at higher levels, they can decrease venous return to the heart and therefore cardiac output. PEEP is used with SIMV and AC, while CPAP is used with PS.

2. **Rate.** After the mode, the next parameter to set is rate, with a normal rate about 10–12 bpm. Higher rates may be necessary to decrease the PCO_2 if higher minute ventilation or lower tidal volumes are required. Remember that if the patient is severely acidotic, he or she may have been compensating with the respiratory system and may require a much higher respiratory rate.

3. **Tidal volume.** Normal tidal volume is 5 mL/kg, but ventilated patients are usually set between 8–10 mL/kg. The higher volumes are needed to overcome dead space and to ensure alveolar filling. However, as compliance of the lungs decreases, especially in patients with ARDS, smaller tidal volumes of 6 mL/kg are beneficial. This volume will need to be adjusted as the patient's condition requires. Occasionally, permissive hypercapnia is beneficial to avoid barotrauma in particularly diseased lungs.

4. With the ventilator settings described previously, one should be able to handle the majority of ventilatory problems. Depending on the patient's condition, there are many other modes used to ventilate patients, but the basic ones that have been listed should suffice for routine ventilatory management. The starting point for most routine ventilator support involves the following:
   a. **Mode:** SIMV; however, if no work of breathing is desired, then use the AC mode
   b. **Rate:** 10–12 bpm
   c. **Tidal volume:** 8–10 mL/kg
   d. **Pressure support:** 5–10 mm Hg
   e. **PEEP/CPAP:** 5 mm Hg
   f. **Fraction of inspired oxygen (FiO_2):** 0.4
   g. The settings described need to be modified for the patient's condition: higher FiO_2 and/or higher PEEP if the patient is hypoxic, lower PEEP if hypotensive, faster rate if acidotic, etc.

5. **Extubation.** Ventilator weaning is the progressive transfer of the responsibility for work of breathing from the ventilator to the patient, eventually leading to the patient being extubated from the ventilator. After a patient is intubated, placed on a ventilator, and stabilized, one should start to think about weaning from the ventilator. Patients placed on a ventilator are usually in a catabolic state and as a result are breaking down muscle protein for fuel and for repair of other damaged proteins elsewhere. If a patient in such a state is placed on complete ventilator support without any work of breathing, the respiratory muscles will rapidly atrophy. Therefore, once the patient is stabilized on the ventilator, the amount of ventilatory support should be adjusted to allow the patient to continue to do a normal amount of the work of breathing in order to keep the respiratory muscles intact. As the patient's condition improves, the respiratory rate delivered by the ventilator is decreased until the patient adequately assumes the work of breathing on an SIMV less than 4 bpm and PS less than 10 mm Hg, have acceptable oxygenation on an FiO_2 of 0.4 and PEEP less than 8 mm Hg, have acceptable weaning parameters as described below, be awake enough to control airway, and have acceptable acid–base balance. When these conditions have been met, the patient is ready for extubation.
   a. **Respiratory rate** less than 30.
   b. Spontaneous **tidal volume** greater than 5 mL/kg.
   c. **Rapid shallow breathing index** (respiratory rate bpm divided by tidal volume in liters) less than 100.
   d. **Vital capacity** or the maximum amount of air that can be moved in and out of the lungs voluntarily of greater than 20 mL/kg. The normal amount is 60–80 mL/kg and represents the reserve ventilation that the patient has to increase his or her minute ventilation.
   e. **Negative inspiratory force (NIF),** or the amount of negative pressure created during a forced inspiration against a closed glottis, of greater than 20 mm Hg. The normal value is 60–80 mm Hg below atmospheric and is a measure of the strength of the patient's respiratory muscles, and as well is another measure of how much reserve the patient has to increase ventilation as needed.
   f. **Arterial blood gases.** In addition to having acceptable spirometry values, the patient must also have acceptable blood gases. The oxygen saturation should be greater than 90% due to the limitations of providing high concentrations of oxygen via a face mask. The PCO_2 should

be between 35 and 45 mm Hg with a corresponding pH between 7.35 and 7.45. Patients with a significant metabolic or respiratory acidosis with or without compensation should not be extubated without careful consideration of the underlying cause and potential future issues.

D **Invasive monitoring**

1. The mainstay of invasive monitoring in modern ICUs is the arterial line for blood pressure, the pulmonary artery catheter for cardiac outputs, pulmonary artery wedge pressures, and mixed venous oxygen saturation and the intracranial catheter for intracranial pressure monitoring .

2. **Arterial catheter**
   a. An **arterial catheter** is usually placed in one of the radial arteries, as these are the most accessible sites. If a radial artery cannot be cannulated, other common sites are femoral, axillary, and brachial arteries. These catheters are slowly flushed with a dilute heparin solution to keep them from clotting. In addition to providing continuous arterial blood pressure monitoring, the arterial line can be used as a simple, nonpainful source for blood sampling.
   b. There are three pressure measurements obtained from an arterial line: systolic, diastolic, and mean. The systolic is the highest pressure recorded during a cardiac cycle, the diastolic is the lowest measured during a cardiac cycle, and the mean is measured by integrating the area under the curve of the cardiac pressure wave. The mean pressure can be indirectly determined as $(BP_{systolic} - 2 \times BP_{diastolic})/3$ and represents the pressure that is available to perfuse the organs.

3. **Pulmonary artery catheter**
   a. The **pulmonary artery catheter** is a flow-directed catheter designed to be inserted into a subclavian or jugular vein, and because of an inflatable balloon on the tip, it can be floated through the heart and into the pulmonary artery. The catheter has an opening (port) in the tip distal to the balloon, another opening in the side of the catheter at a position that rests in the vena cava or right atrium, and a thermistor (a temperature-measuring device) near the distal port; there may also be extra ports for infusion of medications. When the catheter is in position in a distal pulmonary artery, the balloon is inflated and occludes antegrade blood flow, thereby allowing the distal port to measure retrograde pressure from the left atrium. This is referred to as the pulmonary capillary wedge pressure (PCWP) or occlusion pressure (PCOP) and is an indirect measure of left ventricular preload. By assessing ventricular preload, alteration fluid therapy can be made to maximize cardiac output.
   b. Using thermodilution methodology, the pulmonary artery catheter is able to determine cardiac output by accurately measuring changes in blood temperature after introduction of a known thermal challenge. This is accomplished intermittently by injecting a small (10 mL) amount of cold IV fluid in the right atrium or continuously by warming a heating probe and then measuring the temperature change in the pulmonary artery. The less change in temperature, the higher the cardiac output. By using known calibrations, the actual cardiac output can be determined.
   c. By either aspirating blood from the distal port or by using oximetry located on the distal tip, the mixed venous oxygen saturation (SvO_2) can be assessed. The SvO_2 provides a means to determine if the amount of oxygen being pumped by the heart (oxygen delivery) is adequate for the amount of oxygen the body needs (oxygen consumption). The normal mixed venous oxygen saturation is about 70%, and if oxygen consumption is elevated or oxygen delivery is decreased, the saturation will be lower than 70%. The SvO_2, therefore, is one of the best measures readily available to determine if shock is present. If the SvO_2 is persistently low (60% or less), the body is being deprived of sufficient oxygen, and organ dysfunction will begin to appear. Using similar technology, a less invasive but not as accurate method for determining SvO_2 can be obtained from the end of a central venous catheter.
   d. By knowing the cardiac output, the mean arterial pressure, and the central venous pressure, the systemic vascular resistance (SVR) and pulmonary vascular resistance (PVR) can be calculated:

   $SVR = [(MAP - CVP)/CO] \times 80$ normal: 800–1200 dynes·second/cm^5

   $PVR = [(MPAP - PCWP)/CO] \times 80$ normal: 20–120 dynes·second/cm^5

Where MAP is mean airway pressure, CVP is central venous pressure, MPAP is mean pulmonary artery pressure, CO is cardiac output, and 80 is a conversion factor. Low SVR is an indication of systemic inflammation such as in sepsis, and high SVR is an indication of inadequate cardiac output.

   e. In summary, the information gathered from the pulmonary artery catheter is as follows:
      (1) Left atrial and left ventricle preload pressures
      (2) Cardiac output (CO)
      (3) Mixed venous oxygen saturation (SvO_2)
      (4) Systemic vascular resistance (SVR) and pulmonary vascular resistance (PVR)

E Vasoactive medications

1. In the ICU, many patients are on vasoactive medications to affect their hemodynamic parameters; most of the time, this is to increase blood pressure (vasoconstrictors) and cardiac output (inotropes), but there are also times when these parameters need to be decreased. The following medications are the most frequently used, and are all administered in a continuous IV drip.

   a. **Dopamine** has different effects, depending on the concentration used. At a low dose of 1–3 μg/kg/minute, it primarily affects dopamine receptors in the kidneys and intestine, leading to increased blood flow. At doses of 3–10 μg/kg/minute, it is primarily a beta receptor agonist and leads to an increase in cardiac contractility with resulting increase in cardiac output. At doses above 10 μg/kg/minute, it acts primarily as an alpha agonist and vasoconstrictor. Its limiting effect is tachycardia.

   b. **Dobutamine** primarily affects both the beta-1 and beta-2 receptors. As a result, it leads to an increase in cardiac output as well as vasodilatation. This can be beneficial in cases of cardiogenic shock, where an increase in cardiac output and decrease in SVR would be beneficial. The doses are similar to dopamine, but dobutamine does not have the variable dosing effects, and the limiting factor is tachycardia.

   c. **Norepinephrine** is a strong alpha agonist that primarily causes vasoconstriction with mild beta agonist activity that causes some increase in contractility of the heart. Norepinephrine is begun at a concentration of 1–2 μg/kg/minute, and the dose is increased in 1–2 μg/kg/minute increments until the desired effect is reached. The major limiting effect of the medication is the tachycardia that it causes; otherwise, there is really no upper limit.

   d. **Epinephrine** is primarily an alpha agonist but has some beta agonist effect. It is useful for vasoconstriction and increasing cardiac output. It is dosed similar to norepinephrine but causes more tachycardia.

   e. **Phenylephrine** is an alpha agonist that causes pure arterial constriction. It is useful in cases of low SVR with a high cardiac output associated with systemic inflammatory response syndrome (SIRS), as in sepsis. Care must be taken not to use this medication in cases of hypotension associated with low cardiac output, as this would decrease oxygen delivery even more. Phenylephrine is not a very potent medication, and drips are usually begun at about 50 μg/minute and increased in increments of 50 μg/minute until a total dose of 300 μg/minute is reached, and then a more potent vasoconstrictor is needed.

2. While there are more pressors available, thorough knowledge of the indications, actions, and side effects of those discussed previously will suffice in most circumstances. Occasionally, patients will be hypertensive and need their blood pressure lowered, or their SVR will be excessively high and need vasodilation. The following medications are the most commonly used vasodilators:

   a. **Nitroprusside** is primarily an arterial vasodilator. The initial dose of this medication is 0.3 μg/kg/minute, with a maximum dose of 3 μg/kg/minute. Nitroprusside can result in reflex tachycardia, and one of its metabolites is cyanide. If used in large doses for a prolonged period, it can cause cyanide poisoning and acidosis.

   b. **Nitroglycerin** is primarily a venodilator as well as a coronary artery dilator. It is useful in decreasing venous preload to decrease diastolic wall tension and to allow better contraction of the heart if it has been overstretched. Nitroglycerin will also allow better diastolic blood flow to the heart itself and may lead to an increase in cardiac output. Its dosing is begun at

5 μg/minute and increased in 5–20 μg/minute increments until the desired effect is obtained.

VIII SHOCK

A **Definition** Shock is the clinical syndrome resulting from inadequate tissue perfusion to maintain normal cellular metabolism. The definition implies that the normal balance between perfusion and cellular needs becomes disrupted, leading to pathophysiologic changes. Most often, inadequate perfusion is related to decreased oxygen delivery to mitochondria but may also be related to the provision of other nutrients or even the removal of toxins or carbon dioxide from cells.

B **Types of shock** Shock can result from derangement in various fundamental physiologic processes related to volume status, cardiac performance, vascular tone, and cellular metabolism. The physiologic presentation differs depending on the cause of the derangement (Table 1-5).

1. **Hypovolemic shock.** Inadequate blood volume, or hypovolemia, is the most common type of shock, and hemorrhage is the most common reason for hypovolemia. Loss of plasma volume such as with major burns or third spacing can also result in hypovolemia. The perfusion defect is the result of blood volume loss (decreased preload) leading to decreased cardiac output and oxygen delivery to cells. Furthermore, loss of red cell volume reduces hemoglobin levels and oxygen-carrying capacity, worsening oxygen delivery as well. Although hypotension occurs with

TABLE 1-5   Types of Shock Based on Hemodynamic Profile Analysis

Type of Shock	Heart Rate	Blood Pressure	Central Venous Pressure	Systemic Vascular Resistance
Hypovolemic (early)	Increased	Normal systolic Increased diastolic[d]	Decreased	Increased
Hypovolemic (late)	Increased	Decreased	Decreased	Increased
Cardiogenic	Increased	Decreased	Increased	Increased
Neurogenic	Normal or decreased	Decreased	Decreased	Decreased
Septic shock (hypovolemia)	Increased	Decreased	Decreased	Decreased
Septic shock (euvolemia)	Increased	Normal or decreased	Normal or decreased	Decreased
Obstructive	Increased	Decreased	Increased[e]	Increased

Type of Shock	Cardiac Output	Pulmonary Capillary Wedge Pressure	SvO$_2$[a]	(CaO$_2$ – CvO$_2$)[b]	VO$_2$[c]
Hypovolemic (early)	Decreased	Decreased	Decreased	Increased	Normal
Hypovolemic (late)	Decreased	Decreased	Decreased	Increased	Decreased
Cardiogenic	Decreased	Increased	Decreased	Increased	Decreased
Neurogenic	Decreased	Decreased	Normal or decreased	Normal or increased	Normal or decreased
Septic shock (hypovolemia)	Decreased	Decreased	Decreased	Increased	Decreased
Septic shock (euvolemia)	Increased	Normal or increased	Increased	Decreased	Increased
Obstructive	Decreased	Increased or decreased[e]	Decreased	Increased	Decreased

[a]Mixed venous saturation (SvO$_2$).
[b]Arteriovenous oxygen content difference (CaO$_2$ – CvO$_2$).
[c]Oxygen consumption (VO$_2$).
[d]Blood pressure changes are dependent on percentage of blood volume lost.
[e]The specific change is dependent on the type of obstructive shock.

hypovolemia, the important concept is loss of perfusion, not decreased pressure. The clinical presentation and mortality are dependent on the magnitude and duration of volume loss. As blood volume loss increases, peripheral tissue perfusion is decreased to maintain perfusion to key central organs such as the brain, heart, and liver. This is achieved by peripheral vasoconstriction, but as volume loss continues, eventually inadequate perfusion and decreased oxygen delivery affects all organs, leading to cellular damage despite maximal oxygen extraction from hemoglobin. Increased lactate production occurs as normal aerobic cellular metabolism progresses to less energy efficient (fewer ATP produced) anaerobic metabolism, resulting in cellular damage and death. If allowed to progress untreated or if the initial magnitude of volume loss is large, then multisystem organ failure, and eventually death, occurs.

2. **Cardiogenic shock.** Inadequate perfusion can result from inadequate cardiac performance, leading to decreased cardiac output. Most commonly, this is related to myocardial ischemia, but congestive heart failure and valvular diseases can also cause cardiogenic shock. Blood volume remains normal or increased, but loss of adequate pump function results in decreased perfusion. Similar to hypovolemic shock, cardiogenic shock results in decreased oxygen delivery, peripheral vasoconstriction, hypotension, and multisystem organ failure. However, unlike in hypovolemia, the central venous pressures are increased in cardiogenic shock.

3. **Neurogenic shock.** Loss of sympathetic tone leading to peripheral vasodilatation can result in both relative hypovolemia and decreased cardiac performance. This can be a result of vasovagal response, cervicothoracic spinal cord injury, or spinal anesthesia. Hypotension and vasodilatation leading to maldistributive perfusion results in deranged cellular metabolism.

4. **Septic shock.** Toxins released by microbes result in profound hyperinflammatory physiologic derangements, including hypovolemia, cardiac dysfunction, and vasodilatation. The complex nature of this form of shock results in progressive maldistributive hypoperfusion associated with hypovolemia due to decreased blood volume and increased vascular space. Cardiac output may be decreased, normal, or increased, depending on the degree of hypovolemia and the severity of the inflammatory insult. Further, the hyperinflammatory response is characterized by increased cellular metabolism and oxygen demand with decreased efficiency for mitochrondrial oxygen utilization. Cellular hypoperfusion and anaerobic metabolism are common and are associated with organ dysfunction and death.

5. **Obstructive shock.** A physical obstruction resulting in decreased cardiac output is the hallmark of this form of shock. Examples include tension pneumothorax, cardiac tamponade, massive pulmonary embolism, venous air embolism, and severe cardiac valvular stenosis. All result in decreased cardiac output with elevated central venous pressure resulting in tissue hypoperfusion.

   a. **Tension pneumothorax** develops when injured lung develops a one-way valve that allows air into but not out of the pleural space. The trapped air creates an increase in unilateral pleural pressure, causing the heart and other mediastinal structures (e.g., vena cava, aorta) to be displaced to the contralateral side with compression of the vena cava and decreased venous return to the heart. Placement of a chest tube on the affected side relieves the problem and restores perfusion.

   b. **Cardiac tamponade** develops when blood or fluid accumulates around the heart in the pericardium space. The resulting increased pressure in the pericardial sac impairs venous return into the right atrium, and cardiac output is decreased. The treatment is to drain the pericardium, usually operatively, to allow venous return to increase and cardiac output to normalize.

   c. **Pulmonary embolism** causes blockage of blood flow through the pulmonary artery, resulting in decreased cardiac output and hypoxia.

6. **Miscellaneous shock.** Other diverse derangements can result in cellular hypoperfusion and shock. Examples include cyanide toxicity, severe hypoxia, normovolemic severe anemia, profound hypoglycemia, and anaphylaxis. All result in damage to cells and organ dysfunction, leading to death if untreated.

C **Management of shock** Fundamental to the treatment of shock is knowing the underlying etiology. Rapid volume replacement is essential for hypovolemic and vasodilatory shock states. Blood products should be administered if significant blood loss has occurred or when shock is associated with a hematocrit of less than 30%. Inotropic support is indicated if cardiac performance is depressed. Shock related to vasodilatation and unresponsive to volume loading should have vasoconstrictors administered. Caution should be used when administering vasoconstrictors, as perfusion may be negatively affected by these agents. In general, a mean arterial pressure of 65 mm Hg or greater is adequate for tissue perfusion. Monitoring adequacy of resuscitation is critical to correcting shock. Return of normal blood pressure, heart rate, and urine output are simple measures for assessing adequacy. Normalization of lactate levels and mixed venous oxygen saturation are more sophisticated and accurate measures of assessing resuscitation, especially in occult hypoperfusion conditions. Specific management for different shock types include:

a. **Hypovolemic.** Aggressive volume administration, preferably through two large-bore intravenous catheters. Stop ongoing blood loss. Consider central venous access for monitoring and high-flow fluid administration.

b. **Cardiogenic.** Inotropic support with dobutamine or dopamine. Nitroglycerine to reverse cardiac ischemia if blood pressure will tolerate.

c. **Neurogenic.** Volume resuscitation, consider vasoconstrictor administration with phenylephrine or norepinephrine if unresponsive to volume resuscitation.

d. **Septic.** Volume resuscitation, consider placement of central venous access for volume resuscitation and SvO_2 monitoring (goal SvO_2 >70%). Consider dobutamine if adequately volume resuscitated and SvO_2 <70%, consider norepinephrine or dopamine if adequately resuscitated and MAP <65 mm Hg.

e. **Obstructive.** Volume resuscitation and correction of the underlying condition.

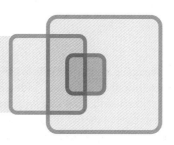

chapter **2**

Essential Topics in General Surgery

MICHAEL J. MORITZ

SECTION A: ESSENTIALS OF NORMAL SURGICAL PRACTICE

I **WOUND CLOSURE**

Wounds, whether traumatic or surgical, must be appropriately closed, layer by layer.

A There are **three types of wound closure and healing;** the choice of technique is determined by the degree of bacterial contamination in the wound (see Chapter 1, V C, D).

1. **Primary intention. Clean** and **clean-contaminated** wounds can be closed in this manner. All layers are closed.
   a. This produces the most cosmetic scar.
   b. With the skin closed, bacteria in the subcutaneous layer can result in a wound infection.

2. **Secondary intention. Infected** wounds are closed in this manner. The deep layers are closed, while the subcutaneous layer and the skin are left open.
   a. Wound care consists of 1 to 3 dressing changes daily, including wound irrigation, packing, and sterile dressings.
   b. The open portion of the wound granulates and slowly re-epithelializes with a broad scar.
   c. Because the skin is not closed, a wound infection cannot occur.

3. **Delayed primary intention. Contaminated** wounds can be closed in this manner. The deep layers are closed, while the subcutaneous layer and skin are left open and packed.
   a. At postoperative day 4 or 5, the wound is unpacked and inspected.
   b. If the subcutaneous tissue is clean and just beginning to granulate, then the skin edges are closed, either with sutures placed and left untied at the initial procedure or with adhesive paper tapes.
   c. If there is purulence in the subcutaneous layer, then the wound is left open to heal by secondary intention.

B **The skin** **The integumentary system** is the largest organ in the body.

1. **Skin layers.** The two principal layers, the dermis and epidermis, have specialized functions.
   a. The **epidermis** is composed of stratified squamous epithelium, which covers the entire body and provides protection. Living cells migrate from the innermost level of the epidermis to the surface to form the dead, desquamating layer. The migration takes approximately 19 days.
   b. The **dermis,** which serves in a nutritive capacity to the epidermis, is itself composed of two layers.
      (1) The **papillary layer** is composed of fine collagen fibers, ground substance, and capillaries.
      (2) The deeper **reticular layer** is composed of dense collagen, hair follicles, sebaceous glands, and sweat glands.
   c. The **hypodermis** or **subcutaneous tissue,** which lies deep to the dermis, contains fat and nutrient vessels and can contain hair follicles and sweat glands.

2. A cosmetically acceptable appearance is a goal of all closures.
  a. Atraumatic handling of tissue minimizes necrosis and decreases scarring.
  b. Eversion of the wound edges results in a level scar with time, whereas inversion of the edges may result in an uneven or concave scar.
  c. Early removal of skin sutures or skin staples decreases the scarring.

C Deeper **fascial layers** vary with location and the type of incision (i.e., transverse vs. vertical).
  1. Fascia generally has greater strength than other layers, and the fascial closure should assume most of the tension distracting the wound, rather than the skin.
  2. Where **multiple deep layers** exist, they can be closed as individual layers or in combination. For example, a transverse abdominal incision will have four deep layers: peritoneum and transversus abdominus, internal oblique, and external oblique muscles. Often, the deepest two or three layers are closed with a single suture line, and the shallowest one or two layers are closed with a second suture line.
  3. When the **integrity** of the deep layers has been violated (or they are at high risk of disruption), as in the case of wound dehiscence, then all layers—deep and superficial, including the skin—can be included in a single suture line, a so-called mass closure, usually using interrupted **retention sutures.**

D **Closure techniques**
  1. Suture lines can either be **interrupted** (a new knot every one or two stitches) or **continuous** (many stitches between knots). Continuous sutures are also called **running** sutures (Fig. 2-1).
    a. Interrupted closures
      (1) The **advantages.** These closures have the potential for better vascular supply to the wound edges.
      (2) The **disadvantages** include the greater time it takes to close with this method, the inconsistency of tension on individual sutures, and the large number of knots required.

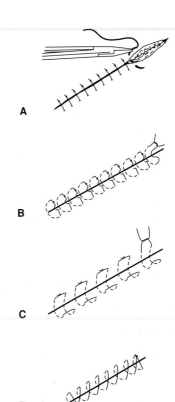

FIGURE 2-1 Suturing techniques. **A:** Simple interrupted suture. **B:** Interrupted vertical mattress suture. **C:** Interrupted horizontal mattress suture. **D:** Continuous (running) simple suture.

    b. Running closures
       (1) The **advantages.** Running closures take less time, have greater water-tightness, and the tension is equal along the entire suture line.
       (2) The **disadvantages** include the potential to strangulate the tissues if the suture is placed too tightly. Also, the integrity of the closure is dependent on one or two sutures and only a few knots, disruption of which will unravel the entire closure.

  2. Sutures, whether continuous or interrupted, can be sewn in a **simple** or a **complex** fashion.
    a. Simple sutures are also called "over and over" sutures.
    b. Complex suture techniques include vertical and horizontal mattress sutures and their variations (Fig. 2-1).

  3. Simple interrupted sutures are created with equal full-thickness bites of tissue.

  4. Vertical mattress sutures are similar to simple sutures, but an additional bite close to each wound edge is used to ensure edge coaptation (far-far, reverse direction, near-near).

  5. Horizontal mattress sutures are similar to simple sutures, but additional parallel bites are taken (far-far, move along incision, and reverse direction, far-far).

  6. Subcuticular sutures are intradermal closures that are usually continuous horizontal mattress sutures; the suture material is usually absorbable. The advantages are the avoidance of suture marks on the skin, and there is no need to remove sutures (especially important in pediatric cases).

E **Knot tying**

  1. The **standard knot** is a **square knot** (overhand throw, then underhand throw).
    a. To create a secure knot, braided sutures (e.g., silk, polyester, polyglycolic acid) require three or four throws, whereas monofilament sutures (e.g., nylon, polypropylene, polydioxanone) require six to eight throws.
    b. More throws are required for thicker suture sizes, running (as opposed to interrupted) closures, and more slippery suture materials (e.g., expanded dedpolytetraflouroethylene [ePTFE]).

  2. When there is **tension on the suture,** a **surgeon's knot** can be used, which begins with a double-overhand throw to secure the first throws. Standard square knot throws follow. This knot is slightly weaker than a square knot.

  3. A **granny knot** begins with overhand throw–overhand throw, creating a slip knot, which is then cinched down to the appropriate tightness. Standard square knot throws follow. This knot is slightly weaker than a square knot.

F **Suture materials**

  1. Strength of tissue. Although the gain in tensile strength varies from one type of tissue to another, as a general principle, the strength of tissue closed primarily returns toward normal, unincised tissue (100%) at the following pace:
    a. At 20 days, 20% of normal.
    b. At 40 days, 40% of normal.
    c. At 90 days, 60% of normal.
    d. At 1 year, 70% of normal.

  2. The first factor in classifying suture material is **nonabsorbable** versus **absorbable** (Table 2-1). The second factor to include is whether the suture material is **braided** or **monofilament.**

  3. Nonabsorbable sutures have enduring strength and last for years. They are **permanent foreign bodies.**
    a. They can serve as a nidus for harboring bacteria, resulting in infection.
    b. When the knots are prominent and just deep to the skin, they are noticeable, and patients may complain.
    c. Examples of situations in which to use nonabsorbable sutures include:
      (1) Prosthetic heart valves
      (2) Vascular suture lines
      (3) Hernia repairs
      (4) Any difficult closure or where the patient's ability to heal at the usual pace is compromised (e.g., radiation therapy, corticosteroid therapy).

TABLE 2-1   Types of Suture Materials

Sutures	Material	Monofilament vs. Braided	Half-life	Natural vs. Synthetic	Comments and Typical Uses
Absorbable sutures					
Gut (catgut)	Collagen from intestine—beef serosa or sheep submucosa	Monofilament	7–10 days	Natural	Originally from cats; packaged in alcohol, must be kept wet; rarely used.
Chromic gut (chromic catgut)	Chromate tanned gut	Monofilament	2 weeks	Natural	Ties well; packaged in alcohol, must be kept wet; less used than in years past.
Polyglactin-910 Poly-glycolic acid	Synthetic polymer	Braided	2–3 weeks	Synthetic	**Bowel, subcutaneous** tissue, fascia
Polydiox-anone Polygly-conate	Synthetic polymer	Monofilament	4 weeks	Synthetic	Fascia, bowel, biliary and **urinary tract**
Poligleca-prone 25	Synthetic polymer	Monofilament	1–2 weeks	Synthetic	Subcuticular skin closure
Permanent sutures					
Silk	Silk-organic protein, fibroin	Braided	~20 years	Natural	Best handling, hemostasis
Polyester	Polyester	Braided	Permanent	Synthetic	Heart valves, fascia; known for potential for harboring infection
Polypropylene	Polypropylene	Monofilament	Permanent	Synthetic	Cardiovascular, hernias, fascia
Nylon	Nylon	1. Monofilament 2. Braided	Permanent	Synthetic	1. Skin 2. Looks and handles like silk
Cotton, linen	Plant-derived	Braided	Permanent	Natural	Obsolete due to extent of resulting tissue reaction
Stainless steel	316L Stainless	Monofilament	Permanent, can fracture after years	Synthetic	Sternum, hernias; difficult to handle, sharp ends
ePTFE*	ePTFE	Porous mono-filament	Permanent	Synthetic	Cardiovascular, hernias; has properties of both braided and mono-filament
Staples	1. Skin-Steel 2. Stapling devices—titanium	Monofilament	Permanent	Synthetic	Skin staples: faster than sutured closures. Stapling devices: used for bowel anastamoses; vascular closures, bronchial closures

*ePTFE, expanded PolyTetraFluoroEthylene.

4. **Absorbable suture materials** degrade completely, last a variable time, and leave no permanent foreign body.
   a. Absorbable sutures are made of collagen or synthetic polymers and degrade by enzymatic digestion or hydrolysis. These sutures cause more tissue reaction than nonabsorbables, especially if enzymatically degraded (collagen).

(1) Absorbable sutures are ideal for the **biliary** and **urinary tracts,** where a permanent suture can serve as a nidus for stone formation.

(2) There may be a **decreased infection risk** without the permanent foreign body to harbor bacteria.

(3) There are **no permanent knots** to bother patients.

    b. If the suture loses strength before wound healing is adequate, the risk of wound disruption or incisional hernia increases.

5. Braided, multistrand sutures tend to be stronger, size for size, than monofilaments.

    a. This is especially true for shear strength (as opposed to tensile strength), which is most important at the knot.

    b. Braided sutures are softer, more flexible, and more pliant and hence are easier to handle, easier to tie, and require fewer throws to form a secure knot.

    c. Because braided sutures have interstices in which bacteria can hide, the risk of infection may be increased.

    d. Braided sutures are coarser, have increased drag on tissue, and can tear fragile tissue.

6. Monofilament sutures have much less drag when pulled through tissue, cause less tissue reaction, and have much less risk of harboring infection.

    a. Because monofilament sutures are stiffer, they require more throws to form a secure knot. The knots can be large and bothersome to the patient.

    b. Monofilament sutures must be handled with greater care; crushing, crimping, twisting, or kinking weakens the strand, which can lead to suture breakage.

7. Sutures can also be **classified as natural materials or synthetic.** Both require extensive processing.

8. Suture size uses a scale with "0" in the middle.

    a. Smaller sizes. As the number of 0's rises, the sutures get finer, e.g., 4-0 (0000) is smaller than 3-0 (000). The smallest standard manufactured suture size is 10-0 (pronounced *ten-oh*).

    b. Larger sizes. The sizes increase with each integer: no. 1 and no. 2. No. 2 is the largest standard manufactured suture size.

9. Usage of types of sutures

    a. Braided permanent sutures are the easiest to handle but are known for their increased risk of harboring infection, and so they have **fallen out of common use** for fascial closures. Examples include silk, polyester, and cotton.

    b. Braided absorbable sutures are the **most used** suture material. They can be used for gastrointestinal (GI) and other visceral surgery and for general closures. Examples include polyglactin-910 and polyglycolic acid.

    c. Monofilament permanent sutures are stiff and harder to work with but are best for **cardiovascular** surgery (in small sizes) and **fascial closures** and **hernias** (in larger sizes). Examples include nylon, polypropylene, and stainless steel.

    d. Monofilament absorbable synthetic sutures are the **latest suture type** to be developed. As both gut and chromic gut degrade quickly, the synthetic sutures have almost replaced the gut materials. They are better than braided absorbables for fascia because they last longer. They are also widely used for **biliary** and **urinary tract** surgery. Examples include polydioxanone and polyglyconate.

    e. ePTFE sutures are a **permanent porous monofilament** with properties of both braided (interstices that can harbor bacteria, easy to handle, soft inconspicuous knots) and monofilament (slippery, requires six to eight throws to secure a knot) sutures.

    f. Stapling devices fire multiple rows of small titanium staples for **GI, vascular,** and **pulmonary** applications. The staples act similarly to permanent monofilament sutures in that they are nonreactive, do not harbor bacteria, and are permanent. Titanium has replaced steel for permanent implantables because of its compatibility with magnetic resonance imaging (MRI).

II   SURGICAL TUBES

A **Drainage tubes**   Various types of tubes are used to drain either normal body fluid that cannot be handled by the body or abnormal material, such as pus. A tube can be mandatory, such as a chest tube for a hemothorax, or optional.

1. **Types of drains**
   a. **Closed drains** are tubes connecting a body cavity to a sealed reservoir.
      (1) **Gravity drainage** allows fluid to drain through the tube into a reservoir at a lower level (e.g., Foley bladder catheter).
      (2) **Underwater-seal drainage systems** prevent air and fluid from re-entering the body. The end of the drainage tube is under water in a sealed drainage bottle at floor level. The water prevents air from re-entering the tube and prevents fluid from siphoning back (e.g., chest tube).
      (3) **Suction drainage** applies suction to a drainage tube and can drain large volumes of fluid, such as fluids that can collect in the GI tract. It also promotes closure of "dead space," allowing a better approximation of tissue surfaces (e.g., Jackson-Pratt drain).
   b. **Sump drains** are double-lumen catheters that allow air or irrigation fluid to enter through one lumen while suction is applied to the other lumen. Sump drains are used to evacuate particulate matter, such as debris from an abscess, or as continuous irrigation catheters (e.g., nasogastric [NG] tube).
   c. **Open drains** are not sealed at either end. They allow bacteria and other materials access to the drained area. Open drains are still used for some contaminated cases (e.g., Penrose drain).

2. **Examples of situations requiring drainage**
   a. Chest tube drainage of the **pleural space** is usually indicated to evacuate air, i.e., **pneumothorax** (simple, tension), and blood, i.e., hemothorax.
   b. A **GI tract** that is nonfunctional for a prolonged period (more than 1 or 2 days) or obstructed requires NG drainage, usually with a sump tube.
      (1) The decompression lessens abdominal distention, intestinal dilatation, nausea, and vomiting.
      (2) Drainage also allows one to determine the amount and type of luminal fluid loss so that appropriate replacement can be made.
   c. Areas where **bodily fluids** (e.g., bile, urine, pancreatic fluid) can collect internally require drainage.
   d. Procedures such as **mastectomies or skin flaps** (see Chapter 1, V D 5) where large raw surfaces are to be kept opposed require suction drainage.
   e. **Deep abscesses** not amenable to simple incision require drainage (e.g., deep cavities such as subphrenic or periappendiceal abscesses). Drains cannot be used to control a generalized infection, such as cellulitis or peritonitis (see VI B 2).

3. **Caveats and complications**
   a. The presence of a drain is **no guarantee that a fluid collection will not form.** The foreign body reaction can isolate a drain from adjacent tissues, preventing fluid from accessing the drain's lumen.
   b. A drain is **not a substitute for hemostasis.** If hemostasis is not adequate, a hematoma will likely develop despite drainage.
   c. Drains can become **colonized by microorganisms** from exogenous sources. Drains, particularly open drains, increase the risk of infection.
   d. **Rigid drains may erode** through the wall of a blood vessel or a hollow intestinal structure. This complication can be minimized by using soft drains and removing drains early.
   e. **Excessive suction on a tube can cause necrosis** of nearby structures. Intermittent or low-level suction or use of a sump tube is safer.
   f. A drain in **direct contact with a fistula** may perpetuate the fistula and delay its healing. The drain must then be withdrawn from the fistula if healing is to occur (see VII E 2).
   g. Drains can **retract into the body.** They must always be firmly attached to the skin and should be marked with a radiopaque marker. A safety pin can be used to keep small drains outside the body.
   h. The **free peritoneal space cannot be drained** because tubes are quickly "walled off." Therefore, diffuse peritonitis cannot be drained. Localized collections can be drained.

4. **Removal.** Drains should be removed when they have fulfilled their purpose.
   a. When the **main risk of leakage has passed,** the drain is removed.
      (1) After a **liver** resection, if a leak from a bile duct is present, it should be evident in 1 or 2 days. Therefore, drains are normally removed by the third day.

(2) After **urinary bladder** procedures, a urine leak would not be noticeable until the bladder catheter is removed. Therefore, drains are removed a day after the catheter is removed.

b. When a drain is used for **postoperative fluid collections** (i.e., blood or lymph), it is removed when no substantial drainage occurs.

c. When the drain is used in a **reconstructive procedure,** it is removed once the repair is safe.

(1) After common duct exploration, a T tube is used to drain the bile duct until spasm of the sphincter of Oddi has resolved. The T tube is removed after a cholangiogram documents free flow of bile into the duodenum.

(2) After gastrectomy and Billroth II reconstruction, a **potential complication** is disruption of the duodenal stump.

(a) A tube may be placed within the duodenal lumen (tube duodenostomy) to prevent overdistension of the proximally closed duodenum and prevent disruption.

(b) Once the patient has recovered from the surgical procedure and if no signs of duodenal leakage have developed, the tube can be removed 2–4 weeks after surgery.

B **Gastrointestinal tubes**

1. **Gastrostomy tubes** are tubes inserted between the stomach and the skin and are used for feeding purposes or for prolonged gastric decompression.

   a. Once the tube is no longer needed, it is removed. The tract formed between the skin and stomach will close in 6–24 hours if a tube is not reinserted.

   b. Tubes may be inserted surgically or via endoscopy (percutaneous endoscopic gastrostomy [PEG]).

2. **Gastroesophageal balloon tamponade tubes (Sengstaken-Blakemore or Minnesota tubes)** are NG tubes with inflatable balloons, which are used to compress and tamponade bleeding esophageal varices (see Chapter 14, II E 3 d).

3. **Long intestinal tubes,** particularly the double-lumen **Miller-Abbott tube** and the single-lumen **Cantor tube,** are introduced through the nose and allowed to pass into the small intestine. These are now used infrequently.

   a. A weight or bag is at the leading tip, allowing peristalsis to carry the tube distally.

   b. Long intestinal tubes can be useful for relieving **small bowel obstruction.**

   (1) They are used for recurrent obstructions. The tubes are not used for a first episode of small bowel obstruction; laparotomy and lysis of adhesions should be performed in such cases.

   (2) Multiple areas of partial obstruction, as with radiation enteritis, are treatable with a long tube.

4. **Baker jejunostomy tubes.** Long intestinal tubes may also be inserted directly into the intestine at the time of laparotomy. The tube most commonly used is the Baker jejunostomy tube, which is brought through the abdominal wall, inserted into the proximal jejunum (jejunostomy), and then passed distally to the cecum. It is used either to splint the bowel in situations where adhesions will recur or to decompress greatly distended bowel encountered at surgery. These are used infrequently.

5. **Jejunostomy tubes** are inserted into the jejunum as a surgical procedure. They exit on the abdominal wall and are used for feeding purposes (see Chapter 1, VI E 3).

6. **Cecostomy tubes** are large-caliber tubes that are surgically inserted into a distended cecum.

   a. Their most common use is in **colonic ileus,** where marked colonic distention produces a cecum that is greater than 12 cm in diameter so that cecal rupture is imminent.

   b. Colonic obstruction is usually better treated with a proximal diverting colostomy than by cecostomy.

7. **Rectal tubes** are large-caliber tubes that are inserted transanally into the rectum.

   a. The most common use is to relieve colonic distention from a colonic ileus. It is the treatment of choice for **sigmoid volvulus,** where the tube is passed through the area of torsion under sigmoidoscopic visualization.

   b. Rectal tubes are best removed after several days, as the thin-walled colon is prone to pressure necrosis.

C Catheters and hemodialysis tubes

1. A **central venous catheter** (slang = central line) is a thin, single- or triple-lumen tube placed via the internal jugular or subclavian vein into the superior vena cava. Uses include administration of fluids, parenteral nutrition, and pressors. The most common complication of central lines is infection, often as bacteremia.
   a. Placement via the femoral vein can be used when necessary.
   b. A larger double-lumen catheter can be placed for brief (less than 2 weeks) hemodialysis access.

2. A **peripherally inserted central catheter** (PICC, slang = pick line) is placed via an antecubital vein and is threaded proximally into an intrathoracic vein. A PICC is used as a central catheter, most often for outpatients.

3. A **port** is equivalent to a central venous catheter or PICC, except there is no external extension, and a port is intended for longer-term use. The catheter is attached to a device with a septum (the port) through which to access the lumen. The port is buried subcutaneously. A port is usually used less often than daily, e.g., for periodic chemotherapy.

4. A **cuffed central venous catheter (Hickman-type catheter)** maintains access to the veins for prolonged time periods.
   a. The catheter has a Dacron felt cuff glued to the catheter. The cuff provokes ingrowth of granulation tissue, which functions to secure the catheter's position and as a mechanical barrier to organisms entering via the skin exit site.
   b. They can function for years. Both single- and double-lumen styles are available; they are inserted percutaneously.
   c. **Typical uses include:**
      (1) **Chemotherapy** and phlebotomy in patients with malignant diseases.
      (2) **Hemodialysis** in patients with problems with standard hemoaccess.
      (3) Long-term **hyperalimentation** in patients with nutritional problems.

5. **Tenckhoff peritoneal dialysis catheters** are inserted into the peritoneal cavity either for long-term dialysis therapy or for management of ascites in patients with malignant disease.
   a. They may be inserted either percutaneously or surgically and can function for years if properly maintained with sterile technique.
   b. Two Dacron cuffs are glued to the catheter: one adjacent to the peritoneum and one adjacent to the skin exit site. The cuffs function as barriers against infection (from the skin side) and leakage (from the peritoneal side).

III HERNIAS

Hernias are the abnormal protrusion of intra-abdominal contents through a defect in the abdominal wall.

A Overview

1. **Frequency of occurrence.** In both men and women, hernias occur most commonly in the **inguinal** region (75%–80% of all hernias). **Incisional** (ventral) hernias occur next in frequency (8%–10%), followed by **umbilical** hernias (3%–8%).

2. **Etiology.** Hernias occur as a result of various factors.
   a. **Congenital defects** include indirect inguinal hernia.
   b. **Loss of tissue strength and elasticity** from aging or repetitive stress may result in herniation, as in hiatal hernia.
   c. **Trauma,** especially **operative trauma** in which normal tissue strength is altered surgically, can lead to the development of hernia. A wound infection greatly increases the risk of late incisional hernia.
   d. **Increased intra-abdominal pressure** as a result of
      (1) Heavy lifting
      (2) Coughing, asthma, and chronic obstructive pulmonary disease (COPD)
      (3) Bladder outlet obstruction (e.g., benign prostatic hypertrophy)

      (5) Prior pregnancy

      (6) Ascites and abdominal distention

      (7) Obesity

  3. Descriptive terms. Hernias may be described according to physical or operative findings.

    a. Reducible. The hernia contents can be pushed back into the abdomen.

    b. Incarcerated. The hernia contents cannot be pushed back.

    c. Obstructing. The hernia contains a loop of bowel that is kinked and obstructs the GI tract.

    d. Strangulated. The tissue contained in the hernia is ischemic and will necrose due to compromise of its blood supply.

    e. Sliding. The wall of the hernia sac, rather than being formed completely by peritoneum, is in part formed by a retroperitoneal structure, such as the colon or the bladder.

    f. Richter's hernia. Only one side of the bowel wall is trapped in the hernia (typically, the antimesenteric side) rather than the entire loop of bowel. This is especially dangerous because the incarcerated portion of bowel can necrose and perforate in the absence of obstructive symptoms.

  4. Complications. Hernias should be repaired electively to prevent the development of major complications.

    a. Intestinal obstruction.

    b. Intestinal strangulation with **bowel perforation.**

B **Inguinal hernias**

  1. Anatomy of the inguinal region (Figs. 2-2 and 2-3)

    a. The **internal inguinal ring** is an opening in the transversalis fascia lateral to the inferior epigastric vessels.

    b. The **external inguinal ring** is an opening in the external oblique aponeurosis.

    c. The **inguinal canal** is the communication between the internal and external rings.

      (1) The **anterior wall** of the canal is formed by the external oblique aponeurosis.

      (2) The **inferior wall** of the canal is formed by the inguinal ligament (**Poupart's ligament**) and its reflection.

      (3) The **roof** of the inguinal canal (**superior**) is made up of fibers of the internal oblique and transversus abdominis muscles, forming a structure termed the **conjoint tendon.**

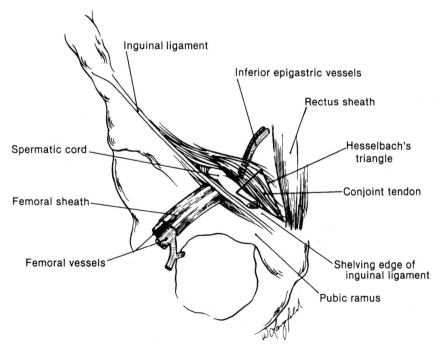

FIGURE 2-2 Anatomy of the inguinal region.

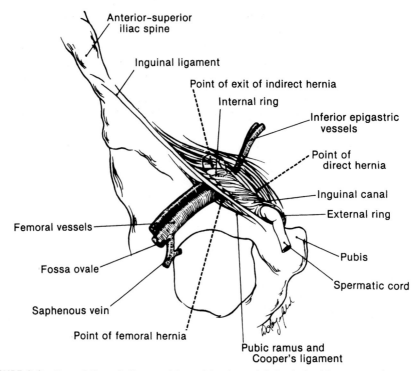

Anterior–superior
iliac spine

Inguinal ligament

Point of exit of indirect hernia

Internal ring

Inferior epigastric
vessels

Point of
direct hernia

Inguinal canal

External ring

Femoral vessels

Pubis

Fossa ovale

Spermatic cord

Saphenous vein

Point of femoral hernia

Pubic ramus and
Cooper's ligament

FIGURE 2-3 Sites of direct, indirect, and femoral hernias and their relationship to anatomic structures.

    (4) The **posterior wall** or **floor** is formed by the transversalis fascia.
        (a) Within the posterior wall of the inguinal canal is **Hesselbach's triangle.**
        (b) The triangle is formed laterally by the inferior epigastric artery, inferiorly by the
            inguinal ligament, and superomedially by the lateral border of the rectus sheath.
  d. In **women,** the **round ligament** traverses the inguinal canal.
  e. In **men,** the **spermatic cord structures** pass into the internal ring, traverse the inguinal
    canal, and pass through the external ring into the scrotum. Structures within the **spermatic
    cord** include:
    (1) **Arteries:** testicular and cremasteric
    (2) **Veins:** pampiniform plexus
    (3) **Vas deferens**
    (4) **Processus vaginalis:** an evagination of peritoneum that accompanies the descent of the
        testicle and gubernaculum through the abdominal wall. Normally obliterated, it remains
        patent in an indirect hernia and forms the hernia sac.
    (5) **Nerves:** the ilioinguinal and genital branch of the genitofemoral nerves are within the
        inguinal canal but are external to the cremasteric fascia, which invests the spermatic cord.

2. Types of hernias
  a. Indirect inguinal hernias
    (1) An indirect inguinal hernia passes from the peritoneal cavity through the **internal
        inguinal ring** (i.e., lateral to the epigastric vessels) and down the inguinal canal (Fig. 2-3).
        It may, on occasion, extend into the scrotum.
    (2) When the processus vaginalis is incompletely obliterated, a **spermatic cord hydrocele**
        may result, with or without an indirect inguinal hernia.
    (3) **Incidence**
        (a) Indirect inguinal hernias are the most common type of hernia in both men and
            women. They are 5 to 10 times more common in men than in women. Approxi-
            mately 5% of men develop an inguinal hernia during their lifetime and require an
            operation.
        (b) Indirect inguinal hernias are five times more common than direct hernias.

(4) Indirect hernias may occur from infancy to old age but generally occur by the fifth decade of life.

(5) A **pediatric inguinal hernia** (see Chapter 29, II) is almost always indirect and has a high risk of incarceration. It is more common on the right (75%) and is often bilateral.

(6) **Potential indirect hernias** are associated with an undescended testis, a testis in the inguinal canal, and a hydrocele.

(7) **Bilateral patent processus vaginalis** occurs in up to 10% of patients with an indirect inguinal hernia.

b. **Direct inguinal hernias.** The inferior epigastric vessels are the anatomic landmarks that distinguish indirect from direct inguinal hernias, which occur **medial** to the epigastric vessels.

(1) A direct inguinal hernia occurs through the floor of the inguinal canal, i.e., through **Hesselbach's triangle** (Fig. 2-2), because of an acquired weakness in the tissue.

(2) The hernia is a direct protrusion of abdominal structures into the floor of the canal posterior to the spermatic cord. It is not contained in the cord as is an indirect hernia, and it does not pass into the scrotum. The sac is a broadly based defect. It is much less often associated with strangulation than an indirect inguinal hernia.

(3) Direct inguinal hernia increases in occurrence with age and is related to physical activity.

c. A **recurrent inguinal hernia** usually recurs as a direct hernia. Most commonly, the defect occurs in the most medial aspect of the repair of the floor of the inguinal canal.

d. **Pantaloon hernias** are combinations of direct and indirect hernias in which the hernia sac passes both medially and laterally to the epigastric vessels.

e. **Femoral hernias**

(1) A femoral hernia occurs along the femoral sheath in the **femoral canal** (Fig. 2-3).

(2) The hernia contents protrude posterior to the inguinal ligament, anterior to the pubic ramus periosteum (i.e., **Cooper's ligament**), and medial to the femoral vein.

(3) The hernia traverses the femoral canal and can present as a mass at the level of the foramen ovale. It may also turn cephalad once it has exited the foramen ovale and can cross anteriorly to the inguinal ligament.

(4) The sac has a narrow neck, and 30%–40% of femoral hernias become incarcerated or strangulated.

(5) Femoral hernias are more common in women than in men.

(6) Femoral hernias are associated with being female, prior pregnancy, and prior inguinal hernia repair.

3. **Diagnosis** of an inguinal hernia is based on history and physical examination.

a. **The history** may include the appearance of a lump in the groin. The mass may be intermittently present and may be painful. Its appearance is often associated with activity.

b. **Physical examination** should be performed with the patient in both the supine and standing positions.

(1) A mass may be visible, and its size and visibility may depend on the patient's position.

(2) The mass may be tender or may be reducible with gentle pressure.

(3) The examining finger should be placed along the spermatic cord at the scrotum and passed into the external ring along the canal.

(a) The mass may become palpable as an impulse felt by the examining finger upon a sudden increase in intra-abdominal pressure, as occurs with a cough.

(b) A **direct hernia** causes a forward bulge low in the canal.

(c) An **indirect hernia** touches the tip of the examining finger.

c. **The differential diagnosis** of an inguinal mass includes a hydrocele, a varix (especially if thrombosed), an inflamed or enlarged lymph node, a lipoma of the spermatic cord, an undescended testicle, or an abscess or tumor.

4. **Repair of inguinal hernias.** Surgery is the only curative procedure for inguinal hernias; there are no lesser therapies that have proved effective. A recent study has reported that the risk of incarceration is low in minimally symptomatic hernias and that observing them is a safe alternative (*JAMA*. 2006 Jan 18;295(3):285–292).

a. **Repair of indirect inguinal hernia** involves

(1) **Return** of the hernia contents into the peritoneal cavity;

(2) Division and/or ligation of the base of the hernia sac at the level of the peritoneal cavity—the sac is **always anteromedial** to the cord at the level of the internal ring;

(3) In **adults,** tightening of the internal ring and **repair** of the **abdominal wall defect** inguinal canal floor to prevent recurrence.

b. Repair of direct inguinal hernia is based on reinforcement of the inguinal canal floor after invaginating the hernia sac.

c. Repair of femoral hernia involves approaching the femoral sheath through the floor of the inguinal canal. The space is closed by apposing the posterior reflection of the inguinal ligament to Cooper's ligament (**Cooper's ligament repair**) or by plugging the space with polypropylene mesh.

d. Repair of the floor of the inguinal canal can be done with many techniques. Two classic techniques used less commonly now are described first, then two newer techniques are described.

(1) Bassini repair

(a) The transversalis fascia and conjoint tendon above are sutured to the reflection of the inguinal ligament (i.e., the shelving edge of Poupart's ligament) below.

(b) In men, the spermatic cord is returned to its normal anatomic location between the reinforced inguinal canal floor and the external oblique aponeurosis.

(c) In women, the round ligament may be ligated and the internal ring closed (true for all inguinal hernia repairs in women).

(2) Cooper's ligament repair (McVay's method)

(a) This method is similar to the Bassini repair except that the transversalis fascia and conjoint tendon are sutured to Cooper's ligament, which is the periosteum of the pubic ramus.

(b) Because Cooper's ligament is more posterior than the inguinal ligament and subjects the repair to increased tension, a "relaxing" incision is often made in the anterior rectus sheath adjacent to the external oblique aponeurosis. This counterincision allows the conjoint tendon to be sutured to Cooper's ligament with less tension.

(c) Tension is the problem with this technique, causing both postoperative pain and early and late recurrences.

(3) Shouldice repair uses the transversalis fascia, which is divided longitudinally and imbricated upon itself in two layers. The internal oblique muscle and conjoint tendon are then sutured to the reflection of the inguinal ligament in two layers (total four suture lines).

(4) Prosthetic mesh repairs (**Lichtenstein repairs**) are supplanting older techniques. These involve repairing the inguinal floor by using mesh to close the space, suturing it (as in a Bassini repair) to the transversalis fascia and conjoint tendon above and to the reflection of the inguinal ligament (i.e., the shelving edge of Poupart's ligament) below.

(5) Open and laparoscopic techniques (Chapter 30) are used to place polypropylene mesh to reinforce the weakened transversalis fascia. Open techniques also place mesh into the defect deep to the transversalis fascia.

(a) For indirect hernia repairs, a cone-shaped polypropylene mesh is placed adjacent to (anteromedial to) the spermatic cord.

(b) For direct hernia repairs, the cone-shaped mesh is used to "plug" the transversalis fascia defect.

e. Recurrence rates after surgical repair vary depending on the type of hernia, but generally, inguinal hernias recur in under 10% of cases. This figure is usually higher for hernias at other sites.

f. Special situations

(1) When **strangulation** or **necrosis of the incarcerated bowel** is suspected but the bowel returns to the peritoneal cavity spontaneously before visual examination by the surgeon, the abdomen should be opened and explored so that any necrotic bowel can be resected.

(2) Recurrent hernias or **hernias with large defects** may require the insertion of prosthetic material such as polypropylene mesh to repair the abdominal wall defect adequately.

(3) Simple high ligation of the hernia sac is used for hernias in the **pediatric age group.** No floor repair is needed.

(4) A **truss** is a device that exerts external compression over the hernia defect, keeping the space compressed. It is used only when surgery cannot be safely performed or when the patient refuses surgery.

C **Other types of abdominal wall hernias**

1. **Umbilical hernias** occur through the defect where the umbilical structures passed through the abdominal wall.
   a. Umbilical hernias occur 10 times more often in women than in men.
   b. The defect is common in children but usually closes by age 2 years, and fewer than 5% of umbilical hernias persist into later childhood and adult life.
   c. In adults, umbilical hernias are often associated with increased intra-abdominal pressure, as with ascites or pregnancy.
   d. Repair of an umbilical hernia consists of a simple transverse repair of the fascial defect.

2. **Epigastric hernias,** also called **epiploceles,** result from a defect in the linea alba above the umbilicus.
   a. They occur more commonly in men (in a 3:1 ratio).
   b. Some 20% of epigastric hernias are multiple at the time of repair.
   c. Repair (simple suturing) is associated with a recurrence rate as high as 10%.

3. **Ventral hernias** occur in the abdominal wall in areas other than the inguinal region.
   a. **An incisional hernia,** the most common type of ventral hernia, results from poor wound healing in a previous surgical incision and occurs in 5%–10% of abdominal incisions.
      (1) **Common causes** include midline incision, wound infection or hematoma, advanced age, obesity, general debilitation or malnutrition, surgical technique, or a postoperative increase in abdominal pressure, as occurs with paralytic ileus, ascites, or pulmonary complications after surgery.
      (2) Incisional hernias are repaired after the patient has recovered from the prior surgery trauma.
      (3) Repair requires definition of the adequate fascial edges surrounding the defect, closure with nonabsorbable sutures, and use of prosthetic mesh (polypropylene or ePTFE) when the defect is too large to be closed primarily.
   b. **Spigelian hernias** protrude through the abdominal wall along the semilunar line (the lateral edge of the rectus muscle) at the semicircular line of Douglas (below the umbilicus where the transversus abdominis and internal oblique aponeuroses change to pass anteriorly to the rectus muscle).
   c. **Obturator hernias** occur in the pelvis through the obturator foramen. The hernia can cause pain along the obturator nerve (mid-anterior thigh), referred to as Howship-Romberg sign.
   d. **Lumbar hernias** occur on the flank and are seen in the superior (Grynfeltt's) and inferior (Petit's) triangles.
   e. **Perineal hernias** occur in the pelvic floor usually after surgical procedures such as an abdominoperineal resection.
   f. **Peristomal hernias** develop adjacent to an intestinal ostomy.

IV **SURGICAL ONCOLOGY**

A **Overview** **Cancer** is a group of diseases caused by unregulated growth and spread of **neoplastic cells. Neoplasias** may be either **benign** (noninvasive growth, no metastases) or **malignant** (invasive growth, metastases).

1. **Types**
   a. **Carcinomas** are malignancies that arise from epithelium.
   b. **Adenocarcinomas** are malignancies that arise from epithelium and have a glandular component.
   c. **Sarcomas** are malignancies that arise from mesodermal tissues.

2. Neoplastic transformation. Neoplastic cells have "escaped" from the normal homeostatic inhibition (or regulation) of cell proliferation. **Causes of neoplastic transformation** are listed next with illustrative examples of human tumors. Because no single etiology exists for most human cancers, remember that multiple factors lead to neoplastic transformation.

    a. Chemical carcinogens. Soot is associated with cancer of the scrotum of chimney sweeps (described by Pott in 1775); asbestos is associated with mesothelioma of the pleura; and smoking tobacco is associated with squamous cell carcinoma of the lung.

    b. Physical carcinogens. Ultraviolet light is associated with basal cell and squamous cell carcinomas of the skin; ionizing radiation is associated with bone cancer in radium-dial workers, lung cancer in uranium miners, and leukemia in atomic bomb survivors (Hiroshima); and papillary thyroid cancer appears in individuals treated with neck irradiation.

    c. Hereditary factors. A few cancers have direct genetic links, such as retinoblastoma, familial adenomatous polyposis, and multiple endocrine neoplasia syndromes (e.g., pheochromocytoma, medullary carcinoma of the thyroid, and other endocrine tumors) (Chapter 17).

    d. Geographic factors are unexplained epidemiologic phenomena whereby a particular cancer is very common in certain locations (e.g., gastric cancer is common in Japan and esophageal cancer in southeastern China).

    e. Oncogenic viruses. Epstein-Barr virus is linked to Burkitt's lymphoma and nasopharyngeal carcinoma; human papilloma virus is linked to cervical and anogenital carcinomas; human T-cell leukemia virus type 1 (HTLV-1) is linked to adult T-cell leukemia; and hepatitis B and C are linked to hepatocellular carcinoma.

B **Epidemiology**   Cancer is the **second** leading cause of death in the United States (20% of all deaths); approximately 1 million new cases are diagnosed annually. One in four U.S. residents will develop cancer during his or her lifetime, with an overall 5-year survival rate of 40%.

    1. Mortality

        a. Overall, the highest number of deaths is caused by **lung cancer** (incidence rising), followed by colon and rectal cancer and breast cancer (incidence stable), and pancreatic cancer (incidence rising). Lung cancer is now the most common cause of cancer death for both sexes (having exceeded breast cancer for women).

        b. A decreasing number of deaths are found from gastric cancer and uterine/cervical cancer. For gastric cancer, the incidence is falling for unknown reasons. For uterine/cervical cancer, early diagnosis (Pap smear) and improved treatments are presumably responsible.

    2. Incidence. Overall, the order is the same as for mortality. However, for women, the most common cancer is breast cancer.

C **Molecular physiology of neoplastic cells**   Neoplastic cells proliferate more rapidly than normal cells and fail to acknowledge signals to stop dividing.

    1. Cancer is caused by a cascade of inherited and acquired **mutations in those genes, which result in unsuppressed cellular proliferation.**

        a. Mutations in DNA produce altered or lost genes: point mutations (altered single base pair), deletions (loss of a DNA segment), and translocations (rearrangements).

        b. Recessive mutations must cause loss of both copies of a growth-regulating molecule to contribute to malignant transformation.

    2. There are at least three **types** of **cancer-causing genes.**

        a. Oncogenes result from mutations of the normal host proto-oncogenes.

            (1) Proto-oncogenes are expressed during cellular proliferation, e.g., during embryonic development or during injury/healing responses.

            (2) Examples of oncogenes:

                (a) The **HER-2/*neu* gene** is a membrane receptor mimic, and it encodes a protein similar to the epidermal growth factor receptor. This gene is amplified (overproduced) in 30% of breast and ovarian carcinomas and independently adversely effects prognosis.

                (b) The ***ras* oncogene** encodes a **signal transduction** protein and is found in 20% of solid tumors and in 50% of colon carcinomas.

        (c) **C-*myc*** is a **nuclear transcription factor** that binds to enhancer and promoter regions of target genes. C-*myc* expression is increased in many solid tumors. In Burkitt's lymphoma, c-*myc* is uniformly translocated adjacent to the immunoglobulin (Ig)G or IgM light chain genes.

    b. **Tumor suppressor genes** function to suppress or regulate cellular proliferation.

        (1) Loss of function results from mutation or deletion in **both** genes.

        (2) p53 is a **tumor suppressor oncogene.** Normally, p53 suppresses DNA replication sites.

            (a) Loss of p53 is the single most common genetic change found in malignancy (75% of colon carcinomas, 90% of hepatocellular carcinomas caused by aflatoxin).

            (b) **Human papilloma virus** gene product E6 binds and inhibits p53.

C **DNA repair genes** encode for proteins that correct most of the errors that creep into replicated DNA. Diminished or lost function of these genes increases the net mutation rate in other genes.

D **Multistep carcinogenesis** Malignancy is the result of the accumulation of critical mutations that produce a cancerous cell.

    1. As a corollary, a single specific oncogene or lost suppressor gene may be necessary but **not sufficient by itself** to produce the malignant phenotype.

    2. An important point is the **diverse functions** of the lost or mutated molecules. The multiplicity of genes and their products and the multitude of possible mutations leads to enormous diversity on every level for human cancers.

    3. **Hereditary factors** are well illustrated by the BRCA-1 and BRCA-2 genes.

        a. BRCA-1 and BRCA-2 are genes, certain mutations of which increase a woman's risks of breast (BRCA-1 only) and ovarian cancers. These mutations are usually inherited and are highly penetrant autosomal dominant traits.

        b. The BRCA-1 gene is a tumor suppressor gene. Mutations are present in 10% of young women (younger than 35 years old) with breast cancer but in 20% of young Jewish women with breast cancer.

        c. For BRCA-1 and BRCA-2, the prevalence of these mutations is 0.0014. The cumulative lifetime risk of breast cancer for carriers is 73.5%, in contrast to a risk of 6.8% for noncarriers.

        (1) For ovarian cancer, the equivalent lifetime risks are 28% for carriers and 2% for noncarriers.

        (2) In the United States, individuals with BRCA-1 mutations account for 3% of breast cancers and 4.4% of ovarian cancers.

    4. The steps in **colon carcinogenesis** are relatively well understood.

        a. APC (adenomatous polyposis coli) gene mutations occur early and may be the first event in tumorogenesis of sporadic cases. APC mutations are typically found in benign calonic adenomatous polyposis.

        (1) When two copies of this recessive gene are inherited, the individual has Familial Adenomatous Polyposis and develops multitudinous colonic polyposis with early cancers.

        b. The DCC (deleted in colorectal carcinoma) gene is typically lost late in adenomatous polyposis. Loss of the DCC gene also plays a role much later, after tumorigenesis, in propensity of a cancer to metastasize.

        c. K-ras, an oncogene, typically mutates in adenomes, perhaps enabling small adenomatous polyposis to enlarge.

        d. p53 is a tumor suppressor gene, and loss of the second normal allele typically occurs at the initiation of malignancy.

        e. For HNPCC (hereditary nonpolyposis colon cancer), a different etiology of carcinogenesis has been described. These patients are hypermutable because of defects in the DNA repair genes. However, the cascade of mutations seen in sporadic colon cancers (APC, DCC, K-ras, p53) also occurs in HNPCC.

    5. Cancerous cells (i.e., growth unregulated cells) are not necessarily capable of metastasis. Further changes are required to produce the metastatic phenotype. Some of these changes may include the following:

        a. Altered or increased **expression of cell adhesion molecules** or their receptors, which allows circulating blood- or lymph-borne cancer cells to adhere to endothelial cells.

    b. Ability to produce **extracellular matrix molecules** for its own milieu or enzymes to degrade the existing matrix, e.g., type IV collagenase to degrade endothelial basement membrane collagen and to gain access to new tissues.

    c. Ability to produce **cytoskeletal proteins** for increased cell motility.

    d. Ability to produce **angiogenic factors** for neovascularization of the new "colony."

E Diagnostics

1. A single malignant cell that undergoes 30 doublings results in 1 billion cells, which creates a **1-cm diameter tumor.**

2. With tumor doubling times of clinical cancers ranging from 20–120 days, one can extrapolate that most human tumors have **been present for 1–10 years to reach clinical detection.**

3. **Flow cytometry** is a test done on tumor cells to detect the relative amount of DNA and the growth rate.

    a. Ploidy describes the amount of DNA.

        (1) **Diploid** signifies a normal amount of DNA (i.e., two copies of each chromosome).

        (2) **Aneuploid** signifies abnormal DNA content.

        (3) **Polyploid** signifies increased DNA content at integer multiples of normal.

    b. S-phase measures the proportion of cells in the S-phase of the cell cycle. When elevated, this indicates more rapid tumor growth and presumably a more aggressive tumor.

4. **Tumor markers** are tests developed to detect tumor or tumor-specific products.

    a. Classification includes tumor-specific antigens, tumor-specific enzymes, and tumor-specific hormones.

    b. Screening. A marker used for screening should possess a high sensitivity for the detection of early, curable lesions in asymptomatic patients. Prostate-specific antigen (PSA) is an example.

    c. Prognosis and detection of residual disease. Carcinoembryonic antigen (CEA) is used as a measure of colorectal malignancy. A rising level of CEA indicates recurrence as well as prognosis (see Chapter 13, IV B 9 c).

5. **Molecular diagnostics** increases the sensitivity of biopsy material.

    a. For more accurate pathology of lymph nodes in **breast cancer, immunohistochemistry** is used to look for **cytokeratin** (an epithelial cell marker) in lymph nodes. Approximately 10%–30% of nodes considered negative with standard pathology will be found positive by the above techniques.

    b. Quantitative **immunohistochemistry** for **oncogene c-*erbB*-2** on frozen sections of **breast cancer** primary tumors correlates increased expression of c-*erbB*-2 with poorer survival.

    c. To increase the sensitivity of **pancreatic** aspiration cytology biopsies, **polymerase chain reaction** (PCR) amplification for the K-ras oncogene has a 96% sensitivity for pancreatic cancer cells.

F Clinical manifestations of cancer

1. **Seven classic symptoms of cancer** spell out the mnemonic "CAUTION:"

    a. Change in bowel or bladder habits

    b. A sore that does not heal

    c. Unusual bleeding or discharge

    d. Thickening or lump in the breast or elsewhere

    e. Indigestion or difficulty swallowing

    f. Obvious change in a wart or mole

    g. Nagging cough or hoarseness.

2. **Other manifestations**

    a. Growth, causing a **mass,** obstruction, or neurologic deficit

    b. Growth into **neighboring tissues** causing pain, paralysis, fixation, or immobility of a palpable mass

    c. Tumor necrosis causing bleeding or fever

    d. Systemic manifestations such as thrombophlebitis, endocrine symptoms due to hormones secreted by the tumor, and cachexia

      e. Extreme **weight loss** over a short period of time

      f. **Metastatic spread** as the first symptom such as enlarged lymph nodes, neurologic symptoms, or pathologic bone fractures.

   3. Screening tests for cancer detection. Asymptomatic cancers detected by screening generally have a better prognosis than symptomatic cancers. Common screening tests and the current American Cancer Society's recommendations for their use include:

      a. Mammography (annually after age 35–40)

      b. Stool for **occult blood** and **digital rectal examination** (annually after age 50)

      c. Pap smear of the cervix (every 3 years after two negative tests 1 year apart)

G **Staging of cancer** The standard staging of most cancers is based on the **tumor, nodes, and metastasis (TNM) system.** Various TNM classes are then grouped into stages. The staging of gastric cancer will be used to exemplify this system (Table 2-2).

   1. T describes the primary **tumor.**

   2. N describes the involvement of lymph **nodes** with metastatic spread.

   3. M describes distant **metastases.**

   4. Stage grouping. Staging is necessary to choose the appropriate therapy and to assess the prognosis. It also allows investigators to report their results in a standardized way so that conclusions regarding treatments and their outcomes are interpretable.

H **Diagnostic procedures**

   1. Biopsy. It is **mandatory** that **tissue be obtained** to prove microscopically that a malignancy is present. Therefore, a biopsy is always obtained in diagnosing and treating cancer. There are several types of biopsy.

      a. Aspiration biopsy or aspiration cytology biopsy. A narrow needle (e.g., 22-gauge needle) is inserted into the lesion, and **cells** are aspirated into the needle and deposited on slides. The specimen is similar to that obtained by a Pap smear and is read by a **cytopathologist.**

TABLE 2-2 Tumor, Nodes, and Metastasis (TNM) Classification System and Stage Grouping for Gastric Adenocarcinoma

Tumor (T)	
T0	No evidence of primary tumor
Tis (in situ)	Tumor limited to mucosa
T1	Tumor limited to mucosa or submucosa
T2	Tumor to but not through the serosa
T3	Tumor through the serosa but not into adjacent organs
T4	Tumor into adjacent organs (direct extension)
Nodes (N)	
N0	No metastases to lymph nodes
N1	Only perigastric lymph nodes within 3 cm of the primary tumor
N2	Only regional lymph nodes more than 3 cm from tumor but removable at operation
N3	Other intra-abdominal lymph nodes involved
Metastases (M)	
M0	No distant metastases
M1	Distant metastases
Stage grouping	
Stage 0	Tis, N0, M0
Stage 1	T1, N0, M0
Stage 2	T2 or T3, N0, M0
Stage 3	T1–3, N1 or N2, M0
Stage 4	Any T4, any T3, any N3, any M1

    b. Needle biopsy. A large needle (e.g., 18-gauge) is inserted into the lesion and a core of tissue is removed for histology. Because a needle biopsy removes more tissue than does aspiration, complications (e.g., bleeding) are more common, but the specimen is larger and the diagnosis obtained is more precise.

    c. Incisional biopsy removes a superficial or accessible portion of the lesion for diagnosis.

    d. Excisional biopsy completely removes a discrete tumor without a wide margin of normal tissue and is not curative for malignancy. It is used when local removal will not interfere with the therapy to be used for definitive local control.

    e. Staging laparotomy for Hodgkin's disease establishes the correct stage.

2. Imaging studies, such as computed tomography (CT) scan, ultrasound, and MRI are useful for assessing the extent of spread when the study is **positive.** A negative imaging study does not exclude the possibility of microscopic disease spread.

    a. Positron emission tomography (PET) scanning is an imaging modality that measures the radiation emitted by radioactive tracer molecules as they are taken up by specific cells.

    b. The data are translated into an image by CT reconstruction.

        (1) Cancer cells exhibit accelerated glucose membrane transport. Administered radio-labeled 2-fluoro-2-deoxy-D-glucose (FDG) is metabolized intracellularly and remains trapped in the cell for essentially all human cancers.

        (2) PET-FDG scanning has been demonstrated to be superior to CT scanning in detecting colorectal cancer both for preoperative staging and post-treatment assessment of recurrence, metastases, etc.

3. Laparoscopy for staging has become standard for **upper abdominal tumors** (gastric, pancreatic, hepatic) to exclude intra-abdominal spread. This decreases the number of laparotomies at which unresectable (i.e., nonsurgical) disease is found.

I Multimodality cancer therapy. Most cancer patients are treated surgically, with radiation, chemotherapy, and immunotherapy playing increasingly important roles. Choice of therapy is based on disease, stage, histologic grade, patient age, other concomitant diseases, and the intent of therapy (i.e., cure vs. palliation).

1. Surgery and radiation therapy are both used for the treatment of the primary tumor and the regional lymph nodes. Neither has any effect on areas of distant spread.

2. Chemotherapy and immunotherapy are systemic therapies with the potential to affect distant areas of spread.

3. Adjuvant therapy is systemic therapy used for patients with local control (e.g., resection) who are at high risk of microscopic disease existing in lymph nodes or distant organs. A high proportion of these patients would develop recurrence at these sites, and adjuvant therapy attempts to destroy these distant, microscopic foci of cancer.

4. Multimodality therapy uses the advantages of each therapy to counteract the shortcomings of others. Examples follow:

    a. Curable breast cancer. Surgery (mastectomy) or surgery (lumpectomy) plus radiation are used for local control. Surgery is used for staging of axillary lymph nodes, and postoperative chemotherapy is used for patients with positive malignancy in the nodes to decrease the chance of metastatic disease.

    b. Pancoast tumor of the lung. Preoperative radiation is used for regional spread into the brachial plexus to decrease the tumor's size and to render the tumor surgically resectable.

    c. Extremity sarcoma. Incisional biopsy is used for diagnosis; preoperative radiation therapy is used to decrease tumor size; radical local resection is used for initial local control; postoperative adjuvant radiation is used for further regional control; and chemotherapy is used for systemic control.

J Cancer surgery. The principles of cancer surgery are based on removing a tumor for cure. To prevent **implantation** of tumor cells at surgery, dissection is done through uninvolved tissue, staying away from the tumor. To prevent **vascular dissemination,** tumors are minimally manipulated, and the vascular pedicle is ligated early. To prevent **lymphatic spread,** the measures described previously are performed, plus the lymph node draining area is removed **in continuity** with the tumor.

1. **Curative resection.** The several types of curative resection vary with the tumor's size, biologic behavior, and location.
   a. **Wide local resection** is adequate for low-grade neoplasms that do not either metastasize to regional lymph nodes or deeply invade surrounding tissue. Examples include basal cell carcinoma of the skin or mixed tumor of the parotid gland.
   b. **Radical local resection** is used for neoplasms that deeply invade surrounding tissue, e.g., extremity sarcoma where the resection includes the entire biopsy incision and the entire muscle compartment where the tumor lies.
   c. **Radical resection with en bloc excision of lymphatic drainage** is used for tumors that usually first metastasize to regional lymph nodes (e.g., colon cancer where the segment of colon plus regional mesentery and lymphatics are removed as one specimen).
   d. **Super radical resections** remove large portions of the body and are reserved for locally extensive disease with low likelihood of metastatic spread. Examples include pelvic exenteration removal of rectum, bladder, uterus [in women], and all pelvic lymphatics and soft tissues) for locally advanced cancers of the rectum, cervix, uterus, or bladder.

2. **Staging procedures** are used to establish the extent of disease to guide treatment.
   a. **Lymph node dissections** for breast cancer and malignant melanoma are important for assessing prognosis and determining treatment. There is significant morbidity associated with lymph node dissection.
   b. **Sentinel lymph node excision** is a less invasive, potentially equally accurate staging technique.
      (1) The tumor or just adjacent to the biopsy site is injected with a **tracer,** which is followed to the first lymph node draining the area.
      (2) The tracer can be a visible dye (isosulfan blue) or a radioactive tracer (technetium-99m[^{99}Tc]-labeled sulfur colloid) visualized with a hand-held gamma probe.
      (3) The **sentinel node** can be identified in about 95% of cases; however, excisional biopsies distort lymphatic drainage and lead to lack of success in identifying the node and also compromise the technique's accuracy.
      (4) The **false-negative rate** for sentinel node biopsy (negative sentinel node but other nodes in the same area positive) is less than 5%.
      (5) The **diagnostic accuracy** depends on precise pathology, often utilizing immunohistochemistry (see IV E 5).

3. **Other surgical resections**
   a. **Resection of recurrent cancer** is occasionally feasible with localized recurrences. Examples include local (anastomotic) recurrence of GI cancer and local recurrence of skin cancer.
   b. **Resection of metastases** is feasible in several circumstances. The two most common are isolated liver metastases from colon cancer and pulmonary metastases (especially from sarcomas sensitive to chemotherapy).
   c. **Palliative surgery** is used to relieve or prevent a specific symptom of a cancer patient but without the intent to cure. An example is removal of an obstructing or bleeding colon cancer in a patient with liver metastases.
   d. **Debulking** is the removal of the majority of a tumor, leaving residual disease. The rationale is that the remaining, smaller number of cancer cells will be more susceptible to chemotherapy or radiation therapy. It appears to be useful for advanced ovarian cancers.

SECTION B: PROBLEMS AND COMPLICATIONS

V **POSTOPERATIVE COMPLICATIONS**

Postoperative complications can be associated with any operation or can be related to a specific kind of surgery. The latter types are discussed in the relevant chapters, whereas general types of complications are discussed here. **Thrombophlebitis and pulmonary embolus,** which are common postoperative complications, are discussed briefly here and in detail in Chapter 8. Most surgical complications develop in relation to some event that occurs in the operating room, emphasizing the fact that prevention is the best form of management.

A **General principles of management** during the postoperative period are important both in preventing potential complications and in allowing early detection of problems that do develop. These principles include:

1. Daily or more frequent **examination of the patient,** including the surgical wound.
2. Removal of all **surgical tubes** as soon as possible.
3. Early **ambulation** of the patient.
4. Close **monitoring** of fluid balance and electrolyte levels.
5. Adequate but not excessive **pain medication.**
6. Good **nursing care.**

B **Postoperative fever** occurs in typical patterns, and the "5W's" mnemonic is useful.

1. **Wind. Pulmonary complications,** which typically occur earliest, on postoperative days **1–3.**
   a. **Atelectasis** is the usual problem and is treated with coughing, deep breathing, ambulation, and incentive spirometry. Antibiotics should not be given unless evidence of infection is present. For a collapsed pulmonary segment or lobe, nasotracheal suction or bronchoscopy is often needed to remove secretions.
   b. **Pneumonia** can supervene if atelectasis is not treated adequately.
   c. **Pulmonary problems** are often related to pre-existing pulmonary dysfunction coupled with incisional pain, depressed respirations and cough from narcotics, and abdominal distention.
2. **Water. Urinary tract infection** typically occurs **3–5** days postoperatively, usually after bladder catheterization.
3. **Wound infections** typically cause fever beginning **5–8** days postoperatively. Only streptococcal and clostridial wound infections cause earlier fever.
4. **Walk. Venous complications** are discussed in greater detail in Chapter 8.
   a. **Deep venous thrombosis** or **phlebitis** usually starts in the lower extremities, can involve more proximal veins, can occur **any time** postoperatively, and causes fever.
   b. **Pulmonary embolism** can also be associated with fever.
   c. **Intravenous (IV) catheter infections** are related to the site and duration of placement.
      (1) **Peripheral IVs,** especially when placed in an antecubital vein or more proximally, can become infected and cause fever. On physical examination, an inflamed IV site that may have purulent drainage is found.
      (2) **Suppurative thrombophlebitis** is an infected thrombosed vein from an IV catheter. Excision of the thrombosed segment of vein is the appropriate treatment.
      (3) **Central catheters** are more prone to infection when placed near a tracheostomy or via the femoral vein.
      (4) **Subclavian** or **internal jugular vein catheters** can result in subclavian vein thrombosis.
5. **Wonder drugs.** In fact, any drug can cause **drug fever.** Be especially suspicious of antibiotics, which are often being used empirically.
6. **Less common sources** of postoperative fever include postpericardiotomy syndrome (see Chapter 6) (occurs 5–7 days postoperatively), anastomotic leak after bowel surgery (7–10 days postoperatively), parotitis, sinusitis, acalculous cholecystitis, pancreatitis, pseudomembranous colitis, and addisonian crisis.

C **Hydration** is in flux postoperatively.

1. **Dehydration (hypovolemia)** is common early after surgery because of third-space sequestration of fluids in the operative site.
   a. Oliguria, tachycardia, and orthostatic hypotension may result.
   b. Treatment is hydration.
2. **Overhydration (hypervolemia).** On the third or fourth postoperative day, the body begins to mobilize the third-space fluid, which increases the intravascular volume until the fluid is excreted by the kidneys. Hypervolemia may thus occur in patients with impaired cardiac or renal function.
   a. Congestive heart failure or pulmonary congestion and impaired oxygenation may result.

b. The intravascular volume increase that results from mobilization of third-space fluid should be anticipated.

c. Attending to fluid balance and weighing the patient daily should prevent this problem.

VI Surgical Infections

Surgical infections can be defined as infections that require surgical intervention to resolve completely or infections that develop as a complication of surgery. Some are in both categories.

A Overview

1. **Characteristics of surgical infections**
   a. They usually involve a penetrating **injury** (e.g., from trauma), a perforating injury (e.g., a perforated ulcer), or an operative site (e.g., the surgical wound).
   b. Multiple **organisms** are often present.
   c. **Treatment** may require surgical drainage of the infection or debridement of necrotic or grossly contaminated tissue; **antibiotics alone will not resolve the infection.**

2. **Surgical wound infections**
   a. **The incidence** of wound infections is related directly to the nature of the surgical procedure performed. The classification of wounds by extent of contamination is described in Chapter 1, V C.
   b. **Clinical presentation.** Wound infection often presents as a spiking fever at approximately the fifth to eighth postoperative day. There may be localized wound tenderness, cellulitis, or drainage from the wound.
   c. **Treatment.** Simple incision and drainage will resolve most postoperative wound infections. Deeper wound infections or extensive necrosis may require operative debridement and antibiotics.

3. **Prosthetic infections.** Prostheses are synthetic implantable devices, including vascular grafts, heart valves, artificial joints, fascial mesh replacements, and metallic bone supports.
   a. **Clinical presentation.** An infected prosthesis usually causes symptoms of either local infection or generalized sepsis. The most common organisms infecting prostheses are **staphylococci; these infections are life threatening.**
   b. **Treatment.** Prophylactic antibiotics are always used when implanting a prosthesis; however, an infected prosthesis usually cannot be sterilized with antibiotics and, therefore, removal of the prosthesis is usually necessary.

4. **Prophylactic antibiotics** are given during the perioperative period to combat bacterial contamination of tissues that occurs during the operative procedure. The general rules for the use of prophylactic antibiotics are:
   a. The operation must carry a significant **risk of a postoperative infection.** A clean procedure would not require prophylactic antibiotics, but the following situations would:
      (1) A procedure in which a prosthesis is to be implanted
      (2) Clean-contaminated procedures, where a nonsterile area is entered; e.g., the respiratory or upper GI tract
      (3) Contaminated procedures, such as colon or rectal surgery
   b. The antibiotics used should be **effective against** the **pathogens** likely to be present in the operative site.
   c. The antibiotics must reach an **effective tissue level** at the time of the incision. Therefore, they should be given 1–2 hours **before** surgery.
   d. The antibiotics should be given for only **6–24 hours after surgery.** Longer-lasting regimens offer no additional protection and carry risks of superinfection.
   e. The **benefits** of the prophylactic antibiotic should **outweigh** its **potential dangers,** such as allergic reactions or the risk of bacterial or fungal superinfections from overgrowth of pathogens.

B Abscesses

1. **Cutaneous abscesses**
   a. **Types**

(1) **Furuncles (boils)** are cutaneous staphylococcal abscesses. They are frequently seen with acne and other skin disorders. Bacterial colonization begins in hair follicles and can cause both local cellulitis and abscess formation.

(2) **Carbuncles** are cutaneous abscesses that spread through the dermis into the subcutaneous region. They are common in individuals with diabetes.

(3) **Hidradenitis suppurativa** is an infection involving the apocrine sweat glands in the axillary, inguinal, and perineal regions. The infection results in chronic abscess formation and often requires complete excision of the apocrine gland-bearing skin to prevent recurrence.

b. **Causative organisms**

(1) **Staphylococcal organisms** (*Staphylococcus epidermidis, Staphylococcus aureus*) frequently infect cutaneous lesions. Staphylococci usually produce **pus,** which must be drained to allow healing.

(2) **Other organisms,** including anaerobic and gram-negative organisms, can also cause cutaneous abscesses. Coliform organisms are often present in axillary, inguinal, and perineal cutaneous abscesses.

c. **Diagnosis.** The microbiologic diagnosis is made by incising the abscess, then culturing and Gram staining the pus. Most staphylococcal organisms are resistant to penicillin; therefore, one of the semisynthetic penicillins, erythromycin, a cephalosporin, or a fluoroquinolone should be used.

d. **Treatment**

(1) Drainage

(2) Appropriate antibiotic therapy

(3) Wound care with irrigation and debridement when necessary

(4) Excision of the involved area when it contains multiple small abscesses, sinus tracts, or necrotic tissue.

2. **Intra-abdominal abscesses**

a. **Causes**

(1) **Extrinsic causes** include penetrating trauma and surgical procedures.

(2) **Intrinsic causes** include perforation of a hollow viscus, such as the appendix or duodenum; seeding of bacteria from a source outside the abdomen, e.g., tubo-ovarian abscess; or ischemia and infarction of tissue within the abdomen.

b. The most common **sites** are the

(1) Subphrenic space

(2) Subhepatic space

(3) Lateral gutters posteriorly

(4) Pelvis

(5) Periappendiceal or pericolonic areas.

(6) Multiple abscesses are present in up to 15% of cases.

c. **Signs and symptoms** of abdominal abscesses are fever, pain, and leukocytosis.

(1) These abscesses may be large and usually produce spiking fevers.

(2) Postoperative abscesses usually produce fever during the second postoperative week.

(3) When there is a delay in seeking medical attention or a delay in diagnosis, patients may present with generalized sepsis.

(4) GI bleeding or pulmonary, renal, or hepatic failure may occur.

d. **Diagnosis.** The key to an expeditious diagnosis is a high index of **suspicion.**

(1) The patient may have tenderness or an abdominal mass, but often no physical findings are present (particularly with a pelvic abscess).

(2) Ultrasonography and CT scan are essential for diagnosis.

e. **Treatment**

(1) The mainstay of intra-abdominal abscess treatment is **drainage.**

(2) Diagnosis and localization with imaging studies allows proper choice of modality.

(3) Unilocular and accessible abscesses can be drained percutaneously with radiologic guidance.

(4) Abscesses that are complex, multilocular, include significant amounts of necrotic debris, or are inaccessible require surgical drainage.

(5) Ideally, drainage is performed without contaminating the general peritoneal cavity.

(a) Pelvic abscesses may be drained transrectally or through the superior vagina.

(b) Subphrenic abscesses may be drained posteriorly through a twelfth rib approach.

C **Cellulitis** is inflammation of the dermal and subcutaneous tissues secondary to **nonsuppurative bacterial invasion.** It may result from a puncture wound or any other type of skin break.

1. **Signs and symptoms**
   a. Cellulitis produces redness, edema, and localized tenderness. Fever and leukocytosis are usually present.
   b. The bacteria may also infect the lymphatics, resulting in red, tender streaks on an extremity (lymphangitis).
   c. A deep abscess can result in overlying cellulitis and should be suspected when a patient does not rapidly respond to antibiotics.

2. **Treatment.** The usual organism is a *Streptococcus,* which is almost always sensitive to penicillin.

D **Tetanus prophylaxis**

1. **Active immunization** with tetanus toxoid injections given in the recommended schedule results in a protective titer within 30 days. This immunization is usually given in infancy (with the diphtheria-pertussis-tetanus shots) or during military induction. A booster dose every 10 years is recommended.

2. **Prophylaxis at the time of injury**
   a. Any person with a penetrating injury must receive tetanus prophylaxis if previous immunization cannot be documented.
      (1) A previously immunized person should be given a booster dose if not given within the past 5 years.
      (2) A patient with a clean injury who has never been immunized may be given the first of three immunizing doses, but the patient must receive the subsequent two doses (4–6 weeks and 6–12 months later, respectively).
      (3) A patient with a dirty wound who has never been immunized should be given **passive immunization** with human tetanus immune globulin intramuscularly.
         (a) The protection lasts approximately 1 month.
         (b) The first dose of tetanus toxoid may be given at the same time, but it should be given at a separate intramuscular site.
   b. Adequate **debridement** of devitalized tissue and removal of all foreign debris are also essential.
   c. The value of **antibiotics,** particularly penicillin, for the prophylaxis of tetanus-prone wounds is unproven. However, for patients who have a suspected *Clostridium tetani* infection or extensive necrosis, prophylactic penicillin should be given in high doses.

E **Necrotizing fasciitis** is a rapidly progressive bacterial infection in which multiple organisms invade fascial planes. The infection travels rapidly and causes vascular thrombosis as it progresses, resulting in necrosis of the tissue involved. The overlying skin may appear normal, leading the clinician to underestimate the severity of the infection. Necrotizing fasciitis may result from a puncture wound, a surgical wound, or open trauma.

1. **Signs and symptoms**
   a. **Hemorrhagic bullae** may develop on the skin, accompanied by edema and redness, and crepitus may be present; however, the skin also may appear normal.
   b. The patient shows signs of **progressive toxicity** (fever, tachycardia) and may have localized wound pain.
   c. The necrotic wound or tissue involved has a foul-smelling serous **discharge.**
   d. A plain radiograph of the wound area may reveal **air** in the **soft tissues.** CT scans will also show air in the tissues.

2. **Diagnosis. Gram stain** reveals multiple organisms, which act synergistically, giving the fasciitis its rapidly progressive and destructive character, including:
   a. Microaerophilic streptococci
   b. Staphylococci
   c. Gram-negative aerobes and anaerobes.

3. **Treatment** is surgical, and early diagnosis is extremely important.
   a. The surgeon attempts to remove all infected or devitalized tissue at the first debridement because remaining necrotic tissue will allow the process to continue.
   b. The removal of large amounts of skin and surrounding tissue and, occasionally, amputation of an extremity may be required.
   c. Daily debridement may be needed.
   d. Appropriate antibiotics in high doses are required.
   e. This infection is **life threatening,** and prompt treatment is essential.

F Clostridial myositis and cellulitis (gas gangrene) is most commonly caused by *Clostridium perfringens.*

1. **Characteristics of wounds susceptible to develop this condition** include the following:
   a. Extensive **tissue destruction** has occurred
   b. Marked impairment of the **local blood supply** from the injury itself, from complications of the injury (e.g., vascular thrombosis), or from iatrogenic causes (e.g., an overly tight orthopedic cast)
   c. The wound is grossly **contaminated**
   d. There has been a **delay in treatment** (usually more than 6 hours)
   e. The patient has a **pre-existing condition** causing immunologic incompetence, such as corticosteroid drug therapy or poorly controlled diabetes.

2. **Clinical presentation**
   a. The **onset of symptoms** is usually 48 hours after injury but may occur as early as 6 hours after injury.
   b. The most common complaint, **severe pain** at the site of injury, is due to the rapidly infiltrating infection. This symptom may be obscured if the patient is receiving narcotics. If a surgical patient requires an increase in narcotics, the wound should be examined before the narcotics are increased.
   c. The **pulse** is rapid and thready. The patient appears diaphoretic, pale, weak, and confused or delirious. The temperature is often, but not always, elevated.
   d. The wound is more **tender to the touch** than is the usual postoperative wound. The skin may appear normal, but the wound usually drains a brownish serous fluid with a foul odor. **Crepitus** may appear around the wound edges but is often a late sign.
   e. **Blood studies** reveal a falling hematocrit and a rising bilirubin from hemolysis. The white blood count may be mildly elevated.
   f. Gram stain of the wound discharge reveals **Gram-positive bacilli with spores.** Numerous red blood cells are present, but few white cells are present.
   g. A plain x-ray of the wound area may reveal **air** in the **soft tissues.**

3. **Treatment.** Adequate **debridement** at the time of initial injury is important for prophylaxis. Treatment for established clostridial infection includes extensive debridement within the tissue planes involved and antibiotics, especially penicillin. If extensive soft tissue necrosis is present in an extremity, amputation may be necessary.
   a. Hyperbaric oxygen therapy is used, but its value is unproven.
   b. Human tetanus immune globulin will not prevent or treat gas gangrene.
   c. Delay in treatment to consider further diagnostic procedures or to observe the patient's course is usually catastrophic.

G Infections after surgery

1. **Gastrointestinal surgery**
   a. **Upper GI tract surgery**
      (1) The rate of serious infections after operations on the upper GI tract is 5%–15%.
      (2) The **oral cavity** is colonized by large numbers of aerobic and anaerobic bacteria. These bacteria are generally killed in the low pH environment of the **stomach.**
      (3) Gastric cultures become positive when obstruction or blood is present; therefore, prophylactic antibiotics should be used in these settings.

(4) Patients without the protective low gastric pH, e.g., those taking antiulcer medications (H_2-blockers, proton pump inhibitors, etc.), achlorhydria, or gastric malignancy also should be given prophylactic antibiotics.

(5) The usual antibiotics are a cephalosporin or a fluoroquinolone to cover both aerobes and anaerobes.

b. Biliary tract surgery

(1) The biliary tree is not colonized with **bacteria** in the normal individual. The colonization rate rises to 15%–30% for patients with chronic calculous cholecystitis and to over 80% in patients with common duct obstruction. Of those patients with positive cultures:

(a) *Escherichia coli* is present in over one half of the cases; other gram-negative organisms account for most of the remainder.

(b) *Streptococcus faecalis,* the aerobic gram-positive enterococcus, may also be present, and *Salmonella* strains are occasionally present. Anaerobic organisms, especially *C. perfringens,* are present in up to 20% of cases.

(2) For elective cholecystectomy, simple prophylaxis with a cephalosporin is adequate.

(3) Therapeutic antibiotics are needed in patients with common duct stones, cholangitis, and empyema or gangrene of the gallbladder. A cephalosporin or penicillin-combination should be given.

c. Colonic and rectal surgery

(1) Wound and intraperitoneal infections often (6%–60%) follow colorectal surgery.

(2) Normal human **colonic flora** is composed of both aerobes and anaerobes.

(a) **Aerobes** are present at levels of 10^8–10^9 bacteria per gram of stool. *E. coli,* the most common aerobe, is the organism most often found in wound infections after colonic surgery.

(b) **Anaerobes** are present at levels of 10^{11} bacteria per gram of stool (1000-fold greater numbers than those for aerobes). Many types are present, but *Bacteroides fragilis* is the most common and is the usual cause of anaerobic wound infections.

(c) Mixed aerobic and anaerobic infections are typical.

(3) An effective **preoperative regimen** combines the removal of gross feces (mechanical preparation of the bowel) with the use of oral nonabsorbable antibiotics.

(a) **Mechanical removal** of the feces is the most important factor in lowering the bacterial counts and the incidence of wound infections. Regimens include aggressive purgation—with potent oral laxatives such as mannitol or polyethylene glycol—plus enemas.

(b) **Antibiotic prophylaxis** will lower the incidence of wound infection only after adequate mechanical preparation. To be effective, the antibiotics must be active against both aerobic and anaerobic organisms.

(i) **Oral antibiotics,** such as neomycin and erythromycin base started 10–22 hours before surgery, result in maximal bacterial suppression at the time of surgery. Longer treatment periods allow resistant bacterial overgrowth.

(ii) IV antibiotics may further lower the incidence of wound infection.

(c) **Preparation of the colon and rectum** should be carried out before all elective operations unless a high-grade (complete) obstruction is present. An obstruction will compromise the mechanical bowel preparation and may require the creation of a proximal stoma to relieve the obstruction.

(d) In **emergency procedures** (e.g., after trauma) when no bowel preparation is possible, IV antibiotics should be given, and the wound should not be closed primarily. Colonic anastomoses are riskier in these situations than in elective situations.

2. Gynecologic surgeries are usually clean-contaminated procedures, and prophylactic antibiotics are appropriate.

3. Urologic surgery

a. Although the normal urinary tract is sterile, the most common **pathogen** encountered is *E. coli,* followed by other gram-negative rods and enterococci.

b. The general principle is that elective surgery should be postponed until any **infection has been successfully treated;** this principle is especially true for urologic surgery.

    c. Chronic indwelling tubes (e.g., suprapubic bladder catheters nephrostomies) are generally colonized with bacteria but do not require antibiotic therapy unless the patient has a symptomatic local infection, generalized sepsis, or catheter obstruction; or unless a urea-splitting organism, such as *Proteus*, is present.

    d. In the presence of urinary tract **pathology**, it may be impossible to sterilize the urine. Therefore, antibiotics are used perioperatively as both treatment and prophylaxis.

4. Vascular surgery

    a. The risk of **vascular prosthetic graft** infection is 1%–6%. Infection may develop early (within months) or years later.

    b. The most common infecting organism is *S. aureus*, followed by coagulase-negative *S. epidermidis*. Coliform infections are becoming more common.

    c. Perioperative prophylactic antibiotics will lower the incidence of graft infection from a high of 6% down to 1%. The recommended antibiotic is a cephalosporin.

    d. Prophylactic antibiotics (amoxicillin) should also be used when a patient with a prosthetic graft undergoes a procedure associated with a transient bacteremia (such as dental extraction).

5. Cardiac surgery. The sources of infection for cardiac surgery are the same as those for vascular surgery. Severe infections include sternal osteomyelitis and dehiscence and prosthetic valve endocarditis.

6. Noncardiac thoracic surgery. Lung surgery has a high risk of infection when the lung is already infected or when a significant volume of lung is removed (as in a pneumonectomy) and a large dead space remains. For elective pulmonary resections, many surgeons use prophylactic antibiotics for the gram-positive cocci that colonize the upper respiratory tree.

7. Orthopaedic surgery. Postoperative infections of bone or implanted prostheses are major **life-threatening** complications (similar to vascular and cardiac surgery). The most common organisms are slime-forming staphylococci. Prophylactic antibiotics against these organisms are used routinely.

H **Infections after trauma**

1. Deep burns (second and third degree). Tetanus prophylaxis must be assured.

    a. Burns are prone to develop **group A streptococcal infection** during the first 5 days. If present, penicillin G or a penicillinase-resistant synthetic penicillin is used. Prophylactic antibiotics are not usually given, however.

    b. To reduce the colonization of injured tissues, topical antibiotics are applied. These antibiotics should be effective against both gram-negative rods and gram-positive cocci.

    c. Purulent infection of IV catheter and cutdown sites is called *suppurative thrombophlebitis* and must be treated by excision of the vein (see V B 4 c [2]).

2. Penetrating abdominal trauma should be treated with an antibiotic regimen that covers both anaerobic and aerobic organisms.

3. Penetrating chest wounds should be treated with antibiotics effective against organisms commonly found in the respiratory tract.

4. Bites. Human bites should be treated with penicillin, as they are likely to contain mixed anaerobic and aerobic organisms. **Animal bites** warrant prophylactic antibiotics if injury is extensive.

VII   GASTROINTESTINAL FISTULAS

A **Definitions**

1. A **fistula** is an abnormal communication between two or more hollow organs or between one hollow organ and a body surface.

2. A fistula is **named** according to the **sites** that are joined. Therefore, a **bronchobiliary fistula** connects the bronchial tree with the biliary tree; a **gastrocutaneous fistula** communicates between the stomach and the skin.

B **Etiologies**

1. Congenital. Distal tracheoesophageal fistula with esophageal atresia is the most important congenital fistula (see Chapter 29, IV).

TABLE 2-3 Approximate Electrolyte Content of Gastrointestinal Secretions

Source	Electrolytes (mEq/L)			
	Na$^+$	K$^+$	Cl$^-$	HCO$_3^-$
Stomach	60	10	50–100	0–20
Duodenum	120	5	100	20
Bile duct	145	5	100	40
Pancreas	140	5	75	100
Ileum	100	5	65	30

2. **Trauma or operative injury.** Traumatic injury or anastomotic breakdown can produce fistulization. Examples include a colocutaneous fistula from an anastomotic leak or a pancreaticocutaneous fistula complicating a splenectomy.

3. **Inflammation.** Crohn's disease can cause many fistulas, including enterovesical (i.e., small bowel to bladder) and ileosigmoid.

4. **Malignancy.** Fistulas can develop when a tumor destroys tissue. For example, a colovesical fistula can occur if a sigmoid colon cancer erodes into the urinary bladder.

5. **Radiation damage.** An enterovaginal fistula can develop after pelvic irradiation for cervical carcinoma.

C **Complications**

1. **Fluid and electrolyte imbalances** are frequent complications of fistulas, especially those involving the proximal bowel or pancreas. The electrolyte content of various GI secretions is shown in Table 2-3. Electrolyte losses can be directly measured from a sample of the fistula drainage. For example, a pancreatic fistula that drains 700 mL of bicarbonate-rich fluid a day can produce dehydration and metabolic acidosis.

2. **Sepsis,** a frequent accompaniment of fistulas, occurs when the contents of an organ leak and contaminate sterile spaces (e.g., peritoneum or pleura).

3. **Skin excoriation** can occur when intestinal secretions drain onto the abdominal skin. This skin disruption can be painful and result in cellulitis or sepsis.

4. **Malnutrition** can develop either from inadequate absorption of nutrients due to short circuiting of the bowel or external loss of ingested food (e.g., gastrocolic fistula and high-output enterocutaneous fistula, respectively) or because of increased caloric needs from associated infection or stress.

5. **Hemorrhage** is an infrequent but potentially life-threatening complication of enteric fistulas. It occurs when a fistula erodes into a mesenteric blood vessel, causing severe bleeding.

D **Evaluation** Management of the patient with an enteric fistula requires knowledge of the anatomy, etiology, and physiology of the defect.

1. **History and physical examination**
   a. The **history** can provide useful etiologic information, e.g., diverticulitis or Crohn's disease, or pneumaturia.
   b. **Examining the patient** provides information about the location of an external fistula and the character of its drainage. The status of hydration and malnutrition should be assessed.
   c. The **volume of drainage** must be determined.

2. **Radiographic studies** are vital in determining the anatomy. Contrast material may be administered by mouth, by rectum, or directly into the fistula (**fistulogram** or **sinogram**).
   a. Ultrasonography, CT scan, and MRI can be useful in locating an undrained collection (i.e., an abscess), which may be associated with the fistula and if undrained could be a source of infection.
   b. Radiographs should also be used to **exclude the presence of obstruction** distal to the fistula (see VII E 6 f).

    3. Laboratory tests on the drainage are useful to determine electrolyte losses from the fistula, and bacteriologic cultures should be obtained in patients with possible sepsis.

E **Management**

    1. Hydration and correction of electrolyte disturbances require urgent attention.

    2. Control of infection requires immediate attention. Antibiotics and drainage of abscesses are usually required before patients improve: A fistula will not heal in the presence of an infected collection.

    3. Control of external drainage helps to minimize further morbidity. Suction catheters, drains, collection bags, or operative diversion may be useful in protecting body surfaces from irritation. Bowel rest, provided by prolonged fasting, often diminishes GI fluid losses.

    4. Correction of malnutrition should begin as soon as the patient is stabilized. Most patients require parenteral nutrition. Occasionally, tube feedings of a low-residue diet, or even oral feedings, will be possible.

    5. Therapy to inhibit organ-specific secretions is used when appropriate.
       a. For the stomach: H_2-blockers or proton pump inhibitors
       b. For the pancreas: octreotide.

    6. "Spontaneous closure" will occur in most patients with conservative therapy to minimize drainage and with appropriate nutrition. Closure with conservative measures takes 2–8 weeks. However, spontaneous closure is unlikely, and operative repair is required when any of the following is present, using the mnemonic "FRIEND":
       a. **F**oreign body at the fistula
       b. **R**adiation injury at the fistula
       c. **I**njured bowel or inflammatory bowel disease at the fistula site
       d. **E**pithelialization of the fistula tract
       e. **N**eoplasia (or cancer) at the fistula
       f. **D**istal obstruction beyond the fistula.

    7. Operative repair is best performed electively in a nonseptic, well-nourished patient. Operation typically involves:
       a. **Identification** of the fistula
       b. **Resection** of the fistula and damaged bowel
       c. **Anastomosis** to restore bowel continuity.

F **Results** Major improvements in fistula management have occurred in the past 2 decades, with resultant increased survival rates.

    1. Mortality rates. Until the mid 1960s, mortality rates were over 50% for gastric, duodenal, or small bowel fistulas.
       a. Management emphasized early attempts at operative repair before malnutrition developed.
       b. Major causes of death were electrolyte and fluid disturbances, malnutrition, and peritonitis.

    2. Current management should lower the mortality rates to 2%–10%, depending on the etiology of the fistula.
       a. Sepsis and renal failure remain significant causes of death.
       b. Malnutrition and electrolyte disturbances have largely been eliminated as causes of death because of improved techniques for venous access, blood chemistry monitoring, and prolonged parenteral feeding.

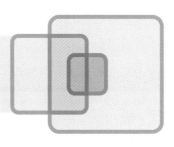

chapter 3

Medical Risk Factors in Surgical Patients

PAULINE K. PARK · HOWARD H. WEITZ · BRUCE E. JARRELL

I GENERAL ASPECTS

Although the natural history of each medical disorder has a pattern of its own, certain considerations apply to most disease processes when evaluating and minimizing operative risk.

A **Overview** Operative risk is a function of many factors, including the **baseline general medical status** of the patient, the **natural history of the disease process** precipitating the need for surgery, and any **alterations of the patient's baseline medical status** by the surgical process.

1. **Elective surgery.** The majority of elective surgery patients undergo preoperative evaluation as an **outpatient,** prior to admission to the hospital. Adequate time should be allowed for a complete assessment.

   a. **Routine preoperative laboratory testing for elective surgery** should be performed **selectively.**

      (1) In low-risk populations, randomly ordered screening studies are not cost effective. In a study of more than 3,000 asymptomatic patients undergoing elective surgery, Perez reported that routine testing led to a change in perioperative management in fewer than 1% of cases (Perez A, Planell J, Bacardaz C, et al. Value of routine preoperative tests: a multicenter study in four general hospitals. *Br J Anaesth.* 1995:74[3]:250–256).

      (2) In a randomized study of 18,198 patients undergoing cataract surgery, perioperative morbidity and mortality was not reduced by the use of routine preoperative testing when patients were stratified by severity of underlying medical illness, American Society of Anesthesiology (ASA) risk class, or history of coexisting medical conditions (Schein OD, Katz J, Bass EB, et al. The value of routine preoperative medical testing before cataract surgery. *N Engl J Med.* 2000;342[3]:168–175).

      (3) While elderly patients have a higher incidence of abnormal laboratory values, routine testing based on age may not impact outcome. In a study of 544 patients greater than 70 years of age undergoing noncardiac surgery requiring anesthesia, only ASA risk class and surgical risk were found to be independently predictive of postoperative adverse events (Dzankic S, Pastor D, Gonzalez C, et al. The prevalence and predictive value of abnormal preoperative laboratory tests in elderly surgical patients. *Anesth Analg.* 2001;93[2]: 249–250).

   b. **Testing should be directed by** the patient's history, examination, and presenting illness (Table 3-1).

2. **Emergency surgery.** Patients requiring emergency surgery are at higher risk **for perioperative morbidity and mortality.** They often have **acute metabolic derangements** and need **prompt, thorough evaluation before surgery** to identify any factors that can be improved preoperatively.

B A careful history helps the physician to ascertain risk factors, including:

1. Underlying medical conditions

2. **Allergies** to medications

TABLE 3-1 Suggested Criteria for Preoperative Testing

Complete blood count
Procedures that may involve substantial blood loss
History or examination suggesting anemias or polycythemia
History of malignancy
Systemic disease associated with anemia or risk from anemia
Chronic renal insufficiency
Cardiac disease
Pregnant women
Populations with a higher prevalence of anemia
Institutionalized elderly (age 75 or older)
Recent immigrants
As a screening test for health maintenance in patients without prior medical care

Electrolytes, glucose, and creatinine
Conditions associated with fluid and electrolyte abnormalities
SIADH
DI
Severe liver disease
Chronic diarrhea
Systemic disease associated with electrolyte abnormalities or risk from electrolyte abnormalities
Cardiac disease
Hypertension
Renal disease
Endocrine disease
Diabetes mellitus
Pancreatic, hypothalamic, adrenal dysfunction
Use of medications associated with fluid and electrolyte abnormalities
Diuretics
Steroids
Inability to provide a history

Liver function tests
Liver/biliary tract disease
History of hepatitis
Known or suspected malignancy

PT/PTT/Platelet count
Current active bleeding
Anticoagulant therapy
History of abnormal bleeding
Liver disease
Malabsorption or malnutrition
Inability to provide a history
Not indicated without a clinical history or evidence of a bleeding disorder

Urinalysis
Surgery in which urinary tract instrumentation is anticipated

Electrocardiogram
Active cardiac disease by history and physical examination
Systemic diseases associated with occult cardiac conditions
Hypertension
Peripheral vascular disease
Diabetes mellitus
Collagen vascular disease
Certain malignancies
Certain infectious disease
Use of medication with potential cardiac toxicity
Doxorubicin

TABLE 3-1 Suggested Criteria for Preoperative Testing (Continued)

Phenothiazines
Tricyclic antidepressants
Consider in:
  Planned intrathoracic, aortic, intraperitoneal, or emergency procedures
  Men >40–45 years of age and women >55 years of age

Chest radiograph
Intrathoracic surgical procedures
Active chest disease on history and physical examination
Elderly patients, selected

DI, diabetes insipidus; SIADH, syndrome of inappropriate secretion of antidiuretic hormone.
Adapted from Ziring BS. In: Merli EJ, Weitz HH, eds. *Medical Management of the Surgical Patient*. Philadelphia: WB Saunders; 1992.

3. **Current medications** (e.g., steroids, diuretics, anticoagulants) as well as **over-the-counter products** (e.g., aspirin) or **alternative medications** that a patient might not consider to be a drug

4. **Prior difficulties with surgical procedures or anesthetics**

5. **Familial disorders,** such as bleeding disorders (e.g., von Willebrand's disease) or anesthetic complications (e.g., malignant hyperthermia)

C **Physiologic parameters**   Attention to certain physiologic parameters in preoperative patients lowers operative risk.

1. **Volume status** (see Chapter 1, I) should be assessed.
   a. **Factors to consider** include:
      (1) Past and current weight
      (2) Skin turgor, mucous membrane moistness, and presence of axillary sweat
      (3) Jugular venous distention or pulmonary rales
      (4) Alterations in vital signs, such as blood pressure and heart rate
   b. In acute situations, volume status abnormalities should be treated promptly (see Chapter 1, I).
      (1) **Orthostatic blood pressure changes** can be determined by a comparison of the supine and the upright blood pressures.
      (2) **Urine output** should be determined **hourly** if time permits.
      (3) Even in urgent cases (e.g., a perforated viscus), it may be beneficial to stabilize volume status preoperatively.

2. **Electrolyte abnormalities** (see Chapter 1, I) should be corrected.
   a. The presence of nausea, vomiting, diarrhea, chronic anorexia, or bowel obstruction can be associated with dehydration and electrolyte shifts.
   b. In **acute situations,** serum electrolyte levels may not reflect the true fluid or metabolic status and should be interpreted with the clinical picture in mind.

3. **Red blood cell (RBC) mass** (see Chapter 1, IV C) should be evaluated.
   a. **Acute blood loss** may not alter the peripheral blood hematocrit for up to 24 hours. Therefore, the need for RBC replacement should be determined from other variables, such as sites of obvious blood loss.
   b. **Chronic anemia** is usually well compensated by an increase in plasma volume.
      (1) The **cause** of the anemia should be determined, because the underlying disease may affect the planned surgery.
      (2) For example, patients with **sickle cell anemia** frequently develop **cholelithiasis.** Hydration and oxygenation should be carefully maintained in these patients during cholecystectomy to avoid precipitating a sickle cell crisis.
   c. Measures to **conserve** or **increase RBC mass** follow.

(1) **Autologous blood donation** can be considered in elective cases with anticipated blood loss in order to reduce the risk of acquiring transmissible disease (see Chapter 1, IV B 3).

(2) Oral or parenteral **iron supplements** should be given to patients who have an iron deficiency and to those undergoing autologous donation or receiving erythropoietin.

(3) Recombinant human **erythropoietin** stimulates RBC production. It may be useful in patients with renal failure–related anemia, anemia of chronic disease, in association with autologous donation, or in patients who refuse transfusion.

(4) **Intraoperative blood salvage** and **autotransfusion** of recovered blood can be utilized if not specifically contraindicated by the presence of infection, contamination, or malignancy.

(5) **Operative blood loss should be minimized** with effective surgical hemostasis.

d. Criteria for **allogeneic RBC transfusion** are not fixed. Consideration must be given to the **patient's medical status** (i.e., the presence of underlying pulmonary, cardiac, and cardiovascular disease), the **duration of anemia,** and the **blood loss anticipated** during the procedure. This must be weighed against the risk; allogeneic transfusion has been associated with increased rates of pneumonia and perioperative infection and increased mortality.

(1) In general,

(a) Patients with hemoglobin greater than 10 g/dL generally do not require transfusion.

(b) Patients with hemoglobin between 7 and 10 g/dL compensate adequately and require an individual assessment of the risks and benefits prior to transfusion.

(c) Patients with hemoglobin less than 7 g/dL generally benefit from transfusion.

(2) Transfusion should be triggered by the presence of **symptomatic anemia,** as manifested by tachycardia, oliguria, hypotension, fatigue, syncope, tachypnea, dyspnea, or transient ischemic attack.

(3) Requirements of **critically ill patients**

(a) May be based on a calculation of oxygen delivery (see Chapter 1, IV C).

(b) A randomized clinical trial demonstrated no difference in overall 30-day mortality between intensive care unit (ICU) patients managed with a restrictive transfusion strategy (transfusion for hemoglobin below 7 mg/dL, goal 7–9 mg/dL) versus a more liberal strategy (transfusion for hemoglobin below 10mg/dL, goal 10–12 mg/dL) (Hebert PC, Wells G, Blajchman MA, et al. A multicenter, randomized, controlled clinical trial of transfusion requirements in critical care. Transfusion Requirements in Critical Care Investigators, Canadian Critical Care Trials Group. *N Engl J Med.* 1999;340:409–417).

4. **Malnutrition,** when severe, can increase the risk of postoperative complications following major elective surgery (see Chapter 1, VI).

5. **Infection** (see Chapter 2, VI) should be controlled before surgery.

a. **Elective procedures** should be postponed until infections are under control.

b. **Prophylactic antibiotics** (see Chapter 2, VI A 4) may reduce the risk of infectious complications.

(1) The antibiotic agent should cover pathogens that are likely to cause surgical site infection.

(2) **Dosing should be timed to establish bactericidal concentrations in serum and tissues at the time of skin incision.**

(3) Redosing should be timed to maintain serum and tissue levels for a few hours after skin closure.

c. **In emergency conditions** that involve **potential contamination,** such as a perforated viscus or penetrating trauma, appropriate antibiotics should be given as early as possible.

D **Surgical outcomes research** The Department of Veteran's Affairs (VA) National Surgical Quality Improvement Program (**NSQIP**) has systematically collected and analyzed risk-adjusted surgical data in VA hospitals since 1991.

1. By **measuring and responding to variations in outcome,** the program succeeded in **reducing 30-day mortality and hospital length of stay due to complications** in a broad range of surgical patients. [Khuri SF, Daley J, Henderson W, et al. The Department of Veterans Affairs' NSQIP: the first national, validated, outcome-based, risk-adjusted, and peer-controlled program for the measurement and enhancement of the quality of surgical care. National VA Surgical Quality Improvement Program. *Ann Surg.* 1998;228(4):491–507].

2. In the initial data set, the **most predictive preoperative risk factors for mortality in noncardiac surgery** patients were:
   a. Admission serum albumin
   b. ASA class
   c. Disseminated cancer
   d. Emergency operation
   e. Age
   f. Blood urea nitrogen (BUN) >40 mg/dL
   g. Do Not Resuscitate orders
   h. Operation complexity score
   i. SGOT >40 IU/mL
   j. Weight loss >10% in 6 months
   k. Functional status
   l. WBC >11,000/mm^3

E **Prevention of complications**   In certain acute conditions, such as appendicitis and small bowel obstruction, the overall prognosis depends on interventions that halt the natural progression of the disease. It is important to establish the diagnosis and to begin treatment before complications develop, even if a surgical procedure is required for diagnosis. For example, the overall mortality rate for simple appendicitis without rupture is lower than 1%, but the rate increases in patients with a ruptured appendix.

F **Patient education**   Ensuring that the patient has a **realistic understanding of the prognosis and the expected outcome** of the operative procedure helps to ensure the patient's cooperation postoperatively and, therefore, improves the operative risk.

II   THE SURGICAL PATIENT WITH CARDIAC DISEASE

Perioperative cardiac mortality is the leading cause of death after anesthesia and surgery. Extensive research has focused on preoperative assessment of cardiac risk and prevention of postoperative complications.

A **American College of Cardiology (ACC)/American Heart Association (AHA) Guidelines (2002)** (Tables 3-2 and 3-3; Fig. 3-1)

1. An ACC/AHA consensus committee has developed a stepwise strategy to estimate coronary risk related to noncardiac surgery. This approach relies on an assessment of clinical markers of risk before coronary evaluation and treatment, functional capacity, and surgery-specific risk.

2. Several findings from the consensus committee follow.
   a. Perioperative and long-term risk is increased in patients with poor exercise tolerance, i.e., unable to reach a 4-MET (Metabolic Equivalents of Exercise, called METS) demand during most activities.
   b. Patients with moderate or excellent functional capacity are at low risk for cardiac complications in the setting of intermediate risk surgery.
   c. Patients with a poor functional capacity or those who have only a moderate functional capacity and are facing high-risk surgery should be considered for further noninvasive testing.
   d. A recent myocardial infarction (MI) within the prior 30 days is a major risk factor for perioperative cardiac complication. A history of an MI more than 30 days before noncardiac surgery is an intermediate risk factor.
   e. Post-MI stress test without reversible ischemia suggests a lower risk of a perioperative MI than if significant inducible ischemia is identified.
   f. In the patient who has undergone a coronary revascularization procedure, it is suggested (but not proved in a controlled, randomized fashion) that coronary artery revascularization may reduce the risk of cardiac complication before vascular surgery. This benefit is probably present in the patient who has undergone complete coronary revascularization 6 months to 5 years before his or her noncardiac surgery and has no symptoms of myocardial ischemia with physical activity greater than 4 METs. Noncardiac surgery should probably be delayed for several days after a coronary angioplasty.

TABLE 3-2   Cardiac Risk* Stratification for Noncardiac Surgical Procedures

High	(Reported cardiac risk often >5%)
	• Emergent major operations, particularly in the elderly
	• Aortic and other major vascular
	• Peripheral vascular
	• Anticipated prolonged surgical procedures associated with large fluid shifts or blood loss
Intermediate	(Reported cardiac risk generally <5%)
	• Carotid endarterectomy
	• Head and neck
	• Intraperitoneal and intrathoracic
	• Orthopaedic
	• Prostate
Low[†]	(Reported cardiac risk generally <1%)
	• Endoscopic procedures
	• Superficial procedures
	• Cataract
	• Breast

*Combined incidence of cardiac death and nonfatal myocardial infarction.
[†]Do not generally require further preoperative cardiac testing.
From Eagle KA, Berger PB, Calkins H, et al. ACC/AHA guideline update for perioperative cardiovascular evaluation for noncardiac surgery: a report of the American College of Cardiology/American Heart Association Task Force on Practice Guidelines (Committee to Update the 1996 Guideline on Perioperative Evaluation for Noncardiac Surgery). 2002. American College of Cardiology website. http://www.acc.org/quality and science/clinical/guidelines/perio/clean/perio_index.htm (Accessed December 15, 2006).

3. **Noninvasive assessment of myocardial perfusion by exercise or pharmacologic stress testing (e.g., radionuclide myocardial imaging, stress echocardiography, dobutamine echocardiography)** in conjunction with clinical predictors is helpful in risk assessment of the intermediate-risk patient.

   a. **Low-risk** patients are younger than 70 years of age; they are physically active; and they have none of the following risk factors: angina, congestive heart failure, MI, diabetes, or ventricular ectopy. No preoperative ischemia testing is necessary; surgery can proceed.

   b. **Intermediate-risk** patients have one or two of the risk factors in the low-risk category or live a sedentary lifestyle. Noninvasive assessment of myocardial perfusion should be done via exercise or via pharmacologic methods if the patient is unable to exercise.
      (1) If **no ischemia is present,** surgery is recommended.
      (2) If **myocardial ischemia is present,** the risk should be determined based on the extent of myocardium that is at risk for ischemia.

   c. **High-risk** patients have three or more risk factors noted in the low-risk category or they have angina with daily activity, progressive angina, angina at rest, or a recent MI. Options depend on the patient's medical status.
      (1) Cardiac catheterization to define the coronary anatomy and to perform a revascularization procedure can be undertaken, if indicated, before vascular surgery.
      (2) A lower-risk vascular surgical procedure can be selected (e.g., axillofemoral bypass in a patient with aortoiliac disease).
      (3) Surgery can proceed, and the patient can be treated with parenteral antianginal therapy while being followed with invasive hemodynamic monitoring.

B Anesthesia principles

   1. All **inhaled general anesthetic agents** are myocardial depressants.
      a. **Myocardial depression** is usually minimized by reflex sympathetic response. For example, when nitrous oxide is administered, the systemic blood pressure usually remains unchanged, despite myocardial depression, as a result of reflex peripheral vasoconstriction.
      b. **Halothane** is also a peripheral **vasodilator.** Myocardial depression and vasodilatation may result in hypotension, which may be further exaggerated if the patient is hypovolemic or is taking vasodilators.

TABLE 3-3   Clinical Predictors of Increased Perioperative Cardiovascular Risk (Myocardial Infarction, Congestive Heart Failure, Death)

Major
Unstable coronary syndromes
- Recent myocardial infarction* with evidence of important ischemic risk by clinical symptoms of noninvasive study
- Unstable or severe† angina (Canadian class III or IV)‡

Decompensated congestive heart failure
Significant arrhythmias
- High-grade atrioventricular block
- Symptomatic ventricular arrhythmias in the presence of underlying heart disease
- Supraventricular arrhythmias with uncontrolled ventricular rate

Severe valvular disease

Intermediate
Mild angina pectoris (Canadian class I or II)
Prior myocardial infarction by history or pathologic Q waves
Compensated or prior congestive heart failure
Diabetes mellitus

Minor
Advanced age
Abnormal ECG (left ventricular hypertrophy, left bundle branch block, ST-T abnormalities)
Rhythm other than sinus (e.g., atrial fibrillation)
Low functional capacity (e.g., inability to climb one flight of stairs with a bag of groceries)
History of stroke
Uncontrolled systemic hypertension

ECG = electrocardiogram.
*The American College of Cardiology National Database Library defines a *recent MI* as greater than 7 days but less than or equal to 1 month (30 days).
†May include "stable" angina in patients who are unusually sedentary.
‡Campeau L. Grading of angina pectoris. *Circulation*. 1976;54:522–523.
From Eagle KA, Berger PB, Calkins H, et al. ACC/AHA guideline update for perioperative cardiovascular evaluation for noncardiac surgery: a report of the American College of Cardiology/American Heart Association Task Force on Practice Guidelines (Committee to Update the 1996 Guideline on Perioperative Evaluation for Noncardiac Surgery). 2002. American College of Cardiology website. http://www.acc.org/quality and science/clinical/guidelines/perio/clean/perio_index.htm (Accessed December 15, 2006).

   2. Regional and general anesthesia are associated with the **same cardiac morbidity and mortality.**
      a. Exceptions follow.
         (1) The **elderly patient undergoing inguinal hernia repair.** Local anesthesia has been found to be associated with a lower risk of cardiovascular complication than regional or general anesthesia.
         (2) The **patient with a history of congestive heart failure.** Regional anesthesia is associated with a lower incidence of perioperative congestive heart failure.
      b. Advantages of regional anesthesia in the cardiac patient follow.
         (1) Less myocardial or respiratory depression occurs than with general anesthesia.
         (2) Autonomic stimulation, which may accompany endotracheal intubation, is avoided.
      c. Disadvantages of regional anesthesia in the cardiac patient include the following:
         (1) The **awake** patient may become **anxious,** which increases circulating catecholamines and can cause myocardial ischemia to develop.
         (2) Spinal anesthesia may result in **vasodilatation and hypotension.**
            (a) A patient with a "fixed" cardiac output (i.e., severe aortic stenosis, severe left ventricular dysfunction) may be unable to compensate.
            (b) Vasodilatation may also be harmful in the patient dependent on preload (e.g., the patient with severe pulmonary hypertension).
   3. Recent data suggest that intensive **perioperative and postoperative epidural analgesia** may be associated with decreased postoperative myocardial ischemia and improved outcome. The mechanism is unclear but may involve a blunting of the sympathetic response to operative stress.

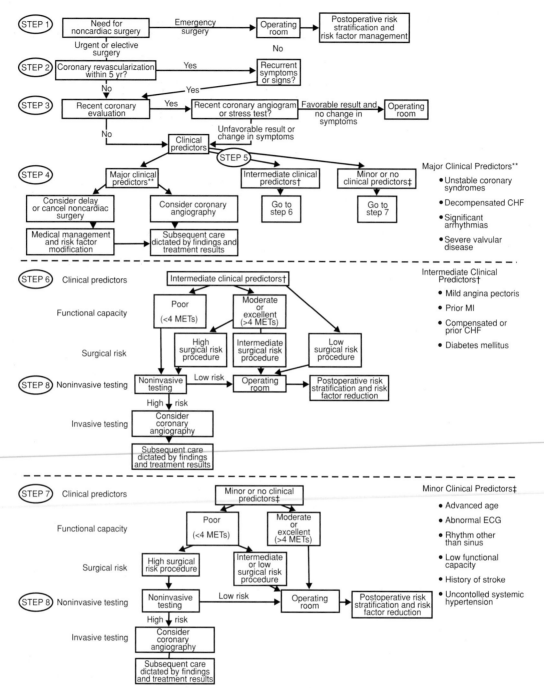

FIGURE 3-1 ASS/AHA risk stratification strategy. (From the American College for Cardiology/American Heart Association Task Force Report: guidelines for perioperative cardiovascular evaluation for noncardiac surgery. *J Am Coll Cardiol.* 1996;27:910–948.)

C **Pre-existing cardiovascular disease**

1. **Hypertension**

   a. **Diastolic blood pressure greater than or equal to 110 mm Hg** is a risk factor for the development of cardiac complications. If possible, surgery should be delayed if the patient with cardiovascular disease presents with preoperative diastolic blood pressure ≥110 mm Hg.

   b. Patients with hypertension have a 25% incidence of either hypotension or an exacerbation of hypertension during the perioperative period.

   c. The risk of a **perioperative MI** is increased if, during surgery, the blood pressure decreases by 50% at any time or by 33% for 10 minutes or longer.

2. **Angina** (Canadian Cardiovascular Society class designations)
   a. **Class 1 or class 2 angina** (**chronic stable angina**) is not a risk factor for perioperative cardiac complications.
   b. **Class 3 angina** (angina walking up one flight of stairs or two blocks) is a cardiac risk factor and poses a risk similar to sustaining an MI during the 6 months before surgery.
   c. **Class 4 angina** (angina on any exertion) indicates twice the risk of class 3 angina.
   d. For patients who are well maintained on an antianginal regimen, care must be taken to ensure effective antianginal therapy in the perioperative period.

3. **Myocardial infarction**
   a. The ACC/AHA consensus guidelines assign a history of MI or pathologic Q waves on the preoperative electrocardiogram (ECG) as intermediate-risk predictors and a recent MI (within the prior 30 days) as a major predictor of perioperative cardiac risk.
   b. The patient who has undergone a **coronary revascularization procedure** may have a **reduced** risk of cardiac complications before vascular or other major surgery. However, this suggestion has not been proven by randomized controlled trials.
      (1) Patients with prior **coronary artery bypass grafting (CABG)** or **percutaneous transluminal coronary angioplasty (PTCA)** are subject to **further coronary artery disease** involving their native coronary arteries as well as bypass grafts.
      (2) Saphenous vein bypass occlusion rates are 12%–20% at 1 year, 20%–30% at 5 years, and 40%–50% at 10 years after CABG.
      (3) The incidence of coronary restenosis after a PTCA is 25%–35% at 6 months.
   c. Most **perioperative MIs** occur during the first 4–5 postoperative days, with a **peak incidence on days 1 and 2.** A mortality rate of up to 69% has been reported.
   d. **Postoperative MIs** are typically *not* associated with anginal pain but rather with new-onset congestive heart failure, arrhythmias, or confusion.

4. **Congestive heart failure**
   a. Congestive heart failure is a risk factor for perioperative cardiac complications. Patients with a **prior history but no preoperative clinical evidence** of heart failure have a 6% incidence of perioperative pulmonary edema compared with a 16% incidence in patients found to have clinical or radiographic evidence of heart failure preoperatively.
   b. Approximately 70% of patients who develop **perioperative pulmonary edema** do so in the first hour after surgery, and the greatest onset occurs during the first 30 minutes. **Causes** include the following:
      (1) Volume overload
      (2) Cessation of positive-pressure ventilation with subsequent increase in preload
      (3) Anesthetic-induced myocardial depression
      (4) Postoperative hypertension

5. **Arrhythmias and conduction abnormalities**
   a. **Incidence**
      (1) Up to 84% of patients who undergo surgery exhibit abnormalities of cardiac rate or rhythm in the perioperative period. Only 5% of these abnormalities are clinically significant.
      (2) The incidence of arrhythmias is highest during surgery that lasts longer than 3 hours, during neurosurgical or thoracic surgery, and during endotracheal intubation.
   b. **Metabolic abnormalities** are the most common cause of arrhythmia (i.e., hypoxia, hypercarbia, hypokalemia, hyperkalemia). Therapy is aimed at reversal of these abnormalities.
   c. **Electrocautery used during surgery can affect the performance of cardiac pacemakers and implanted cardiac defibrillators (AICD)**
      (1) The electromagnetic interference generated by electrocautery may be "sensed" by a pacemaker as intrinsic cardiac electrical activity and inhibit cardiac pacemaker activity. This inhibition may be prevented by temporarily programming the pacemaker to a fixed rate mode. In the operating room, placing a pacemaker magnet on the pacemaker during the surgical procedure will make the pacemaker operate in a fixed rate mode.
      (2) An AICD may interpret the electromagnetic interference of electrocautery as ventricular tachycardia or ventricular fibrillation, which would trigger the AICD to deliver a

defibrillating shock. This may be prevented by turning off the AICD immediately prior to surgery and turning on the AICD on completion of the surgical procedure.

6. **Valvular heart disease**
   a. **Critical aortic stenosis** is associated with an increased risk of perioperative cardiac complications.
      (1) These patients typically cannot increase cardiac output because an outflow obstruction is present at the site of the aortic valve.
      (2) Therefore, any hemodynamic changes that could result in a need for increased cardiac output (e.g., vasodilatation) should be avoided.
   b. **Aortic or mitral regurgitation.** Operative risk is related to the status of left ventricular function rather than to the degree of valvular regurgitation.
   c. **Mitral stenosis.** Volume status and heart rate are key factors in the perioperative period.
      (1) **Tachycardia** decreases diastolic filling time and may result in pulmonary edema.
      (2) **Small fluid shifts** may result in marked hemodynamic abnormalities.
   d. **Prosthetic heart valves.** Patients with prosthetic heart valves are at risk for **valve thrombosis** and **thromboembolic complications** if anticoagulants are withheld for an excessive period preoperatively.
      (1) For most patients, anticoagulants can be discontinued up to 3 days before surgery and restarted 2–3 days after surgery without thromboembolic complications.
      (2) Patients with **caged-disk prosthetic mitral valves** have a high risk of valve thrombosis when they are not receiving anticoagulation.
         (a) For these patients, warfarin anticoagulation should be stopped 3 days before surgery and replaced with full-dose intravenous heparin, which is stopped 12 hours before surgery.
         (b) Once hemostasis is stable after surgery (usually at 12–24 hours postoperatively), heparin therapy is resumed. Warfarin therapy is started again once oral intake is begun.

7. **Hypertrophic cardiomyopathy.** Patients with hypertrophic cardiomyopathy with left ventricular outflow tract obstruction are at risk for worsening of left ventricular outflow tract obstruction in the perioperative period. Factors that may lead to worsening of the left ventricular outflow tract gradient include excessive preload or afterload reduction, which may occur with volume depletion or vasodilator therapy. Perioperative catecholamine release may directly act on the left ventricular outflow tract to increase myocardial contractility and increase the outflow tract gradient.

D **Approaches to reduction of perioperative cardiac risk**

1. **Perioperative beta blocker therapy**
   a. Data from small clinical trials suggest that beta blockers decrease the risk of cardiac complications in the perioperative period.
   b. An observational study has found that perioperative beta blockers have their greatest benefit in preventing cardiac complications in patients at increased cardiac risk, i.e., those having three or more of the following clinical features: (a) ischemic heart disease, (b) cerebrovascular disease, (c) renal insufficiency, (d)diabetes mellitus, (e) undergoing high-risk surgery.
   c. **The American College of Cardiology/American Heart Association 2006 Update on Perioperative Beta Blocker Therapy** recommends that beta blockers be continued in patients already receiving beta blockers and initiated in patients undergoing vascular surgery who are estimated to be at high cardiac risk as determined by the presence of ischemia on preoperative testing. This guideline states that beta blockers are **probably recommended** for patients who undergo vascular surgery with a history of coronary artery disease or who have multiple coronary artery disease risk factors and for patients with multiple cardiac risk factors who undergo intermediate-risk or high-risk surgical procedures. Beta blockers **may be considered** for patients who undergo intermediate-risk or high-risk surgical procedures who have a single clinical cardiac risk factor and may also be considered for patients who undergo vascular surgery who have no cardiac risk factors.
   d. Beta blocker therapy should be titrated to achieve a heart rate of 60–70 beats per minute in the perioperative period.

    e. For the patient who requires perioperative beta blocker therapy but does not have indications for the long-term use of beta blockers, we typically continue beta blockers for 30 days following surgery.

  2. Perioperative alpha adrenergic agonists (clonidine, mivazerol) have been demonstrated to decrease perioperative ischemia and mortality following vascular surgery. This approach is not commonly used in the United States.

  3. Anesthetic agents

    a. Meta-analyses suggest that neuraxial anesthetic techniques (epidural, spinal anesthesia) is associated with a lower risk of pulmonary or thrombotic complications compared with general anesthesia. While these techniques were initially thought to also lower the risk of perioperative cardiac complications, recent meta-analysis has not confirmed that finding.

  4. Prophylactic coronary artery revascularization

    a. There is no evidence that coronary artery revascularization is indicated "just to get the patient through a noncardiac surgical procedure." Coronary artery revascularization should be done prior to noncardiac surgery following the same guidelines and indications that would be followed if the patient were not undergoing noncardiac surgery.

  5. Maintenance of normothemia in the postoperative period has been shown to decrease cardiac complications in patients at increased cardiac risk. This impact is primarily related to a reduction in postoperative ventricular arrhythmias.

  6. HMG-CoA reductase inhibitors in observational studies have been shown to be associated with a reduced incidence of postoperative cardiac complications. Data from prospective studies is necessary before these agents can be recommended to reduce perioperative cardiac risk.

E The patient who has had coronary artery angioplasty with placement of a coronary artery stent needs attention placed to the antiplatelet regimen utilized with stent placement.

  1. A drug-eluting stent is the most commonly used coronary artery stent in the United States. It is essential that the patient's antiplatelet regimen (apirin and clopidogrel) be continued for at least 3 months following placement of a sirolimus-coated stent and for at least 6 months following placement of a paclitaxol-coated stent. Premature discontinuation of this antiplatelet regimen may result in acute stent thrombosis with subsequent MI.

  2. If surgery cannot be performed in the presence of aspirin and clopidogrel, delay elective surgery until the patient's antiplatelet course is completed.

  3. If emergency surgery is required and the patient has not completed a poststent placement antiplatelet regimen, consider each case on an individual basis. For most patients, proceed to surgery, and utilize platelet transfusions in the event that excessive bleeding occurs.

  4. If a patient presents for coronary artery angioplasty and it is known that he or she is to have subsequent noncardiac surgery in less than 3 months, consider the use of a bare-metal stent, which requires 1 month of antiplatelet therapy (aspirin and clopidogrel).

F **Invasive hemodynamic monitoring** No well-designed, randomized, prospective study has been undertaken on the impact of invasive hemodynamic monitoring in the perioperative period. Examples of intuitive indications for invasive hemodynamic monitoring include the following:

  1. Anticipation of fluid shifts in the patient with left ventricular dysfunction or fixed cardiac output

  2. Major vascular surgery in the patient with left ventricular dysfunction

Surgery in the patient with a recent MI or unstable angina

G **Bacterial endocarditis prophylaxis** (Tables 3-4–3-8) is indicated for procedures associated with **bacteremia** for patients with

  1. Prosthetic heart valves

  2. Rheumatic or other acquired valvular abnormalities

  3. Mitral valve prolapse with mitral regurgitation

TABLE 3-4 Cardiac Conditions Associated with Endocarditis

Endocarditis prophylaxis recommended
High-risk category
  Prosthetic cardiac valves, including bioprosthetic and homograft valves
  Previous bacterial endocarditis
  Complex cyanotic congenital heart disease (e.g., single ventricle states, transposition of the great
    arteries, tetralogy of Fallot)
  Surgically constructed systemic pulmonary shunts or conduits
Moderate-risk category
  Most other congenital cardiac malformations (other than above and below)
  Acquired valvar dysfunction (e.g., rheumatic heart disease)
  Hypertrophic cardiomyopathy
  Mitral valve prolapse with valvar regurgitation or thickened leaflets

Endocarditis prophylaxis not recommended
Negligible-risk category (no greater risk than the general population)
  Isolated secundum atrial septal defect
  Surgical repair of atrial septal, ventricular septal defect, or patent ductus arteriosus (without residua
    beyond 6 months)
  Previous coronary artery bypass graft surgery
  Mitral valve prolapse without valvar regurgitation
  Physiologic, functional, or innocent heart murmurs
  Previous Kawasaki disease without valvar dysfunction
  Previous rheumatic fever without valvar dysfunction
  Cardiac pacemakers (intravascular and epicardial) and implanted defibrillators

From Dajani AS, Taubert K, Wilson W, et al. Prevention of bacterial endocarditis: recommendations by the American Heart Association. *JAMA.* 1997;277:1794–1801.

TABLE 3-5 Dental Procedures and Endocarditis Prophylaxis

Endocarditis prophylaxis recommended*
Dental extractions
Periodontal procedures including surgery, scaling and root planing, probing, and recall maintenance
Dental implant placement and reimplantation of avulsed teeth
Endodontic (root canal) instrumentation or surgery only beyond the apex
Subgingival placement of antibiotic fibers or strips
Initial placement of orthodontic bands but not brackets
Intraligamentary local anesthetic injections
Prophylactic cleaning of teeth or implants where bleeding is anticipated

Endocarditis prophylaxis not recommended
Restorative dentistry[†] (operative and prosthodontic) with or without retraction cord[‡]
Local anesthetic injections (nonintraligamentary)
Intracanal endodontic treatment; postplacement and buildup
Placement of rubber dams
Postoperative suture removal
Placement of removable prosthodontic or orthodontic appliances
Taking of oral impressions
Fluoride treatments
Taking of oral radiographs
Orthodontic appliance adjustment
Shedding of primary teeth

*Prophylaxis is recommended for patients with high- and moderate-risk cardiac conditions.
†This includes restoration of decayed teeth (filling cavities) and replacement of missing teeth.
‡Clinical judgment may indicate antibiotic use in selected circumstances that may create significant bleeding.
From Dajani AS, Taubert K, Wilson W, et al. Prevention of bacterial endocarditis: recommendations by the American Heart Association. *JAMA.* 1997;277:1794–1801.

TABLE 3-6   Other Procedures and Endocarditis Prophylaxis

Endocarditis prophylaxis recommended
Respiratory tract
Tonsillectomy or adenoidectomy
Surgical operations that involve respiratory mucosa
Bronchoscopy with a rigid bronchoscope
Gastrointestinal tract*
Sclerotherapy for esophageal varices
Esophageal stricture dilation
Endoscopic retrograde cholangiography with biliary obstruction
Biliary tract surgery
Surgical operations that involve intestinal mucosa
Genitourinary tract
Prostatic surgery
Cystoscopy
Urethral dilatation

Endocarditis prophylaxis not recommended
Respiratory tract
Endotracheal intubation
Bronchoscopy with a flexible bronchoscope, with or without biopsy[†]
Tympanostomy tube insertion
Gastrointestinal tract
Transesophageal echocardiography[†]
Endoscopy with or without gastrointestinal biopsy[†]
Genitourinary tract
Vaginal hysterectomy[†]
Vaginal delivery[†]
Cesarean section
In uninfected tissue:
   Urethral catheterization
   Uterine dilatation and curettage
   Therapeutic abortion
   Sterilization procedures
   Insertion or removal of intrauterine devices
Other
Cardiac catheterization, including balloon angioplasty
Implanted cardiac pacemakers, implanted defibrillators, and coronary stents
Incision or biopsy of surgically scrubbed skin
Circumcision

*Prophylaxis is recommended for high-risk patients; it is optional for medium-risk patients.
[†]Prophylaxis is optional for high-risk patients.
From Dajani AS, Taubert K, Wilson W, et al. Prevention of bacterial endocarditis: recommendations by the American Heart Association. *JAMA.* 1997;277:1794–1801.

4. Most congenital cardiac defects

5. Surgically constructed systemic-pulmonary shunts

6. Hypertrophic obstructive cardiomyopathy

7. Prior history of bacterial endocarditis

III   **THE SURGICAL PATIENT WITH CHRONIC LUNG DISEASE**

Chronic lung disease is common and affects surgical patients of all ages and diagnoses. It has multiple causes and, when severe, increases the risk of surgery. The disease may be symptomatic (in the form of dyspnea) or totally asymptomatic. In addition, an acute infectious process may be superimposed on a chronic disorder.

TABLE 3-7   Prophylactic Regimens for Dental, Oral, Respiratory Tract, or Esophageal Procedures

Situation	Agent	Regimen
Standard general prophylaxis	Amoxicillin	Adults: 2 g; children: 50 mg/kg orally 1 hour before procedure
Unable to take oral medications	Ampicillin	Adults: 2 g IM or IV; children: 50 mg/kg IM or IV within 30 minutes before procedure
Allergic to penicillin	Clindamycin **or**	Adults: 600 mg; children: 20 mg/kg orally 1 hour before procedure
	Cephalexin† or cefadroxil† **or**	Adults: 2 g; children; 50 mg/kg orally 1 hour before procedure
	Azithromycin **or** clarithromycin	Adults: 500 mg; children: 15 mg/kg orally 1 hour before procedure
Allergic to penicillin and unable to take oral medications	Clindamycin **or**	Adults: 600 mg; children: 20 mg/kg IV within 30 minutes before procedure
	Cefazolin†	Adults 1 g; children: 25 mg/kg IM or IV within 30 minutes before procedure

IM, intramuscularly; IV, intravenously.
*Total child's dose should not exceed the adult dose.
†Cephalosporins should not be used in individuals with an immediate-type hypersensitivity reaction (urticaria, angioedema, or anaphylaxis) to penicillins.
From Dajani AS, Taubert K, Wilson W, et al. Prevention of bacterial endocarditis: recommendations by the American Heart Association. *JAMA.* 1997;277:1794–1801.

A **Assessment of pulmonary risk**

1. **History**
   a. A history of **pulmonary symptoms and disorders** should alert the physician that further intervention and evaluation may be necessary.
      (1) Dyspnea
      (2) Sputum production
      (3) Chronic cough
      (4) Exercise intolerance
   b. **Prior medical conditions**
      (1) Recurrent bronchitis or pneumonia
      (2) Chronic obstructive pulmonary disease (COPD)
      (3) Emphysema
      (4) Systemic disease with potential pulmonary involvement
      (5) Previous lung surgery
      (6) Exposure to environmental toxins
   c. **Cigarette smoking,** the most common cause of chronic lung disease, is toxic to the respiratory epithelium and cilia and results in impaired transport of mucus, with consequent impaired resistance to infection.

2. **Physical examination.** Abnormal findings follow.
   a. **Anatomic abnormalities** (e.g., scoliosis or chest wall abnormalities)
   b. **Findings on auscultation of the chest** (e.g., decreased breath sounds, wheezing, and rhonchi or rales)
   c. **Signs of inadequate oxygenation** (e.g., cyanosis, finger clubbing, and use of accessory muscles for breathing)

3. **Chest radiograph.** Abnormal findings include blebs, pneumonitis, consolidation, pleural effusion, and hyperaeration with flattening of the diaphragm.

4. **Laboratory studies**
   a. **Arterial blood gases** provide information on the adequacy of ventilation and oxygenation. Abnormal laboratory values include hypoxemia and hypercarbia.
   b. **Secondary polycythemia** may also be seen in patients with chronic hypoxia.

TABLE 3-8 Prophylactic Regimens for Genitourinary/Gastrointestinal (Excluding Esophageal) Procedures

Situation	Agent*	Regimen†
High-risk patients	Ampicillin plus gentamicin	Adults: ampicillin 2 g IM or IV plus gentamicin 1.5 mg/kg (not to exceed 120 mg) within 30 minutes of starting the procedure; 6 hours later, ampicillin 1 g IM/IV or amoxicillin 1 g orally Children: ampicillin 50 mg/kg IM or IV (not to exceed 2 g) plus gentamicin 1.5 mg/kg within 30 minutes of starting the procedure; 6 hours later, ampicillin 25 mg/kg IM/IV or amoxicillin 25 mg/kg orally
High-risk patients allergic to ampicillin/amoxicillin	Vancomycin plus gentamicin	Adults: vancomycin 1 g IV over 1–2 hours plus gentamicin 1.5 mg/kg IV/IM (not to exceed 120 mg); complete injection/infusion within 30 minutes of starting the procedure Children: vancomycin 20 mg/kg IV over 1–2 hours plus gentamicin 1.5 mg/kg IV/IM; complete injection/infusion within 30 minutes of starting the procedure
Moderate-risk patients	Amoxicillin or ampicillin	Adults: amoxicillin 2 g orally 1 hour before the procedure, or ampicillin 2 g IM/IV within 30 minutes of starting the procedure Children: amoxicillin 50 mg/kg orally 1 hour before the procedure, or ampicillin 50 mg/kg IM/IV within 30 minutes of starting the procedure
Moderate-risk patients allergic to ampicillin/amoxicillin	Vancomycin	Adults: vancomycin 1 g IV over 1–2 hours; complete infusion within 30 minutes of starting the procedure Children: vancomycin 20 mg/kg IV over 1–2 hours; complete infusion within 30 minutes of starting the procedure

IM, intramuscularly; IV, intravenously.
*Total child's dose should not exceed the adult dose.
†No second dose of vancomycin or gentamicin is recommended.
From Dajani AS, Taubert K, Wilson W, et al. Prevention of bacterial endocarditis: recommendations by the American Heart Association. *JAMA.* 1997;277:1794–1801.

5. **Pulmonary function tests.** The correlation between preoperative pulmonary function tests and postoperative complication rates is controversial. No single pulmonary function test absolutely contraindicates an operation; however, abnormal results on several pulmonary function tests are thought to be associated with an increased probability of postoperative pulmonary complications.

   a. In the absence of symptoms or significant history, routine preoperative spirometry is *not* indicated in extrathoracic surgery.

   b. **Preoperative spirometry and arterial blood gases** may be considered in patients with

      (1) **Planned thoracic procedures,** with or without pulmonary resection

      (2) Productive cough and dyspnea

      (3) A history or physical findings of cardiopulmonary disease

      (4) A history of more than 20 pack-years of cigarette smoking

      (5) Abnormal chest radiograph findings

      (6) Morbid obesity

6. **The ASA risk classification,** when greater than class I or II, in combination with other risk factors, may predict the occurrence of pulmonary complications.

7. For patients with **planned thoracic surgery,**
   a. Specific criteria have been published for the minimum pulmonary function necessary to tolerate varying degrees of **pulmonary resection** (Table 3-9).
   b. Pulmonary function tests may be repeated after **bronchodilator therapy** to assess improvement after treatment. Failure to improve after therapy may be an indication of high risk.
   c. **Ventilation-perfusion scans, quantitation of carbon dioxide diffusion capacity, exercise testing,** and determinations of **pulmonary artery pressures** may be performed in borderline cases.
   d. **Split-lung pulmonary function tests** may be required in pulmonary resections because the segment to be resected may be diseased and may not contribute significantly to pulmonary function.
   e. **Lung volume reduction surgery** may be considered to improve postoperative pulmonary function in patients undergoing resection sufficient to raise concerns of inadequate reserve.

B **Pre-existing pulmonary disease** Patients with chronic lung disease are thought to be at increased risk for complications after surgery and may benefit from a preoperative pulmonary evaluation and an education in incentive spirometry.

1. **Cigarette smoking**
   a. A history of **20 pack-years** or consumption of **more than 20 cigarettes per day** increases the risk of postoperative pulmonary complications.
   b. **Cigarette smoking should be stopped at least 6–8 weeks** preceding elective surgery to demonstrate any statistically significant decrease in complication rate.

2. **COPD**
   a. **Antibiotics** should be administered before surgery in patients with **acute bronchitis, productive cough,** or **purulent sputum production.** If an elective procedure is planned, it should be delayed until after treatment.
   b. **Aerosol β_2-agonists** and **mucolytic drugs** (e.g., acetylcysteine) relieve bronchospasm and may help to liquefy and mobilize retained secretions. **Postural drainage** and **chest physiotherapy** can be used to expedite this in selected cases.

TABLE 3-9   Pulmonary Function Ranges Suggesting Increased Operative Risk

Forced vital capacity (FVC)	<50%–75% predicted
	<1.7–2 L
Forced expiratory volume in 1 second (FEV₁)	<35%–70% predicted
	<0.6 L*
	<1 L†
	<2 L‡
Forced expiratory flow (FEF)	<50% predicted
	<0.6 L*†
	<1.6 L‡
Maximum voluntary ventilation (MVV)	<35%*†–<55%‡ predicted
Maximum expiratory flow rate (MEFR)	<200 L/min
Residual volume (RV)	<47%
Diffusion capacity of carbon monoxide (Dco)	<50%
Arterial partial pressure of carbon dioxide (Paco₂)	>45 mm Hg
Pulmonary artery pressure (PAP)	>22–35 mm Hg
Pulmonary vascular resistance (PVR)	>190 dynes/cm/sec
	<1 L/min
Oxygen uptake (Vo₂)	15 mL/kg/min

*Criteria for a wedge excision or a segamentectomy.
†Criteria for a lobectomy.
‡Criteria for a pneumonectomy.
From Pett SB, Wernly JA. Respiratory function in surgical patients: perioperative evaluation and management. *Surg Annual.* 1988;20:36.

    c. Bronchodilators (e.g., aminophylline) may also have an inotropic effect on respiratory muscles.

    d. Steroids should be used preoperatively, when necessary, to improve pulmonary function; however, they have adverse effects on wound healing and resistance to infection.

3. Asthma

    a. Poorly controlled asthmatics are at increased risk for pulmonary complications. The risk of pulmonary complications is reduced by medical management (e.g., use of antibiotics, bronchodilators, β_2-agonists, steroids) to **eliminate wheezing preoperatively.**

    b. Peak expiratory flow may be measured before and after bronchodilator therapy to assess the presence, severity, and reversibility of bronchospasm.

    c. Muscle relaxants with muscarinic activity (e.g., d-tubocurare) may stimulate bronchospasm and should be avoided.

    d. Propofol may reduce airway irritation during instrumentation.

4. Obesity increases the work of ventilation and impairs the function of the chest wall, leading to a restrictive respiratory pattern. **Postoperative atelectasis** is common in obese patients.

    a. Morbidly obese patients may suffer from **sleep apnea** or **oropharyngeal obstruction.**

    b. Consideration should be given to using a **transverse rather than vertical surgical incision.**

    c. Ambulation and **mobilization** must be encouraged early in the postoperative period.

5. Age. A slight decrease in pulmonary function is associated with increasing age. Age >70 years has been identified as an independent risk factor for postoperative complications but should not contraindicate surgery in otherwise healthy patients.

6. Restrictive lung disease, neuromuscular disorders, or pulmonary vascular disease. These patients have an impaired ventilatory reserve as a result of weak muscles or abnormal mechanics of ventilation.

C **Operative variables**

1. The type of surgery influences the pulmonary risk.

    a. Thoracotomy and **upper abdominal surgery** are associated with the most marked changes in postoperative functional residual capacity (FRC).

        (1) Chest wall and diaphragmatic excursion mechanics are altered, leading to decreased total lung capacity (TLC), decreased FRC, and decreased tidal volume (TV), which may persist for 1–2 weeks postoperatively.

        (2) Postoperative pain causes hypoventilation and a poor cough reflex, leading to retention of secretions and ventilation-perfusion mismatch.

        (3) Risk factors for postoperative complications after laparotomy [Hall JC, Tarala RA, Hall JL, et al. A multivariate analysis of the risk of pulmonary complications after laparotomy. *Chest.* 1991;99(4):923–927]:

            (a) ASA class >II

            (b) Upper abdominal procedures

            (c) Residual intraperitoneal sepsis

            (d) Age greater than 59 years

            (e) A body mass index (BMI) higher than 25 kg/m^2

            (f) Preoperative stay for longer than 4 days

            (g) Colorectal or gastroduodenal surgery

    b. Lower abdominal surgery is associated with fewer pulmonary complications than thoracic and upper abdominal surgery.

    c. Extremity surgery rarely affects postoperative pulmonary function.

    d. Minimally invasive surgery

        (1) May reduce postoperative pulmonary complications by improving the forced expiratory volume in 1 second (FEV_1), FRC, oxygenation, and ventilation. Definitive improvements in outcome have not been demonstrated, and the site of surgery (i.e., upper abdominal) may be more important than the specific operative technique.

        (2) Requires intraperitoneal insufflation and may be associated with intraoperative CO_2 retention.

2. Vertical incisions are more susceptible to respiratory complications when compared with transverse, muscle-splitting incisions.

3. Length of surgery. Surgical procedures lasting longer than 3.5 hours are associated with increased pulmonary complications.

4. Anesthesia
   a. General anesthesia may decrease the FRC for up to 1–2 weeks postoperatively.
      (1) Endotracheal intubation and **inhalational anesthetics** may exacerbate bronchospasm.
      (2) Mechanical ventilation impairs many protective mechanisms, such as ciliary function and mucus transport. It also increases the risk of pneumothorax secondary to barotrauma.
   b. Spinal anesthesia shows no difference from general anesthesia in terms of pulmonary morbidity.
   c. Regional block is associated with lower pulmonary risk than either general or spinal anesthesia.

D Perioperative management

1. Preoperative education. Controlled studies in elective surgical patients demonstrate that the **maximal reduction in pulmonary complications** is obtained when interventions are begun preoperatively.
   a. Incentive spirometry and **deep-breathing exercises** are inspiratory maneuvers to recruit alveoli and to counteract the postoperative reduction in FRC. The most effective and simplest intervention is the instruction to cough, deep breathe (5 deep breaths, holding each at full inspiration for 5–6 seconds), and change position hourly while awake.
   b. Other modalities
      (1) Continuous positive airway pressure (CPAP) has been demonstrated to improve pulmonary function values, but it is not clear that use of this modality leads to a reduction of pulmonary complications.
      (2) Postural drainage and chest physiotherapy are useful in mobilizing secretions but should be reserved for patients with lobar collapse or high sputum production because they may exacerbate bronchospasm. In addition, these maneuvers are often difficult to do during the postoperative period because of patient discomfort.

2. Extubation. Discontinuation of mechanical ventilatory support after general anesthesia should be performed only after the patient is awake, is hemodynamically stable, and has full respiratory muscle strength.
   a. Parameters for extubation follow (Table 3-10).
      (1) Assess for adequate oxygenation.
      (2) Assess for adequate ventilation.
      (3) Other considerations (Table 3-10).
   b. Protocol-based weaning of mechanical ventilation has been shown to decrease the time on mechanical ventilator support and to reduce the incidence of ventilator-associated pneumonia.
   c. Once criteria for weaning have been met, tolerance of a **30-minute spontaneous breathing trial** has been associated with **decreased time to extubation when compared with intermittent mandatory ventilation (IMV) or pressure support modes.**
   d. In patients who require mechanical ventilation >24 hours, **causes of ventilator dependency** should be identified and all possible contributing factors reversed.
   e. After extubation, respiratory sufficiency should be carefully observed and evaluated. If in doubt about the patient's respiratory sufficiency, the physician should perform a **physical examination,** followed by arterial blood gases and chest roentgenography, if indicated.
   f. Noninvasive ventilation (CPAP, bilevel positive airway pressure [BiPAP]) may provide respiratory support and lower reintubation rates in patients managing only borderline function following extubation.

3. Early mobilization. Patients should be out of bed and upright as much as possible because this simple maneuver improves the FRC between 10% and 20%. This action allows gravity to assist more in respiration and also helps to minimize the retention of secretions.

4. Oxygen should be administered if necessary but with caution in patients with COPD. The oxygen should be heated and humidified.

TABLE 3-10 Criteria for Weaning Mechanical Ventilation	
Measurements of Oxygenation	**Measurements of Ventilation**
Pao_2/Fio_2 ratio >150–200	$Paco_2$ <50 mm Hg
Arterial saturation >90%	Arterial pH >7.25
Fio_2 ≤40%–50%	Respiratory rate <24 breaths/min
PEEP ≤5–8 cm H_2O	Tidal volume 6–8 mg/kg
Alveolar-arterial oxygen tension	Vital capacity 10–15 mL/kg
(AAo_2) <300–350 mm Hg	Minute volume <10 L/min
Other Considerations	**Negative respiratory force >–20 cm H_2O**
Hemodynamic stability not requiring	Dead space-to-tidal volume ratio <0.6
significant vasopressor support	
Adequate inspiratory effort and cough	
Absence of excessive secretions	
Absence of active myocardial ischemia	
Absence of neurologic impairment	
Absence of airway compromise	

Fio_2, fraction of inspired oxygen; $Paco_2$, partial pressure of carbon dioxide in arterial blood; Pao_2, partial pressure of oxygen in arterial blood.
Summarized from MacIntyre NR, Cook DJ, Ely EW Jr, et. al. Evidence-based guidelines for weaning and discontinuing ventilatory support: a collective task force facilitated by the American College of Chest Physicians; the American Association for Respiratory Care; and the American College of Critical Care Medicine. *Chest.* 2001;120(6)(suppl): 375S–395S; Coates NE, Weigelt JA. Weaning from mechanical ventilation. *Surg Clin North Am.* 1991;74(4):860.

5. **Narcotics** should be used judiciously to avoid oversedation and respiratory depression.
   a. The use of **regional or epidural anesthesia** can provide excellent perioperative analgesia, reduce respiratory depression secondary to parenteral narcotics, and allow improved pulmonary toilet.
   b. Inducing **respiratory depression** must be avoided when using parenteral or epidural narcotics.

E **Pulmonary complications** occur in the perioperative period in up to 50% of patients with chronic lung disease and in up to 70% of patients with abnormal pulmonary function tests.

1. **Atelectasis** is the most common complication, followed by **pulmonary infection,** both of which may lead to pulmonary failure. Pulmonary secretions tend to accumulate after hypoventilation secondary to decreased FRC and splinting from pain.

2. **Aspiration of gastric contents** occurs in up to 25% of emergency cases but may occur in as many as 8%–10% of elective cases. The main causes of aspiration are the diminished loss of consciousness and abnormal motility of the gastrointestinal tract during anesthesia.
   a. **Acid aspiration** alone causes an inflammatory pulmonary reaction, even in the absence of bacterial contamination. **Histamine (H_2) blockers or proton pump inhibitors (PPI)** are often administered preoperatively in patients who have a high risk of aspiration or gastroesophageal reflux.
   b. **Bronchoscopy** is indicated only for removal of large aspirated particulate matter.
   c. **Steroid therapy** is *not* indicated after aspiration.
   d. A **nasogastric tube** should be placed for gastric decompression if an ileus is present. Once gastric emptying is satisfactory, the nasogastric tube should be removed promptly to allow the patient to cough more effectively.

3. **Other** significant postoperative complications include the following:
   a. Bronchospasm
   b. Pulmonary edema
   c. Pneumothorax
   d. Pulmonary embolism
   e. Adult respiratory distress syndrome

IV THE SURGICAL PATIENT WITH CHRONIC RENAL FAILURE

The preoperative condition of patients with chronic renal failure is strongly dependent on the **residual glomerular filtration rate (GFR)** and the presence of underlying disease. **Volume and electrolyte homeostasis** is altered. **The metabolism or excretion of medications** (especially many antibiotics and radiopaque, iodinated angiographic dye) is impaired.

A **Assessment of renal function**

1. History
   a. **Congenital abnormalities; obstructive uropathy; polycystic kidney disease; and chronic, recurrent urologic infection** may be associated with significant renal dysfunction.
   b. The presence of **underlying systemic disease** (e.g., diffuse arteriosclerosis, diabetes mellitus, hypertension, autoimmune diseases, collagen vascular disease) should alert the physician to the possibility of associated renal disease.
   c. **Known renal insufficiency** should be carefully investigated, including fluid and dietary restrictions, as well as the requirement for dialysis.

2. **Physical examination.** Careful attention should be paid to the following:
   a. **Volume status**
      (1) **Intravascular volume overload** is common; manifestations include pulmonary rales, jugular venous distention, and peripheral edema.
      (2) Certain renal diseases (e.g., chronic pyelonephritis, medullary cystic disease, other interstitial disease) may result in **salt wasting** and **subsequent dehydration.**
   b. **Evidence of coagulopathy** includes petechiae and ecchymoses.
   c. **Central nervous system changes** include lethargy and altered mental status.
   d. **Pericardial or pleural rubs** and effusions may occur.

3. **Laboratory studies**
   a. Serum electrolytes, BUN, and creatinine allow assessment of the **volume and electrolyte and acid–base status** of the patient.
   b. The **hematocrit** is decreased in renal failure secondary to decreased production of erythropoietin.
   c. **Urinalysis** should be performed to evaluate the ability of the kidneys to concentrate and acidify the urine and also to assess for proteinuria and glucosuria as well as for microscopic evaluation.
   d. Calculation of the **creatinine clearance** and **fractional excretion of sodium** gives objective evidence of the underlying GFR and the degree of parenchymal function.
   e. **A chest radiograph** and **an ECG** should be performed to assess the patient's volume status and degree of cardiac dysfunction.

B **Pre-existing renal disease**

1. **If the GFR is 25% of normal,** the kidney loses its ability to correct many different abnormalities.
   a. **Fluid and electrolyte homeostasis** is altered, which results in
      (1) Hypertension
      (2) Peripheral edema
      (3) Salt retention
      (4) Hyponatremia, as a result of fluid retention
      (5) Hyperkalemia
      (6) Metabolic acidosis, as a result of failure to excrete organic acids (e.g., phosphates, sulfates)
   b. **Hematologic functions** are altered.
      (1) **Anemia** occurs as the GFR drops, and it becomes profound as the GFR approaches zero.
      (2) **Coagulation defects** occur as a result of altered platelet adhesion and aggregation as well as abnormalities in the coagulation cascade (see Chapter 1, III A).
   c. **Altered calcium metabolism and altered parathyroid hormone metabolism** result in secondary hyperparathyroidism and bone disease with hypocalcemia and hyperphosphatemia.
   d. **Cardiac and other vascular abnormalities** develop, including
      (1) Increased incidence of atherosclerosis
      (2) Pericarditis and pericardial effusions

   e. Nutritional status is impaired, secondary to
      (1) Proteinuria, which may be as high as 25 g/day
      (2) Decreased body stores of nitrogen, which are catabolized as uremia progresses
      (3) Decreased dietary intake, which may result from anorexia, nausea, malabsorption, or dietary restrictions placed by the physician
   f. Immune function disorders can result in
      (1) Increased urinary tract infections caused by oliguria
      (2) Impaired mucocutaneous barriers, which may be secondary to pruritus or epidermal atrophy
      (3) Increased pulmonary infections, which are related in part to decreased pulmonary clearance mechanisms
      (4) Increased incidence of malignancies
      (5) Impaired phagocytosis
      (6) Mildly impaired response to vaccines
      (7) Impaired elimination of certain viruses, such as hepatitis B virus. This impairment is a major problem in dialysis patients because as many as 60% of these patients become chronic antigen carriers once they contract the infection.

2. If the GFR is less than 5% of normal, dialysis is required for maintenance of bodily functions.
   a. Dialysis corrects or improves many of the uremic symptoms and abnormalities (e.g., fluid and electrolyte problems, hypertension, nutritional problems related to dietary intake).
   b. Complications related to dialysis
      (1) Peritoneal dialysis is associated with an increased risk of peritonitis.
      (2) Hemodialysis requires systemic heparin levels that may worsen the coagulopathy of chronic renal failure. In addition, the vascular access necessary for dialysis is associated with blood-borne infections, especially staphylococcal infections.

C **Dialysis**

1. Preoperative dialysis
   a. Routine dialysis should be undertaken **24 hours before elective surgery** both to minimize the effects of the intravenous heparin given with dialysis and to allow the patient to stabilize after treatment.
   b. More emergent treatment is required for the following conditions:
      (1) Hyperkalemia must be addressed expeditiously.
         (a) A reading of the potassium level must be obtained immediately preceding surgery, and treatment must be instituted if the level is **greater than 5 mEq/L.**
         (b) ECG changes (e.g., a tall, peaked T wave, loss of P waves, and widened QRS complexes) require immediate treatment. **Intravenous calcium** will block the effect of excess potassium at the cellular level.
         (c) Sodium bicarbonate or a combination of **insulin** and **glucose** may be administered intravenously to temporarily shift potassium to the intracellular compartment.
         (d) Exchange resins, such as sodium polystyrene sulfonate (Kayexalate), can control potassium levels and may be given as an enema.
         (e) Emergent dialysis may also be required.
      (2) Metabolic acidosis should be corrected by either bicarbonate administration or dialysis therapy.
      (3) Coagulopathy of chronic renal failure is best controlled preoperatively by **adequate dialysis. Heparin may be withheld** during emergency treatment. Bleeding tendencies during or after surgery may also be controlled by the administration of **fresh frozen plasma** or **deamino-8-D-arginine vasopressin (DDAVP).**
      (4) Pericarditis and pericardial effusion should be resolved before the administration of a general anesthetic because of impaired cardiac output and the risk of pericardial tamponade.

2. Postoperative dialysis
   a. Dialysis should be **withheld for 24 hours postoperatively, if possible,** because it requires the use of heparin, acutely lowers the platelet count, and causes transient **hypotension** and **hypoxia** during treatment.

    b. Dialysis should be performed **emergently** for the following:

      (1) Hyperkalemia unresponsive to medications

      (2) Metabolic acidosis with the inability to give sodium bicarbonate

      (3) Severe volume overload

      (4) Signs of uremia (e.g., pericarditis, mental status changes, asterixis)

    c. **Peritoneal dialysis** patients require temporary vascular access for hemodialysis following abdominal procedures.

    d. **Continuous arteriovenous or venovenous hemofiltration** may be indicated in patients with massive volume overload. This treatment modality uses hydrostatic transport through a semipermeable membrane to permit water and solute removal. The filtrate composition is similar to that of plasma.

D **Operative management** follows the same basic principles as those for any surgical patient. Patients with renal failure are susceptible to appendicitis, cholecystitis, diverticulitis, and peptic ulcer disease. In addition, they may require surgery for problems related specifically to their disease, such as vascular access procedures and urologic procedures.

1. Fluid and electrolyte management must be monitored closely.

2. Anesthesia. The altered metabolism and excretion in chronic renal failure must be taken into consideration.

    a. **Benzodiazepines** with a long half-life may tend to accumulate and lead to prolonged sedation.

    b. **Muscle relaxants**

      (1) **Succinylcholine** administration leads to increases in serum potassium and is contraindicated in hyperkalemic patients.

      (2) Certain antibiotics and diuretics may further prolong drug action at the neuromuscular junction; this situation can lead to postoperative recurarization (recurrent paralysis) with catastrophic results.

      (3) **Atracurium** undergoes enzymatic degradation independent of renal function and may be the agent of choice in patients with renal failure.

    c. All currently used **inhalational agents decrease GFR** and urinary excretion of sodium, with variable effects on renal blood flow.

E **Perioperative management**

1. Residual renal function, which may be adversely affected by a surgical procedure, is best protected by the following maneuvers:

    a. **Correction of volume excess or deficits and any accompanying electrolyte disorder** can be achieved by either medical management or the use of dialysis.

    b. Avoid **intraoperative hypotension.**

    c. Once adequate intravascular volume resuscitation is ensured, **maintenance of diuresis** may simplify fluid management in perioperative patients with preservable renal function.

    d. **Infections,** especially urinary tract infections, should be treated.

    e. **Nephrotoxic drugs** (e.g., aminoglycosides, vancomycin, intravenous contrast, angiotensin-converting enzyme inhibitors) should be avoided when possible.

2. Dialysis patients with no preservable renal function should be treated similarly.

    a. Nephrotoxic drugs may be used safely if blood levels are followed and other side effects (e.g., ototoxicity) are monitored.

    b. A urinary bladder catheter should not be used in patients with oliguria or with no preservable renal function.

3. General medical management

    a. **Medication dosages** should be carefully adjusted for the level of renal function.

    b. Anemia is well tolerated by these patients.

      (1) A hematocrit of 20%–25% (i.e., 7–8 g/dL) is adequate for most major surgical procedures.

      (2) Perioperative transfusions should be given during dialysis to minimize hyperkalemia.

    c. Supplemental **steroids** should be given in the perioperative period to patients on long-term steroid therapy (e.g., renal transplant patients).

    d. Persistent **coagulopathy** may be addressed with DDAVP, conjugated estrogens, or transfusion of cryoprecipitate.

    e. Malnutrition

        (1) Elective surgery for patients with malnutrition should be postponed until their nutritional status improves.

        (2) After emergency surgery, nutritional requirements should be supplied intravenously, adhering to appropriate volume and protein restrictions until adequate oral intake is possible.

    f. Systemic disorders, such as diabetes mellitus or a thyroid disorder, should be controlled.

F **Postoperative complications** are more common in patients with chronic renal failure and may include labile blood pressure, impaired wound healing, postoperative hematomas, and shunt thrombosis.

V THE SURGICAL PATIENT WITH LIVER DISEASE

Hepatic insufficiency increases the risk of complications and death in the postoperative period. The recognition and management of liver disease preoperatively can minimize the postoperative problems.

A **Assessment of hepatic function** Liver disease should be suspected, based on the history and physical examination.

  1. History

    a. A prior history of jaundice, hepatitis, hemolytic anemia, parasitic infection, biliary stone disease, pancreatitis, enzyme deficiencies (e.g., α_1-antitrypsin deficiency), or prior malignancy (e.g., gastrointestinal or breast cancer) should be considered.

    b. A history of **drug or alcohol abuse** and **possible exposure to infectious hepatitis** agents (e.g., via tattoos, blood transfusions) or to environmental or other hepatotoxins suggest the possibility of hepatic parenchymal disease.

    c. A history of prior hepatotoxicity after inhalational anesthesia is a risk factor for future exposure to halogenated anesthetics.

  2. The physical examination should include an assessment of

    a. Clinically evident features (e.g., jaundice, ascites, peripheral edema, muscle wasting, testicular atrophy, palmar erythema, spider angiomas, gynecomastia) should be examined.

    b. Stigmata of **portal hypertension,** including caput medusae (dilated periumbilical vessels) or splenomegaly, should be assessed.

    c. The presence of upper gastrointestinal bleeding, delirium tremens, or encephalopathy suggests the presence of portal hypertension and underlying cirrhosis.

    d. Evidence of **bleeding disorders** should be sought.

    e. Evidence of **encephalopathy** or asterixis should also be checked.

    f. Liver size. Hepatomegaly or a shrunken liver (especially a shrunken liver with a rounded edge or with palpable nodules on its surface) may be present in liver disease. Hepatic tenderness to percussion should be assessed.

  3. Laboratory tests can confirm the diagnosis but may be normal despite the presence of significant liver disease.

    a. The most useful tests are **aspartate aminotransferase (AST), alanine aminotransferase (ALT), bilirubin, alkaline phosphatase, albumin, and prothrombin time.**

    b. Platelet count and **bleeding time** may be abnormal in patients with significant liver disease.

    c. Hepatitis B surface antigen and hepatitis C serology should be sought if their presence is suspected, given the potential for hospital staff exposure.

  4. A **liver biopsy** may be necessary preoperatively if an acute hepatitis is suspected.

B **Operative risk factors** and their management in patients with pre-existing liver disease have not been fully defined, but several generalizations are useful.

  1. Acute hepatitis. It is advisable to delay elective surgery in the patient with acute hepatitis until the hepatitis is resolved.

a. **Acute alcoholic hepatitis**
  (1) Abstinence from alcohol for 6–12 weeks before elective surgery has been recommended.
  (2) General anesthesia is associated with an operative mortality rate of 50% or higher when portal decompressive surgery is performed.
b. **Acute drug-induced hepatitis.** The results of studies have ranged from no increase in risk to as high as a 20% morbidity and mortality rate.
c. **Acute viral hepatitis.** Elective surgery should be deferred for at least 1 month after the acute illness.

2. **Chronic liver disease.** Patients with chronic liver disease can tolerate most surgical procedures well if they are in a relatively compensated state preoperatively.
   a. The risk appears similar to that of patients undergoing portal decompressive procedures (see **Childs-Pugh** classification in Table 14-1).
   b. **Emergency or abdominal surgery** increases surgical risk.
   c. Patients with **decompensated cirrhosis (Childs C)** have significant surgical morbidity and mortality.
   d. **Management of portal hypertension** may include *β*-**blockers, octreotide, and transvenous intrahepatic portosystemic shunting (TIPS).**

3. **Obstructive jaundice** is associated with increased operative risk, especially in the presence of biliary tract infection. The increased intestinal absorption of enteric endotoxin in the absence of luminal bile salts may lead to systemic endotoxemia and a higher rate of complications.
   a. **Cholangitis** mandates prompt decompression by **endoscopic retrograde cholangiopancreatography (ERCP) with sphincterotomy and biliary stenting** or **transhepatic cholangicography with drainage (THC)** to effectively treat sepsis.
   b. **Coagulation disorders** are common secondary to diminished intestinal absorption of **vitamin K. Disseminated intravascular coagulation** may be present, especially in association with biliary sepsis.
   c. **Acute renal failure** with renal tubular dysfunction has been reported in approximately 10% of postoperative patients, and the risk is apparently related to the degree of jaundice.
   d. **Gastrointestinal hemorrhage,** especially stress gastritis, occurs in 5%–14% of postoperative patients.
   e. **Delayed wound healing** and **wound infection** are likely to be exacerbated by associated malnutrition, malignancy, and sepsis.
   f. **Risk factors for postoperative complications in patients with obstructive jaundice** [Friedman LS. The Risk of Surgery in Patients with Liver Disease. *Hepatology.* 1999;29:1617–1623]
     (1) Hematocrit <30%
     (2) Bilirubin >11 mg/dL
     (3) Malignancy
     (4) Hypoalbuminemia
     (5) Cholangitis
     (6) Azotemia

C **Anesthetics** The liver is the primary site of much first-pass metabolism. Impaired function leads to altered drug pharmacokinetics and prolongation of effects.

1. All **inhalational anesthetics** reduce splanchnic perfusion and hepatic blood flow to some extent.
   a. **Isoflurane** is associated with minimal hepatic metabolism and therefore may be the inhalational anesthetic of choice.
   b. **Halogenated inhalational agents** should be avoided in patients with a history of hepatotoxicity after inhalation anesthesia.

2. **Muscle relaxants**
   a. **Neuromuscular blockade** may be prolonged after the administration of nondepolarizing muscle relaxants to patients with chronic liver failure.
   b. **Atracurium** undergoes peripheral enzymatic degradation, and its metabolism is unaffected by hepatic dysfunction.

D **Perioperative management** should be aimed at the treatment of potentially correctable factors.

1. **Fluid and electrolyte balance**
   a. Care must be taken to **avoid hypotension,** as the compromised liver is sensitive to further ischemic insults.
   b. Patients with cirrhosis may be in **high-output cardiac failure** secondary to volume overload and peripheral arteriovenous shunting.
   c. **Hypokalemia** and **alkalosis** must be corrected.
   d. **Hypomagnesemia** and **hypophosphatemia** are common in alcoholics and should be identified and corrected.
   e. Impairment of **lactate metabolism** may result in significant acid–base disturbances.

2. **Coagulopathy**
   a. The **prothrombin time** may be elevated secondary either to **vitamin K deficiency** in patients with obstructive jaundice or to failure of synthetic function in patients with parenchymal disease. Treatment may be instituted with **vitamin K** or **fresh frozen plasma.**
   b. **Thrombocytopenia** may be present in patients with portal hypertension secondary to splenomegaly. The response to platelet transfusion may be lessened.

3. **Prophylactic antibiotics** should include coverage of biliary and enteric flora.

4. **Stress gastritis** prophylaxis should be administered.

5. **Narcotics and sedatives** that may precipitate hepatic encephalopathy must be avoided. The half-life of **meperidine** is significantly prolonged in patients with hepatic failure.

6. **Hypoxemia** may be present secondary to increased intrapulmonary shunting.

7. **Encephalopathy** should be treated with dietary **protein restriction** and the administration of intestinal antibiotics (i.e., **neomycin**) and **lactulose.**

8. **Ascites** may be controlled with diuresis, sodium and water restriction, and judicious paracentesis.

9. **Malnutrition,** with its attendant increased risks of infection and wound complications, should be improved by adequate nutrition and treatment of current infections.

VI THE SURGICAL PATIENT WITH DIABETES MELLITUS

Diabetes mellitus affects 2%–10% of the general population. As many as one half of these patients have no symptoms until a stressful situation (e.g., sepsis, surgery) results in overt manifestations of hyperglycemia.

A **Assessment of risk**   There is increasing awareness that tighter glycemic control can limit long-term complications of the disease. The patient with diabetes frequently requires surgery for **complications of the diabetes** as well as for nondiabetic surgical problems. The patient history should emphasize the diabetes and its management, and the physical examination should focus on evidence of systemic complications.

1. **History**
   a. The type of diabetic control used, the dosage schedule, and the adequacy of control for the patient should be determined.
   b. The propensity to develop ketosis, ketoacidosis, hyperglycemia, or hypoglycemia and a history of "brittleness" (i.e., unpredictable wide swings in blood glucose level) should be assessed.
   c. Specific questions related to the **complications of diabetes** (e.g., peripheral vascular and coronary artery disease, nephropathy, neuropathy, hypertension, and retinopathy) should be answered.

2. **The physical examination** should be directed at identifying target organ involvement.
   a. **Associated cardiovascular disease,** with silent myocardial ischemia, may be present.
   b. **Retinopathy** is associated with diffuse small-vessel disease.
   c. **Autonomic neuropathy** occurs as a result of diabetic degeneration of the autonomic nervous system. This neuropathy may manifest as the following conditions:

        (1) Postural hypotension

        (2) Bladder-emptying problems

        (3) Impaired intestinal motility

        (4) Gastroparesis

        (5) Impotence

        (6) Cardiac autonomic dysfunction

    d. Somatic neuropathy, with "stocking-glove" loss of sensation, increases the risks of injury (of which the patient may not be aware) to an insensate foot.

    e. Patients with uncontrolled diabetes are susceptible to **infections,** and the presence of an ongoing infection should be investigated.

3. Laboratory studies

    a. Elevated **HbA1c levels** are correlated with increased cardiovascular complications.

    b. The patient's **volume and electrolyte status** should be assessed, especially in relation to the acuteness of the disease requiring surgery.

    c. **Serum glucose level** and the degree of **glucosuria** should be determined.

    d. The **anion gap** should be determined, and if it is elevated, arterial blood gases should be tested. The usual finding is low serum bicarbonate and a decreased pH secondary to

        (1) Diabetic ketoacidosis

        (2) Lactic acidosis

        (3) Retained organic acids containing phosphates and sulfates secondary to chronic renal failure

    e. Radiopaque dye studies performed on patients with diabetes increase the risk of acute renal failure, especially when patients are older than 40 years of age or have a creatinine level higher than 2 mg/dL.

B **Perioperative management** of the patient with diabetes depends on the severity of the acute disease as well as on the severity of the diabetes. Insulin requirements increase with the stress of surgery, and noninsulin-dependent diabetics may transiently require supplemental insulin for adequate glucose control.

1. Perioperative glucose control is aimed at maintaining normoglycemia. Careful attention must be paid to avoid overly aggressive glycemic control while the patient is under or recovering from anesthesia, as the patient may not be able to relate symptoms of hypoglycemia.

2. Elective surgery

    a. Surgery should be deferred until blood glucose control is adequate.

    b. Surgery should be scheduled for the first case in the morning, if possible.

    c. Patients with diabetes often have **gastroparesis,** and they should fast at least 12 hours before elective surgery. **Metoclopamide** may be administered to promote gastric emptying.

3. Patients with diet-controlled diabetes do not usually require any specific perioperative measures other than glucose monitoring.

4. Oral agents

    a. Orally administered hypoglycemic agents should not be given on the day of surgery.

    b. Sulfonylurea drugs should be withheld at least 2–3 days before surgery, based on the half-life of the specific agent (e.g., the half-life of the long-acting agent chlorpropamide is 38 hours).

    c. Metformin should be held 24 hours prior to surgery because of the risk of **lactic acidosis.**

5. Insulin may be administered by either a subcutaneous route or a continuous intravenous infusion.

    a. Preoperatively, one half to two thirds of the daily dose of insulin is usually given **as NPH insulin.**

        (1) On the morning of the surgery, an intravenous drip of glucose-containing solution should be administered to maintain glucose metabolism and to prevent ketoacidosis.

        (2) Postoperatively, **intermittent doses of regular insulin** can be titrated to frequently determined blood glucose levels until the patient can tolerate a regular diet and can resume the previous stable regimen.

    b. Alternatively, an **insulin-dextrose infusion** can be titrated to maintain normoglycemia.

6. In cardiac surgery and surgical ICU patients, **tight glycemic control** to blood glucose levels between 80 and 110 mg/dL has been associated with decreases in morbidity and mortality.

C **Emergency surgery**   Patients with diabetes and emergent surgical conditions (e.g., perforated viscus, acute cholecystitis) may develop extremely high glucose levels secondary to stress or ongoing infection.

1. These patients require **correction of the acute disease process** before the diabetes can be controlled. Nevertheless, intraoperative management is often improved with a brief period to stabilize fluid and electrolyte balance.

2. Hyperglycemia. The serum glucose level should be monitored, and abnormalities should be treated promptly. Perioperatively, the serum glucose should be stable and **within normal range, if possible.**

3. Diabetic ketoacidosis. Patients with diabetic ketoacidosis are hyperglycemic, ketotic, and acidotic. They are also dehydrated and have decreased body stores of potassium and sodium. They may exhibit Kussmaul's respirations (rapid deep breaths).

   a. Measured serum sodium levels decrease 1.7 mEq/dL for each 100 mg/dL that the glucose is elevated.

   b. Massive free water deficits may occur secondary to osmotic diuresis from glucosuria.

   c. Ketoacidosis is best corrected by the administration of intravenous fluids, insulin, bicarbonate, and potassium.

   d. Surgery should be postponed until the ketoacidosis is at least partially resolved, as measured by an improvement in pH, hydration, and correction of electrolyte abnormalities and serum glucose levels.

4. Hyperosmolar nonketotic states. The stress of surgery, infection, or the high glucose load of hyperalimentation may induce a nonketotic, hyperglycemic, hyperosmolar coma in patients with adult-onset diabetes mellitus.

   a. The hyperosmolar nonketotic state is not associated with acidosis but is otherwise very similar to diabetic ketoacidosis.

   b. Management principles include administering intravenous fluids, insulin, and potassium as necessary as well as correcting any underlying cause.

D **Operative complications**

1. Infections. Patients with out-of-control diabetes tend to have an increased rate of infectious complications both at the surgical site and elsewhere. Complications from infections account for up to 20% of perioperative deaths in diabetic patients.

2. Wound healing is likely to be impaired in patients with poor glucose control secondary to changes in soft tissue matrix, granulation tissue, and microvascular disease.

3. If **macrovascular disease** is present, impaired wound healing is more likely than in patients without diabetes. However, if peripheral blood flow is adequate, wound healing is likely to proceed.

4. Mortality rates
   a. The **overall mortality rate for surgery in patients with diabetes** is approximately 2%.
      (1) Almost 30% of deaths are a direct result of **cardiovascular** complications.
      (2) Almost 16% of deaths are related to **sepsis,** particularly from staphylococcal infections.
   b. The **mortality rate for emergency surgical procedures in patients with diabetes** is several times higher than the mortality rate for elective procedures. For example, in patients with diabetes, the mortality rate for emergency cholecystectomy for acute cholecystitis is as high as 22%, compared with a mortality rate lower than 1% for elective cholecystectomy.

VII   **THE SURGICAL PATIENT WITH BLOOD-BORNE PATHOGENS—PREVENTION OF TRANSMISSION**

The operative management of patients with blood-borne pathogens requires vigilant adherence to protocols to reduce the risk of occupational exposure.

A Because the serologic status of a patient may not be known before surgery, the Centers for Disease Control and Prevention (CDC) have recommended that all patients be **assumed** to be infectious and be handled with appropriate precautions (i.e., universal precautions).

B **Blood** is the single most important source of HIV and viral hepatitis exposure in the workplace. Other **high-risk fluids** are cerebrospinal, synovial, pleural, peritoneal, pericardial, and amniotic fluid as well as semen and vaginal secretions.

C **Occupational transmission** has been documented by percutaneous inoculation or by contact with an open wound, nonintact (e.g., chapped, abraded, weeping, dermatitic) skin, or mucous membranes by blood, blood-contaminated body fluids, tissue, or concentrated virus.

D **Prevention is the primary means of preventing occupational exposure.**

1. **Proper protective** attire should be donned before any procedure with the possibility of exposure to blood or body fluids, including:
   a. **Gloves**
   b. **Eyewear**
   c. **Mask**
   d. **Gown.** This garment should be disposable and impermeable to large quantities of blood or splashes.

2. **Techniques that minimize percutaneous injury**
   a. Careful handling and disposal of sharp objects are essential.
   b. Good lighting and a carefully organized operative field minimize accidental exposures.
   c. Tissue retraction should be performed with instruments rather than by hand.
   d. The presence of unnecessary personnel in the operating room should be minimized.
   e. Inexperienced operators should not be permitted to perform exposure-prone procedures.

E **Postexposure prophylaxis**   The CDC recommends prompt evaluation for postexposure prophylaxis following occupational exposure. Treatment regimens are based on the extent of exposure and the serologic status of the patient.

Study Questions for Part I

Directions: *Each of the numbered items in this section is followed by several possible answers. Select the ONE lettered answer that is BEST in each case.*

1. A healthy adult presents for a pre-employment physical. What will be the largest component of his or her body by mass?

- [A] Protein
- [B] Water
- [C] Calcium
- [D] Sodium
- [E] Potassium

2. An 80-year-old man with a history of ischemic cardiomyopathy is hypotensive and oliguric after major abdominal surgery. Initial fluid resuscitation produces only transient improvements. He is transferred to the intensive care unit for further management. A pulmonary artery catheter could be used to measure all of the following *except:*

- [A] Left atrial filling pressure
- [B] Cardiac output
- [C] Ejection fraction
- [D] Mixed venous oxygen saturation
- [E] Systemic vascular resisitance

3. A 25-year-old man is injured in the arm with a knife. What is the first mechanism responsible for hemostasis?

- [A] Extrinsic clotting system
- [B] Vessel constriction
- [C] Intrinsic clotting system
- [D] Platelet activation
- [E] Fibrinolytic system

4. A 27-year-old woman is experiencing perioral and extremity numbness the morning after a neck operation. What is the cause of her symptoms?

- [A] Hypokalemia
- [B] Hypercalcemia
- [C] Hypocalcemia
- [D] Hypochloremia
- [E] Hyperkalemia

5. A 55-year-old woman undergoes laparotomy for small bowel obstruction. During lysis of adhesions, an enterotomy is made in the obstructed, but viable, bowel, and a large amount of fecal-looking bowel contents are spilled into the abdomen. The incision would now be considered what kind of wound?

- [A] Clean contaminated
- [B] Secondary
- [C] Infected
- [D] Contaminated
- [E] Clean

6. A critically ill 55-year-old man is in septic shock in the intensive care unit after removal of a nonviable small bowel. What is the most reliable measurement of arterial blood pressure?

- [A] Arterial line diastolic
- [B] Noninvasive systolic

C. Arterial line mean
D. Arterial line systolic
E. Noninvasive mean

7. Delayed primary closure would be the most appropriate wound closure technique for which of the following procedures?

A. Removal of perforated appendix
B. Repair of wound dehiscence 1 week after elective left colectomy
C. Emergency drainage of a diverticular abscess with sigmoid resection and end colostomy
D. Vagotomy and pyloroplasty for bleeding duodenal ulcer
E. Repair of an incisional hernia 12 weeks after an elective left colectomy complicated by a wound infection and a resultant incisional hernia.

8. A 55-year-old man with insulin-dependent diabetes presents to the emergency department with acute abdominal pain. His heart rate is 130 beats per minute, his blood pressure is 90/60 mm Hg, and his oral temperature is 101.8°F. His respiratory rate is 28 breaths per minute. The abdominal examination demonstrates diffuse peritonitis. What should be the first step in the evaluation and management of this patient?

A. Volume resuscitation
B. Abdominal radiograph
C. Intravenous antibiotics
D. Computed tomography (CT) scan
E. Immediate laparotomy

9. A 57-year-old man underwent a laparoscopic splenectomy for idiopathic thrombocytopenic purpura (ITP). He subsequently develops a persistent output of 100 cc daily of amylase-rich fluid from a drain placed at the time of surgery. All of the following would be expected to prevent spontaneous resolution of this problem *except:*

A. Octreotide administration
B. Pancreatic duct stricture
C. Infection
D. Nonabsorbable suture in distal pancreatic duct
E. Epithelialization of the tract

10. For appropriate procedures, antibiotic prophylaxis for bacterial endocarditis should be administered in patients with a history of which of the following?

A. Mitral valve prolapse without regurgitation
B. Automatic implantable cardiac defibrillator placement
C. Aortic valve replacement
D. Coronary artery bypass graft
E. Surgically repaired ventricular septal defect

11. Which of the following procedures would be expected to have the greatest impact on postoperative pulmonary function?

A. Low anterior resection
B. Femoropopliteal bypass
C. Subtotal gastrectomy
D. Open cholecystectomy
E. Total abdominal hysterectomy

12. Which of the following is a criteria for emergent preoperative dialysis?

A. Potassium (K^+) 5.0, without arrhythmia
B. Arterial pH 7.30, anion gap 8
C. Pericardial friction rub

[D] Blood urea nitrogen 105
[E] Creatinine 5.5

13. Preoperative coagulation studies should be obtained on which of the following patients?

[A] A 35-year-old woman on aspirin, prior to varicose vein surgery
[B] A 65-year-old diabetic man, prior to inguinal hernia repair
[C] A 70-year-old jaundiced woman, prior to choledochojejunostomy
[D] A 45-year-old woman prior to bilateral prophylactic mastectomy with transverse rectus abdominus myocutaneous flap reconstructions
[E] A 50-year-old man with stable angina, prior to coronary artery bypass

Directions: *The group of items in this section consists of lettered options followed by a set of numbered items. For each item, select the lettered option(s) that is(are) most closely associated with it. Each lettered option may be selected once, more than once, or not at all.*

QUESTIONS 14–17

Match the clinical situation with the appropriate type of drain.

[A] Jackson-Pratt closed drain
[B] No drain
[C] Underwater-seal drain
[D] Sump drain

14. Nasogastric decompression

15. Spontaneous pneumothorax

16. Diffuse peritonitis from perforated duodenal ulcer

17. Splenectomy for ruptured spleen

Answers and Explanations

1. The answer is B (Chapter 1, I A 1). The normal adult human body is made up of 50%–70% water. The water is contained in three primary compartments of the body: intracellular, extracellular, and intravascular. On average, two thirds of the body is made of water; in the hypothetical 70-kg man, this is 46 L. Of this 46 L, two thirds is intracellular (30 L), and one third is extracellular (16 L). Of the extracellular portion, two thirds is extravascular (10.5 L), and one third is intravascular (5.5 L). This approximation gives a good starting point when beginning to estimate fluid resuscitation, replacement, and maintenance.

2. The answer is C (Chapter 1, VII D). A pulmonary artery catheter can be useful in distinguishing cardiac dysfunction from other causes of shock in certain patients. It will allow the treating physician to measure left atrial filling pressure from the port in the tip via back pressure through the lungs. Cardiac output is measured via thermal dilution. Mixed venous oxygen saturation can be measured by drawing a sample from the catheter. Systemic vascular resistance can be calculated from the cardiac output, mean arterial pressure, and central venous pressure.

3. The answer is B (Chapter 1, III A). The first mechanism activated when there is damage to a vessel is constriction, which is an effort to stop blood flow. This is followed by platelet activation, which produces a platelet plug. The intrinsic and extrinsic pathways are then activated to form a fibrin clot. The fibrinolytic system is the body's mechanism to dissolve established clots.

4. The answer is C (Chapter 1, II B). Hypocalcemia can induce neuromuscular irritability, including perioral and extremity numbness. This can progress to carpopedal spasm and tetany. The most common cause of hypocalcemia is parathyroid surgery to treat hypercalcemia, resulting in rebound hypocalcemia.

5. The answer is D (Chapter 1, V C). The wound described is a contaminated wound due to the gross spill of contaminated material. A clean wound is one made through normal, antiseptically prepared skin and encounters no infected or colonized areas. A clean-contaminated wound is similar to a clean wound except that a contaminated or potentially contaminated area (e.g., bowel, bronchus, urinary tract), which has been prepared to the best of one's ability and presents minimal contamination, has been opened. An infected wound is one that already has an established infection present. Secondary is a type of wound closure and not a classification of a wound.

6. The answer is C (Chapter 1, VII D 2 b). The arterial line mean pressure is the most accurate and is the most physiologically useful measurement of blood pressure. It may be very accurate but often has limited clinical usefulness and must be used cautiously. Noninvasive blood pressures are not very accurate in critically ill patients. Noninvasive blood pressure measurements are notoriously high in hypotensive patients and low in hypertensive patients.

7. The answer is A (Chapter 1, V C, D 3; Chapter 2, I A 3). Delayed primary closure is appropriate for contaminated wounds, such as a ruptured appendix without abscess formation. Wound dehiscences are closed with retention sutures that include all layers, including the skin, because the fascial strength has been compromised. Infected wounds are packed open to heal by secondary intention, as with drainage of a diverticular abscess. Clean and clean-contaminated wounds can be closed primarily, as with incisional hernia repair (clean) and vagotomy/pyloroplasty (clean contaminated).

8. The answer is A (Chapter 3, VI C a). Intra-abdominal sepsis in a diabetic patient may be complicated by the development of ketoacidosis and dehydration. The patient presents with a condition that will likely require emergent surgical intervention. Initial management should be directed at restoration of the patient's circulating blood volume and optimization of his physiologic status prior to possible laparotomy. The serum glucose, electrolytes, and pH should be determined and abnormalities corrected. Measurement of hourly urine output will allow assessment of the adequacy of resuscitation.

Abdominal radiographs should be obtained to look for free intraperitoneal air, and broad spectrum intravenous antibiotics should be administered, but fluid resuscitation takes top priority. A computed tomography scan may not be indicated in the patient who, on physical examination and history, clearly has peritonitis.

9. The answer is A (Chapter 2, VII D). Enterocutaneous fistulas typically respond to conservative management and spontaneously close when conditions are favorable. Octreotide has been shown to decrease pancreatic fistula output and clearly does not inhibit resolution. Distal obstruction (pancreatic duct stricture), infection, foreign body (nonabsorbable suture), and epithelialization all inhibit resolution.

10. The answer is C (Chapter, 3 II D; Table 3-5). In 1997, the American Heart Association updated guidelines to clarify recommendations for antibiotic prophylaxis for the prevention of bacterial endocarditis. In general, appropriate prophylaxis should be given to patients with underlying structural cardiac defects (e.g., prosthetic cardiac valves, significant valvular disease, hypertrophic cardiomyopathy, complex congenital heart disease, surgically constructed systemic-pulmonary shunts) who undergo procedures leading to bacteremia with organisms likely to cause endocarditis (e.g., major dental work or invasive procedures of the respiratory, gastrointestinal, or genitourinary tracts).

11. The answer is C (Chapter 3, III C). Major upper abdominal surgery performed via a vertical midline incision would be expected to have the greatest impact on postoperative pulmonary function. Other operative factors would include thoracotomy, residual intraperitoneal sepsis, age greater than 59 years, prolonged preoperative hospitalization, colorectal or gastroduodenal surgery, procedure longer than 3.5 hours, and higher body mass index. Lower abdominal and extremity surgery are associated with fewer pulmonary complications when compared with thoracic and upper abdominal surgery.

12. The answer is C (Chapter 3, C 1 b). Indications for emergent dialysis include life-threatening hyperkalemia, severe metabolic acidosis secondary to retained organic acids, uremic pericarditis, and volume overload. The serum creatinine and blood urea nitrogen levels reflect the underlying renal dysfunction but will not necessarily mandate emergent preoperative dialysis.

13. The answer is C (Chapter 3, I C; Table 3-1). Preoperative evaluation with routine coagulation studies is neither cost effective nor routinely indicated. Patients with a history of postsurgical bleeding or ongoing acute hemorrhage, patients on oral anticoagulation, patients with liver disease or hepatobiliary obstruction, malnourished patients, and patients unable to give an adequate history should have prothrombin time, partial thromboplastin time, and platelet counts checked preoperatively.

14–17. The answers are 14-D, 15-C, 16-B, and 17-A (Chapter 2, II A; II A 1 b). Sump drains are needed to adequately decompress the stomach. When the pleural space requires drainage, a chest tube is placed and connected to an underwater seal so that air and fluid cannot reflux into the chest. This is needed because of the negative intrathoracic pressure generated with each inspiration. Diffuse peritonitis cannot be drained, as the peritoneal contents quickly "wall off" foreign bodies such as drains; discrete intraperitoneal collections can be drained. Splenectomy jeopardizes the pancreatic tail, which is in close proximity to the splenic hilum. When the area is obscured, as with the hematoma accompanying splenic rupture, the integrity of the pancreas cannot be assured, and the potential pancreatic fluid leak is drained with a closed-suction drain such as a Jackson-Pratt drain.

PART **II**

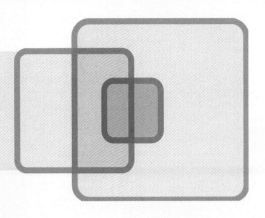

Thoracic Disorders

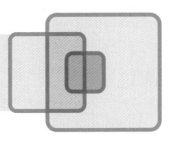

chapter 4

Principles of Thoracic Surgery

D. BRUCE PANASUK • WILLIAM R. ALEX • RICHARD N. EDIE

I GENERAL PRINCIPLES OF THORACIC SURGERY

A Anatomy of the thoracic cavity

1. The **chest wall** (Fig. 4-1) is formed by the sternum, ribs, vertebral column, intercostal muscles, intercostal vessels (that run on the undersurface of the ribs), and nerves. Its inferior border is the diaphragm. It is lined internally by the parietal pleura.

2. The **mediastinum** (Fig. 4-2) is the anatomic region between the pleural cavities for the length of the thorax.
   a. The **anterior compartment** extends from the undersurface of the sternum to the pericardium and contains the thymus gland, lymph nodes, ascending and transverse aorta, and great veins.
   b. The **visceral compartment** extends from the pericardium to the anterior longitudinal spinal ligament and and contains the pericardium, heart, trachea, hilar structures of the lung, esophagus, phrenic nerves, and lymph nodes.
   c. The **paravertebral sulci** are actually potential spaces that contain the sympathetic chains, intercostal nerves, and descending thoracic aorta.

3. **Lungs and tracheobronchial tree** (Fig. 4-3)
   a. The **right lung** has three lobes—the upper, middle, and lower—separated by two **fissures.**
      (1) The **major (oblique) fissure** separates the lower lobe from the upper and middle lobes.
      (2) The **minor (horizontal) fissure** separates the upper lobe from the middle lobe.
   b. The **left lung** has two lobes—the upper and the lower. The **lingula** is a portion of the upper lobe. The lobes are separated by a **single oblique fissure.**
   c. **Bronchopulmonary segments** are intact sections of each lobe that have a separate blood supply, allowing segmental resection. There are ten bronchopulmonary segments on the right and eight bronchopulmonary segments on the left.
   d. The **tracheobronchial tree** (see Chapter 5, IX A) is formed from respiratory epithelium with reinforcing cartilaginous rings; the branching **bronchial tubes** are progressively smaller, down to a diameter of 1–2 mm.
   e. The blood supply is dual.
      (1) **Pulmonary artery** blood is **unoxygenated.**
      (2) **Bronchial artery** blood is **oxygenated.**
   f. **Lymphatic vessels** are present throughout the parenchyma and toward the hilar areas of the lungs.
      (1) Lymphatic flow in the pleural space is from parietal pleura to visceral pleura.
      (2) Lymphatic drainage within the mediastinum is cephalad, flowing along the paratracheal areas toward the scalene nodal areas.
      (3) Generally, lymphatic drainage affects ipsilateral nodes, but contralateral flow often occurs from the left lower lobe.

B General thoracic procedures

1. **Radiologic diagnostic procedures.** The standard procedures consist of the **chest radiograph** and **computed tomography (CT) scan.** These studies are very useful in localizing a process anatomically as well as delineating cavitation, calcification, lymphadenopathy, or multiple lesions. **Magnetic resonance imaging (MRI)** may be used when a vascular lesion is suspected or if vascular involvement is anticipated.

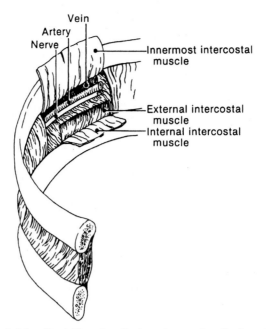

FIGURE 4-1 Chest wall. (Adapted from Way L. Thoracic wall, pleura, lung, and mediastinum. In: Way LW, ed. *Current Surgical Diagnosis and Treatment.* 10th ed. Stamford, CT: Appleton & Lange; 1983:319.)

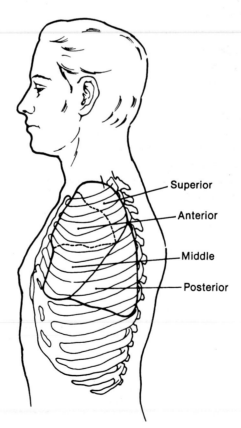

FIGURE 4-2 The anatomic compartments of the mediastinum.

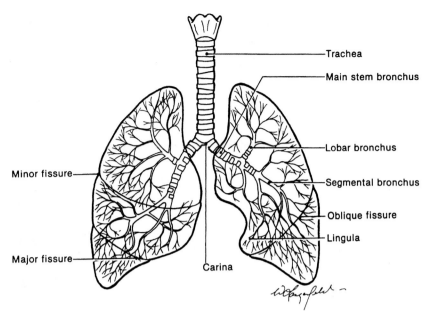

FIGURE 4-3 Lungs and tracheobronchial tree. (Courtesy of Thomas C. King and Craig R. Smith. Columbia Presbyterian Hospital, New York.)

2. **Endoscopy**
   a. **Laryngoscopy** is occasionally an important procedure when carcinoma of the lung is suspected. Tumor involvement of the recurrent laryngeal nerves (signifying inoperability) can be diagnosed via laryngoscopy when suspicion is raised by vocal cord paralysis with resultant hoarseness.
   b. **Bronchoscopy** is useful in many diseases of the tracheobronchial tree for both diagnostic and therapeutic purposes.
      (1) **Diagnostic uses**
         (a) To confirm a lung or tracheobronchial tumor suggested by history, physical examination, or chest radiograph
         (b) To identify the source of hemoptysis
         (c) To obtain specimens for culture and cytologic examination from an area of persistent pulmonary atelectasis or pneumonitis
         (d) To obtain tissue biopsy
      (2) **Therapeutic uses**
         (a) To remove a foreign body
         (b) To remove retained secretions (e.g., after administration of general anesthesia or from aspiration of gastric contents)
         (c) To drain lung infections, such as abscesses
      (3) **Types**
         (a) **Rigid bronchoscopy** allows visualization of the trachea and main bronchi to the individual lobes.
            (i) It is excellent for biopsies of endobronchial lesions and for clearing of thick secretions and blood.
            (ii) The performance of rigid bronchoscopy under local anesthesia requires considerable skill.
         (b) **Flexible fiberoptic bronchoscopy** is used more frequently.
            (i) It is particularly helpful for visualizing lobar bronchi and small bronchopulmonary segments and for the biopsy of lesions in that area.
            (ii) Although not as effective as rigid bronchoscopy, it may also be used for clearing secretions.

(iii) It is especially useful when the patient is intubated, allowing the broncho-scope to be introduced through the endotracheal tube, thus retaining the airway.

(4) Specific advantages

(a) Biopsy for suspicion of endobronchial or parenchymal tumor may be performed transbronchially via the bronchoscope in approximately one third of cases. Pneumothorax is a rare complication that occurs in fewer than 1% of cases.

(b) Parenchymal biopsies are also useful if an infection is suspected. Infections, such as those caused by *Pneumocystis carinii,* can be diagnosed with fixed tissue specimens and may require biopsy.

(c) Widening of the tracheal carina in patients with lung tumors can be seen on bronchoscopy. It suggests distortion of the tracheal anatomy by subcarinal nodes and is a poor prognostic sign.

c. **Mediastinoscopy** is a procedure in which a lighted hollow instrument is inserted behind the sternum at the tracheal notch and directed along the anterior surface of the trachea in the pretracheal space.

(1) Diagnostic uses

(a) Direct biopsy of paratracheal and subcarinal lymph nodes. Positive nodes may either indicate the need for preoperative chemotherapy or unresectability.

(b) It is also useful for diagnosing other pulmonary problems, such as sarcoidosis, lymphoma, and various fungal infections.

(2) Mortality rate is less than 0.1%.

(3) Complications include hemorrhage, pneumothorax, and injury to the recurrent laryngeal nerves, although the incidence is extremely low.

3. Scalene node biopsy

a. The scalene node-bearing fat pad is located behind the clavicle in the region of the sternocleidomastoid muscle. This area should be palpated in patients suspected of having lung tumors and should be biopsied if nodes are palpable.

b. Tumor is found in 85% of patients with palpable nodes but in fewer than 5% of patients with nonpalpable nodes.

c. The scalene nodes are surrounded by important structures, including the pleura, subclavian vessels, thoracic and other large lymph ducts, and phrenic nerves. The main **complications** of scalene node biopsy result from injury to these structures (e.g., pneumothorax, hemorrhage, chyle leak, and diaphragmatic paralysis).

4. Diagnostic pleural procedures

a. **Thoracentesis.** Pleural effusions are examined for organisms in suspected infections and are examined cytologically in suspected malignancies. Positive cytologic findings prove a tumor to be inoperable. Pneumothorax is the main complication of this procedure.

b. **Pleural biopsy.** Either percutaneous or open pleural biopsy yields a positive diagnosis in 60%–80% of patients with tuberculosis or cancer when a pleural effusion or pleural-based mass is present. Pneumothorax is the main complication of this procedure.

5. Lung biopsy

a. **Diagnostic uses.** Percutaneous lung biopsy may be used for either a localized peripheral lesion or a diffuse parenchymal process.

b. **Types**

(1) CT—directed fine needle aspiration biopsy is an excellent method for obtaining tissue for tumor diagnosis. However, sampling errors do exist, and a biopsy negative for a tumor **does not** rule out the existence of a tumor. Needle biopsy may also be useful for the diagnosis of infections and inflammatory processes.

(a) Complications of needle biopsy are pneumothorax and hemorrhage.

(2) Open lung biopsy is necessary if needle biopsy fails to diagnose the problem. Open biopsies or resections are ultimately necessary for many lesions of the chest.

6. Thoracic exposure for various diseases is provided by different **thoracic incisions,** for example:

a. **Median sternotomy** (Fig. 4-4) for exposure of the heart, pericardium, and structures in the anterior mediastinum

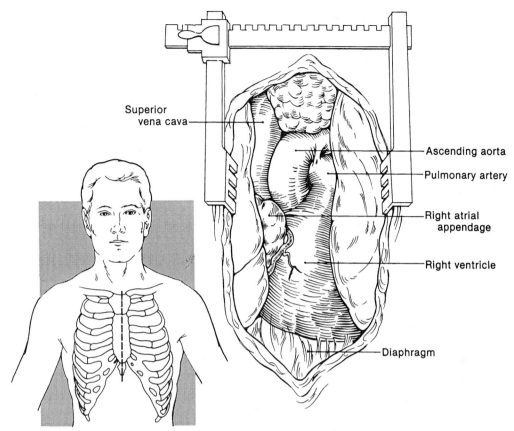

Superior
vena cava

Ascending aorta

Pulmonary artery

Right atrial
appendage

Right ventricle

Diaphragm

FIGURE 4-4 Median sternotomy. (Adapted from Kirklin JW, Barratt-Boyes BG. Hypothermia, circulatory arrest, and cardiopulmonary bypass. In: *Cardiac Surgery.* New York: Wiley; 1986:62.)

    b. Posterolateral thoracotomy (Fig. 4-5) for exposure of the lung, esophagus, and posterior mediastinum

    c. Axillary thoracotomy (Fig. 4-6) for limited exposure of the upper thorax during procedures such as upper lobe biopsy or sympathectomy

    d. Anterolateral thoracotomy (Fig. 4-7) for rapid exposure in patients with thoracic trauma or in patients with a very unstable cardiovascular status who cannot tolerate a lateral incision. This type of procedure also allows for excellent control of the airway during the incision.

    e. Anterior parasternal mediastinotomy (Chamberlain procedure), a 2–3 cm parasternal incision that allows insertion of a mediastinoscope into the mediastinum or, more commonly, direct visualization and biopsy of mediastinal lymph nodes

7. Video-assisted thoracic surgery (VATS) has become a frequently performed and well-tolerated procedure for numerous pleural and pulmonary diseases.

    a. Procedure. A lighted rigid scope connected to a video display is passed into the pleural space, providing comprehensive intrathoracic visualization. This technique permits major procedures to be performed through minor incisions, using a combination of conventional and unique instrumentation. However, the greatest advantage of VATS is the avoidance of a rib-spreading thoracotomy.

    b. Applications of VATS include the diagnosis or management of

        (1) Idiopathic exudative pleural effusion

        (2) Known malignant pleural effusion

        (3) Diffuse interstitial lung disease

        (4) Recurrent pneumothorax or persistent air leak

        (5) Indeterminate peripheral solitary pulmonary nodules

        (6) Mediastinal cyst

        (7) Anatomic lobectomy (in experienced hands only)

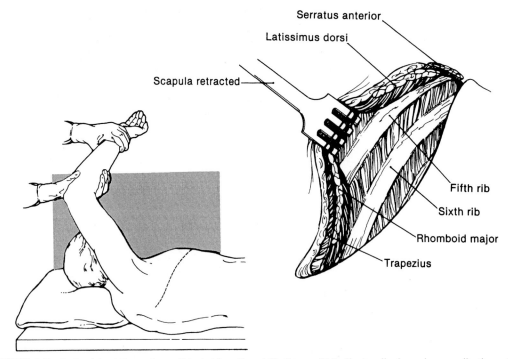

FIGURE 4-5 Posterolateral thoracotomy. (Adapted from Bryant LR, Morgan CV Jr. Chest wall, pleura, lung, mediastinum. In: Schwartz SI, Shires GT, Spencer, FC. eds. *Principles of Surgery*. 5th ed. New York: McGraw-Hill; 1989:634.)

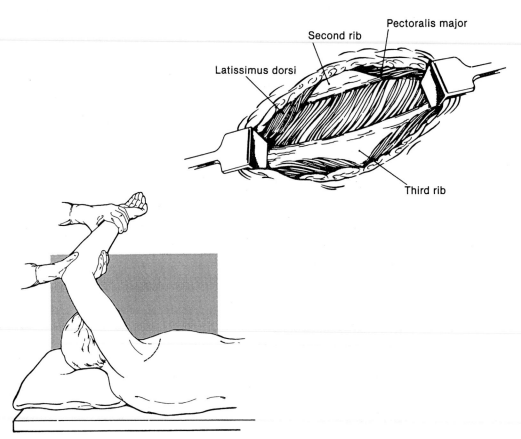

FIGURE 4-6 Axillary thoracotomy. (Adapted from Bryant LR, Morgan CV Jr. Chest wall, pleura, lung, and mediastinum. In: Schwartz SI, Shires GT, Spencer, FC, eds. *Principles of Surgery*. 5th ed. New York: McGraw-Hill; 1989:637.)

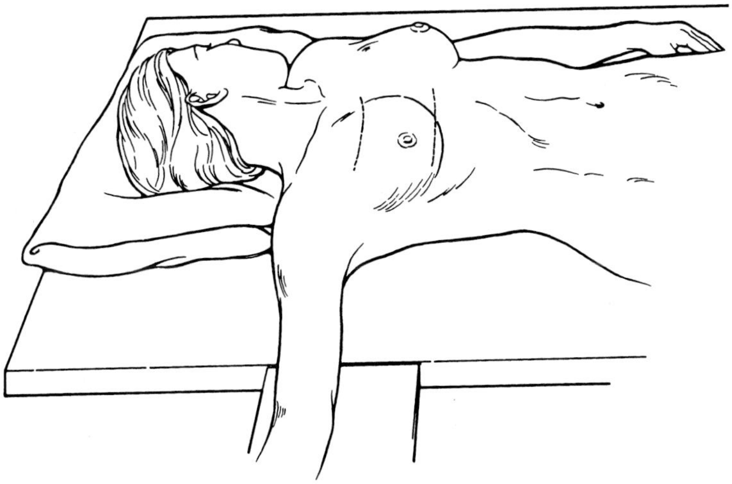

FIGURE 4-7 Anterolateral thoracotomy.

II ▪ THORACIC TRAUMA

Most thoracic trauma can be managed nonoperatively, using expeditious control of the airway and thoracostomy tube drainage of the pleural space. Less than 25% of chest injuries require surgical intervention. Thoracic trauma can be divided into immediate life-threatening injuries and potentially life-threatening injuries, according to the designation by the American College of Surgeons Committee on Trauma.

A **Immediate life-threatening injuries** are those that can cause death in a matter of minutes and, therefore, must be rapidly identified and treated during the initial evaluation and resuscitation.

1. **Airway obstruction** quickly leads to hypoxia, hypercapnia, acidosis, and cardiac arrest. The highest priority is rapid evaluation and securing the upper airway by clearing out secretions, blood, or foreign bodies; endotracheal intubation; or cricothyroidotomy.

2. **Tension pneumothorax** implies that the pleural air collection is under positive pressure that is significant enough to cause a marked mediastinal shift away from the affected side.
   a. **Causes.** Tension pneumothorax is caused by a check-valve mechanism in which air can escape from the lung into the pleural space but cannot be vented. It is a cause of **sudden death.**
   b. **Clinical presentation.** The collapsed lung results in chest pain, shortness of breath, and decreased or absent breath sounds on the affected side. Hypotension results from mediastinal shift to the contralateral side, which compresses and distorts the vena cavae and obstructs venous return to the heart.
   c. **Treatment.** The thorax must be decompressed with a needle, which is replaced by an intercostal tube with underwater seal and suction.

3. **Open pneumothorax** describes an injury in which an open wound in the chest wall has exposed the pleural space to the atmosphere.
   a. **Clinical presentation.** The open wound allows air movement through the defect during spontaneous respiration, causing ineffective alveolar ventilation.
   b. **Treatment** involves covering the wound and inserting a thoracostomy tube. Later, debridement and closure of the wound may be necessary.

4. **Massive hemothorax** occurs with the rapid accumulation of blood in the pleural space, which causes both compromised ventilation as well as hypovolemic shock.
   a. **Treatment** entails securing intravenous access and beginning volume restoration followed immediately by placement of a thoracostomy tube.
   b. **Complications**
      (1) If the hemothorax is inadequately drained, the patient may develop an empyema or fibrothorax, both of which would require subsequent thoracotomy and decortication.

(2) Initial drainage of at least 1000 mL or continued hemorrhage at the rate of 200 mL/hour for 4 hours is an indication for prompt surgical exploration.

5. Cardiac tamponade occurs with the rapid accumulation of blood in the pericardial sac, which causes compression of the cardiac chambers, decreased diastolic filling, and thus, decreased cardiac output.

  a. Clinical presentation includes hypotension with neck vein distention.

  b. Treatment is prompt **pericardial** decompression either by pericardiocentesis (if in extremis) or via median sternotomy or left anterior thoracotomy (if more stable).

6. Flail chest. Blunt chest trauma, causing extensive anterior and posterior rib fractures or sternocostal disconnection, results in paradoxical chest wall movement.

  a. Clinical presentation. Paradoxical chest wall movement interferes with the mechanics of respiration and, if severe, causes acute alveolar hypoventilation. Morbidity is also related to underlying lung injury.

  b. Treatment includes adequate pain control (intercostal blocks or epidural narcotics) and aggressive pulmonary toilet. Mechanical ventilation may be required in severe cases.

B **Potentially life-threatening injuries** are those that, left untreated, would likely result in death, but that usually allow several hours to establish a definitive diagnosis and institute appropriate treatment.

1. Tracheobronchial disruption usually occurs within 2 cm of the carina.

  a. Diagnosis is made by bronchoscopy and is suspected when a

  (1) Collapsed lung fails to expand, following placement of a thoracostomy tube

  (2) Massive air leak persists

  (3) Massive progressive subcutaneous emphysema is present

  b. Treatment is by primary repair.

2. Aortic disruption is the result of a deceleration injury in which the mobile ascending aorta and arch move forward while the descending thoracic aorta remains fixed in position by the mediastinal pleura and intercostal vessels. This movement causes a tear at the aortic isthmus, just distal to the takeoff of the left subclavian artery.

  a. Clinical presentation. The aortic injury usually results in **fracture** of the **intima** and **media** with the adventitia remaining mainly intact. However, complete disruption of all layers can occur with the hematoma contained only by the intact mediastinal pleura.

  b. Chest radiograph findings include:

  (1) Widened mediastinum

  (2) Indistinct aortic knob

  (3) Depressed left main stem bronchus

  (4) Apical cap

  (5) Deviation of trachea to the right

  (6) Left pleural effusion

  c. Diagnosis is confirmed by an aortogram.

  d. Treatment involves repair by interposition graft with or without some method of distal perfusion.

3. Diaphragmatic disruption results from blunt trauma to the chest and abdomen, producing a radial tear in the diaphragm, beginning at the esophageal hiatus.

  a. Diagnosis is by chest radiograph, which shows evidence of the stomach or colon in the chest.

  b. Treatment

  (1) The immediate placement of a nasogastric tube (if not already in place) will prevent acute gastric dilatation, which can produce severe, life-threatening respiratory distress. This is followed by urgent transabdominal repair with simultaneous treatment of any associated intra-abdominal injuries.

  (2) If rupture is not diagnosed until 7–10 days later, transthoracic repair is recommended to free any adhesions to the lung that might exist.

4. Esophageal disruption usually results from penetrating trauma rather than blunt trauma.

  a. Clinical presentation. It causes rapidly progressive mediastinitis.

b. Treatment is wide mediastinal drainage and primary closure with tissue reinforcement (pleura, intercostal muscle, or stomach).

5. **Cardiac contusion** results from direct sternal impact. It ranges in severity from subendocardial or subepicardial petechiae to full-thickness injury.
   a. **Functional complications**
      (1) Arrhythmias (i.e., premature ventricular contractions, supraventricular tachycardia, and atrial fibrillation)
      (2) Myocardial rupture
      (3) Ventricular septal rupture
      (4) Left ventricular failure
   b. **Diagnosis** is made by an electrocardiogram, isoenzymes, and two-dimensional (2D) echocardiogram.
   c. **Treatment** includes cardiac and hemodynamic monitoring, appropriate pharmacologic control of arrhythmias, and inotropic support if cardiogenic shock develops.

6. **Pulmonary contusion** is the most common injury seen in association with thoracic trauma (30%–75% of all patients have a major chest injury).
   a. **Causes.** It is caused by blunt trauma, which produces capillary disruption with subsequent intra-alveolar hemorrhage, edema, and small airway obstruction.
   b. **Diagnosis** is made by chest radiograph, arterial blood gas, and clinical symptoms of respiratory distress.
   c. **Treatment** includes fluid restriction, supplemental oxygen, vigorous chest physiotherapy, adequate analgesia (epidural narcotics), and prompt chest tube drainage of any associated pleural space complication.

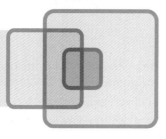

chapter 5

Chest Wall, Lung, and Mediastinum

D. BRUCE PANASUK • WILLIAM R. ALEX • RICHARD N. EDIE

I DISORDERS OF THE CHEST WALL

A **Chest wall deformities**

1. **Pectus excavatum (funnel chest).** An exceedingly depressed sternum is the **most common chest wall deformity.** It is usually asymptomatic, but it may cause some functional impairment. **Surgery** is indicated for moderate to severe deformities and is performed at 4–5 years of age. The operation involves
   a. Subperichondrial resection of all involved costal cartilages
   b. An osteotomy of the sternum
   c. Overcorrection of the sternal defect with a bone wedge
   d. Use of a retrosternal support (optional)

2. **Pectus carinatum (pigeon breast).** An overly prominent sternum is less likely to cause functional impairment than a depressed sternum. The repair is similar to that used for pectus excavatum.

3. **A distal sternal defect** occurs as part of the **pentalogy of Cantrell** (see Chapter 29, III A 2 d).

4. **Poland's syndrome** is a unilateral absence of costal cartilages, pectoralis muscle, and breast. **Surgery** is indicated for protection of the underlying thoracic structures and for cosmetic reasons.

5. **Thoracic outlet syndrome (TOS)**
   a. **Clinical presentation**
      (1) **Compression of the neurovascular bundle** at the thoracic outlet (by fibromuscular bands, the anterior scalene muscle, the first rib, or the cervical ribs) causes pain and paresthesia in the neck, shoulder, arm, and hand.
      (2) **Brachial plexus compression (neurogenic TOS)** occurs most often. Pain affects the neck, shoulder, anterior chest wall, and arm. Paresthesia predominantly affects the hand, often in an ulnar nerve destination.
      (3) **Vascular compression (vasculogenic TOS)** occurs much less frequently.
   b. **Diagnosis** is **clinical** and is based on a careful history and detailed physical examination. Electrodiagnostic studies provide little help in establishing brachial plexus compression, although these studies more reliably rule out peripheral neuropathies. Cervical disk disease must be ruled out by magnetic resonance imaging (MRI).
   c. **Treatment** is initially conservative, using a focused **physical therapy** program for 3–6 months. Patients with refractory symptoms can be offered surgery, which involves brachial plexus decompression by way of **supraclavicular scalenectomy, brachial plexus neurolysis,** or **first rib resection.**

B **Chest wall tumors**

1. **Benign tumors**
   a. **Fibrous dysplasia of the rib** occurs posteriorly or on the lateral portion of the rib. It is not painful, and it grows slowly. It may occur as part of Albright's syndrome.

b. **Chondroma** is the most common benign tumor of the chest wall. It occurs at the costo-chondral junction.

c. **Osteochondroma** occurs on any portion of the rib.

2. **Malignant tumors** include fibrosarcoma, chondrosarcoma, osteogenic sarcoma, myeloma, and Ewing's sarcoma.

3. **Treatment** of chest wall tumors involves wide excision and reconstruction, using autologous grafts, prosthetic grafts, or both.

II DISORDERS OF THE PLEURA AND PLEURAL SPACE

A **Spontaneous pneumothorax** occurs when a **subpleural bleb** ruptures into the pleural space with resultant loss of negative intrapleural pressure, allowing the **lung** to **collapse.**

1. **Incidence.** Young adults 18–25 years of age are most commonly affected, although older persons with asthma or chronic obstructive pulmonary disease are also susceptible.

2. **Symptoms** include chest pain, cough, and dyspnea and range from mild to severe.

3. **Diagnosis** is made by physical examination and chest radiograph.

4. **Treatment** is achieved by chest tube drainage of the pleural space.
   a. **Indications for surgery**
      (1) Recurrent pneumothorax (ipsilateral or contralateral)
      (2) Persistent air leak for 3–5 days
      (3) Incomplete lung expansion
      (4) **Hemopneumothorax**
   b. **Procedure** is stapling of apical blebs and pleural abrasion. This is an excellent indication for **videothoracoscopy** and repair.

B **Pleural effusions**

1. **Transudative effusions** result from systemic disorders that alter hydrostatic or oncotic pressures, allowing the accumulation of **protein-poor** plasma filtrate in the pleural space.
   a. **Treatment** is directed toward the underlying systemic process. Thoracentesis may be helpful for both diagnosis and symptomatic relief. Tube thoracotomy should be avoided if possible.

2. **Exudative effusions** result from the local pleural pathology, which alters the permeability characteristics of the pleura, allowing accumulation of a *protein-rich* plasma filtrate within the pleural space.
   a. **Treatment** usually requires tube thoracostomy, videothoracoscopy, or thoracotomy to resolve effusion.

C **Pleural empyema**   Pus in the pleural space usually accumulates secondary to pulmonary infection.

1. Pathophysiology of empyema evolves in three stages.
   a. **Acute or serous phase** (onset to 7 days) during which pleural fluid is initially produced
   b. **Transitional or fibrinopurulent phase** (7–21 days) during which fluid gravitates to dependent areas and undergoes septation and loculation
   c. **Chronic or organized phase** (>21 days) in which fibrin and pleura fuse and thicken around the periphery of the fluid, resulting in frank abscess formation

2. **Diagnosis** is made by thoracentesis in a patient with pleural effusion and fever.
   a. The aspirated fluid is sent for laboratory studies. If organisms are seen on a Gram stain, if organisms are cultured out, or if the pH is below 7.4, the diagnosis is probably an empyema.
   b. On gross examination, if the fluid is very cloudy or smells foul, an empyema is likely to be present.

3. **Treatment**
   a. **Early empyemas** associated with pneumococcal pneumonia may be treated with repeated aspiration and antibiotics.

b. Established empyemas, which usually have thicker fluid, need continuous closed drainage. If the empyema is loculated and, therefore, not completely drained by the intercostal tube, then thoracotomy, debridement, and decortication are necessary.

c. Small, dependent empyemas that do not respond to chest tube drainage may require open drainage via localized rib resection, especially in poor-risk patients.

d. Recent use of **computed tomography (CT)–guided catheters followed by pleural lytic therapy using TPA** has demonstrated impressive results in successfully draining empyemas and avoiding surgical intervention.

D **Pleural tumors and mesothelioma**

1. **Localized benign mesotheliomas** are *not related* to asbestos exposure. They usually arise from the **visceral** pleura and are treated by local excision.

2. **Malignant mesothelioma** is *related* to prior asbestos exposure, arises in the **parietal** pleura, and presents with a pleural effusion. It is almost always a fatal disease. The role of surgery is primarily for diagnosis and palliation of symptomatic malignant effusion—usually by way of thoracoscopy and talc sclerosis.

III PULMONARY INFECTIONS

A **Lung abscess**

1. **Etiology.** An abscess of the lung usually occurs in patients subject to aspiration (altered sensorium, e.g., alcoholics, drug overdose, elderly, debilitated). It occurs in the dependent segments of the lung (i.e., the posterior segment of the upper lobe or the superior segment of the lower lobe). These infections are most often mixed, but anaerobic organisms may predominate.

2. **Treatment**

a. **Intravenous antibiotics** are the usual treatment; more than 90% of acute lung abscesses resolve with antibiotic therapy. **Penicillin** is the most effective mode of treatment. There is no proven efficacy of intracavitary antibiotic instillation.

b. **Transbronchial drainage** via a rigid or flexible bronchoscope is occasionally successful.

c. **CT-directed catheter drainage** of large abscesses is often effective.

d. **Indications for surgery**

(1) Failure of the abscess to resolve with adequate antibiotic therapy

(2) Hemorrhage

(3) Inability to rule out carcinoma

(4) Giant abscess (>6 cm in diameter)

(5) Rupture with a resultant empyema. This can be treated initially by chest tube drainage of the pleural space but may require open drainage and decortication with or without actual resection.

B **Bronchiectasis** is a complication of repeated pulmonary infections, which causes bronchial dilatation. The disease usually affects the lower lobes. It occurs in adults and children who present with a chronic illness accompanied by excessive production of sputum.

1. **Diagnosis.** High-resolution CT scanning has replaced bronchography as the definitive diagnostic study. **Bronchoscopy** may also be helpful to determine the specific segmental location of secretions and to identify foreign bodies, bronchial stenosis, or neoplasms.

2. **Treatment**

a. **Medical treatment.** Antibiotics and pulmonary toilet resolve most cases.

b. **Surgical treatment** involves segmental resection of the affected area, and best results are obtained in patients with localized disease.

C **Tuberculosis**

1. **Incidence.** Approximately 25,000 new cases of tuberculosis are diagnosed each year in the United States.

2. **Treatment**
   a. **Chemotherapeutic agents** are used to treat this disease. Fewer than 5% of patients require pulmonary resection as part of their therapeutic regimen, and this is usually performed after a course of chemotherapy.
   b. **Indications for surgery**
      (1) Bronchopleural fistula with empyema
      (2) Destroyed lobe or lung
      (3) Persistent open cavities with positive sputum
      (4) Post-tubercular bronchial stenosis
      (5) Pulmonary hemorrhage
      (6) Suspected carcinoma
      (7) Aspergilloma
      (8) Bronchiectasis

IV SOLITARY PULMONARY NODULES (COIN LESIONS)

Solitary pulmonary nodules are well-circumscribed, peripheral nodules that are manifestations of neoplastic disease (e.g., bronchogenic carcinoma) or of granulomatous or infectious processes (e.g., fungus or tuberculosis).

A General characteristics

1. Solitary pulmonary nodules are usually asymptomatic.
2. They occur more often in men than in women.

B Benign versus malignant etiology

1. When no other tumor is known to be present, the solitary pulmonary nodule is rarely a sign of metastatic disease.
2. If the patient is younger than 40 years of age, there is a two-thirds chance that the lesion is benign.
3. The likelihood of cancer is higher in men than in women.
4. **Radiographic evidence** of a benign lesion includes the following:
   a. Calcification is present, particularly concentric, heavy, or popcornlike calcification (if the calcification appears as small flecks, a malignant lesion should be suspected).
   b. Radiographs taken at least 2 years apart show no growth in the size of the lesion.
   c. The lesion's size is less than 1 cm in diameter. (The larger the lesion, the greater is the chance of a malignancy.)
   d. CT scan demonstrates a well-circumscribed lesion. (Multiple lesions that are demonstrated on a CT scan but are not seen on plain film suggest either metastatic disease or satellite lesions from carcinoma or granulomas.) There is no advantage of MRI over a CT scan for imaging of solitary pulmonary nodes.
5. Because **no radiographic characteristic other than dense calcification absolutely indicates a benign lesion,** tissue biopsy is mandatory for diagnosis.

V BRONCHOGENIC CARCINOMA

A Overview

1. **Incidence**
   a. Bronchogenic carcinoma is the **leading cause of cancer death in the United States.**
   b. Approximately 180,000 new cases are diagnosed each year in the United States.
   c. **About 95%** of lung cancers occur in patients who are older than 40 years of age.
2. **Etiology**
   a. **Ninety-five percent** of all lung carcinomas are **related to smoking;** affected individuals usually have a history of smoking one or more packs of cigarettes daily for 20 years.

b. There is no known environmental cause. However, chronic exposure to various substances may play a role; nickel, asbestos, arsenic, radioactive materials, and petroleum products have all been implicated.

B **Pathology**

1. **Adenocarcinoma** is now the **most common lung carcinoma,** representing 30%–45% of all malignant lung cancers. It is less strongly associated with smoking and occurs more commonly in women.
   a. **Histology** reveals distinct acinar formation of cells, which arise from the subsegmental airways in the periphery of the lung.
   b. **Characteristics**
      (1) Many of these tumors are formed in conjunction with lung scars, representing a response to chronic irritation.
      (2) Growth may be slow, but the cancer metastasizes readily by a vascular route. It may spread diffusely throughout the lung via the tracheobronchial tree.
   c. **Variants. Bronchoalveolar carcinoma** is a variant of adenocarcinoma, which represents a highly differentiated form that spreads along alveolar walls.
      (1) Its three forms consist of a solitary nodule, a multinodular form, and a diffuse/pneumonic form.
      (2) It has the best prognosis of all the cell types.

2. **Squamous cell carcinoma** is the second most common carcinoma of the lung, representing 25%–40% of all malignant tumors. It is associated with smoking.
   a. **Histology** reveals intercellular bridge formation and cell keratinization. It is thought to arise from squamous metaplasia of the tracheobronchial tree.
   b. **Characteristics**
      (1) Approximately two thirds of squamous cell carcinomas occur centrally in the lung fields.
      (2) The tumor is bulky and is associated with bronchial obstruction.
      (3) It is characterized by slow growth and late metastasis.
      (4) It undergoes central necrosis and cavitation.

3. **Small cell anaplastic (oat cell) carcinoma,** which is highly malignant, represents approximately 15%–25% of all malignant lung tumors.
   a. **Histology** reveals clusters, nests, or sheets of small, round, oval, or spindle-shaped cells with dark, round nuclei and a scanty cytoplasm.
      (1) Electron microscopy reveals the presence of neurosecretory cytoplasmic granules.
      (2) This finding, together with observed production of biologically active substances, has led to their classification as neuroendocrine tumors of the amine precursor uptake and decarboxylation (APUD) system.
   b. **Characteristics**
      (1) It is usually centrally located.
      (2) It metastasizes early by the lymphatic and vascular routes.
   c. **Treatment** involves a combination of chemotherapy and radiotherapy. Surgery may be indicated in a few patients who have early lesions.
   d. **Prognosis** overall is quite poor.

4. **Undifferentiated large cell carcinoma** is the rarest of the major cell types of lung cancer.
   a. **Histology** reveals anaplastic, large cells with abundant cytoplasm and no apparent evidence of differentiation.
   b. **Characteristics**
      (1) It may be located either centrally or peripherally.
      (2) It is a highly malignant lesion that spreads early.
   c. **Prognosis.** It has a poorer prognosis than the more differentiated nonsmall cell carcinomas.

5. **Other tumors,** such as bronchial adenoma, papilloma, and sarcomas, are rare.

C **Clinical presentation**

1. **Pulmonary symptoms** include cough, dyspnea, chest pain, fever, sputum production, and wheezing. Patients may be **asymptomatic,** which is the only clue to the cancer producing an abnormal chest radiograph.

2. **Extrapulmonary symptoms**
   a. **Metastatic extrapulmonary manifestations** include weight loss, malaise, symptoms referable to the central nervous system, and bone pain.
   b. **Nonmetastatic extrapulmonary manifestations** (paraneoplastic syndromes) are secondary to hormonelike substances that are elaborated by the tumor. These include Cushing's syndrome, hypercalcemia, myasthenic neuropathies, hypertrophic osteoarthropathies, and gynecomastia.

3. **Pancoast's tumor,** which involves the superior sulcus, may produce symptoms related to brachial plexus involvement, sympathetic ganglia involvement, or vertebral collapse secondary to local invasion. This may result in pain or weakness of the arm, edema, or **Horner's syndrome** (i.e., ptosis, miosis, enophthalmos, and anhidrosis).

D **Diagnosis and staging**

1. **Abnormal chest radiograph** is the most common finding.
   a. The tumor may present as a nodule, an infiltrate, or as atelectasis.
   b. An abnormal chest radiograph is more likely to represent carcinoma in patients older than 40 years of age.

2. **CT scan** reveals the extent of the tumor and the possibility of mediastinal lymph node metastasis.

3. **Positron emission tomography (PET) scan** is routinely used to assess the primary tumor, the mediastinal lymph nodes, and to screen for metastatic disease.

4. **Bronchoscopy** assesses for bronchial involvement and resectability in central lesions, and tissue is obtained for cytologic examination.

5. **Mediastinoscopy or mediastinotomy** obtains mediastinal lymph nodes for pathologic examination and aids in the staging of the disease. Positive findings may or may not preclude a curative resection, depending on the pathologic cell type, the extent of nodal involvement, and the condition of the patient.

6. **Percutaneous needle biopsy** may be used for peripheral lesions to obtain tissue for cytologic examination.

E **Staging** of lung carcinoma is fundamental for the evaluation of treatment protocols (Table 5-1). It is based on information obtained during the preoperative evaluation, findings at mediastinoscopy (see V D 4), thoracotomy, and pathologic findings of the surgical specimens. Definitions of tumor size (T), lymph node metastasis (N), and distant metastasis (M) comprise the **TNM classification of carcinoma of the lung** by the revised International Clinical Staging System.

TABLE 5-1   Stage Grouping in Cancer of the Lung

Stage Grouping	Tumor	Nodal Involvement	Distant Metastasis
Occult carcinoma	TX	N0	M0
Stage 0	TIS	CIS	—
Stage Ia	T1	N0	M0
Stage Ib	T2	N0	M0
Stage IIa	T1	N1	M0
Stage IIb	T2	N1	M0
	T3	N0	M0
Stage IIIa	T3	N1	M0
	T1–3	N2	M0
Stage IIIb	Any T	N3	M0
	T4	Any N	M0
Stage IV	Any T	Any N	M1

T, tumor size; N, lymph node metastasis; M, distant metastasis.
Reprinted with permission from the American Joint Committee for Cancer Staging (AJCC), 1998.

1. **T (primary tumors)**
   a. **TX:** The tumor is proved by the presence of malignant cells in bronchopulmonary secretions but is not visualized on a radiograph or by bronchoscopy, or any tumor that cannot be assessed, such as one in a retreatment staging.
   b. **T0:** No evidence of primary tumor
   c. **TIS:** Carcinoma in situ
   d. **T1:** A tumor that is 3 cm or less in greatest dimension, surrounded by lung or visceral pleura and with no evidence of invasion proximal to a lobar bronchus at bronchoscopy
   e. **T2:** A tumor more than 3 cm in greatest dimension or a tumor of any size that either invades the visceral pleura or has associated atelectasis or obstructive pneumonitis that extends to the hilar region. At bronchoscopy, the proximal extent of demonstrable tumor must be within a lobar bronchus or at least 2 cm distal to the carina. Any associated atelectasis or obstructive pneumonitis must involve less than an entire lung.
   f. **T3:** A tumor of any size with direct extension into the chest wall (including superior sulcus tumors), diaphragm, mediastinal pleura, or pericardium without involving the heart, great vessels, trachea, esophagus, or vertebral body or a tumor in the main bronchus within 2 cm of the carina without involving the carina
   g. **T4:** A tumor of any size with invasion of the mediastinum or involving the heart, great vessels, trachea, esophagus, vertebral body, or carina or the presence of malignant pleural effusion. In addition, satellite tumor nodules can occur within the ipsilateral primary tumor lobe of the lung.

2. **N (nodal involvement)**
   a. **N0:** No demonstrable metastasis to regional lymph nodes
   b. **N1:** Metastasis to lymph nodes in the peribronchial or the ipsilateral hilar region, or both, including direct extension
   c. **N2:** Metastasis to ipsilateral mediastinal lymph nodes and subcarinal lymph nodes
   d. **N3:** Metastasis to contralateral mediastinal lymph nodes, contralateral hilar lymph nodes, ipsilateral or contralateral scalene or supraclavicular lymph nodes

3. **M (distant metastasis)**
   a. **M0:** No (known) distant metastasis
   b. **M1:** Distant metastasis present or separate metastatic tumor nodules in the ipsilateral non-primary tumor lobes of the lung.

F **Treatment**

1. **Surgical treatment**
   a. **Pulmonary resection** (i.e., lobectomy, extended lobectomy, or pneumonectomy) is the only potential cure for bronchogenic carcinoma. The surgical approach is to resect the involved lung, regional lymph nodes, and involved contiguous structures, if necessary.
      (1) Lobectomy is used in disease localized to one lobe.
      (2) Extended resections and pneumonectomy are used when the tumor involves a fissure or is close to the pulmonary hilus.
      (3) Wedge resections or bronchial segmentectomy may be used in localized disease in high-risk patients.
   b. **Contraindications for thoracotomy.** One half of all patients with lung carcinomas are not candidates for thoracotomy at the time of diagnosis.
      (1) Extensive ipsilateral mediastinal lymph node involvement (N2 disease), particularly high paratracheal and subcarinal
      (2) Any contralateral mediastinal lymph node involvement (N3 disease)
      (3) Distant metastases
      (4) Malignant pleural effusion
      (5) Superior vena cava syndrome
      (6) Recurrent laryngeal nerve involvement
      (7) Phrenic nerve paralysis
      (8) Poor pulmonary function (relative contraindication)

2. **Adjuvant therapy.** Further treatment using radiotherapy, chemotherapy, or both is indicated for some advanced-stage tumors.
   a. **Postoperative adjuvant chemotherapy** is now indicated in all resected nonsmall cell lung cancer patients **Stage Ib** and higher, demonstrating a small but statistically significant survival benefit.
   c. **Preoperative chemotherapy** (with or without radiation therapy) in patients with stage IIIa (N2) disease has been used in an attempt to convert advanced local disease into a resectable lesion. However, the efficacy of this therapy has yet to be determined, although early results appear promising.

G **Prognosis** depends primarily on cell types and on the stage of disease at the time of diagnosis.
   1. Five-year survival based on **cell type**
      a. Bronchoalveolar carcinoma, 30%–35%
      b. Squamous cell carcinoma, 8%–16%
      c. Adenocarcinoma, 5%–10%
      d. Small cell carcinoma, <3%
   2. Five-year survival based on **postoperative pathologic stage**
      a. Stage I, 60%–80%
      b. Stage II, 40%–55%
      c. Stage IIIa, 10%–35%

VI BRONCHIAL ADENOMAS

The term **adenoma** is an unfortunate misnomer because these lesions are all **malignant neoplasms,** albeit relatively low grade in character. They arise from the epithelium, ducts, and glands of the tracheobronchial tree and include the carcinoid tumor, adenoid cystic carcinoma (cylindroma), and mucoepidermoid carcinoma.

A **Carcinoid tumors,** which comprise 80%–90% of bronchial adenomas, occur mainly in the **proximal bronchi** (20% main stem bronchi, 60% lobar or segmental bronchi, and 20% peripheral parenchyma).
   1. **Characteristics**
      a. Carcinoid tumors arise from basal bronchial stem cells, which in the process of malignant transformation differentiate in the direction of **neurendocrine** tissue. These tumors are seen most commonly in the fifth decade of life.
      b. They grow slowly and protrude endobronchially, often causing some degree of bronchial obstruction.
      c. Regional lymph node metastases occur in 10% of patients, mainly in those with the **atypical variant** of carcinoid tumor, which is characterized by pleomorphism, increased mitotic activity, disorganized architecture, and tumor necrosis. Of these patients, 70% present with metastases.
   2. **Signs and symptoms** include cough (47%), recurrent infection (45%), hemoptysis (39%), pain (19%), and wheezing (17%). Approximately 21% are asymptomatic.
   3. **Chest radiograph** may reveal evidence of atelectasis or pulmonary nodule.
   4. **Treatment** for carcinoid tumor is surgical excision.
      a. **Lobectomy** is the most commonly performed procedure.
      b. **Wedge excision** or **segmentectomy** can occasionally be used for peripheral typical carcinoids.
      c. **Pneumonectomy** should rarely be required, especially since the introduction of **bronchoplastic techniques,** which allow **sleeve resection** of lesions involving the main stem bronchi or bronchus intermedius.
   5. **Prognosis** should be more than 90% 5-year survival for typical carcinoid tumors, decreasing to less than 50% for the atypical variant.

B **Adenoid cystic carcinoma (cylindroma)** comprises approximately 10% of bronchial adenomas.
1. **Characteristics**
   a. They **occur more centrally** in the lower trachea/carina area and in the orifices of the main stem bronchi.
   b. Although considered a low-grade malignancy, the adenoid cystic carcinoma is more aggressive than is the carcinoid tumor.
   c. Metastases tend to occur late, but about one third of patients present with metastases, commonly along perineural lymphatics to regional lymph nodes but also distantly to liver, bone, and kidneys.
2. **Treatment** is by generous en bloc excision of the tumor, including peribronchial tissue and regional lymph nodes. This may require lobectomy, sleeve resection, or both. **Radiation therapy** should be considered in all inoperable patients and in those in whom residual tumor remains after resection.
3. **Prognosis** is less favorable than in the case of a carcinoid tumor, with approximately 50% having a 5-year survival rate.

C **Mucoepidermoid carcinoma** accounts for less than 1% of bronchial adenomas.
1. **Characteristics**
   a. The location and distribution in the tracheobronchial tree are similar to those found with carcinoid tumors
   b. High-grade and low-grade variants exist, although the latter type predominates.
2. **Treatment** principles that are outlined for carcinoid tumors apply to low-grade mucoepidermoid carcinoma. High-grade variants should be approached and managed like other bronchial carcinomas.

VII HAMARTOMAS

A **Pathology** These pulmonary tumors are benign and are classified histologically as adenochondromas. They occur within the substance of the lung and usually present as solitary pulmonary nodules.

B **Treatment** involves removal during a diagnostic thoracotomy for evaluation of the solitary nodule.

VIII METASTATIC TUMOR

A Metastatic tumors are common to the lung, which may be the only site of metastases from a nonpulmonary primary tumor.

B **Treatment**
1. Single or multiple metastatic tumors can be removed from the lung as part of the treatment protocol (Table 5-2).
2. The best treatment results are obtained with metastatic tumors that can be completely resected and in those patients with less than three to five metastatic nodules.

TABLE 5-2 Common Metastatic Pulmonary Tumors	
Primary	**Five-Year Survival (%)**
Colorectal	13–38
Breast	27–50
Melanoma	13 months
Renal	24–54

IX DISORDERS OF THE TRACHEA

A Anatomy

1. **Structure**
   a. The trachea is 11 cm from the cricoid to the carina with a range in the adult of about 10–13 cm in length and 1.8–2.3 cm in diameter.
   b. The trachea is encircled by 18–22 cartilaginous rings. The **cricoid cartilage** is the only complete tracheal ring. The remaining rings are incomplete and have a membranous portion posteriorly.
   c. The trachea is vertically mobile. When the neck is extended, one half of the trachea is in the neck; when the neck is flexed, the entire trachea is behind the sternum.

2. **Relationship to other organs**
   a. The thyroid isthmus is at the second or third tracheal ring.
   b. The innominate artery crosses the trachea in its midportion.
   c. The aorta arches over the trachea in its distal portion.
   d. The esophagus is posterior to the trachea throughout its course.

3. **Blood supply** is segmental and is shared with the esophagus. Blood is supplied by the inferior thyroid artery, the subclavian artery, the superior intercostal artery, the internal mammary artery, the innominate artery, and the bronchial circulation.

B Congenital lesions

1. **Types**
   a. **Stenosis.** The three types of tracheal stenosis are generalized, funnel, and segmental. The bronchi may be small in congenital tracheal stenosis, and an associated pulmonary artery sling, in which the artery tethers the trachea, may be present. **Webs** may also be present.
   b. **Congenital tracheomalacia. Cartilaginous softening** is caused by compression of the trachea by vascular rings, which are anomalies of the aortic arch. These anomalies include a double aortic arch, a right arch with a left ligamentum arteriosum, an aberrant subclavian artery, or an aberrant innominate artery. The diameter of the trachea is normal, but the wall is collapsible.

2. **Diagnosis**
   a. **Signs and symptoms**
      (1) Inspiratory and expiratory wheezing, or stridor, which may be paroxysmal
      (2) Feeding problems
      (3) Frequent infections
   b. **Diagnostic studies**
      (1) Air tracheography (tomography)
      (2) Bronchoscopy
      (3) Angiography to assess vascular anomalies

3. **Treatment**
   a. **Stenosis and webs** are usually **treated conservatively** because of the difficulty in performing tracheal reconstruction in infants.
      (1) A web may be removed endoscopically.
      (2) Tracheostomy may be helpful and should be performed in a narrow area to avoid injury to normal parts of the trachea.
   b. **Chondromalacia** is treated by **aortopexy** and is performed under bronchoscopic guidance to maximize the tracheal lumen. The patient may still have some airway problems for a period of time postoperatively.

C Neoplasms of the trachea

1. **Types**
   a. **Primary neoplasms** are rare.
      (1) **Squamous cell carcinomas** are the most common neoplasms of the trachea. They may be exophytic, may cause superficial ulceration, or may be multiple lesions with interposed

areas of normal trachea. The tumor spreads through the regional lymph nodes and by direct extension to mediastinal structures.

(2) **Adenoid carcinoma** grows slowly and has a prolonged course.

(3) **Other primary tracheal neoplasms** include carcinosarcomas, pseudosarcomas, mucoepidermoid carcinomas, squamous papillomas, chondromas, and chondrosarcomas.

b. **Secondary tumors** to the trachea are usually from the lung, the esophagus, or the thyroid gland.

2. Diagnosis

a. **Radiographic studies** include a chest radiograph, tracheal tomogram, and fluoroscopy for evaluation of the larynx. Instillation of contrast medium is rarely necessary for the evaluation of tracheal tumors.

b. **Bronchoscopy** is deferred until the final operation because the biopsy may be hazardous due to bleeding or obstruction of the airway. Frozen section examination is adequate for assessment of the tracheal tumor.

c. **Pulmonary function testing** is mandatory if carinal or pulmonary resection is contemplated.

3. **Treatment** is by tracheal resection.

a. **Overview**

(1) **Preoperative antibiotics** are selected on the basis of preoperative tracheal cultures.

(2) When there is an airway obstruction, **anesthesia** should be induced with halothane.

(3) High-frequency **ventilation** may be helpful, and it may be possible to pass a small tube beside the tumor.

(4) In the **resection procedure,** up to one half of the trachea may be removed.

(a) Adequate mobilization can usually be obtained simply by flexing the patient's neck, although laryngeal or hilar release techniques are sometimes necessary.

(b) An **end-to-end anastomosis** is performed.

b. **Incisions used**

(1) A cervical incision is used for resection of the upper half of the trachea.

(2) A posterolateral thoracotomy is used for the lower portion of the trachea.

(3) The entire trachea can be exposed via a combined cervical incision and median sternotomy.

4. **Prognosis** is similar to that for resectable carcinoma of the lung (see V G 2).

X **LESIONS OF THE MEDIASTINUM (see Chapter 4, I A 2)**

A **Anterior compartment lesions**

1. **Thymomas** (see Chapter 16, IV B 1)

2. **Teratomas**

a. **Incidence.** Teratomas occur most frequently in adolescents, and 80% of these tumors are benign.

b. **Etiology.** They originate from the branchial cleft pouch in association with the thymus gland. All tissue types are present in these tumors, including ectodermal, endodermal, and mesodermal elements.

c. **Diagnosis.** Teratomas are diagnosed radiographically and may appear as smooth-walled cystic lesions or as lobulated solid lesions. Calcification is often present.

d. **Treatment** is total surgical excision.

3. **Lymphomas.** Fifty percent of patients with lymphomas (including those with Hodgkin's disease) have mediastinal lymph node involvement; however, only 5% of patients with lymphomas have *only* mediastinal disease.

a. **Symptoms** of mediastinal lymphoma include cough, chest pain, fever, and weight loss.

b. **Diagnosis** is by chest radiograph and lymph node biopsy, using either mediastinoscopy or anterior mediastinotomy.

c. **Treatment** is nonsurgical.

4. **Germ cell tumors.** These tumors are rare and occur with an incidence of less than 1% of all mediastinal tumors. They metastasize to pleural lymph nodes, the liver, bone, and the retroperitoneum.

    a. Histologic types

      (1) Seminoma

      (2) Embryonal cell carcinoma

      (3) Teratocarcinoma

      (4) Choriocarcinoma

      (5) Endodermal sinus tumor

    b. Symptoms include chest pain, cough, and hoarseness caused by invasion of the vagus nerves.

    c. Diagnosis. These tumors are diagnosed by a combination of radiographs and serum tumor markers (**β-human chorionic gonadotropin** and **α-fetoprotein**)

    d. Treatment

      (1) Seminomas are treated by complete surgical resection followed by postoperative radiotherapy.

      (2) Nonseminomas are treated by combination chemotherapy.

    e. Adjuvant therapy. Seminomas are very radiosensitive, and the other cell types may benefit from chemotherapeutic agents.

B **Visceral compartment lesions** are usually cystic. The two most common types are pericardial cysts and bronchogenic cysts.

    1. Pericardial cysts are usually asymptomatic and are seen on a chest radiograph. They are smooth walled and occur most commonly in the cardiodiaphragmatic angle. Surgery is usually done as a diagnostic procedure to identify the lesion.

    2. Bronchogenic cysts generally arise posterior to the carina. They may be asymptomatic, or they may cause pulmonary compression, which can be life threatening, particularly in infancy. The usual **treatment** is surgical excision.

    3. Ascending aortic aneurysms are also included as middle mediastinal masses due to the location of the great vessels in this compartment.

C **Paravertebral sulcus lesions** are neurogenic tumors located in the paravertebral gutter. Approximately 10%–20% are malignant.

    1. Incidence. Seventy-five percent of these neurogenic tumors occur in children younger than 4 years of age. A malignancy is most likely to occur if the tumor begins during childhood.

    2. Histologic types

      a. Neurilemomas, which arise from the Schwann cells of the nerve sheath

      b. Neurofibromas, which can degenerate into neurosarcomas

      c. Neurosarcomas

      d. Ganglioneuromas, which originate from sympathetic ganglia

      e. Neuroblastomas, which also arise from the sympathetic chain. Neuroblastomas may have **metastasized** to bone, liver, and regional lymph nodes by the time that the diagnosis is made. Also, direct extension to the spinal cord may occur.

    3. Pheochromocytomas occur in the mediastinum, although rarely; they behave similarly to the usual intra-adrenal pheochromocytomas.

    4. Symptoms

      a. Symptoms include chest pain secondary to compression of an intercostal nerve. If the tumor grows intraspinally, it may cause symptoms of spinal cord compression. Rarely, these tumors have an endocrine function and can secrete catecholamines.

      b. The symptoms of neuroblastoma include fever, vomiting, diarrhea, and cough.

    5. Diagnosis is by chest radiograph and CT scan.

    6. Treatment is by surgical excision. Postoperative radiation is helpful in the treatment of malignant tumors.

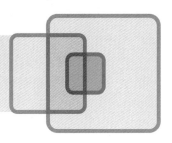

chapter **6**

Heart

D. BRUCE PANASUK · WILLIAM R. ALEX · RICHARD N. EDIE ·
JAMES S. GAMMIE

I **ACQUIRED HEART DISEASE**

A **Overview**

1. **Epidemiology**
   a. Heart disease is the leading cause of death in North America, responsible for 38% of all deaths. Three million myocardial infarctions are recorded annually in the United States, with an accompanying mortality rate of 10%–15%.
   b. Heart valve disease is less frequent than coronary artery disease but still accounts for significant morbidity and mortality. Surgical interventions for heart valve disease are growing 5% per year, primarily due to the ageing of the population and an increased incidence of aortic stenosis.

2. **Signs and symptoms**
   a. **Dyspnea** is caused by pulmonary congestion, which is the result of increased left atrial pressure.
   b. **Peripheral edema** may be the result of significant right-sided congestive heart failure.
   c. **Chest pain** may be caused by angina pectoris, myocardial infarction, pericarditis, aortic dissection, pulmonary infarction, or aortic stenosis.
   d. **Palpitations** may indicate a serious cardiac arrhythmia.
   e. **Hemoptysis** may be associated with mitral stenosis or pulmonary infarction.
   f. **Syncope** may result from mitral stenosis, aortic stenosis, or heart block.
   g. **Fatigue** is the result of decreased cardiac output.

3. **Physical examination** should include:
   a. **Blood pressure,** which should be measured in both arms and legs
   b. **Peripheral pulses.** The quality and regularity of pulses are important.
      (1) Pulsus parvus et tardus may be seen with aortic stenosis.
      (2) A wide pulse pressure with a "water-hammer pulse" is seen with aortic insufficiency
   c. **Neck veins.** Central venous pressure may be indirectly inferred from the height of the internal jugular vein filling. Jugular venous distention may be caused by cardiac tamponade, tricuspid regurgitation, or right heart failure.
   d. **Heart**
      (1) **Inspection and palpation** of the precordium
         (a) Normally, the apical impulse is appreciated at the midclavicular line, fifth intercostal space. In left ventricular hypertrophy, the apical impulse is increased and displaced laterally.
         (b) With right ventricular hypertrophy, a parasternal heave is appreciated.
         (c) Thrills from valvular disease may be felt.
      (2) **Auscultation.** The quality of heart tones, type of rhythm, murmurs, rales, and gallops are all important.

4. **Preoperative management**
   a. **A baseline chest radiograph** and **electrocardiogram should be obtained.**
   b. **Echocardiography** can define ventricular ejection performance. Color doppler echocardiography can demonstrate valvular stenosis or insufficiency.
   c. **Cardiac catheterization** remains the gold standard for defining coronary artery anatomy and assessing the presence of coronary artery disease. Right heart catheterization is used to

determine pulmonary artery pressure, cardiac output, pulmonary capillary wedge pressure, and the presence of left to right shunts ("step up"). Left heart catheterization includes coronary artery angiography and ventriculography (to determine ejection fraction).

   d. Pulmonary function studies are important in patients with known pulmonary disease.

5. Cardiac arrest

   a. Causes of cardiac arrest include:

     (1) Anoxia

     (2) Coronary thrombosis

     (3) Electrolyte disturbances

     (4) Myocardial depressants: anesthetic agents, antiarrhythmic drugs, or digitalis

     (5) Conduction disturbances

     (6) Vagotonic maneuvers

   b. Immediate cardiopulmonary resuscitation is critical, as brain injury results after 3–4 minutes of diminished perfusion.

   c. Treatment should include the following measures:

     (1) Airway: best accomplished by endotracheal intubation

     (2) Breathing: ventilatory support with an Ambu-bag or a ventilator

     (3) Circulation:

       (a) Cardiac massage. Closed-chest cardiac massage is usually appropriate. In the patient with cardiac tamponade, acute volume loss, an unstable sternum, or an open pericardium, open-chest massage is usually required.

       (b) Electrical defibrillation should be performed if cardiac arrest is the result of ventricular fibrillation.

       (c) Drug therapy. Commonly used agents include:

         (i) Epinephrine, for its cardiotonic effect

         (ii) Calcium, also for its cardiotonic effect

         (iii) Sodium bicarbonate, to treat associated acidosis

         (iv) Vasopressor agents, to support blood pressure

         (v) Atropine, to reverse bradycardia

       (d) Replacement of **blood volume,** if necessary

6. Extracorporeal circulation (cardiopulmonary bypass). The rationale for using extracorporeal circulation is to provide the surgeon with a motionless heart and a bloodless field in which to work while simultaneously perfusing the different organ systems with oxygenated blood.

   a. Technique. Blood is drained from the right atrium, passed through an oxygenator and a heat exchanger, and pumped back to the aorta.

   b. Protection of the myocardium during the ischemia induced by the procedure is accomplished by **hypothermia** and **cardioplegia.**

   c. Pathophysiologic effects of extracorporeal circulation include:

     (1) Widespread total body inflammatory response with initiation of humoral amplification systems, including:

       (a) Coagulation cascade

       (b) Fibrinolytic system

       (c) Complement activation

       (d) Kallikrein-kinin system

     (2) Release of vasoactive substances

       (a) Epinephrine

       (b) Norepinephrine

       (c) Histamine

       (d) Bradykinin

     (3) Retention of both sodium and free water, causing diffuse edema

     (4) Trauma to blood elements, resulting in hemolysis of red blood cells and destruction of platelets

7. Prosthetic valves. The two general categories are tissue valves and mechanical valves,.

   a. Tissue valves are made from porcine aortic valves or bovine pericardial tissue. These valves do not require long-term anticoagulation. Tissue valves have a limited life span and will fail

TABLE 6-1 Mitral Valve Repair versus Mitral Valve Replacement

	Repair	Replacement
Operative mortality	1%	6%
Anticoagulation	Not required	Mandatory for 3 months for tissue, life for mechanical
Reoperation	<10% at 20 years	10–15 years for tissue
Stroke risk	0.04%/year	1%–2%/year

gradually over time, exposing patients to the risk of a second operation. Aortic tissue valves can be expected to last 17 years, while mitral tissue valves had a durability of 10–15 years.

 b. **Mechanical valves** require lifetime anticoagulation therapy to prevent thrombosis/embolism but typically last for life.

 c. Both mechanical (with anticoagulation) and tissue (without anticoagulation) prosthetic heart valves are associated with a risk of stroke of 1%–2% per year. The risk of stroke is higher for mitral valves than aortic valves. Both tissue and mechanical valves have a similar risk of prosthetic valve endocarditis.

 d. The choice between a mechanical and a tissue valve for a patient depends on the risk of long-term anticoagulation versus the risk of a reoperation.

8. Heart valve repair is possible for the majority of patients undergoing mitral valve surgery. Repair is superior to replacement (Table 6-1).

B **Aortic valvular disease**

1. Aortic stenosis

 a. Etiology

  (1) **Congenital.** Bicuspid aortic valves occur in 1%–2% of the population. These usually develop calcific changes by the fourth decade and symptoms by the sixth decade.

  (2) **Acquired** stenosis is the most common heart valve disease requiring surgery. It results from progressive degeneration and calcification of the valve leaflets.

  (3) Patients with a history of **rheumatic fever** rarely have isolated stenosis but usually have a mixed lesion of stenosis and insufficiency.

 b. Pathology

  (1) **Thickening and calcification of the leaflets** result in a decreased cross-sectional area of the valve. Symptoms usually begin when the valve area is less than 1 cm^2 (the normal aortic valve is 2.5–3.5 cm^2).

  (2) Critical aortic stenosis imposes a significant **pressure load** on the left ventricle, which increases left ventricular work, resulting in concentric left ventricular hypertrophy (without associated dilatation). Eventually, myocardial decompensation occurs.

 c. Clinical presentation

  (1) Classic symptoms are angina, syncope, and dyspnea.

  (2) **Patients with asymptomatic aortic stenosis have a low likelihood of sudden death.**

  (2) Survival is poor after the development of symptoms

  (3) The presence of symptoms is the indication for surgery (Fig. 6-1).

 d. Diagnosis

  (1) **Physical examination**

   (a) The classic systolic crescendo–decrescendo murmur is heard best in the second right intercostal space. Radiation of the murmur to the carotid arteries is common.

   (b) An associated thrill is often appreciated.

   (c) A narrowed pulse pressure along with pulsus parvus et tardus is frequently found.

  (2) **Chest x-ray** usually shows a heart of normal size. Calcification of the aortic valve may be seen.

  (3) **Electrocardiogram** demonstrates left ventricular hypertrophy.

  (4) **Echocardiography** estimates the degree of stenosis, any associated insufficiency, and quality of left ventricular function.

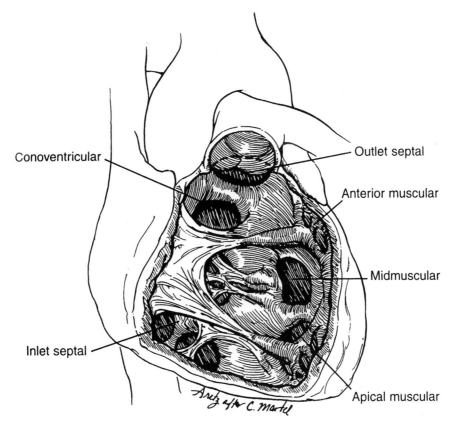

Conoventricular

Outlet septal

Anterior muscular

Midmuscular

Inlet septal

Apical muscular

FIGURE 6-1 Location of congenital ventricular septal defects (Reprinted with permission from Kaiser LR, Kron IL, Spray TL. *Mastery of Cardiothoracic Surgery.* Philadelphia: Lippincott-Raven; 1998:688.)

     (5) Cardiac catheterization is important to identify the presence of concomitant coronary artery disease, which is present in 50% of patients requiring surgery. (Crossing the stenotic aortic valve with a catheter to measure pressure gradients can cause stroke and does not provide additional information to that available from the echocardiogram.)

  e. Treatment

    (1) Surgical correction is recommended for patients with symptoms.

    (2) Surgery consists of **excision** of the diseased valve and replacement with a prosthetic valve.

2. Aortic insufficiency

  a. Etiology. Myxomatous degeneration, aortic dissection, bacterial endocarditis, rheumatic fever, and aortic root aneurysm are common causes.

  b. Pathology

    (1) The underlying pathologic process may be a fibrosis and shortening of the valve leaflets (which occurs in rheumatic fever), a dilatation of the aortic annulus (as occurs in Marfan's syndrome), or myxomatous degeneration of the leaflets.

    (2) Aortic insufficiency imposes a significant **volume load** on the left ventricle in accordance with Starling's law of the heart. This extra load leads to early left ventricular dilatation. If left uncorrected, this dilatation may lead to left ventricular failure with pulmonary congestion. Secondary mitral insufficiency may occur at this stage.

  c. Clinical presentation

    (1) There is a greater variability in time between the onset of aortic insufficiency and the appearance of symptoms than occurs with aortic stenosis.

    (2) Early symptoms include palpitations secondary to ventricular arrhythmias and dyspnea on exertion.

    (3) Later, severe congestive heart failure is seen. Death results from progressive cardiac failure.

d. Diagnosis
  (1) **Physical examination**
    (a) The characteristic diastolic murmur is heard along the left sternal border. The duration of the murmur during diastole often correlates with the severity of the aortic insufficiency. The murmur radiates to the left axilla.
    (b) The pulse pressure is often widened. Short, intense peripheral pulses (**"water-hammer pulses"**) are characteristic.
  (2) **Chest x-ray** shows left ventricular dilatation.
  (3) **Echocardiography** is used to quantitate the degree of aortic insufficiency and to assess left ventricular ejection performance.
  (4) **Cardiac catheterization** is used to determine the presence of associated coronary artery disease.

e. Treatment
  (1) Aortic valve replacement surgery is recommended for patients with severe aortic insufficiency and:
    (a) Symptoms
    (b) Left ventricular systolic dysfunction (ejection fraction <50%)
    (c) Severe left ventricular dilation (end-systolic dimension >55 mm, end-diastolic dimension >75 mm)

C Mitral valve disease

1. Mitral stenosis
  a. Etiology. Although only 50% of patients report a history of rheumatic fever, this condition is thought to be the cause of mitral stenosis in almost all cases.
  b. Pathology
  (1) The time interval between the episode of rheumatic fever and the manifestation of mitral stenosis averages between 10 and 25 years.
  (2) The underlying pathologic changes are fusion of the commissures and thickening of the leaflets with or without shortening of the chordae tendineae.
  (3) The normal **cross-sectional area** of the mitral valve is 4–6 cm^2. In mild mitral stenosis, the area is reduced to 2–2.5 cm^2; in moderately severe stenosis, to 1.5–2 cm^2; and in severe stenosis, to 1–1.5 cm^2.
  (4) **Pathophysiologic changes** include:
    (a) Increased left atrial pressure
    (b) Pulmonary hypertension
    (c) Atrial fibrillation
    (d) Decreased cardiac output
    (e) Increased pulmonary vascular resistance
  c. Clinical presentation
  (1) Dyspnea is the most significant symptom. It indicates pulmonary congestion secondary to increased left atrial pressure.
  (2) Other manifestations include:
    (a) Paroxysmal nocturnal dyspnea and orthopnea
    (b) Chronic cough and hemoptysis
    (c) Pulmonary edema
    (d) Systemic arterial embolization, usually from a left atrial thrombus
  (3) Long-standing pulmonary hypertension may result in right ventricular failure and secondary tricuspid regurgitation.
  d. Diagnosis
  (1) **Physical examination.** The typical patient is thin and cachectic. Auscultation reveals the **classic triad** of an apical diastolic rumble, an opening snap, and a loud first heart sound.
  (2) **Chest x-ray** typically shows a prominent pulmonary vasculature in the upper lung fields. The cardiac silhouette may be normal or may show a double density of the right heart border. A lateral chest x-ray with a barium swallow may detect left atrial enlargement.
  (3) **Electrocardiogram** may be normal or may show P-wave abnormalities, signs of right ventricular hypertrophy, and right axis deviation.

(4) **Echocardiography** is used to determine the morphology of the valve and the severity of the mitral stenosis.

(5) **Cardiac catheterization** is used to calculate the mitral valve cross-sectional area, the mitral valve end-diastolic pressure gradient, pulmonary artery pressure, and any associated valvular or coronary artery disease.

e. **Treatment.** Surgery is recommended for all patients with symptomatic mitral stenosis. The choice of operative approach depends on the extent of these changes.

(1) **Commissurotomy** (opening of the fused commissures) can be accomplished under direct vision during surgical mitral valve repair or percutaneously by balloon mitral valvuloplasty. For patients with pliable leaflets, minimal mitral regurgitation, and minimal valvular calcification, results with balloon mitral valvuloplasty are equivalent to those with open mitral commissurotomy.

(2) **Mitral valve replacement** is required for patients with severe disease of the chordae tendineae and papillary muscles.

2. **Mitral insufficiency**

a. **Etiology**

(1) Degenerative mitral valve disease

(2) Altered valvular geometry resulting from ventricular dilation (also called functional mitral regurgitation). Dilatation occurs with ischemic or idiopathic cardiomyopathy.

(3) Infective endocarditis

(4) Rheumatic fever

b. **Pathology**

(1) "Myxomatous degeneration" is the most common cause of degenerative mitral valve disease. It is characterized by leaflet thickening and chordal elongation. There are structural alterations of collagen in the leaflet and chordae as well as an abnormal accumulation of proteoglycans in the leaflet tissue.

(2) Mitral valve prolapse is present when one or both leaflets of the mitral valve rise more than 2 mm above the plane of the annulus on echocardiography (in the long-axis view). Mitral valve prolapse is present in 2%–3% of the population. The vast majority of patients with mitral valve prolapse do not progress to develop significant mitral regurgitation and do not require surgery.

(3) The pathogenesis in mitral insufficiency secondary to rheumatic fever is similar to that in mitral stenosis. Why insufficiency predominates in some patients and stenosis in others is not understood.

(4) Pathophysiologic changes include:

(a) Increased left atrial pressure during systole

(b) Late-appearing pulmonary vascular changes, including increased pulmonary vascular resistance

(c) Increased left ventricular stroke volume

c. **Clinical presentation**

(1) Many years may elapse between the first evidence of mitral insufficiency and the development of symptoms.

(2) Symptoms include dyspnea on exertion, fatigue, and palpitations.

(3) Atrial fibrillation can occur as a result of distention and enlargement of the left atrium caused by elevated left atrial pressure. Approximately one third of patients undergoing surgery for mitral regurgitation have atrial fibrillation.

d. **Diagnosis**

(1) **Physical examination** reveals a holosystolic blowing murmur at the apex that radiates to the axilla, accompanied by an accentuated apical impulse.

(2) Echocardiography is the single most important diagnostic test for patients with clinical evidence of mitral regurgitation. Color Doppler echocardiography can accurately quantitate the degree (mild, moderate, severe) of mitral regurgitation. Echocardiography can demonstrate underlying anatomic abnormalities of the valve (e.g., leaflet prolapse, ruptured chordae tendinae, annular dilation, leaflet restriction, annular calcification, presence of vegetations, etc.), degree of left atrial enlargement, extent of left ventricular dysfunction, and the presence of associated tricuspid regurgitation.

(3) **Cardiac catheterization** is important to determine if coronary artery disease is present.

e. **Treatment**

(1) There is no effective medical therapy for mitral regurgitation.

(2) Only patients with severe mitral regurgitation should be considered for surgery. Careful echocardiographic assessment of the degree of mitral regurgitation by a skilled echocardiographer is essential to quantitate the amount of mitral regurgitation. If transthoracic echocardiography is inadequate, a transesophageal echocardiogram should be performed.

(3) **Surgical indications** include:

(a) Symptoms

(b) Evidence of left ventricular dysfunction, including:

(i) Ejection fraction <60% (mitral regurgitation allows ventricular ejection into the low-pressure left atrium and results in significantly decreased afterload; as a result, ejection fraction below 60% is abnormal)

(ii) Ventricular dilation (end-systolic dimension >45 mm)

(c) Development of atrial fibrillation or significant pulmonary hypertension

(d) There is growing evidence that asymptomatic patients with severe mitral regurgitation enjoy improved long-term survival with early operation.

(4) When possible, **mitral valve repair** is performed.

(5) Commonly used techniques for repair include:

(a) Quadrangular resection of the posterior leaflet

(b) Insertion of an annuloplasty ring (a cloth-covered ring that stabilizes and sometimes decreases the size of the mitral valve annulus)

D Tricuspid valve, pulmonic valve, and multiple valvular disease

1. **Tricuspid stenosis and insufficiency**

a. **Etiology**

(1) Organic tricuspid stenosis is almost always caused by rheumatic fever and is most commonly found in association with mitral valve disease. Isolated tricuspid disease is rare.

(2) Functional tricuspid insufficiency is the result of right ventricular dilatation secondary to pulmonary hypertension and right ventricular failure. Functional insufficiency is more common than organic tricuspid valve disease. The most common cause of functional tricuspid insufficiency is mitral valve disease.

(3) Tricuspid insufficiency is sometimes seen in the carcinoid syndrome, secondary to blunt trauma or secondary to bacterial endocarditis in drug addicts.

b. **Pathology**

(1) The pathogenesis in tricuspid stenosis secondary to rheumatic fever is similar to that in mitral valve disease.

(2) Elevation of right atrial pressure secondary to tricuspid stenosis leads to peripheral edema, jugular venous distention, hepatomegaly, and ascites.

c. **Clinical presentation**

(1) Moderate isolated tricuspid insufficiency is usually well tolerated.

(2) When right-sided heart failure occurs, symptoms (e.g., edema, hepatomegaly, ascites) develop.

d. **Diagnosis**

(1) **Physical examination**

(a) **Tricuspid insufficiency** produces a systolic murmur at the lower end of the sternum.

(b) **Tricuspid stenosis** produces a diastolic murmur in the same region.

(c) A prominent jugular venous pulse may be observed.

(d) The liver may be pulsatile in tricuspid insufficiency.

(2) **Chest x-ray** shows enlargement of the right side of the heart, which may also be reflected on the electrocardiogram.

(3) **Echocardiography** estimates the amount of tricuspid valve pathology. It should include an evaluation of any associated aortic or mitral valve lesions.

(4) **Cardiac catheterization** is the most accurate guide to diagnosing tricuspid disease.

e. Treatment

(1) Isolated tricuspid disease, especially tricuspid insufficiency, may be well tolerated without surgical intervention.

(2) In mild to moderate tricuspid insufficiency associated with mitral valve disease, opinion varies concerning the need for tricuspid surgery.

(3) In the case of extensive tricuspid insufficiency associated with mitral valve disease, the consensus is that either **tricuspid repair** or (rarely) **tricuspid valve replacement** is appropriate. Usually, the tricuspid valve can be repaired with an annuloplasty ring.

(4) Tricuspid stenosis, when significant, is remedied by a **commissurotomy** or **valve replacement.**

2. Pulmonic valve disease

a. **Pathology.** Acquired lesions of the pulmonic valve are uncommon. The carcinoid syndrome, however, may produce pulmonic stenosis.

b. **Treatment.** Surgical **repair** or **replacement of the valve** is carried out when warranted by the degree of dysfunction.

3. Multiple valvular disease

a. **Pathology.** More than one valve may be involved in rheumatic fever, as indicated in the foregoing discussions. Abnormal physiologic responses to multivalvular disease may be additive but usually reflect the most severely affected valve.

b. **Treatment** involves **repair** or **replacement of all valves** with significant dysfunction.

E **Coronary artery disease**

1. Etiology and epidemiology

a. **Atherosclerosis** is the predominant pathogenetic mechanism underlying obstructive disease of the coronary arteries. Uncommon causes of coronary artery disease include vasculitis (occurring with collagen vascular disorders), radiation injury, and trauma.

b. **Atherosclerotic heart disease** represents the most common cause of death in the United States and most other developed nations.

c. **Coronary artery disease** is four times more prevalent in men than in women, although the incidence in women is rapidly increasing.

d. **Risk factors** for coronary artery disease that have been identified by epidemiologic studies include:

(1) Hypertension

(2) Smoking

(3) Hypercholesterolemia

(4) Family history of heart disease

(5) Diabetes

(6) Obesity

2. Pathophysiologic effects of ischemic coronary artery disease of the myocardium include:

a. Decreased ventricular compliance

b. Decreased cardiac contractility

c. Myocardial necrosis

3. Clinical presentation. Coronary artery disease may take the form of:

a. **Angina pectoris**

(1) Angina pectoris typically presents as substernal chest pain lasting 5–10 minutes. The pain may be precipitated by emotional stress, exertion, or cold weather and is relieved by rest.

(2) Angina may be characterized by its patterns of occurrence.

(a) Stable angina: angina that is unchanged for a prolonged period

(b) Unstable angina: angina that shows a recent change from a previously stable pattern, including new-onset angina

(c) Angina at rest

(d) Postinfarction angina

b. Myocardial infarction

c. Congestive heart failure

d. Sudden death

4. **Diagnosis**
    a. **History.** The diagnosis of angina pectoris due to coronary artery disease is most often made from the patient's history.
    b. **Electrocardiogram**
        (1) The electrocardiogram is normal in up to 75% of patients when they are at rest without pain.
        (2) ST-segment changes and T-wave changes may be seen.
        (3) Evidence of a previous infarction may be apparent.
    c. **Exercise stress testing** helps to evaluate the induction of angina and associated electrocardiographic changes.
    d. A **radio thallium scan** of the heart delineates ischemic and infarcted areas of myocardium.

5. **Treatment**
    a. **Medical treatment.** Management of coronary artery disease is initiated with medical therapy in patients with stable angina and with no evidence of congestive heart failure.
        (1) Drugs used include nitrates, aspirin, ß-blockers, digitalis derivatives, and calcium channel blockers.
        (2) In addition, the patient is encouraged to adopt a low-fat diet, stop smoking, and begin a graded exercise program.
    b. **Cardiac catheterization** and **coronary angiography** provide the most accurate means of determining the extent of coronary artery disease. An obstruction is considered physiologically significant when the diameter of the vessel on angiography is narrowed by 50%. In addition, left ventricular function may be assessed by the ventriculogram and hemodynamic measurements.
    c. **Treatment**
        (1) Catheter-based coronary interventions: A catheter is threaded through an artery from the arm or grain and into the coronary arteries. A balloon (angioplasty) is expanded in the diseased segment to push the vessel wall out and to relieve the obstruction. In most cases, a wire tube (stent) is placed in the artery to keep it from closing over time ("restenosis"). The stent may be "bare metal" or may be coated with a drug (e.g., sirolimus) that elutes over time to prevent restenosis.
        (2) Coronary artery bypass surgery (CABG). Not all patients can be treated with a catheter-based intervention. Most commonly, anatomic considerations including chronic total occlusions, left main stenosis, and extensive lesions preclude a catheter-based approach.
            Coronary bypass surgery involves construction of bypass grafts to downstream segments of the affected coronary arteries to re-establish normal blood flow to the myocardium. Most commonly, the left anterior descending coronary artery is bypassed with the left internal mammary artery, and other target vessels are bypassed with reversed saphenous vein grafts constructed from the ascending aorta to the target vessel.
            There is strong evidence that CABG surgery increases survival in patients with left main disease, in those with "three-vessel disease" and decreased ventricular function, and in diabetics with three-vessel disease. CABG is highly successful at relieving angina pectoris: More than 90% of patients are free of angina 1 year after surgery.
    d. **Prognosis after bypass surgery**
        (1) The results of coronary artery revascularization depend on multiple factors. Risk is increased in patients with renal failure, urgency of operation, the presence of peripheral vascular disease, etc.
        (2) Overall mortality for CABG in North America is between 2% and 3%.
        (3) Ten-year patency rates for internal mammary artery (IMA) grafts are more than 90%, whereas vein graft patency is only 50% at 10 years. Therefore, the IMA is the conduit of choice for coronary artery bypass.

6. **Surgical treatment of myocardial infarction complications.** Myocardial infarction and many of its complications are treated medically, but some complications warrant surgery. These complications include the following:
    a. **Ventricular aneurysms.** The scarred myocardium may produce either akinesia or dyskinesia of ventricular wall motion, decreasing the ejection fraction.

(1) This decrease may result in congestive heart failure, ventricular arrhythmias, or rarely, systemic thromboembolization.

(2) Surgical correction of the aneurysm is undertaken when these problems occur.

(3) Coronary revascularization may also be warranted at the same time.

b. **Ruptured ventricle** is rare, and the mortality rate is approximately 100% without surgery.

c. **Rupture of the interventricular septum** (postinfarct ventricular septal defect) carries a high mortality rate. Again, early operative repair is important.

d. **Mitral valve papillary muscle dysfunction or rupture**

(1) The posterior papillary muscle is usually involved.

(2) Treatment is by mitral valve replacement or repair.

(3) Long-term survival depends on the extent of myocardial damage.

F **Cardiac tumors**

1. **Types of tumors**

   a. **Benign tumors**

   (1) **Myxomas,** which account for 75%–80% of benign cardiac tumors, may be either pedunculated or sessile. Most are pedunculated and are found in the left atrium attached to the septum.

   (2) Other benign tumors include rhabdomyomas (most common in childhood), fibromas, and lipomas.

   b. **Malignant tumors.** Overall, primary malignant tumors account for 20%–25% of all primary cardiac tumors. The various types of sarcomas are the most common.

   c. **Metastatic tumors** occur more frequently than primary cardiac tumors (benign or malignant).

   (1) Autopsy studies show cardiac involvement by metastatic disease in about 10% of patients who have died of malignancy.

   (2) Melanoma, lymphoma, and leukemia are the tumors that most often metastasize to the heart.

2. **Clinical presentation.** Cardiac neoplasms may be manifested by pericardial effusion, which results in cardiac tamponade. The neoplasms may also be manifested by congestive heart failure, arrhythmias, peripheral embolization (especially with myxomas), or other constitutional signs and symptoms.

3. **Treatment** is by **surgical excision** if possible.

G **Cardiac trauma**   Injuries to the heart may be divided into several categories.

1. **Penetrating injury** may involve any area of the heart, although the anterior position of the right ventricle makes it the most commonly involved chamber.

   a. Penetrating wounds may result from gunshots, knives, and other weapons. In addition, penetrating injury may be iatrogenic, as a result of catheters or pacing wires.

   b. Bleeding into the pericardium is common. **Pericardial tamponade** may result, manifested by:

   (1) Distended neck veins

   (2) Hypotension

   (3) Pulsus paradoxus

   (4) Distant heart sounds

   c. Small wounds may spontaneously seal, in which case pericardiocentesis may suffice; however, open thoracotomy may be required.

2. **Blunt trauma** may be more extensive than is usually appreciated.

   a. **History** of a significant blow to the chest, with or without fractured ribs or sternum, should create a high index of suspicion of a cardiac contusion or infarction. A patient with such a history should be observed and monitored in a manner similar to a patient with myocardial infarction because the trauma is likely to cause a similar myocardial injury.

   (1) Serial electrocardiograms and cardiac enzyme studies should be obtained.

   (2) Echocardiography may be helpful in determining myocardial injury.

   (3) The appearance of new murmurs should be investigated and may require cardiac catheterization.

b. Treatment. Blunt trauma may cause rupture of a tricuspid, mitral, or aortic valve, requiring treatment by valve replacement or repair.

H Pericardial disorders

1. Pericardial effusion

a. The pericardium responds to noxious stimuli by an increased production of fluid.

b. A pericardial effusion volume as small as 100 mL may produce symptomatic tamponade if the fluid accumulates rapidly, whereas larger amounts may be tolerated if the fluid accumulates slowly.

c. Pericardial effusion is treated by pericardiocentesis or by tube pericardiostomy via a subxiphoid approach.

d. Chronic effusions, such as those that occur with malignant involvement of the pericardium, may require pericardiectomy via left thoracotomy or sternotomy.

2. Pericarditis may be acute or chronic.

a. Acute pericarditis

(1) Causes of acute pericarditis include:

(a) Bacterial infection, as from staphylococci or streptococci. Acute pyogenic pericarditis is uncommon and is usually associated with a systemic illness.

(b) Viral infection

(c) Uremia

(d) Traumatic hemopericardium

(e) Malignant disease

(f) Connective tissue disorders

(2) Treatment consists of managing the underlying cause. Open pericardial drainage may be required. Most cases of acute pericarditis resolve without serious sequelae.

b. Chronic pericarditis may represent recurrent episodes of an acute process or undiagnosed long-standing viral pericarditis. The etiology is often impossible to establish. It may go unnoticed until it results in the chronic constrictive form, causing chronic tamponade.

c. Chronic constrictive pericarditis presents with dyspnea on exertion, easy fatigability, marked jugular venous distention, ascites, hepatomegaly, and peripheral edema.

(1) The pericardium may become calcified, which is evident on a chest x-ray.

(2) Cardiac catheterization may be needed to confirm the diagnosis.

(3) Once the diagnosis has been established in the symptomatic patient, **pericardiectomy** should be undertaken with or without the use of cardiopulmonary bypass.

II CONGENITAL HEART DISEASE

A Overview

1. The incidence of congenital heart disease is approximately 3 in 1000 births.

2. Etiology. In most cases, the etiology is unknown.

a. Rubella occurring in the first trimester of pregnancy is known to cause congenital heart disease (e.g., patent ductus arteriosus).

b. Down's syndrome is associated with endocardial cushion defects.

3. Types. The most common forms of congenital heart disease are in decreasing order:

a. Ventricular septal defect

b. Transposition of the great vessels

c. Tetralogy of Fallot

d. Hypoplastic left heart syndrome

e. Atrial septal defect

f. Patent ductus arteriosus

g. Coarctation of the aorta

h. Endocardial cushion defects

4. History

a. The mother should be questioned about difficulties during the pregnancy, especially in the first trimester.

b. The mother often states that the child shows the following symptoms, which indicate pulmonary overcirculation and congestive heart failure:

   (1) Easy fatigability and decreased exercise tolerance

   (2) Poor feeding habits and poor weight gain

   (3) Frequent pulmonary infections

c. A history of cyanosis should be sought, as this indicates a right-to-left shunt.

5. Physical examination

   a. Abnormalities in growth and development should be identified.

   b. Cyanosis and clubbing of the fingers may be noted.

   c. Examination of the heart should proceed in the same manner as in the adult.

   (1) Systolic murmurs are frequently found in infants and small children and may not be clinically significant.

   (2) A gallop rhythm is of great clinical importance.

   (3) Congestive heart failure in children is frequently manifested by hepatic enlargement.

6. Diagnosis

   a. History and physical examination suggest the presence of a cardiac abnormality.

   b. Echocardiogram is the mainstay of diagnosis and can define abnormal anatomy and physiology.

   c. Cardiac catheterization may be required.

B **Patent ductus arteriosus**

1. Pathophysiology

   a. **Hypoxia** and **prostaglandins E_1** (PGE_1) and **E_2** (PGE_2) act to keep the ductus open in utero.

   b. In the normal infant born at term, circulation of the blood through the pulmonary vascular bed results in elevated oxygen levels and breakdown of the prostaglandins, which results in closure of the ductus within a few days.

   c. The **natural history** of patent ductus arteriosus is variable.

   (1) A few patients experience heart failure within the first year of life.

   (2) Many patients remain asymptomatic and are diagnosed on routine examination.

   (3) Some patients eventually develop pulmonary vascular obstructive disease, which can lead to elevated pulmonary vascular resistance.

   d. Patent ductus arteriosus may be seen in combination with other defects, such as ventricular septal defect and coarctation of the aorta.

2. Clinical presentation. Common presenting complaints are dyspnea, fatigue, and palpitations, signifying congestive heart failure.

3. Diagnosis is based primarily on the physical findings.

   a. Physical examination

   (1) The classic continuous "machinerylike" murmur is usually heard, but it may be absent until 1 year of age.

   (2) Other signs include a widened pulse pressure and bounding peripheral pulses.

   (3) Cyanosis may be seen in patent ductus arteriosus, which is associated with other anomalies or in right-to-left shunt from pulmonary vascular disease.

   b. Echocardiography can define a patent ductus arteriosus and other associated anatomic abnormalities.

4. Treatment

   a. Surgical management consists of **ligation of the ductus.** This is reserved for:

   (1) Premature infants with severe pulmonary dysfunction

   (2) Infants who suffer from congestive heart failure within the first year of life

   (3) Asymptomatic children with a patent ductus that persists until 2 or 3 years of age

   b. Indomethacin, a prostaglandin inhibitor, has been used with some success to close the ductus in premature infants with symptomatic simple patent ductus arteriosus.

C **Coarctation of the aorta**

1. Overview. Coarctation, a severe narrowing, is found twice as often in male children as in female children.

   a. It is commonly located adjacent to the ductus arteriosus.

    b. Coarctation may be fatal in the first few months of life if not treated.

    c. Associated intracardiac defects, present in up to 60% of patients, include patent ductus arteriosus, ventricular septal defect, and bicuspid aortic valve.

2. Clinical presentation

    a. Some children are asymptomatic for varying periods of time.

    b. In others, symptoms suggesting congestive heart failure are present shortly after birth.

    c. Headaches, epistaxis, lower extremity weakness, and dizziness may be seen in the child with symptomatic coarctation.

3. Diagnosis

    a. Physical findings include:

        (1) Upper extremity hypertension

        (2) Absent or diminished pulses in the lower extremities

        (3) A systolic murmur

    b. Chest x-ray may reveal "rib notching" in older children, representing collateral pathways via intercostal arteries.

    c. Echocardiography suggests the degree of flow limitation and other associated anomalies.

    d. Cardiac catheterization is usually recommended to define the location of the coarctation and any associated cardiac defects.

4. Treatment

    a. Surgical correction of the coarctation is indicated for all patients and may be delayed until 5 or 6 years of age in asymptomatic patients.

    b. Operative procedures include:

        (1) Resection and **end-to-end anastomosis**

        (2) Prosthetic patch graft

        (3) A **subclavian flap procedure**

            (a) The distal subclavian artery is transected.

            (b) A proximal-based subclavian artery flap is used to enlarge the aorta at the level of the coarctation.

    c. Any associated defects must also be corrected.

5. Complications

    a. Residual hypertension may be a problem postoperatively.

    b. Spinal cord injury due to ischemia during surgery rarely occurs.

    c. Postoperative mesenteric ischemia is seen in a small but significant number of patients and is related to postoperative hypertension.

    d. Postoperative aneurysm may develop at the site of the operative repair.

D **Atrial septal defects**

1. Classification. Atrial septal defects occur twice as frequently in female children as in male children. Three types are commonly seen:

    a. Ostium secundum defects, which account for most atrial septal defects, are found in the midportion of the atrial septum.

    b. Sinus venosus defects are located high up on the atrial septum and are often associated with anomalies of pulmonary venous drainage.

    c. Ostium primum defects are components of atrioventricular septal defects and are located on the atrial side of the mitral and tricuspid valves.

    d. A **patent foramen ovale** is **not** considered an atrial septal defect.

2. Pathophysiology

    a. Atrial pressures are equal on both sides of a large atrial septal defect.

    b. Since atrial emptying occurs during ventricular diastole, the direction of shunt at the **atrial level** is determined by the relative compliances of the **right** and **left ventricles** (diastolic phenomena). Because the right ventricle is more compliant than the left ventricle, the **flow is left to right across an atrial septal defect.**

    c. This results in a modest increase in pulmonary blood flow, which causes mild growth retardation.

d. If left uncorrected, **pulmonary vascular obstructive disease** may develop. This condition results in the right ventricle becoming less compliant than the left, with blood flow shunting right to left across the atrial septal defect.

3. Clinical presentation

    a. Mild dyspnea and easy fatigability are seen in infancy and early childhood.

    b. If left untreated, symptoms may progress to congestive heart failure as an adult.

    c. Initially, patients may present with neurologic symptoms, including cerebrovascular accident or transient ischemic attack.

4. Diagnosis

    a. Physical examination reveals a systolic murmur in the left second or third intercostal space and a fixed, split, second heart sound.

    b. Chest x-ray reveals moderate enlargement of the right ventricle and prominence of the pulmonary vasculature.

    c. Electrocardiogram reveals right ventricular hypertrophy.

    d. Echocardiography can define the atrial septal defect and note the direction of shunting.

    e. Cardiac catheterization can make the diagnosis from the "step-up" in oxygen saturation in the right atrium. The amount of left-to-right shunt may be calculated.

5. Treatment is based on the size of the left-to-right shunt.

    a. Some atrial septal defects may close spontaneously.

    b. Closure of the defect is indicated if the pulmonary blood flow is 1-1/2 to 2 times greater than the systemic blood flow. In addition, patients with documented neurologic events should undergo atrial septal defect closure.

    c. Closure may be attempted via a percutaneous approach in the catheterization laboratory.

    d. Surgery carries a mortality risk of less than 1%.

    e. Ideal time for closure is age 4 or 5, before the child goes to school.

E Ventricular septal defects

1. Classification. Ventricular septal defects are the most common congenital heart defects. Associated anomalies, such as coarctation of the aorta, are common. They may be classified according to their location in the ventricular septum (Fig. 6-1).

    a. Conoventricular defect is the most common ventricular septal defect and occurs in 70%–80% of cases.

    b. Muscular defects may be single or multiple (occurring in 10%–15%).

    c. Inlet septal defect (atrioventricular canal type) occurs in 5% of isolated defects.

    d. Conoseptal defects (outlet defect) constitute 5%–10% of defects (also called supracristal or infundibular defects).

2. Pathophysiology

    a. Ventricular **pressures** are **equal** on either side of a large ventricular septal defect.

    b. Because ventricular emptying occurs during systole, the direction of the shunt at the ventricular level is determined by the **relative resistances** of the **pulmonary** and **systemic circuits** (systolic phenomena).

        (1) Because the pulmonary vascular resistance is much less than the systemic vascular resistance, **flow is left to right across a ventricular septal defect.**

        (2) This causes greatly increased pulmonary blood flow, which imposes a volume load on the left ventricle and may lead to early congestive heart failure.

    c. Other adverse effects of pulmonary overcirculation include:

        (1) Poor feeding

        (2) Failure to thrive

        (3) Frequent respiratory tract infections

        (4) Increased pulmonary vascular resistance

        (5) Development of irreversible pulmonary vascular obstructive disease

            (a) This condition results in a higher pulmonary vascular resistance than systemic resistance and leads to reversal of flow across the ventricular septal defect (**Eisenmenger's syndrome**).

            (b) At this point, the patient cannot be operated on.

3. **Clinical presentation**
   a. Small ventricular septal defects rarely cause significant symptoms in infancy or early childhood, and these defects may close spontaneously before they are recognized.
   b. Symptoms are usually seen with ventricular septal defects, which are approximately the diameter of the aortic root.
      (1) Children with large defects usually have dyspnea on exertion, easy fatigability, and an increased incidence of pulmonary infections.
      (2) Severe cardiac failure may be seen in infants but is less common in children.

4. **Diagnosis**
   a. **Physical examination** reveals a harsh pansystolic murmur.
   b. **Chest x-ray and electrocardiogram,** especially in large ventricular septal defects, show evidence of biventricular hypertrophy.
   c. **Cardiac catheterization** is essential for delineating the severity of the left-to-right shunt, pulmonary vascular resistance, and the location of the defects.

5. **Treatment**
   a. Surgical closure of the defect should be performed in:
      (1) Infants with significant cardiac failure or increased pulmonary vascular resistance
      (2) Asymptomatic children with significant shunts who have not had spontaneous closure by 2 years of age
      (3) Patients with pulmonary blood flow 1-1/2 to 2 times greater than systemic blood flow
   b. Operative mortality risk ($<5\%$) is related to the degree of preoperative pulmonary vascular disease.

F **Tetralogy of Fallot**

1. **Pathophysiology**
   a. Tetralogy of Fallot, one of the most common **cyanotic congenital heart disorders,** consists of:
      (1) Obstruction to right ventricular outflow
      (2) A ventricular septal defect
      (3) Hypertrophy of the right ventricle
      (4) An overriding aorta
   b. The addition of an atrial septal defect (which is of little further physiologic significance) turns the condition into the **pentalogy of Fallot.**
   c. Because resistance to right ventricular outflow exceeds the systemic vascular resistance, the shunt is right to left, resulting in desaturation of the blood and cyanosis.
   d. Exercise tolerance is limited because of the inability to increase pulmonary blood flow.

2. **Clinical presentation**
   a. Cyanosis and dyspnea on exertion are routinely seen in patients with tetralogy of Fallot. Children soon learn that by squatting, they can temporarily alleviate these symptoms.
      (1) Squatting increases the systemic vascular resistance, which decreases the magnitude of right-to-left shunt and causes an increase in pulmonary blood flow.
      (2) The cyanosis is seen at birth in 30% of the cases, by the first year in 30%, and later in childhood in the remainder. Polycythemia and clubbing accompany the cyanosis.
   b. Cerebrovascular accidents and brain sepsis constitute the major threats to life because cardiac failure is rare.

3. **Diagnosis**
   a. **Physical examination** reveals clubbing of the digits and cyanosis. A harsh systolic murmur of pulmonary stenosis is often heard.
   b. **Cardiac catheterization** is important for determining the level of pulmonic outflow obstruction and the size of the main and branch pulmonary arteries.

4. **Treatment** depends on many variables, including the anatomy of the defect and the age of the child.
   a. Total correction is undertaken after 2 years of age.
   b. Controversy exists over whether the defect should be corrected before this age. Many believe that a palliative **systemic-to-pulmonary** (Blalock-Taussig) **shunt** should be done initially, followed by definitive correction later on.

c. The risk of surgery depends on the age of the patient and the degree of cyanosis.

d. After correction, a dramatic improvement is usually seen.

G **Transposition of the great arteries**

1. **Pathophysiology**

   a. Transposition of the great arteries (TGA) occurs when the **aorta** arises from the morphologic **right ventricle** and the **pulmonary artery** arises from the morphologic **left ventricle.** This results in two independent parallel circuits.

   b. Survival depends on a **communication** between the right and left sides of the heart to allow mixing of oxygenated and unoxygenated blood. This communication usually occurs across an atrial septal defect, although a patent ductus arteriosus or ventricular septal defect could also be present.

2. **Diagnosis**

   a. Echocardiogram demonstrates a posterior vessel dividing into the right and left pulmonary arteries arising from the left ventricle.

   b. Cardiac catheterization is reserved for infants with additional intracardiac or extracardiac anomalies or inadequate shunting.

3. **Treatment**

   a. When inadequate shunting exists, **balloon atrial septostomy** is performed to increase the size of the interatrial communication and facilitate mixing of blood. Septostomy is followed by definitive surgical correction.

   b. Operative procedures include:

   (1) **Arterial switch** division of the great arteries with transfer of the coronaries and proper anastamoses of the aorta to the left and pulmonary artery to the right ventricles.

Study Questions for Part II

Directions: *Each of the numbered items in this section is followed by several possible answers. Select the ONE lettered answer that is BEST in each case.*

1. A 50-year-old man is brought to the emergency room after falling 20 feet from a roof. He is complaining of dyspnea, and his blood pressure is 70/50 mm Hg. Breath sounds are diminished on the left, and there is tracheal deviation to the right. What is the best initial treatment for this patient?

- A Chest radiograph
- B Close observation
- C Needle decompression of the left chest
- D Computed tomography (CT) scan of the thorax
- E Emergent surgical exploration

2. A patient undergoes a left scalene node biopsy to rule out carcinoma of the lung. One hour later, the patient is cyanotic and dyspneic; a marked tachycardia is accompanied by decreased breath sounds on the left. Which step is most likely to improve the patient's condition?

- A Blood transfusion
- B Insertion of a right subclavian catheter and administration of intravenous fluids
- C Endotracheal intubation
- D Insertion of a left chest tube
- E Re-exploration of the wound

3. A patient is brought to the emergency department with a stab wound to the right chest in the fourth intercostal space in the midaxillary line. The patient is hypotensive, complains of shortness of breath, and is found to have absent breath sounds on the right side of the chest. Which step should come next in the management of this patient?

- A Chest radiograph
- B Chest tube insertion
- C Needle thoracentesis
- D Local wound exploration
- E Pericardiocentesis

4. A tall, thin 19-year-old male presents to the emergency department with sudden onset of chest pain, cough, and shortness of breath. Breath sounds are absent in the left chest. Which of the following is an indication for surgery?

- A Family history of recurrent spontaneous pneumothorax
- B Persistent air leak after 3 days of chest tube drainage
- C Identification of an apical bleb on chest CT
- D Evidence of life-threatening respiratory compromise on initial presentation
- E History of one prior episode successfully treated with conservative management on the contralateral side

QUESTIONS 5–6

A chest radiograph of a 55-year-old man involved in a high-speed motor vehicle accident shows a widened mediastinum and pneumomediastinum. Electrocardiogram shows sinus tachycardia with frequent premature ventricular contractions.

5. All of the following maneuvers are appropriate at this time *except*

- A Aortogram
- B Bronchoscopy

    ☐C Continuous cardiac monitoring

    ☐D Left thoracotomy

    ☐E Endotracheal intubation

6. Expected physiologic changes due to blunt chest trauma include all but which of the following?

    ☐A Elevated PCO_2

    ☐B Increased compliance

    ☐C Elevated A-a gradient

    ☐D Decreased ventricular contractions

    ☐E Elevated shunt fractions

QUESTIONS 7–8

A 70-year-old patient on antibiotic therapy for necrotizing bacterial pneumonia is found to have a large pleural effusion.

7. In addition to continued antibiotics, what should be the next step in management of this patient?

    ☐A Sputum culture and sensitivity

    ☐B Chest tube insertion

    ☐C Thoracentesis

    ☐D Thoracotomy and decortication

    ☐E Rib resection and open drainage

8. A sample of pleural fluid is cloudy and thick, with a pH of 7.2. What should be the next therapeutic step?

    ☐A Video-assisted thorascopic surgery with talc pleurodesis

    ☐B Chest tube drainage

    ☐C Repeat thoracentesis

    ☐D Thoracotomy and decortication

    ☐E Rib resection drainage

9. A routine chest radiograph for a 55-year-old man with a 50 pack-year smoking history shows a peripherally located 1.5-cm, noncalcified lesion of the upper lobe of the left lung. No evidence of this lesion appeared on a chest radiograph 5 years earlier. What should be the next step in this patient's management?

    ☐A Observation with serial chest radiographs

    ☐B Thoracotomy

    ☐C Bronchoscopy

    ☐D Biopsy

    ☐E Sputum cytology

10. A 35-year-old man is involved in a high-speed motor vehicle collision. He arrives in the emergency room in respiratory distress. Radiographs taken during the initial evaluation reveal an air-fluid level in the left chest. Management includes all of the following *except*

    ☐A Establishment of a secure airway

    ☐B Immediate placement of a nasogastric tube

    ☐C Urgent thoracotomy to repair the injury

    ☐D Placement of adequate peripheral vascular access

    ☐E Urgent laparotomy to repair injury

11. Which of the following forms of congenital heart disease is most common?

    ☐A Transposition of the great vessels

    ☐B Tetralogy of Fallot

    ☐C Atrial septal defect

D Patent ductus arteriosus

E Ventricular septal defect

12. A 32-year-old man is referred for a 1.0-cm lesion of the right upper lobe of the lung. The lesion appears calcified. Previous chest radiograph taken 1 year prior demonstrates the lesion to be present at the same size. Further workup and treatment would include which of the following?

A CT scan–guided biopsy

B Radiation therapy

C Surgical excision

D Antibiotics

E Observation with repeat chest x-ray

13. A 57-year-old male patient with a 60 pack-year smoking history is referred for a 1.5-cm solitary mass in the right upper lobe. CT scan demonstrates no evidence of lymph node involvement. What should further workup or treatment include?

A Radiation therapy

B Open lung biopsy

C Chemotherapy

D Right upper lobectomy

E Repeat chest x-ray in 6 months

14. A 22-year-old female is referred for evaluation of a 2-cm posterior mediastinal mass discovered on routine chest radiograph. What is the most likely diagnosis?

A Bronchogenic cyst

B Lymphoma

C Neurogenic tumor

D Thymoma

E Adenocarcinoma

15. A 78-year-old previously healthy man is admitted to the emergency department complaining of angina, dyspnea, and near syncope. Electrocardiogram is normal, and a loud systolic murmur is heard in the second right interspace with radiation to the carotids. What is the most likely diagnosis in this patient?

A Myocardial infarction

B Pericarditis

C Mitral regurgitation

D Aortic stenosis

E Aortic insufficiency

16. Which of the following is not a risk factor for coronary artery disease?

A Hypertension

B Smoking

C Diabetes

D Renal failure

E Hypercholesterolemia

17. A 72-year-old female patient is admitted with unstable angina. Cardiac catheterization reveals severe triple-vessel coronary artery disease. The optimal treatment of this patient would include which of the following?

A Coronary artery bypass surgery

B Observation

C Medical management (nitrates, β-blockers)

D Coronary angioplasty

E Tissue plasminogen activator

18. A 72-year-old patient with a history of syncope and dyspnea presents for evaluation for peripheral vascular surgery. Physical examination reveals a systolic crescendo–decrescendo murmur that radiates to the carotid arteries. As he is symptomatic, his diseased valve would typically have an area of less than which of the following?

- A 1 cm^2
- B 1.5 cm^2
- C 2 cm^2
- D 3 cm^2
- E 4 cm^2

19. A 29-year-old man is evaluated for a cerebral vascular accident. Physical examination reveals a systolic ejection murmur at the left second interspace and a fixed split second heart sound. What is the most likely diagnosis?

- A Ventricular septal defect
- B Atrial septal defect
- C Mitral stenosis
- D Aortic insufficiency
- E Ventricular aneurysm

Answers and Explanations

1. The answer is C [Chapter 4, II A 2]. Hypotension, diminished breath sounds, and tracheal deviation are clinical signs of tension pneumothorax. This represents a surgical emergency and without treatment may rapidly become fatal. In this scenario, prompt needle decompression of the left chest is indicated, prior to chest x-ray or other diagnostic studies that could delay treatment.

2. The answer is D [Chapter 4, I B 3 c]. Insertion of a left chest tube will most likely improve the patient's condition. The pleura of the lung lies immediately adjacent to the scalene fat pad. If the pleura is injured during scalene node biopsy, a resultant pneumothorax can cause the symptoms that developed in the patient described. Scalene node biopsy can also injure other nearby structures; for example, lymph duct structures, the brachial plexus, the vagus and phrenic nerves, and the subclavian vessels, resulting in corresponding symptoms.

A large wound hematoma could cause tracheal compression and airway compromise, but this is not described. Intubation with positive pressure ventilation will make the pneumothorax worse without a chest tube. While injury to the subclavian vessels could cause a hemothorax, a chest tube still needs to be inserted for evaluation. A pneumothorax is the more likely injury. With a suspected left-sided pneumothorax, a subclavian line should be inserted on the left because of the risk of producing a second right-sided pneumothorax.

3. The answer is C [Chapter 4, II A 2 b–c]. The patient has signs and symptoms consistent with a tension pneumothorax. This life-threatening situation should be treated immediately by needle thoracentesis. A chest tube insertion should follow this maneuver. A chest radiograph is not necessary to confirm the diagnosis and will only delay treatment. Local wound exploration has no role in the management of stab wounds of the chest. Pericardiocentesis is the choice when evidence indicates pericardial tamponade.

4. The answer is E [Chapter 5, II B]. Indications for definitive surgical management of spontaneous pneumothorax include recurrence (ipsilateral or contralateral), persistent air leak greater than 7–10 days, and incomplete expansion of lung.

5–6. The answers are 5-D [Chapter 4, II A 5, 6; B 1, 2, 5, 6] **and 6-B** [Chapter 4, II A 6]. Causes for the chest radiograph and electrocardiographic findings are multiple and include aortic rupture, cardiac tamponade, tracheobronchial disruption, hypoxia, and cardiac contusion. A more precise diagnosis would be mandatory before undertaking thoracotomy because operative strategy would depend on which injury is present.

Blunt thoracic trauma with or without flail chest results in chest wall muscle damage and pain, with resultant splinting and loss of chest wall elasticity. Intra-alveolar hemorrhage and interstitial edema reduce pulmonary parenchymal elasticity. Therefore, both lung and chest wall compliance decrease. PCO_2, A-a gradient, and shunt fractions would probably be elevated, and ventricular contractions would probably be decreased.

7–8. The answers are 7-C [Chapter 5, II B 2] **and 8-B** [Chapter 5, II C 2–3]. The patient developing a pleural effusion in the setting of an underlying pneumonia requires thoracentesis for diagnosis. The character of the fluid described is consistent with that present in an empyema. Initial treatment of an empyema should involve closed chest tube drainage. Thoracotomy and decortication or rib resection may be required when the empyema is not adequately drained by the chest tube or is otherwise not amenable to closed drainage. Video-assisted thorascopic surgery pleurodesis is not standard treatment for an empyema.

9. The answer is D [Chapter 5, IV B 5]. The patient has a solitary pulmonary nodule. He is older than age 40, and the characteristics do not favor a benign lesion, such as concentric calcification. In addition, the lesion was not present on the chest radiograph 5 years earlier. Diagnosis is mandatory for determining whether the lesion is malignant. This can be done by needle biopsy or thoracoscopic biopsy.

10. The answer is C [Chapter 4, II B]. This patient is presenting with a diaphragmatic disruption, as evidenced by the identification of the stomach in the chest. Treatment involves standard resuscitation principles, (Airway, Breathing, Circulation), placement of a nasogastric tube to prevent acute gastric dilitation (which can produce severe, life-threatening respiratory distress), and urgent transabdominal repair of the diaphragmatic defect. If diagnosis is delayed by 7–10 days, transthoracic repair is preferred to facilitate the freeing of any adhesions to the lung.

11. The answer is E [Chapter 6, II A]. The most common forms of congenital heart disease are, in decreasing order: ventral septal defect, transposition of the great vessels, tetralogy of Fallot, hypoplastic left heart syndrome, atrial septal defect, and patent ductus arteriosus.

12. The answer is E [Chapter 5, IV B]. Isolated lung nodules less than 1.0 cm are known as coin lesions. Workup should include a detailed history, noting any use of tobacco products or previous malignancy. Any prior chest radiographs should be obtained. A calcified lesion that has not enlarged over a 2-year period suggests a benign process. In this patient, observation with follow-up x-ray is indicated. Any change in the lesion is an indication for biopsy.

13. The answer is D [Chapter 5, V F]. The appropriate treatment is surgical lobectomy. Observation with repeat chest x-ray is not warranted with a smoking history.

This patient is in clinical stage I, based on tumor size and nodal status. There is no clear benefit in biopsying the lesion. Chemotherapy and radiation may be indicated in certain stage IIIa lesions or in locally advanced disease.

14. The answer is C [Chapter 5, X C]. The most common posterior mediastinal mass is a neurogenic tumor. Seventy-five percent of neurogenic tumors occur in children under 4 years of age. Childhood tumors are more likely to be malignant. Lymphoma, thymoma, and germ cell tumors are commonly located in the anterior mediastimun. Middle mediastinal lesions include bronchogenic and pericardial cysts. Metastatic adenocarcinoma may involve the pleural surfaces; however, lesions are often small and multiple.

15. The answer is D [Chapter 6, I B]. Angina, syncope, and dyspnea are the classic symptoms of aortic stenosis. Physical examination generally reveals a systolic ejection murmur in the second right intercostal space. An electrocardiogram and serial cardiac enzymes should be obtained to rule out cardiac ischemia. The murmur of aortic insufficiency is diastolic with a clinical picture of heart failure.

16. The answer is D [Chapter 6, I E]. Risk factors for coronary artery disease are the same as those for vascular disease in general—smoking, diabetes, obesity, hypertension, and hypercholesterolemia. While renal failure is often associated with coronary artery disease, this is because of the frequent association with other risk factors, such as hypertension and diabetes.

17. The answer is A [Chapter 6, I E]. This patient has severe triple-vessel coronary disease. Studies have shown a significant survival advantage for patients in this category who are treated with surgical revascularization, rather than with medical management or angioplasty. Additional benefit may be realized in patients with compromised ventricular function.

18. The answer is A [Chapter 6, I B]. This patient has aortic stenosis. Symptoms usually begin when the valve area is less than 1 cm^2.

19. The answer is B [Chapter 6, II D]. Echocardiogram searching for thrombus or septal defect should be obtained in a younger patient who suffers from a cerebral vascular accident. A second interspace murmur and fixed splitting of the second heart sound are classic findings in atrial septal defect. Anticoagulation for 4–6 weeks with elective repair of the atrial septal defect is the indicated treatment.

PART **III**

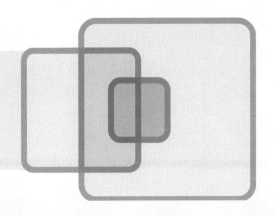

Vascular Disorders

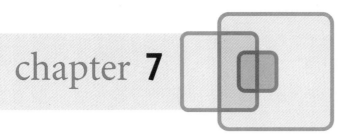

chapter 7

Peripheral Arterial Disease

JOSEPH V. LOMBARDI • PAUL J. DIMUZIO • R. ANTHONY CARABASI III

I · GENERAL PRINCIPLES OF PERIPHERAL ARTERIAL DISEASE

Atherosclerosis is the most common cause of arterial occlusive disease in humans. Arterial lesions occur at certain locations within the vascular tree, such as the proximal internal carotid artery, the infrarenal aorta, and the superficial femoral artery (SFA); the supraceliac aorta and the deep femoral artery are rarely diseased. Atherosclerotic plaques typically occur at arterial bifurcations (branch points), suggesting that their formation may be related to shear stress phenomena.

A **Pathology**   Atherosclerosis occurs within the arterial tree as three types of lesions.

1. **Fatty streaks** are discrete, subintimal lesions that are composed of cholesterol-laden macrophages and smooth muscle cells. These streaks may occur early in life and are not hemodynamically significant.

2. **Fibrous plaques** are more advanced lesions and also contain an extracellular matrix.

3. **Complex plaques** are characterized by intimal ulceration or intraplaque hemorrhage.

B **Pathophysiology**   Atherosclerotic lesions may cause symptoms via two different mechanisms.

1. **Stenosis/occlusion:** As the lesions become more advanced, stenoses (partial luminal blockages) develop, resulting in decreased blood flow distally. If the stenosis becomes severe, blood flow may be diminished to the point where thrombosis occurs, resulting in an occlusion. Distal blood flow is maintained by collateral circulation.

2. **Embolism:** A complex plaque may lose its fibrous cap and discharge debris within the lesion distally (atheroembolism). Additionally, a plaque may have deep ulceration, which acts as a nidus for platelet formation or local thrombus. These platelets or clots may then embolize distally.

C **Collateral circulation** refers to multiple arterial pathways that develop around a stenosis as it progresses over time. These pathways maintain blood flow distally. Resistance in collateral pathways is always higher than in the previously nonoccluded vessels. Symptoms develop if collateral circulation is poorly developed or is compromised by atherosclerosis or multilevel disease. When an artery occludes acutely, collateral circulation does not have time to develop, leading to acute ischemia and distal tissue loss (see IIB). Examples of important collateral circulation beds include:

1. The **external carotid artery** helps to maintain blood flow around a diseased internal carotid artery.

2. The **internal iliac** and **lumbar arteries,** as well as the **internal mammary artery** (via the **superior** and **inferior epigastric arteries),** can form a collateral bed to help supply the leg in aortoiliac occlusive disease.

3. The **profunda (deep) femoral artery** collaterals supply the popliteal artery in the case of SFA disease.

4. The **geniculate** collaterals around the knee supply the lower leg in the case of popliteal disease.

D **Risk factors** for peripheral arterial disease secondary to atherosclerosis include:

1. **Tobacco abuse**

2. **Diabetes mellitus**

   3. Hyperlipidemia

   4. Family history of atherosclerosis

   5. Hypertension

II   **LOWER EXTREMITY OCCLUSIVE DISEASE**

Lower extremity occlusive disease includes occlusive disease of the femoral, popliteal, and tibial arteries (Fig. 7-1).

A   **Pathology**   The most common cause of lower extremity disease is **atherosclerosis,** although other less common conditions can also cause occlusive disease.

   1. The **SFA** is the artery most frequently involved. Disease usually occurs at the adductor muscle hiatus (Hunter's canal), where the SFA passes through the adductor muscle group to form the popliteal artery. When focal stenoses become critical, the entire SFA occludes; the profunda (deep) femoral artery provides collateral blood flow to maintain flow to the popliteal artery distally.

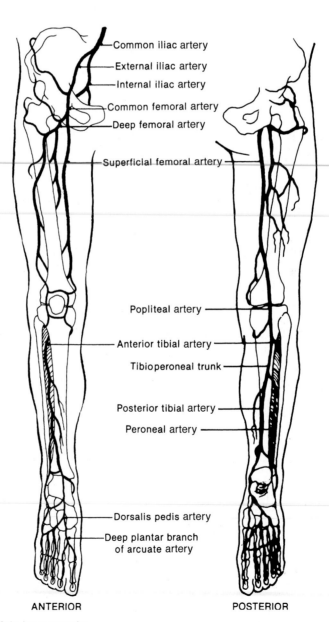

Common iliac artery
External iliac artery
Internal iliac artery
Common femoral artery
Deep femoral artery
Superficial femoral artery
Popliteal artery
Anterior tibial artery
Tibioperoneal trunk
Posterior tibial artery
Peroneal artery
Dorsalis pedis artery
Deep plantar branch of arcuate artery

ANTERIOR   POSTERIOR

FIGURE 7-1   Arteries of the lower extremity.

2. The **profunda (deep) femoral artery** supplies blood to the thigh. The origin of this vessel may be involved with atherosclerosis, but the remaining distal vessel is usually spared. A heavily diseased distal profunda is typical in diabetic patients.

3. The **popliteal artery** frequently harbors atherosclerosis. Other causes of occlusive disease in this artery include entrapment by the gastrocnemius muscle (**popliteal entrapment**) and cysts in the adventitia of the artery (**cystic adventitial disease**). These latter two conditions, which are more rare, may be found in younger patients.

4. **Tibial artery** atherosclerosis is common in elderly patients and in those with diabetes mellitus.

B **Clinical presentation**   Atherosclerosis of the lower extremities is frequently asymptomatic, provided that the collateral flow around the existing lesions is good. When collaterals are inadequate or are compromised by atherosclerosis or multilevel disease, symptoms occur in a predictable pattern.

1. **Claudication** is pain felt in the large muscle groups distal to an arterial lesion after exercise. Given that the most common site of atherosclerosis in the lower extremity is the SFA, claudication typically occurs in the calf after walking. Key features of vascular claudication are its **reproducible** occurrence at a consistent walking distance and its prompt **relief** by rest (within minutes). It is caused by muscle group exertion, not by standing or sitting for prolonged periods. The patient is asymptomatic at rest because the blood flow through collaterals is adequate at rest, but blood flow is inadequate for the increased metabolic demands of exercise.
   a. **Natural history.** Claudication is not considered a limb-threatening condition. The prognosis of the affected limb is relatively good, with only 10% of patients progressing to severe ischemia or limb loss in 10 years.
   b. **Survival.** Patients with claudication frequently have diffuse atherosclerosis. The long-term survival of these patients is more guarded, being 73% at 5 years and 38% at 10 years. The most common cause of death is associated atherosclerotic heart disease.

2. **Ischemic rest pain** results from severe compromise of arterial flow. Here, the collateral blood supply is inadequate to supply the metabolic demands of the tissues, even at rest. Patients describe intense pain across the distal foot and arch, exacerbated by elevating the foot (e.g., while trying to sleep in bed). Patients will typically try to obtain relief of pain by placing the foot in a dependent position or by walking slowly. **Natural history:** Rest pain is considered a limb-threatening condition because most patients (85% at 5 years) will suffer limb (i.e., major) amputation if revascularization is not performed or is not possible.

3. **Gangrene** refers to tissue necrosis and occurs when blood flow is inadequate to maintain tissue viability. The term **wet gangrene** refers to the presence of infection within nonviable tissue (as opposed to **dry gangrene**). Tissue loss typically begins with a nonhealing ulcer located in the most distal vascular bed, i.e, the toes. These ulcers are generally painful and well demarcated. **Natural history:** Like rest pain, gangrene is a limb-threatening condition. Necrotic tissue, especially if infected, should be debrided, and revascularization should be performed to avoid major amputation.

C **Evaluation**   As with most disease processes in medicine and surgery, diagnosis of lower extremity peripheral vascular disease begins with a sound history and physical examination. Noninvasive laboratory testing follows to confirm the diagnosis or establish current patient baselines. Invasive testing (e.g., arteriography) is generally reserved for revascularization planning and is not used for simple diagnosis.

1. **History.** The various clinical presentations are described previously. Detailed characterization of these presentations should include:
   a. **Claudication:** major muscle groups involved (buttock, thigh, and/or calf), distance required to reproduce it, time of rest required for relief, how long it has been present, and whether its onset was acute or gradual. Differential diagnosis includes neurogenic claudication, which is lower extremity pain produced by lumbar spinal stenosis and subsequent nerve irritation. A history of back pain, associated with burning or electric-type pain shooting down the posterior leg, which may be combined with numbness/paresthesias, is characteristic of neurogenic claudication.

b. **Ischemic rest pain:** location and characterization of pain within the foot, what is done for relief, how long the pain has been present, and whether its onset was acute or gradual. Differential diagnosis includes arthritic pain and diabetic peripheral neuropathy.

c. **Gangrene:** location of the tissue loss, history of local trauma, evidence of infection (fevers, purulent drainage, local pain), and how long it has been present. Differential diagnosis of nonhealing foot ulcers in diabetic patients includes neuropathic ulceration and underlying osteomyelitis.

d. **Risk factors for atherosclerosis:** detailed questioning regarding history of diabetes mellitus, hypertension, tobacco abuse, hypercholesterolemia, and family history of atherosclerosis.

e. **Cardiopulmonary assessment:** thorough history and review of systems concerning the patient's cardiac and pulmonary history, including history of myocardial infarction, congestive heart failure, arrhythmia, chronic obstructive pulmonary disease, and exercise tolerance. Results of recent cardiac stress testing, catheterization procedures, and pulmonary function tests, if available, should be reviewed.

f. **Neurological assessment:** History of cerebrovascular accident, transient ischemic attack, or amaurosis fugax (see VII A 3) should be obtained as well as the results of recent carotid duplex imaging tests, if available.

g. **Renal assessment:** History of chronic renal insufficiency and prior blood urea nitrogen/creatinine levels should be reviewed, especially for patients who may need arteriographic assessment.

2. **Physical examination.** A thorough physical examination should be performed for general evaluation as well as for specific vascular diagnosis.

a. **General evaluation.** All patients with peripheral vascular disease should be assessed for neurological, cardiac, and pulmonary disease. Complete neurological assessment includes auscultation of carotid bruits as well as cranial nerve, sensory, and motor examinations. Diabetic patients should undergo two-point discrimination or light touch testing of the feet to rule out peripheral neuropathy. Cardiopulmonary examination should rule out evidence of active congestive heart failure, cardiac valvular disease, or evidence of chronic obstructive pulmonary disease.

b. **Specific vascular evaluation.** The pulse examination, performed by an experienced clinician, is the most important part of the physical examination for diagnosing peripheral vascular disease. The presence of normal, diminished, or absent pulses should be noted at the femoral, popliteal, and pedal (dorsalis pedis and posterior tibial) levels. Auscultation of abdominal, pelvic, and femoral bruits indicates turbulent blood flow, and hence atherosclerotic stenoses, at the aortoiliac and femoral arterial segments. Additional note should be made of enlarged abdominal aortic pulsations as well as popliteal pulsations, suggesting aneurysmal disease at these levels. Lower extremity skin changes should be carefully documented, including:

(1) **Ischemic ulcerations.** These usually are punctate and located distally in the foot.

(2) **Elevation pallor/dependent rubor,** noted in the foot. These indicate severe chronic peripheral vascular disease.

(3) **Trophic changes,** noted in the skin. These include a shiny appearance to the skin, loss of hair, and diminished nail growth.

3. **Noninvasive vascular laboratory testing.** When history and physical examination suggest the presence of vascular disease, noninvasive testing is performed to confirm the diagnosis and to establish current patient baselines.

a. **Segmental arterial blood pressures** are obtained at each arterial segment within the lower extremity, namely the thigh, calf, ankle, and toes. Systolic pressures obtained at each of these levels correspond to the pressure within underlying arterial segments, namely the aortoiliac, femoral-popliteal, tibial, and digital segments, respectively. The brachial pressure is obtained as a reference.

(1) In the supine position, each of the lower extremity pressures should be greater than or equal to the brachial pressure. A pressure drop >20 mm Hg between segments indicates arterial obstruction within the underlying segment.

(2) The **ankle brachial index (ABI)** is the ankle pressure compared with that of the brachial artery (i.e., ABI = ankle systolic pressure divided by the highest brachial systolic pressure). In general, a patient's ABI correlates with his or her functional status.

(a) **1.00** represents a normal ABI.

     (b) 0.5–0.99 is consistent with a history of claudication.

     (c) 0.2–0.49 is consistent with a history of ischemic rest pain.

     (d) <0.20 represents impending tissue loss.

(3) Exercise testing can be used to increase the sensitivity of ankle pressure testing. After exercise, the ankle pressure (or ABI) should remain normal or increase. In a patient who has claudication but is found to have a normal ABI at rest, a decrease of ABI >0.20 after exercise indicates that symptoms may be due to peripheral vascular disease.

(4) Sources of error in segmental pressure testing include:

     (a) Abnormal cuff width. The ideal cuff width is 1.2 times the limb diameter.

     (b) Noncompressible arteries. Vessels that are calcified will not compress normally using the standard blood pressure cuff and will yield falsely elevated pressures. The tibial vessels of diabetic patients commonly are noncompressible.

  b. Segmental waveform analysis. Similar to pressure measurements, two types of waveforms can be obtained from each arterial segment, namely **Doppler waveforms** and **pulse-volume recordings.**

    (1) Doppler waveforms are obtained by recording the Doppler signal over each of the lower extremity arteries. A normal waveform, indicating normal blood flow up to that segment, is polyphasic. As blood flow diminishes to a segment, it becomes monophasic.

    (2) Pulse-volume recordings measure the volume change in a limb under an inflated cuff with each cardiac cycle. A normal waveform has a sharp upstroke, with a dicrotic notch in diastole. As blood flow diminishes to a segment, the notch disappears, and the upstroke diminishes.

    (3) The **morphology** of these waveforms is generally not influenced by compressibility of the vessels. Waveform analysis, therefore, serves as a complementary test to segmental pressure testing.

4. Arteriography. Invasive testing, as mentioned previously, is reserved for patients who are intended to undergo some form of arterial revascularization (see Treatment, II D). Because of the invasive nature of the test, it is generally not used solely to make the diagnosis of peripheral vascular disease.

  a. Technique. During conventional arteriography of the lower extremity, contrast media is injected into the abdominal aorta by utilizing catheters placed through a femoral artery puncture. As the media flows distally within the arterial tree, images are recorded either fluoroscopically (**digital subtraction arteriography**) or on conventional film (**cut film arteriography**).

  b. Complications. Arteriography generally can be performed with a low rate of complications.

    (1) Contrast media complications

      (a) Dye-induced nephrotoxicity may cause acute tubular necrosis following an arteriogram. Risk factors include diabetes mellitus, dehydration, advanced age, elevated creatinine level, and total dye load. It generally presents 1–2 days after the examination and may produce a high-output renal failure. Prevention with periprocedure hydration and limiting the dye load (using CO_2 as a contrast agent and digital subtraction techniques) are helpful. Treatment is supportive.

      (b) Dye allergy may result in cutaneous flushing and itching, but if serious, it can cause cardiovascular collapse. Risk factors include prior history of dye allergy and shellfish sensitivity. Preprocedural steroid and antihistamine administration, as well as using low-ionic contrast media, are helpful in avoiding this complication.

    (2) Arterial complications

      (a) Arterial thrombosis may result from pericatheter thrombus formation or direct trauma to the diseased arterial wall (i.e., dissection).

      (b) Atheroembolization during an arteriogram refers to the disruption of an arterial plaque by a catheter, with subsequent discharge of debris distally. This may result in ischemic "blue" toes after the examination. Treatment is supportive.

    (3) Puncture site complications

      (a) Hematoma, if large, may result in adjacent nerve compression and damage or in necrosis of the overlying skin. The brachial plexus is at particular risk if hematoma forms within the axillary sheath following an axillary artery approach for arteriography. Treatment under these conditions is prompt surgical decompression.

(b) Pseudoaneurysm may also result if hemostasis is not properly achieved. False aneurysms larger than 2 cm are at risk for rupture. **Ultrasound-guided compression** of the neck of the pseudoaneurysm is used to produce thrombosis within the false cavity; those arteries not successfully treated by this method are repaired surgically.

5. **Magnetic resonance angiography (MRA)** is rapidly becoming a more accurate and common method of assessing the arterial circulation. Its main advantage over conventional arteriography is that MRA avoids the invasive complications noted previously. Successful MRA requires radiologists with specific training in this area as well as special hardware designed for angiographic imaging.

D **Treatment** options for lower extremity occlusive disease are generally based on the patient's symptoms. Asymptomatic patients with arterial occlusions do not require surgery. The decision to perform a revascularization procedure on a symptomatic patient depends on the natural history of the present symptom. **Claudication** is not considered a limb-threatening condition; revascularization is considered only in patients with incapacitating symptoms. The presence of **ischemic rest pain** or **tissue loss** is considered a limb-threatening condition, and revascularization needs to be considered strongly for limb salvage.

1. **Medical treatment.** In patients without limb threat (i.e., claudication), medical treatment is most appropriate.
   a. **Risk factor modification.** The **cessation of tobacco** abuse represents the most important risk factor to control. Treatment of hyperlipidemia, hypertension, and diabetes mellitus is generally important for long-term prognosis.
   b. **Pentoxifylline** is approved for the treatment of intermittent claudication. It reduces whole blood viscosity by decreasing plasma fibrinogen and platelet aggregation. After a 6–8 week course of treatment, approximately one half of patients will double their walking distance. If a positive effect is gained, the medication is continued indefinitely. One of the few adverse effects is gastrointestinal upset.
   c. **Exercise program.** A walking program for patients with claudication, during which they attempt increasingly farther walking distances, has been successful in alleviating some symptoms. Improved collateral circulation and modification of muscle group usage are proposed but unproven mechanisms for this effect.

2. **Percutaneous intervention.** For patients who are intended to undergo revascularization, arteriography is performed. Those who are found to have focal stenoses or occlusions, generally in the iliac or femoral vessels, are considered candidates for percutaneous procedures at the time of the arteriogram.
   a. **Percutaneous transluminal angioplasty (PTA).**
      (1) **Technique.** An inflatable balloon catheter is fluoroscopically guided over a wire through the stenotic area. The balloon is then inflated to 4–8 atm to fracture the plaque, restoring patency to the artery.
      (2) **Results.** Patency rates vary with the anatomic location and character of the stenosis. The larger, proximal arteries, such as the common iliac arteries, show more durable results than the distal femoral, popliteal, or tibial vessels. Lesions that are focal, short, and concentric also have better long-term results.
   b. **Stents** may be used as an adjunct to percutaneous angioplasty. They are expandable metal mesh conduits inserted over a balloon catheter. The balloon is inflated within the lesion to expand the stent, is deflated, and then is withdrawn. Stents are indicated to prevent recoil of a lesion after angioplasty and to "tack down" an area of dissection. Currently, drug-eluting stents are used in the coronary circulation to impede the process of restenosis. Similarly, investigation is under way to evaluate this technology in larger circulatory beds where stents have been less durable, such as the SFA.
   c. **Complications**
      (1) **Atheroembolism.** Clinically significant embolism of atherosclerotic debris follows this procedure in less than 3% of cases. Small vessel atheroembolism (e.g., "blue toe syndrome") is treated conservatively. Large vessel embolism may be treated with thrombolytic therapy or operative intervention.

(2) Intimal hyperplasia. As with any form of arterial injury, lesions treated with angioplasty may produce an exuberant healing response, resulting in restenosis of the lesion. These lesions are generally responsible for failures within 2 years of the angioplasty. It is not proven that stents prevent this occurrence. Repeat angioplasty can be successful in treating this event.

(3) Thrombosis. Acute thrombosis of the artery may occur secondary to in situ thrombus formation or dissection of the treated lesion. Treatment may involve thrombolytic therapy, stenting, or operative intervention.

(4) Rupture. With careful measurements of the lumen of the artery to undergo angioplasty, this complication can be kept to a minimum.

3. **Surgical interventions.** For patients intended to undergo revascularization, arteriography is performed. If a percutaneous intervention is not suitable, surgical revascularization methods are used, provided the patient is a suitable medical risk for surgery.
   a. **Indications.** The indications for surgery are the same as the indications for revascularization in general.
   (1) **Incapacitating claudication.** Because the natural history of claudication is generally benign, without limb loss, surgery to relieve this symptom is considered solely elective. If the symptoms interfere with a patient's desired lifestyle or ability to work, surgery may be offered. Ideally, the patient should be a good medical risk, having undergone a period of failed medical therapy (exercise program, risk factor modification).
   (2) **Rest pain.** Presentation with rest pain suggests severe arterial insufficiency. Surgical revascularization is considered for limb salvage and should be offered to all, except those with prohibitive medical comorbidities.
   (3) **Tissue loss.** Like rest pain, tissue loss is considered a limb-threatening condition. Surgical revascularization is offered, unless specific contraindications exist.
   b. **Contraindications.** Surgical therapy is indicated for the previously noted symptoms, unless the following conditions exist.
   (1) **Nonambulatory status**
   (2) **Nonreconstructible vessels.** When arteriography does not reveal a patent distal vessel (popliteal, tibial, or dorsalis pedis) with adequate runoff to support a graft, surgical reconstruction should not be attempted.
   (3) **Extensive tissue loss.** If the foot is not considered salvageable because of either extensive gangrene precluding an appropriate foot amputation or extensive infection such as widespread osteomyelitis, amputation at the below-knee or above-knee level is indicated.
   (4) **Prohibitive medical comorbidities.** If coexisting medical conditions make an extensive revascularization procedure too risky, the patient may undergo amputation or medical therapy for the rest pain or tissue loss.
   c. **Operative procedures.** Because the most common lesions of lower extremity occlusive disease involve long segment occlusions of the femoral-popliteal system, **bypass** of the occluded arteries is the most common procedure. For the rarer focal lesions in the femoral system, **local endarterectomy** accompanied by a patch angioplasty may be appropriate.
   (1) **Inflow vessel.** The most common site for proximal anastomosis in constructing a bypass is the common femoral artery. In the diabetic population, in which the occlusive disease may be isolated to the tibial vessels, the popliteal artery may be a suitable inflow vessel.
   (2) **Outflow vessel.** The most appropriate outflow vessel in constructing a bypass is the artery with the best unobstructed distal outflow. The above-knee and below-knee popliteal arteries, each of the three tibial vessels (posterior, anterior, and peroneal), and the dorsalis pedis artery all are used for distal anastomosis. The **name** of a specific bypass is derived by using the names of the inflow and outflow vessels (e.g., femoral-popliteal bypass).
   (3) **Conduit.** Many types of conduits have been used, depending on the availability of ipsilateral greater saphenous vein.
   (a) **Greater saphenous vein (GSV).** The ipsilateral greater saphenous vein is the conduit of choice in lower extremity revascularization procedures. It is generally excised and placed in a **reversed** position, without the need for lysing the valves. For femoral-tibial bypasses, reversal of the vein creates a size discrepancy at each anastomosis. In this situation, the GSV is left **in situ,** and the valves are lysed and the vein branches ligated.

(b) Other autogenous veins. In the absence of usable GSV, the **lesser saphenous vein** as well as **arm veins** may be used with acceptable results.

(c) Prosthetic conduits. Polytetrafluoroethylene and Dacron bypass grafts have been used with near-equal success to the GSV in the above-knee position. Prosthetic grafts overall have poor patency rates when used in vessels below the knee. Adjuncts to prosthetic grafting to the tibial vessels designed to improve patency rates include the creation of an **arteriovenous fistula** as well as a venous cuff (**Miller cuff**) or patch (**Taylor patch**) at the distal anastomosis.

(4) Results

(a) Primary patency of a bypass refers to the length of time the graft remains patent without any type of intervention, either surgical or percutaneous. The primary patency rates of most GSV bypass grafts range between 65%–80% at 5 years. Limb salvage rates are even higher, generally being 90% at 5 years.

(b) Assisted primary patency refers to a graft that has always remained patent but has required some sort of intervention, either surgical or percutaneous, to maintain adequate blood flow through it.

(c) Secondary patency refers to a graft that has thrombosed and has had patency restored with either thrombolytic therapy or operative thrombectomy.

4. Amputation. Without revascularization, most patients with severe limb-threatening ischemia eventually suffer limb loss.

a. Indications. Patients with rest pain or tissue loss who are **not** candidates for revascularization are generally treated medically, unless one of the following conditions exists:

(1) Intractable rest pain. If ischemic rest pain cannot be managed with a reasonable amount of pain medication, amputation is appropriate.

(2) Sepsis. Patients with tissue loss, complicated by systemic sepsis, undergo amputation to remove the source of infection.

b. Level. In general, the more distal the amputation is, the more functional the patient's gait will be. The more proximal the amputation, however, the better chance it will have to heal without significant complications. Clinical evaluation by an experienced surgeon is the best predictor of amputation-level healing. Clinical indicators of healing include:

(1) Pulses. In general, there should be a palpable pulse at least one level above the proposed amputation site (e.g., present femoral pulse for healing a below-knee amputation).

(2) Skin temperature and capillary refill. The skin of the proposed amputation site should be soft, warm, and well perfused. The presence of gangrenous changes or dependent rubor precludes healing at that level.

(3) Noninvasive tests. A good pulse-volume recording waveform or pressure >50 mm Hg at the level of the amputation predicts healing.

c. Procedures

(1) Digital amputation transects the proximal phalanx and is associated with minimal gait disturbance.

(2) Ray amputation refers to the amputation of a single digit and its metatarsal head and is associated with minimal gait disturbance.

(3) Transmetatarsal amputation refers to the amputation of the forefoot, transecting the five metatarsal bones midshaft, with a posteriorly based flap. There is minimal gait disturbance postoperatively.

(4) Below-knee amputation transects the tibia and fibula a palm's breadth below the tibial plateau, with coverage achieved by a longer posterior flap. Ambulation with a unilateral below-knee amputation can be achieved in 70%–100% of patients. Energy expenditure for ambulation is increased 10%–40% over bipedal gait.

(5) Above-knee amputation transects the femur at the distal third of the shaft. The anterior and posterior flaps are generally equal. Ambulation with a unilateral above-knee amputation can be achieved in 10%–40% of patients. Energy expenditure for ambulation is increased 70%–100% over bipedal gait, approaching that of crutch walking. Patients with bilateral above-knee amputations are uniformly rendered nonambulatory.

d. Prognosis. Patients who undergo a major limb amputation (below-knee amputation, above-knee amputation) for vascular disease have a significant **perioperative mortality rate** of up to 10%, predominantly for cardiac disease. Up to 50% of patients will also undergo **contralateral amputation** within 3 years. The **long-term mortality** rate following amputation is 50% at 3 years and 70% at 5 years.

III AORTOILIAC OCCLUSIVE DISEASE

A Pathology Aortoiliac occlusive disease is caused by atherosclerosis extending from the distal aorta through the iliac system down to the femoral level (Fig. 7-2). Less commonly, atherosclerosis is isolated to the distal aorta and common iliac arteries.

B Clinical presentation

1. **Symptoms**
   a. **Claudication** most commonly involves the buttock, thigh, and calves. Distal ischemic rest pain and tissue loss is rarely encountered unless more distal disease is present. **Leriche syndrome,** originally described as hypoplasia of the distal aorta, refers to the triad of buttock and thigh claudication, absent femoral pulses, and impotence (males).
   b. **Distal atheroembolism** refers to the rupture of atherosclerotic plaques and subsequent microembolism of the distal circulation. In aortoiliac disease, this may result in **"blue toe syndrome."** The syndrome may be unilateral or bilateral in aortic atherosclerosis; for disease isolated to an iliac vessel, the syndrome is unilateral.

2. **Physical examination** reveals diminished or absent femoral (and subsequently distal) pulses. Bruits of the pelvis may be heard. In cases of atheroembolism, the pulses generally remain intact, with painful, tender, dysvascular toe(s).

C Evaluation The evaluation for aortoiliac occlusive disease is similar to that for lower extremity occlusive disease, outlined previously.

1. **Noninvasive testing.** In patients presenting with claudication, segmental pressure and waveform analysis reveal abnormalities beginning at the thigh level. In cases of atheroembolism, pressures and waveforms may be normal throughout, with the exception of blunted waveforms in the affected toes.

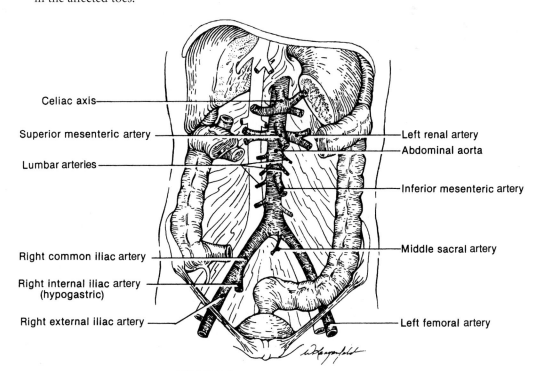

FIGURE 7-2 Arteries of the abdomen.

2. Arteriography. Similar to the evaluation for symptomatic lower extremity occlusive disease, conventional arteriography is reserved for patients who are intended to undergo revascularization, either surgical or percutaneous. Often, arteriography requires a brachial artery approach because the cannulation of the aorta may be difficult from one of the common femoral arteries. Arteriography is indicated in most cases of spontaneous atheroembolism, despite the presence of distal pulses, to identify and treat the offending lesion.

D **Treatment**   The treatment algorithm for aortoiliac disease is similar to that for lower extremity occlusive disease, outlined previously. Patients with asymptomatic atherosclerosis of the aortoiliac segment do not require treatment. For patients with claudication, an attempt at medical therapy, involving an exercise program, risk factor modification, and pentoxifylline, should be instituted prior to consideration for revascularization.

1. **Revascularization is indicated** in patients with aortoiliac disease, via either percutaneous or surgical means, for the same reasons as lower extremity occlusive symptoms:
   a. **Incapacitating claudication**
   b. **Ischemic rest pain**
   c. **Tissue loss**

2. **Percutaneous intervention.** Angioplasty and stenting of aortoiliac segment is the preferred procedure for focal, short-segment stenoses or occlusions. Bilateral lesions can generally be treated via a single common femoral artery approach. In cases of distal aortic stenosis or high-grade bilateral common iliac artery lesions, simultaneously inserted **"kissing" stents** are placed at the same level of the distal aorta through each common iliac artery.

3. **Operative procedures.** Symptomatic patients who are not candidates for percutaneous interventions may be offered surgical therapy for relief, provided they are good risks for surgery. Two techniques are available to improve inflow in one or both lower extremities.
   a. **Aortoiliac endarterectomy.** For patients with shorter-segment occlusion/stenosis of the distal aorta and common iliac arteries, open surgical removal of the plaque and adjacent medial layers will restore patency to the system. Concomitant diffuse disease of the external iliac arteries warrants against endarterectomy and necessitates bypass. Many patients with localized disease who previously were treated with endarterectomy or bypass now undergo percutaneous procedures, obviating the need for this extensive surgery.
   b. **Bypass procedures.** In patients with diffuse disease of the aorta, iliac, and femoral systems not amenable to angioplasty and stenting, a bypass procedure is the **treatment of choice.** In each of these procedures, unlike the infrainguinal bypasses described previously, **prosthetic conduits** (either polytetrafluoroethylene or Dacron) are preferred.
      (1) **Aortobifemoral bypass** represents the gold standard in revascularization procedures for inflow disease.
         (a) **Proximal anastomosis.** Ideally, this is placed as close to the renal arteries as possible to avoid proximal anastomotic failure should the disease progress proximally. The anastomosis is generally performed **end-to-end;** in this case, the pelvis is perfused retrograde back up the external iliac systems. In situations in which the pelvic blood flow would be compromised by an end-to-end configuration, an **end-to-side** aortic anastomosis is created, maintaining antegrade flow to the pelvis. There is no proven difference in long-term graft function between the two techniques.
         (b) **Distal anastomoses.** Because of the diffuse nature of the disease, the bifurcated graft limbs are tunneled retroperitoneally, behind the ureters, and down to the common femoral arteries. Distal anastomoses are then performed in an **end-to-side** fashion. On occasion, anastomoses may be made to the iliac systems; in these cases, the advantage lies in avoiding groin wounds and possible future graft infection.
      (2) **Extra-anatomic bypass.** The contralateral common femoral artery and the axillary artery may be used as alternate inflow sources for aortoiliac disease. These procedures avoid the morbidities associated with aortic cross clamping and laparotomy.
         (a) **Femoral-femoral bypass** may be the preferred procedure for patients with unilateral iliac disease. The cross-femoral prosthetic conduit is tunneled subcutaneously or in the **space of Retzius** (behind the rectus muscles).

      (b) **Axillobifemoral bypass** is preferred in patients with extensive, bilateral aortoiliac disease who otherwise could not tolerate aortobifemoral bypass. The conduit is tunneled subcutaneously. The procedure can be performed with low mortality rates by using local anesthesia with sedation. This procedure may also be used for treatment of **aortic graft infection** in combination with removal of the infected abdominal graft.

    (3) **Results.** The best results are achieved with aortic grafting, yielding up to 85% 10-year primary patency rates. Femoral-femoral grafts can achieve up to 75% 5-year primary patency rates. Axillobifemoral grafts achieve more variable 5-year patencies, between 50% and 70%, depending on patient selection.

IV ACUTE ARTERIAL INSUFFICIENCY OF THE LOWER EXTREMITY

Acute limb ischemia, unlike chronic ischemia, may lead to irreversible tissue loss within hours if rapid diagnosis and restoration of flow are not achieved.

A **Pathology**   These are two general causes of limb ischemia.

  1. **Embolism** refers to the translocation of material within the arterial stream to a more distal site, resulting in the acute interruption of blood flow at that level. Larger (**macro**) emboli will lodge at a distal bifurcation, the most common site being the common femoral artery, followed by the aortoiliac system and popliteal arteries. Smaller (**micro**) embolic debris generally lodges in the distal tibial system or digital arteries (**"blue toe syndrome"**). **Sources** of emboli include:

    a. **Cardiac pathology.** Eighty-five percent of cases originate from the heart.

      (1) **Atrial thrombus.** Patients with atrial fibrillation may develop thrombus within the atria, especially in the atrial appendage. This arrhythmia is present in 50% to 80% of patients diagnosed with embolism. Atrial cardiac myxoma may also embolize distally.

      (2) **Ventricular thrombus.** Mural thrombus may form following a myocardial infarction or within a ventricular aneurysm.

      (3) **Valves** damaged from rheumatic heart disease may produce microemboli.

      (4) **A patent foramen ovale** may allow a paradoxical embolism to travel from the venous circulation into the arterial circulation.

    b. **Proximal arterial pathology.** Arterial-arterial embolism may also occur from several sources.

      (1) **Atherosclerotic plaques** may serve as a nidus for thrombus or platelet aggregates that embolize distally, or they may rupture, discharging smaller debris (**atheroembolization**).

      (2) An **aneurysm** of an arterial segment, most commonly the infrarenal aorta or popliteal arteries, may harbor a mural thrombus that may embolize distally.

  2. **In situ thrombosis** of an arterial segment may result in acute ischemia. This may occur in two settings.

    a. **Thrombosis** of a chronically diseased vessel, most commonly the SFA or popliteal arteries, may cause acute ischemia if collateral circulation is poorly developed or compromised by the in situ thrombosis.

    b. **Hypercoagulable states** may cause arterial thrombosis, even if the arterial segment is normal. This generally occurs in the more distal segments, such as the tibial vessels or pedal arches.

B **Clinical presentation** of acute lower extremity ischemia is generally dramatic because the patient generally can identify the exact moment of sudden change in his or her arterial circulation. The "**5 Ps**" define this syndrome:

  1. **Pain** is characteristic of essentially all patients with acute ischemia. It is distinguished from chronic ischemic pain because of its acute onset and unrelenting severity. Over several hours of acute ischemia, the limb may become anesthetic as neural function is lost.

  2. **Pallor** associated with coolness of the extremity usually occurs at one level below the acute arterial occlusion. Additional signs may include mottling of the extremity and flat veins.

  3. **Paralysis** of the limb results, as muscle function is severely compromised. This finding may occur several hours after the acute event and heralds limb loss if blood flow is not restored promptly.

4. Paresthesias signify severe neural dysfunction and also herald impending limb loss. An insensate limb is generally considered nonviable.

5. Pulselessness. The absence of pulses, especially if the contralateral limb has intact pulses, may help to identify the level of occlusion. Patients with chronic limb ischemia will also have absent pulses but will generally have Doppler signals distally. In contrast, patients with severe acute ischemia usually will not have detectable Doppler signals distally because their collaterals may not be developed enough to support distal flow.

C Evaluation Rapid assessment of the level of acute occlusion is generally performed via physical examination. Comparison with the contralateral extremity, involving level of pulselessness, temperature, and mottling, is generally useful, especially if the contralateral examination is normal. Documentation of motor and sensory examination results are critical; if these results are present, further workup is not performed and the patient is taken directly to the operating room for treatment.

1. Noninvasive examinations. Other than the documentation of the lowest level of signals measurable by Doppler, noninvasive examinations generally are not performed in the interest of time.

2. Arteriography. If the motor and sensory systems are intact, the patient might benefit from arteriographic information defining the level of occlusion and distal reconstitution. This is especially true in the patient with evidence of chronic arterial insufficiency (by history or examination of the contralateral limb) with an acute change because in situ thrombosis may be the cause of the acute ischemia.

D Treatment Management of acute arterial occlusion includes rapid diagnosis and expeditious surgical correction of the occlusion.

1. Heparin therapy. Initial therapy for patients with acute arterial ischemia is intravenous anticoagulation with heparin, unless there is a specific contraindication to heparin (such as heparin-induced thrombocytopenia). This should be given as a bolus of 100 U/kg and continued empirically at 1,000 U/hour up to the time of surgery.

2. Hydration. Patients should be given adequate hydration to maintain high urine output (preferably 100 mL/hour). Alkalinization of the urine and osmotic diuresis (mannitol) are used to protect the kidney from damage due to myoglobinuria in patients with prolonged, severe ischemia.

3. Revascularization. Restoration of blood flow to an ischemic extremity provides definitive treatment. In severe ischemia of the lower limb, this ideally is performed within 6 hours of the onset of the acute event to avoid irreparable nerve and muscle damage.

   a. Surgical therapy. Following heparinization, the patient is generally taken directly to the operating room for revascularization, especially if motor and sensory changes are present.

   (1) Embolectomy is the procedure of choice in cases of macroembolism to a larger artery, such as the common femoral artery. It is performed by introducing a balloon-tipped catheter through a transverse arteriotomy at the level of the occlusion. The catheter is advanced through the embolus (and trailing thrombus). Inflation of the balloon and withdrawal of the catheter extracts the thrombus. Completion arteriography determines the adequacy of the thromboembolectomy procedure. Morbidity and mortality are generally related to the patient's underlying medical problems.

   (2) Bypass. In cases of thrombosis, or when adequate thromboembolectomy cannot be performed, surgical bypass as described previously for chronic arterial insufficiency is necessary for revascularization. If preoperative arteriography has not been performed, intraoperative arteriography is performed to determine the level of distal arterial runoff.

   b. Thrombolytic therapy. In selected patients, such as those with prior vascular interventions, lytic therapy may be used for revascularization. Agents such as **tissue plasminogen activator** and **urokinase** have been used in this setting to dissolve the acutely formed thrombus. Advantages include the possibility of correcting the underlying cause of the thrombosis with angioplasty (avoiding surgery altogether) or with a more limited surgical procedure. **Contraindications** include the presence of sensory and motor changes on presentation (because lytic therapy frequently requires >24 hours of treatment), recent (<2 weeks) surgery, and known intracranial pathology.

4. **Postoperative care.** Patients who have suffered an embolic event should have a complete cardiac evaluation (echocardiogram and Holter monitor) to search for an embolic source. These patients should receive anticoagulation therapy to reduce the incidence of recurrent embolic events. Those with in situ thrombosis who undergo bypass are generally treated without further anticoagulation unless a hypercoagulable state is suspected. **Complications** of the treatment of acute ischemia include:

   a. **Compartment syndrome.** Reperfusion injury to the muscle may result in swelling and increased compartment pressures within the fascial spaces of the calf. If untreated, capillary perfusion is cut off, resulting in neurological injury (usually foot drop) and/or further tissue loss. Clinical presentation includes calf pain, especially with passive stretch; tenderness; and loss of sensation in the first digital web space. Performing four compartment **fasciotomies** is the treatment of choice.

   b. **Myoglobinuria.** With severe ischemia, necrosis of muscle leads to the release of myoglobin into the bloodstream. Myoglobin is filtered by the kidneys and is nephrotoxic. Diagnosis is suggested by the presence of heme on urine dipstick in the absence of red blood cells by microscopic urinalysis. Definitive diagnosis is made by detection of myoglobin in the urine. **Treatment** is generally supportive, maintaining high urine output while the urine is positive for myoglobin.

V MESENTERIC VASCULAR DISEASE

Mesenteric vascular disease may present as an acute life-threatening emergency or as a chronic debilitating problem. The involved arteries include the **celiac axis (CA), superior mesenteric artery (SMA)** and **inferior mesenteric artery (IMA)** arising from the anterior surface of the abdominal aorta.

A **Acute mesenteric ischemia** is a surgical emergency with an 80% mortality rate. Classically, severe abdominal pain out of proportion to physical findings suggests the diagnosis. In the early stages of acute mesenteric ischemia, these patients are often writhing in agony without evidence of peritonitis. If diagnosis or treatment is delayed, transmural infarction of bowel results in peritoneal irritation and more pronounced physical signs.

1. **Etiology.** Acute occlusion of the mesenteric arteries may result from:

   a. **Embolization.** The usual site of distal embolization is the SMA, generally several centimeters distal to the origin (at the level of the middle colic artery). As with lower extremity embolism, the source of embolism is usually the heart (atrial fibrillation or myocardial infarction).

   b. **Thrombosis.** Sudden occlusion of pre-existing atherosclerotic lesions of the visceral vessels may cause acute mesenteric ischemia. Because mesenteric atherosclerosis usually involves the origin of the artery, thrombosis also begins at the origin of the vessel. These patients will frequently admit to the presence of pre-existing symptoms of chronic mesenteric ischemia.

   c. **Nonocclusive mesenteric ischemia** is due to states of low flow to the mesenteric arteries, as seen in cardiogenic shock. It has been recognized in patients after cardiopulmonary bypass and in patients requiring high doses of intravenous vasoconstrictors and inotropes (e.g., epinephrine).

2. **Diagnosis and treatment.** Saving these patients depends on a high index of suspicion and prompt diagnosis and treatment. All patients suspected of acute mesenteric ischemia should have their cardiac status optimized while being aggressively volume resuscitated and treated with broad-spectrum antibiotics.

   a. **Angiography** of the abdominal aorta and mesenteric arteries is performed if acute mesenteric ischemia is suspected. Subsequent treatment is based on the arteriographic findings.

      (1) If embolus is found (usually involving the SMA), prompt surgical **embolectomy** is performed. Subsequent anticoagulation is given, assuming a cardiac source.

      (2) If thrombosis is found (usually involving the origins of the CA and SMA), urgent **aortomesenteric bypass** is performed. A prosthetic bypass is usually used, except in the presence of bowel infarction (then, GSV is preferred).

      (3) The treatment of nonocclusive mesenteric ischemia involves direct **arterial infusion of vasodilators** (i.e., papaverine or nitroglycerine) into the SMA. Supportive care to optimize cardiac output and reverse the low-flow state is critical.

   b. Following embolectomy or reconstruction, the bowel is assessed for viability. Overtly necrotic bowel is resected. If marginal viability is present in the remaining bowel, it should be left in place. A **second-look laparotomy** should be done in 24 hours to ensure viability of the residual bowel. Patients with nonocclusive mesenteric ischemia who develop peritoneal signs should undergo laparotomy to rule out necrotic bowel.

B **Chronic mesenteric ischemia** results from slowly progressive stenosis/occlusion of the visceral vessels (CA, SMA, and IMA) (Fig. 7-2). Atherosclerotic lesions generally involve the anterior abdominal aorta and the origins of these vessels.

   1. **Clinical presentation.** The triad of symptoms suggesting chronic mesenteric ischemia includes:
      a. Postprandial abdominal pain, occurring in the epigastrium, generally 0.5–2 hours after a meal
      b. "Food fear," resulting from the chronic association of eating with subsequent pain
      c. Weight loss

   2. **Diagnosis.** The diagnosis of chronic mesenteric ischemia is suggested by the clinical triad noted previously. Additional symptoms might include gastrointestinal dysmotility. Definitive diagnosis is often delayed for up to 1–2 years, unless a high index of suspicion is maintained.
      a. Recently, **duplex scanning** of the visceral vessels has been used to screen patients with suspected chronic mesenteric ischemia. Elevated velocities within the CA and superior mesenteric vessels may be seen.
      b. Arteriography is the most useful diagnostic study. Both anterior-posterior and lateral views of the aorta must be used to visualize the origins of the visceral vessels. When symptoms occur, two of the three vessels are usually occluded and the remaining one is highly diseased. A rich collateral blood supply between the CA and SMA (pancreatoduodenal arcade) and the SMA and IMA (Riolan's arch) may be seen.
      c. Computed tomography (CT) of the abdomen, as well as upper and lower intestinal endoscopy, is performed to rule out other causes for the patient's symptoms prior to recommending treatment of mesenteric occlusive disease.

   3. **Treatment.** Surgery is recommended if severe mesenteric occlusive disease is found in a patient with the clinical presentation noted previously. In well-selected patients, the results of surgery are excellent, with 90% of patients cured of their symptoms.
      a. Aortomesenteric bypass, usually involving the CA and SMA, is performed with a short prosthetic graft. The bypass can be constructed in an **antegrade** format from the supraceliac aorta or a **retrograde** approach from the infrarenal aorta or iliac system.
      b. Transaortic mesenteric endarterectomy directly removes the atherosclerotic lesions from the aorta and origins of the mesenteric vessels, restoring patency without prosthetic grafting.

C **Mesenteric venous thrombosis** may present more insidiously than acute mesenteric ischemia. Typically, it causes progressive abdominal pain and distention and may be confused with intestinal obstruction.

   1. **Etiology.** It is frequently associated with hypercoagulable states, including patients with a neoplasm or hematologic abnormality.

   2. **Diagnosis** is suggested by CT scan that reveals concentration of contrast in the wall of the mesenteric vein without luminal flow.

   3. **Treatment**
      a. Nonoperative treatment is anticoagulation (intravenous heparin) and treatment of the underlying disorder.
      b. Celiotomy may be necessary if peritonitis develops, but 75% of patients can be treated nonoperatively if the diagnosis is made promptly and appropriate treatment is given.

VI **RENAL ARTERY STENOSIS**

Renal artery stenosis (RAS). Significant stenosis of the renal arteries decreases perfusion pressure to the kidney. This reduction stimulates the juxtaglomerular apparatus to release **renin,** initiating the formation of angiotensin. **Angiotensin** is a potent vasoconstrictor and stimulates adrenal aldosterone production, resulting in sodium retention. Systemic **hypertension, renal insufficiency,** and **pulmonary edema** may result from this cascade of events.

A **Causes** The two most common causes of RAS are **atherosclerosis** and **fibromuscular dysplasia.** Atherosclerosis occurs in older adults and involves the orifices of the renal arteries. Fibromuscular dysplasia generally affects younger women and results in multiple stenoses of the mid and distal renal arteries.

B **Clinical presentation** Renovascular hypertension is a relatively rare cause of hypertension (less than 5% of all patients with hypertension). The diagnosis should be suspected in patients with the following characteristics:

1. Sudden onset of severe hypertension in patients less than 35 or more than 55 years of age

2. Sudden worsening of hypertension in a patient with previously well-controlled disease

3. Inability to control blood pressure despite multiple-drug therapy

4. The presence of abdominal or flank bruits associated with any of the preceding characteristics

C **Diagnosis** **Laboratory tests** may be helpful to confirm the presence of hypertension caused by RAS, although no test is completely reliable.

1. **Captopril renal scan** noninvasively screens for reduced blood flow to each kidney. The administration of the angiotensin-converting enzyme inhibitor increases the sensitivity of this test to detect RAS based on the suppression of glomerular filtration in the presence of significant stenoses.

2. **Duplex scanning** of the renal arteries is another noninvasive screening test for RAS. An increase in renal artery blood flow velocity compared with aortic velocity suggests significant stenosis.

3. The **renal/systemic renin index** documents the contribution of each kidney to plasma renin and also documents suppression of the contralateral kidney in unilateral disease.
   a. The formula is:

$$\frac{(\text{Renal vein renin level} - \text{Infrarenal venacaval renin level})}{\text{Systemic renin level}}$$

   b. An index over 0.48 indicates hypersecretion by that kidney.
   c. An index approaching 0 indicates suppression in that kidney.

4. **Selective renal arteriography** remains the definitive examination to demonstrate stenotic lesions of the renal arteries and is essential in planning therapy.

5. **Computed tomographic angiography (CTA)** and **magnetic resonance angiography (MRA)** are two widely used, noninvasive imaging modalities that have come into favor. Excellent resolution has been obtained with these modalities; however, they are very institution dependent when comparing one with the other.

D **Treatment** of RAS depends on the etiology and location of the lesion, the status of the involved kidney, and the clinical status of the patient. Options include percutaneous dilation, endarterectomy, bypass, and nephrectomy.

1. **PTA** is a very effective treatment for patients with lesions in the midportion of the renal artery. The lesions frequently occur in this location in patients with fibromuscular dysplasia. Early and late results in well-selected patients are excellent. **Stent** placement (in combination with angioplasty) is being used successfully in patients with stenosis of the renal artery orifice. When applicable, this is now the preferred mode of treatment.

2. **Renal artery endarterectomy** can be used for unilateral or bilateral localized atherosclerosis of the renal artery orifices.

3. **Aortorenal artery bypass** distal to the lesion is the most commonly performed procedure.
   a. The saphenous vein in adults and the hypogastric artery in children are the preferred conduits.
   b. The aorta above or below the renal artery is usually used as the origin of the graft. Other sources of inflow are the hepatic, splenic, and iliac arteries.
   c. A small percentage of patients have multiple lesions, involving both the main renal artery and the hilar branches. In these patients, the kidney can be removed, cooled, and repaired **ex vivo.** The kidney is then replaced in its anatomic location or is transplanted to the pelvis.

4. **Nephrectomy** is an alternative in patients with a unilateral vascular lesion and a normal contralateral kidney. The indication would be refractory hypertension with elevated renin from the involved kidney and suppression of the normal kidney. Nephrectomy is usually chosen for small, nonfunctioning kidneys.

5. **Medical treatment. Antihypertensive drugs** can be used to control mild to moderate hypertension from RAS (when the diastolic blood pressure is in the 90–100 range).
   a. The risks of medical management are higher when blood pressure is erratic or difficult to control.
   b. Medical management is a more reasonable approach than surgery in patients with generalized atherosclerosis.
   c. Medical management is less desirable than surgery in children and in patients with fibromuscular dysplasia.

6. **Results of treatment** depend on the disease process, the accuracy of preoperative testing, and the ability to completely repair the arterial lesions.
   a. Fibromuscular dysplasia with localized arterial lesions do very well, with improvement or cure of hypertension in 90% of patients.
   b. Repair of isolated atherosclerotic lesions also yields good results if the distal renal artery is normal.
   c. Nonlocalized lesions in patients with widespread atherosclerosis yield the poorest results.

VII ▪ EXTRACRANIAL CEREBROVASCULAR DISEASE

A **Overview** **Cerebrovascular accident** (stroke) is an injury to the central nervous system that results in death of brain tissue. It can be a silent event or can result in temporary or permanent loss of function.

1. **Epidemiology**
   a. Of approximately 600,000 new strokes per year in the United States, approximately 150,000 result in death (25% mortality).
   b. Cerebrovascular accidents are the third leading cause of death in the United States.
   c. Recurrent stroke is the leading cause of death in stroke patients and occurs at the rate of 9% per year.

2. **Causes** of cerebrovascular accidents include:
   a. **Cerebral artery thrombosis** (85% of cases) due to:
      (1) **Embolization** (most common) from a cardiac source or the carotid arteries (Fig. 7-3).
      (2) **Primary vessel occlusion** (due to intracranial atherosclerosis)
   b. **Hemorrhage** (15% of cases) involving:
      (1) **Intracerebral hemorrhage** (most common)
      (2) **Subarachnoid hemorrhage** (usually due to rupture of an intracranial aneurysm)

3. **Symptoms.** Atherosclerosis of the carotid arteries usually involves the origin of the internal carotid artery. Embolization of atherosclerotic debris, fibrin, or platelets from a carotid plaque is the most common cause of ischemic insult to the brain. Alternatively, the stenosis may result in thrombosis of the internal carotid artery, acutely diminishing blood flow distally if collaterals are not well developed.
   a. **Transient ischemic attacks (TIA)** are episodes of focal neurologic symptoms. The classic TIA syndrome is characterized by abrupt onset, with the maximal symptoms occurring in less than 5 minutes. Rapid resolution usually occurs within 15 minutes but within 24 hours by definition. Neurologic symptoms correspond to a specific hemispheric arterial distribution. Symptoms include:
      (1) **Motor deficit** contralateral to the involved carotid artery
      (2) **Sensory deficit** contralateral to the involved carotid artery
      (3) **Aphasia,** expressive or global
   b. **Amaurosis fugax** is transient monocular blindness caused by an embolus to a retinal vessel. Examination of the retina may show a gray or a bright-yellow (Hollenhorst) cholesterol plaque within a retinal artery.

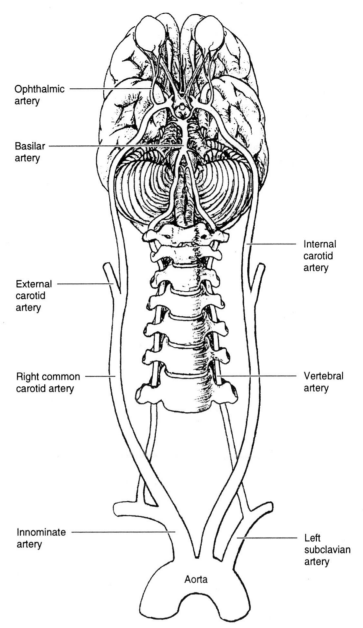

FIGURE 7-3 Diagram of major extracranial components of cerebral and ocular arterial supply. (Adapted with permission from Wylie EJ, Ehrenfeld WK. *Extracranial Occlusive Cerebrovascular Disease*. Philadelphia: WB Saunders; 1970.)

    c. Cerebrovascular accident, or completed stroke, refers to a neurologic deficit that persists for more than 24 hours. In the case of carotid disease, this again may involve a sensory or motor deficit contralateral to the diseased carotid artery or aphasia.

B **Vertebrobasilar artery disease**   The vertebrobasilar arteries (Fig. 7-3) comprise the posterior circulation of the brain. Symptoms of vertebrobasilar insufficiency may occur in the form of a TIA or stroke. These symptoms may include:

1. Loss of vision, diplopia

2. Ataxia or gait disturbance

C **Carotid bruits** are caused by turbulent blood flow within the carotid system. Because most atherosclerotic lesions occur at the bifurcation, bruits originating in the carotid artery are usually heard under the angle of the jaw. They may be confused with transmitted heart murmurs; heart murmurs, however, are usually heard bilaterally and more loudly in the lower neck.

1. Carotid bruits are **not reliable indicators of severe carotid artery disease.** Approximately 60% of patients with bruits have some carotid disease; only 35% of patients with bruits have hemodynamically significant disease. Of all patients with hemodynamically significant stenosis, only 50% have bruits.

2. The presence of a carotid bruit is **more predictive of a myocardial infarction** than of an ipsilateral stroke. Therefore, carotid bruits should alert the examiner to generalized atherosclerotic disease (especially coronary artery disease), not just carotid disease.

D **Workup of cerebrovascular disease**   Patients who present with neurologic symptoms or who are found to have a carotid bruit should be carefully evaluated.

1. **Duplex imaging** of the carotid arteries is the primary screening modality for lesions in the neck.

2. **CT** or **magnetic resonance images** of the brain should be obtained in symptomatic patients to look for cerebral infarction, hemorrhage, or other intracranial pathology.

3. **Cardiac evaluation** should include an electrocardiogram, echocardiogram if a cardiac source is suspected, and a Holter monitor if a rhythm disturbance is suspected. If a patient is considered a surgical candidate, cardiac stress testing may be indicated to screen for significant coronary artery disease.

4. **Cerebral angiography,** performed conventionally, or CT or MRA techniques may be used to confirm the results of duplex imaging if surgery is contemplated.

E **Medical treatment** of cerebrovascular disease primarily involves formal anticoagulation or antiplatelet therapy.

1. **Warfarin.** Anticoagulation with warfarin is useful primarily in patients who have suffered a cerebral embolus originating in the heart. This embolus occurs most commonly after a myocardial infarction (mural thrombus) in patients with rheumatic heart disease or chronic atrial fibrillation.

2. **Aspirin** is an antiplatelet agent that is beneficial in patients with cerebrovascular disease and is used to reduce the risk of cerebrovascular symptoms, myocardial infarction, and death.

3. **Ticlopidine** is an antiplatelet agent that has been shown to be effective in reducing the risk of stroke in patients who have had a TIA or previous stroke. Ticlopidine is considered modestly superior to aspirin in reducing risk. It is, however, associated with significant side effects (e.g., reversible neutropenia in 2.4% of patients) and a high rate of intolerance (20.9%). It is currently recommended for symptomatic patients who are not considered candidates for surgery or who do not respond to aspirin, who cannot tolerate it, or who have had major strokes.

F **Surgical treatment** of cerebrovascular disease has been shown to be effective in reducing the risk of stroke in patients with symptomatic (North American Symptomatic Carotid Endacterectomy Trial) and asymptomatic (Asymptomatic Carotid Artery Surgery Trial) carotid disease.

1. **Indications for surgery** center around the patient's presentation and the degree of stenosis determined by preoperative testing.
   a. **Symptomatic** patients (nondisabling stroke, TIA, or amaurosis) with a 50%–99% stenosis in the ipsilateral carotid artery have a beneficial effect from carotid endarterectomy. The 2-year risk of an ipsilateral stroke is 9% in symptomatic patients with a high-grade stenosis treated with surgery and aspirin. Similar patients treated nonsurgically with aspirin alone have a 26% chance of having an ipsilateral stroke.
   b. **Asymptomatic** patients with a 60%–99% stenosis may also benefit from carotid repair. An asymptomatic, high-grade carotid stenosis is associated with a stroke rate of approximately 10.6% over 5 years. If the surgery is performed with an operative morbidity and mortality of <3%, the 5-year risk of stroke can be reduced to 4.8%.
   c. **Contraindications** to carotid repair include:
      (1) Disabling stroke, especially with altered level of consciousness
      (2) Totally occluded internal carotid artery
      (3) Severe medical illness, which will substantially shorten life expectancy

2. **Carotid endarterectomy** is the procedure of choice.
   a. The surgery removes the diseased inner portions of the common, internal, and external carotid arteries.
   b. During the surgery, the artery is clamped, resulting in decreased blood flow to the brain. **Cerebral protection,** using a shunt, is used routinely by some surgeons and selectively by others. If selective shunting is chosen, the need for shunting can be assessed by:
      (1) Measuring the **back pressure** in the internal carotid artery after clamping the common and external carotid arteries. If the mean arterial pressure is more than 50 mm Hg, shunting is not necessary.
      (2) Observing the **electroencephalogram** for changes after clamping the common and external carotid arteries. If slowing occurs, a shunt should be used.
      (3) Performing the surgery using **regional cervical block** with local anesthesia. This choice allows the neurologic status of the awake patient to be assessed during the case and avoids the risks of general anesthesia. If a change in neurologic status occurs while the artery is clamped, the shunt is inserted.
   c. The blood pressure should be carefully monitored during and after the procedure because these patients are prone to wide pressure swings, which can cause neurologic dysfunction or injury.
   d. **Complications** of the procedure include stroke; transient cerebral ischemia; bleeding; cranial nerve injury, particularly to cranial nerves X and XII; and those related to other medical conditions, especially myocardial infarction.

3. **Carotid angioplasty and stenting** is gaining significant ground in treatment of carotid artery occlusive disease among vascular interventionalists. Currently, clinical trials are investigating the efficacy of PTA/stenting versus traditional endarterectomy. Although this treatment is considered investigational for de novo lesions, there are accepted indications for using PTA/stenting in the carotid artery:
   a. Reccurent stenosis
   b. Anatomically difficult lesions (high bifurcations)
   c. Irradiated necks

VIII ANEURYSMS

A **Abdominal aortic aneurysms (AAA)** An aneurysm is an abnormal dilatation of the wall of an artery. Generally, an aneurysm is considered significant if its diameter is twice that of the normal proximal artery. An aneurysm of the aorta may rupture and cause death and should be repaired when detected. The cause of AAAs is multifactorial. Age, smoking, hypertension, and family history are all predisposing factors for aneurysm formation. Aneurysms are more common in men (4:1).

1. **Diagnosis.** AAAs most often occur below the level of the renal arteries. They are usually discovered on physical examination or during evaluation of an unrelated abdominal condition for which the patient has had a CT scan, ultrasound examination, or abdominal x-rays (**incidentaloma).**
   a. **X-ray.** Calcification of part of the abdominal aorta seen on posterior-anterior or lateral abdominal radiograph is present in 60% of patients (**"eggshell sign").**
   b. **Ultrasonography** and **CT scan** of the abdomen are the most accurate tests for determining aneurysm size (reported as anterior-posterior or lateral diameter). CT is especially useful because it gives details about the relationship of the aneurysm to the renal and visceral vessels and demonstrates venous anomalies, which may be present.
   c. **Angiography** is useful for patients with hypertension (to evaluate RAS), distal arterial occlusive symptoms, or suspected mesenteric ischemia.

2. **Management.** The decision to repair an AAA or to observe it for growth is dependent on aneurysm size and growth rate and the presence of symptoms.
   a. **Size.** Patients with AAA <5 cm who are without symptoms are followed up with serial ultrasound examinations (every 3–12 months) to determine growth. AAA >5 cm are considered for elective repair depending on the medical condition of the patient.

b. **Growth rate.** The natural history of AAA is growth ranging from 2 to 8 mm/year. Expanding aneurysms with growth >4 mm/year are considered for elective repair.

c. **Symptoms.** The vast majority of AAAs are asymptomatic. The presence of symptoms (rupture, unexplained abdominal/back/flank pain, or distal embolization) mandates repair.

3. **Surgical repair**

a. **Preoperative evaluation.** All patients undergoing elective repair should have careful preoperative medical screening, including a cardiac evaluation. Patients with severe or unstable coronary artery disease should undergo coronary catheterization and, if necessary, aortocoronary bypass preoperatively.

b. **Technique.** Surgical repair involves **endoaneurysmorrhaphy.** This involves opening the aneurysm sack and suturing a prosthetic graft to the normal aorta within the aneurysm. The aneurysm wall is then wrapped around the graft following repair.

c. **Endovascular repair.** New techniques for the exclusion of aneurysms are now being developed. They involve the placement of the graft within the aneurysm via remote sites of access, most commonly the common femoral artery. The need for extensive laparotomy is thus avoided. The long-term results of these procedures are revealing acceptable durability with newer technologies emerging routinely. Currently, it is estimated that over 60% of AAAs worldwide are repaired through endovascular means. Criteria for placement of an endograft for AAA repair is as follows:

(1) **Suitable infrarenal neck:** 1–1.5 cm with minimal angulation

(2) **One adequate common iliac artery:** for distal fixation. Unilateral common iliac aneurysms can be excluded by embolizing the hypogastric artery and landing in the external iliac.

B **Ruptured AAA** is the eleventh leading cause of death in the United States. The mortality of rupture is reported as high as 75% because many patients will not survive to receive medical care, and those who do undergo repair still have a high perioperative mortality rate.

1. **Risk factors for rupture** include:

a. **Aneurysm size.** Approximate rates of rupture in 5 years are:

(1) If less than 4.5 cm in diameter, 9%

(2) If 4.5–7 cm in diameter, 35%

(3) If more than 7 cm in diameter, 75%

b. **Expansion rate** of an aneurysm >0.4 cm in diameter per year

c. The presence of **hypertension** and **chronic obstructive pulmonary disease**

2. **Diagnosis** of a ruptured AAA involves a triad of clinical findings. For patients who are hemodynamically stable (without any history or suspicion of shock) and in whom the diagnosis is questionable, CT imaging of the abdomen will reveal the presence of an aneurysm and rupture.

a. **Severe pain** located in the abdomen, flank, or back

b. **Pulsatile, tender abdominal mass**

c. **Shock,** presenting with elevated pulse rate, unstable blood pressure, or syncope. Some patients with a small, contained rupture may have a stable blood pressure, but they are at risk for catastrophic decompensation and should be treated urgently.

3. **Management. Surgical repair** of a ruptured aortic aneurysm must be performed as soon as the diagnosis is suspected. Patients with the previously noted triad are taken to the operating room without further testing. The **technique** for repair is similar to that for elective repair, although emergency proximal aortic control is generally obtained in the supraceliac position, just below the level of the diaphragm.

4. **Surgical complications** may occur in either elective or emergency aortic surgery. Many of these complications can be minimized by careful management, and if recognized early, some can be successfully treated, preventing major morbidity and mortality.

a. **Postoperative acute renal failure** occurs in 21% of cases of ruptured aneurysms and in less than 2% of aneurysms treated by elective surgery. If hemodialysis is required, the risk of mortality increases to approximately 50%.

b. **Ischemic colitis,** usually involving the sigmoid colon, may result from ligation of a patent IMA in both elective and emergent surgery. It occurs to some degree in 6% of elective cases but results in full-thickness injury with necrosis in <1% of cases. Ischemic colitis should be suspected in any patient with postoperative diarrhea, especially when the stools are heme positive. It can usually be diagnosed with sigmoidoscopy. The mortality rate can reach 50% if diagnosis and treatment are delayed. Treatment consists of resection of necrotic colon, proximal colostomy, and closure of the distal colon (Hartmann's procedure).

c. **Acute leg ischemia** can occur postoperatively and is suspected if pulses that were present previously are absent. It is caused by clamp injury to the iliac arteries or distal embolization of the aneurysm thrombus. Treatment is repair of the injury or embolectomy.

d. **Spinal cord ischemia** is a **rare complication** (0.25% of cases) of aortic aneurysm surgery but is most common in cases of ruptured aneurysms. The **artery of Adamkiewicz** supplies the spinal cord and arises from the aorta usually between thoracic levels 8 and 12; occasionally, however, it arises as low as lumbar level 4. Spinal cord ischemia results from diminished flow through this artery due to systemic hypotension, clamping of the aorta, or ligation of the intercostal/lumbar arteries. The **classic anterior spinal artery syndrome** is characterized by:

(1) Paraplegia

(2) Rectal and urinary incontinence

(3) Loss of pain and temperature sensation but preservation of vibratory and proprioceptive sensation (due to the independent anterior and posterior circulation of the middle and lower spinal cord)

e. **Aortic graft infection** is generally a late complication of repair. It can occur in the body of the graft or at the anastomoses. It may **result from bacterial seeding,** either at the time of graft implantation or at a later date as a result of bacteremia. The most common infecting organism is *Staphylococcus aureus,* but *Staphylococcus epidermidis* is not infrequently found.

(1) **Incidence** of infection is 1%–4% of all grafts used. It may be decreased significantly by the perioperative use of antibiotics. First-generation cephalosporins (i.e., cefazolin) are the drugs of choice.

(2) **Timing.** Prosthetic grafts may become infected at any time after implantation, even many years after the surgery.

(3) **Presentation.** Infected grafts can present in several ways.

(a) **Fever** accompanied by **abdominal discomfort** is the usual presentation of infected prostheses contained within the abdomen. If the graft goes to the femoral arteries, the most common presenting sign is an **inflammatory mass or draining sinus in the groin.**

(b) **Gastrointestinal bleeding.** Erosion of the graft into the bowel (usually the duodenum) may result in occult bleeding from the bowel wall or massive bleeding if the anastomosis is involved (**aortoenteric fistula**).

(4) **Diagnosis**

(a) If gastrointestinal bleeding is present, **endoscopy** of the esophagus, stomach, and duodenum should be done to search for bleeding sites, such as an ulcer. The distal duodenum should be visualized because the aortoenteric fistula may be visible in this location.

(b) **CT scan** may demonstrate air or fluid around an infected graft or may show a false aneurysm.

(c) An **indium-tagged white blood cell scan** may localize the area where the graft is infected.

(d) An **aortogram** may demonstrate a false aneurysm and also will guide the surgeon regarding vessels available for reconstruction at surgery.

(e) A **sinogram,** which outlines the graft, is diagnostic if a draining sinus is present.

(5) **Treatment.** Traditional surgical treatment involves **total graft excision** (via a laparotomy) and **extra-anatomic bypass.** In hemodynamically stable patients, the extra-anatomic bypass may be performed prior to graft excision and generally involves an axillobifemoral bypass.

f. **Sexual dysfunction.** The sympathetic nerves controlling ejaculation cross the left common iliac artery near the aortic bifurcation. Injury during aortic repair may result in retrograde ejaculation. Additionally, disturbance of pelvic blood flow during aortic reconstruction may result in vasculogenic impotence. Perfusion of at least one hypogastric artery should be maintained in planning the method of graft placement.

C **Atypical aneurysms of the abdominal aorta**

1. **Inflammatory aneurysms** are characterized by a dense fibrotic reaction primarily involving the anterior and lateral walls of the aneurysm and the surrounding tissues.
   a. The duodenum is often densely adherent to the aneurysm wall and can be severely injured if attempts are made to mobilize the aneurysm. The aneurysm is repaired by dissecting the neck above the area of inflammation for proximal control, frequently above the duodenum near the renal vein. Control of the iliac vessels is often obtained after the aneurysm has been opened by using balloons to occlude the lumens from within.
   b. If the diagnosis is suspected preoperatively, a retroperitoneal approach may be used.
   c. The inflammatory reaction frequently recedes after the aneurysm is repaired.

2. **Mycotic AAAs** are caused by bacterial inflammation of the arterial wall. In the infrarenal aorta, the most common organism found is *Salmonella*.
   a. Mycotic aneurysms usually are saccular, occur in atypical locations, and lack calcification of the wall.
   b. Patients present with fever, elevated white blood cell counts, and positive blood cultures. Evidence of septic embolization may also be present.
   c. Treatment begins with culture and sensitivity-directed antibiotics. The aneurysm is then surgically explored.
      (1) If there is no periaortic purulence and Gram stain of the proximal and distal artery is negative, the aneurysm is repaired with an interposition graft.
      (2) If gross purulence is present, the aneurysm and surrounding tissue are resected, the aorta is closed, and an extra-anatomic bypass (i.e., axillobifemoral bypass) is constructed.
   d. Long-term antibiotic therapy is indicated in these patients.

D **Other arterial aneurysms**

1. **Iliac artery aneurysms** usually involve the common and internal iliac arteries; the external iliac artery is rarely involved. These aneurysms are typically extensions of aortic aneurysms but may occur as isolated aneurysms. They may be diagnosed as pulsatile masses palpable on abdominal or rectal examinations.

2. **Splenic artery aneurysms** are the most common type of aneurysm involving the splanchnic circulation. Causes include fibrous dysplasia, portal hypertension, multiparity, and inflammation (secondary to pancreatitis).
   a. **Diagnosis** is frequently incidental and is suggested on imaging of the abdomen by a left upper quadrant ring-shaped calcification.
   b. **Rate of rupture** of bland splenic aneurysms in nonpregnant women is 2%. The mortality of rupture is 25%. The rate of rupture in a pregnant woman is 90%.
   c. **Indications for repair** include rupture, symptoms (pain in left upper quadrant), the presence of an aneurysm in a woman of childbearing age, and size >2 cm.
   d. **Repair** involves ligation of the splenic artery proximal and distal to the aneurysm, with or without splenectomy. Endovascular embolization may also be performed in selected cases.

3. **Peripheral arterial aneurysms.** The **popliteal artery** is the most common location for peripheral aneurysms. The usual cause is atherosclerosis.
   a. **Clinical presentation**
      (1) Approximately 50% are bilateral. Of these, 25% have associated AAAs.
      (2) Embolization and thrombosis are the most common complications. These aneurysms should be repaired when discovered because ischemic complications frequently lead to limb loss. Rupture is extremely rare.
   b. **Diagnosis.** Physical examination detects prominent popliteal pulses. Duplex ultrasound should be performed to determine the presence and size of the aneurysm. An arteriogram guides reconstruction.

c. Treatment. Indications for surgical repair include any symptomatic popliteal aneurysm and those >2 cm. Popliteal aneurysms are treated by ligation and bypass because attempts to remove the aneurysm may injure the adjacent nerves and veins.

IX VASOSPASTIC DISEASES

Vasopastic diseases chiefly affect the small digital arteries and arterioles of the upper and lower extremities. Common symptoms include pain, numbness, coldness, and occasionally, skin ulcers. In general, bilateral hand symptoms predominate, with sparing of the thumbs. Vasospasm may be associated with collagen vascular disease, atherosclerosis, trauma, and embolism from peripheral arterial lesions or may be without an identifiable associated disease.

A **Raynaud's phenomenon** is episodic vasoconstriction, most commonly of the fingers but occasionally of the feet. It is usually initiated by cold exposure or emotional stimuli and occurs mainly in women.

1. The affected digits may go through a classic sequence of color changes, including:
   a. **Pallor** due to severe vasospasm in the dermal vessels
   b. **Cyanosis** due to sluggish blood flow and resultant marked blood desaturation
   c. **Rubor** due to the reactive hyperemia

2. **Symptoms** begin with **numb discomfort** that is usually localized in the fingers. The prognosis is guarded because patients may then develop small vessel occlusions, leading to digital **ulceration** or **gangrene.**

3. **Associated local or systemic disease.** Raynaud's phenomenon is considered a disorder that occurs secondary to other diseases, most commonly scleroderma and collagen vascular diseases.

4. **Management** of Raynaud's phenomenon includes a number of different modalities.
   a. Cold should be avoided. Hands should be protected by gloves or hand warmers in extremely cold weather.
   b. Tobacco should be avoided because it stimulates vasoconstriction.
   c. Calcium channel blockers, such as nifedipine, are the drugs of choice. Use of phenoxybenzamine for alpha blockade may be therapeutic.
   d. Cervical sympathectomy is not recommended in these patients unless digital ulceration is present.

B **Raynaud's disease** is similar to Raynaud's phenomenon; however, the condition shows no association with a systemic disease. The prognosis is benign, without significant threat of tissue loss. Seventy percent of patients are young women who usually have bilateral and symmetrical symptoms. **Treatment** is similar to that for Raynaud's phenomenon. Sympathectomy is not indicated.

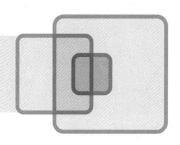

chapter **8**

Venous Disease, Pulmonary Embolism, and Lymphatic System

BRUCE E. JARRELL • R. ANTHONY CARABASI III • MARK B. KAHN • ROBERT A. LARSON

I   **VENOUS DISEASE OF THE LOWER EXTREMITIES**

A Disorders

1. **Superficial thrombophlebitis** is inflammation or thrombosis of the superficial veins.
   a. **Clinical presentation**
      (1) A tender, palpable cord along the course of a superficial vein
      (2) A red, warm, indurated vein
   b. **Treatment**
      (1) Bed rest and elevation of the extremity
      (2) Local application of heat for relief of pain
      (3) Gradient compression stockings
      (4) Nonsteroidal anti-inflammatory drugs
   c. **Complications. Chronic recurrent superficial thrombophlebitis** may require antibiotic therapy due to a streptococcal lymphangitis.
   d. **Suppurative thrombophlebitis** usually is associated with intravenous infusions in immunocompromised or burn patients. It is treated by **excision of the infected vein and antibiotics.**

2. **Varicose veins**
   a. **Clinical presentation**
      (1) Local pain and edema
      (2) Local inflammation
      (3) Local hemorrhage into the surrounding tissue
      (4) Dilated superficial veins
   b. **Diagnosis**
      (1) **Trendelenburg test:** Elevate the leg with the patient supine to exsanguinate the superficial veins, then place an elastic tourniquet below the saphenofemoral junction. Have the patient stand, and observe vein refilling. Normal venous filling is slow; early refilling indicates deep venous insufficiency. Rapid refilling after tourniquet removal indicates saphenofemoral junction (superficial venous) insufficiency.
      (2) **Vascular laboratory**
         (a) **Venous duplex** will identify the presence of deep venous thrombosis (DVT) as well as document venous reflux.
         (b) **Air plesmythography** documents ambulatory venous hypertension and calf muscle pump function.
   c. **Treatment**
      (1) **Nonoperative management:** leg compression with gradient compression stockings and leg elevation

(2) **Operative management**
   (a) **Indications** for surgery
      (i) **Previous or impending hemorrhage:** usually controlled by a combination of elevation and direct compression
      (ii) **Recurrent pain** over the varicosity or **recurrent superficial phlebitis** of the varicosity
      (iii) **Cosmetic considerations**
   (b) **Surgical procedures**
      (i) **Greater saphenous ligation and perforator phlebectomy.** Surgical excision of the individual varicosities through small (>1 cm) incisions (the "stab avulsion technique"), with ligation of proximal incompetent perforators. The greater saphenous vein (GSV) is not removed distal to the knee due to risk of saphenous nerve injury.
      (ii) **Minimally invasive procedures. Thermal ablation** uses radio frequency or laser coagulation and causes GSV thrombosis and fibrosis, eliminating reflux. **Transilluminated powered phlebectomy** is used for subcutaneous perforator vein removal under direct vision. These procedures offer equivalent results with improved recovery time and cosmesis (fewer incisions).

3. **DVT** occurs in approximately 500,000 individuals per year. About 10% of cases end in death from pulmonary embolism (PE). The incidence of DVT following major abdominal surgery is estimated at 30% and is even higher following open prostate surgery (38%) or orthopaedic procedures (50%–70%).
   a. **Etiology**
      (1) DVT usually originates in the lower extremity venous system, starting at the calf vein level and progressing proximally. Approximately 80%–90% of **pulmonary emboli** originate here. The treatment of calf vein clot is controversial. Most surgeons recommend a follow-up scan in 1 week because up to 30% of patients will propagate proximally. Anticoagulation for 3 months helps to reduce the severity of post-thrombotic symptoms.
      (2) Other veins in which thrombi occasionally develop include:
         (a) Pelvic veins, especially during pregnancy and pelvic surgery and from gynecologic cancer
         (b) Renal veins, especially when intrinsic renal disease is present
         (c) Inferior vena cava
         (d) Ovarian veins
         (e) Upper extremity and neck veins, especially with athletic activity or the use of intravenous cannulas
         (f) The right atrium in the presence of intrinsic cardiac disorders
   b. **Clinical presentation**
      (1) The classic clinical syndrome includes calf or thigh pain, edema, tenderness, and a positive **Homans' sign** (calf pain on dorsiflexion of the foot). Only 40% of patients with DVT are symptomatic. Physical exam has only a 50% accuracy rate, and confirmatory testing is required. PE is the presenting symptom in some patients.
   c. **Diagnosis** of DVT is made by means of **laboratory tests.**
      (1) **Duplex ultrasound** has become the standard initial test. It has a 95% sensitivity/specificity for proximal DVT. Diagnosis of iliac vein DVT is less reliable.
      (2) **Venography** of the ascending venous system is the **traditional diagnostic method for DVT.** It can be useful for evaluating the pelvic veins. Twenty to 40% of studies are technically inadequate.
      (3) **Magnetic resonance venography.** Excellent sensitivity and specificity; especially useful for diagnosis of pelvic DVT
   d. **Treatment**
      (1) Continuous **heparin** infusion is given for 5–10 days, followed by administration of warfarin or subcutaneous administration of heparin for 3–6 months. Low molecular weight heparin (LMWH) can be used to initiate outpatient treatment of uncomplicated DVT.
      (2) **Thrombolytic therapy** with urokinase or t-PA is used if extensive DVT results in impaired perfusion of the extremity. It is recommended for extensive iliofemoral DVT to reduce post-thrombotic sequelae.

(3) Inferior venacaval filter or interruption is used if heparin is contraindicated or if a pulmonary embolus occurs despite adequate anticoagulation therapy.

e. Prevention

  (1) Simple preventive measures include leg elevation, early mobilization after surgery, and the use of gradient compression stockings.

  (2) Intermittent calf compression by means of a pneumatic cuff increases leg blood flow velocity and helps to prevent stasis as well as causing a poorly defined systemic lytic effect.

  (3) Preoperative and postoperative administration of **prophylactic heparin** is effective in preventing deep thrombosis. An intermittent subcutaneous dose of 5,000 U is given every 8–12 hours. The risk of perioperative bleeding complication is slightly increased with heparin prophylaxis (6% vs. 4% of controls), but the risk of major hemorrhage is only about 2%.

  (4) LMWH is thought to cause fewer bleeding complications than unfractionated heparin.

f. Complications of DVT

  (1) Postphlebitic syndrome is a common late complication of DVT, often occurring several years after the acute event.

   (a) Clinical presentation: swelling and ulceration

    (i) Chronic valvular incompetence occurs because of damage incurred during the acute episode.

    (ii) Leg edema usually is worse as the day progresses and as the leg is dependent. It usually improves with elevation and rest.

    (iii) Ambulatory venous hypertension, due to reflux or venous occlusion, leads to edema and interstitial exudation of plasma, cells, and protein.

    (iv) This edema and exudation then lead to **brawny induration from hemoglobin metabolism.** Tissue necrosis and skin ulceration result from poor oxygen diffusion in the edematous tissues.

   (b) Treatment

    (i) Gradient compression stockings must be worn continually. If swelling can be prevented, most ulcers can be prevented.

    (ii) An **Unna boot,** a medicated pressure bandage, is applied weekly or biweekly until the ulcer heals. Compression therapy will heal most ulcers.

  (2) Phlegmasia alba dolens is caused by acute occlusion of the iliac and femoral veins due to DVT.

   (a) Clinical presentation. This phlebitis results in a **pale cool leg** with a diminished arterial pulse due to spasm.

   (b) Treatment is **thrombolytic therapy** followed by **heparin administration** to prevent progression to phlegmasia cerulea dolens.

  (3) Phlegmasia cerulea dolens is secondary to acute and nearly total venous occlusion of the extremity outflow, including the iliac and femoral veins. It is more common in the left leg.

   (a) Clinical presentation

    (i) Physical findings include cyanosis of the extremity with massive edema, severe pain, and absent pulses, followed by venous gangrene.

    (ii) Shock may occur as a result of sequestration of a significant amount of blood in the leg.

   (b) Treatment

    (i) Thrombolytic therapy followed by heparin administration

    (ii) Thrombectomy occasionally if nonoperative therapy is unsuccessful

    (iii) Bed rest with leg elevation

II PULMONARY EMBOLISM

A Overview   PE is one of the most common causes of **sudden death in hospitalized patients.**

  1. Patients with pre-existing cardiac or pulmonary disease tolerate even smaller PEs poorly.

  2. Ninety percent of deaths occur within 2 hours after the onset of the initial symptoms. Therefore, if the patient lives longer than 2 hours, the chance of survival is very high.

3. PE develops in about 10%–40% of patients with **DVT**. However, approximately 33% of patients with PE have no antecedent symptoms of DVT.

B **Risk factors**

1. **Surgery and critical illness**

2. **Pregnant and postpartum women** have a five times increased incidence of PE.

3. **Estrogen therapy** is associated with a four to seven times increased risk of PE. The risk is dose dependent and is eliminated within several weeks after cessation of therapy.

4. **Heart disease** is associated with a three to four times higher risk of pulmonary embolus formation. This risk is directly related to the severity of the heart disease.

5. **Obesity** is associated with a 1.5–2 times greater risk of PE.

6. **Carcinoma** is associated with a two to three times greater risk of PE.

7. **Major trauma,** especially spinal cord injury and pelvic or femoral shaft fractures, carries an increased risk of pulmonary embolus formation.

8. A **history of PE** increases the risk of later pulmonary embolus formation, especially after surgery.

9. **Varicose veins** are associated with a two times greater risk of PE.

10. **Older age groups** are associated with an increased risk of developing pulmonary emboli.

C **Symptoms** of PE range from none to severe cardiopulmonary dysfunction. In general, the more complicated the symptoms, the more unreliable the clinical diagnosis.

1. **Classic signs include hemoptysis, pleural friction rub, cardiac gallop, cyanosis, and chest splinting**, which are present in only 24% of patients.

2. **Nonspecific findings,** including **tachycardia** (in 60% of patients), **tachypnea** (in 85% of patients), and **dyspnea** (in 85% of patients), are common. **Bronchospasm** and **pleuritic chest pain** also occur frequently.

3. **Electrocardiographic changes,** including **arrhythmias** and evidence of **right ventricular strain,** may appear.

4. **Chest radiograph** may be abnormal or totally normal.
   a. Occasionally, a **marked diminution of the pulmonary vasculature** produces increased radiolucency in the area of the embolus (**Westermark's sign**).
   b. **Pleural effusion,** which is usually hemorrhagic, or **pulmonary infiltration** may be present, especially in cases of pulmonary infarction, which occurs in 10%–25% of cases of PE.

5. **Arterial blood gases** frequently show hypoxemia with a low carbon dioxide partial pressure (PCO_2) associated with hyperventilation. A normal PO_2 does not eliminate the possibility of PE.

D **Diagnosis** of PE is based on the results of several tests.

1. **Pulmonary arteriogram** is the gold standard. This test is virtually 100% accurate, but it is invasive.

2. **Pulmonary radioisotope scanning** is less invasive than arteriography.
   a. **Perfusion lung scan.** A radioactive particle, small enough to block a small number of pulmonary capillaries temporarily, is injected. A camera records different views of the uptake in the vasculature.
      (1) A major difficulty with this test is that many acute and chronic pulmonary diseases can result in similar perfusion defects. It is critical to compare the chest x-ray with the scan to determine the presence of other abnormalities.
      (2) A normal scan is very reliable in determining the absence of a pulmonary embolus.
         (a) The presence of segmental or large defects predicts PE in 71% of patients.
         (b) A subsegmental or small perfusion defect is associated with PE in only 27% of patients.
   b. **Ventilation scan** performed simultaneously with the perfusion lung scan improves the accuracy of the latter. An inert radioactive gas, such as xenon, is inhaled, and the patency and ventilation of the bronchial tree are assessed.

(1) **Ventilation-perfusion mismatch** occurs when a perfusion defect is present but the ventilation scan is normal. **Matched ventilation-perfusion defect** occurs when a defect in the same location is revealed by both tests.

    (a) A segmental or large perfusion defect mismatched with a normal ventilation scan is associated with PE in 91% of patients.

    (b) A subsegmental or small perfusion defect mismatched with a normal ventilation scan is associated with PE in only 27% of patients.

    (c) A perfusion defect matched with a ventilation defect is associated with PE in 23% of patients.

(2) When pulmonary embolus is clinically suspected but the lung scan is equivocal, an additional test should be performed to increase the reliability of those results. A **pulmonary arteriogram** is most reliable. A **venous duplex** is also useful in documenting the presence of DVT in this situation and, therefore, the likelihood of PE.

E **Treatment** of PE includes both supportive measures to maintain circulatory function and administration of heparin for systemic anticoagulation.

1. **Cardiovascular support** is frequently necessary in patients with significant PE and should be instituted immediately. The supportive measures include oxygen administration, assisted ventilation, correction of cardiac arrhythmias, and treatment of shock by means of adequate hydration and vasopressors.

2. **Heparin as an anticoagulant** should be administered in an initial bolus of 10,000–20,000 U to halt the thrombotic process and to stabilize platelets in the embolus to prevent the release of vasoactive and bronchoactive substances. Administration begins with a continuous intravenous drip of heparin at approximately 1000 U/hour; the dosage is then adjusted to maintain the partial thromboplastin time at 1.5–2 times the control time. Heparin is continued for a minimum of 7 days and is followed by long-term anticoagulation therapy for 3–6 months.

3. **Thrombolytic therapy** with urokinase or tissue plasminogen activator may be used in cases of acute life-threatening PE when cardiopulmonary function is severely compromised as evidenced by shock, profound hypoxemia, or elevated pulmonary arterial pressure. Thrombolysis is **contraindicated** in patients with recent intracranial hemorrhage, recent surgery, or conditions associated with bleeding, such as peptic ulcer disease.

4. **Pulmonary embolectomy** is reserved for very ill patients who cannot endure the several hours required for thrombolysis. A closed embolectomy using a suction catheter or open embolectomy on cardiopulmonary bypass are the two most common methods.

5. **Long-term anticoagulation** may be maintained by either oral administration of warfarin to an international normalized ratio (INR) of two to three times control or subcutaneous intermittent administration of heparin.

F Complications of anticoagulation therapy

1. **Major hemorrhage** requiring transfusions occurs in 1%–2% of patients on anticoagulants, **minor bleeding episodes** are common in more than 16%, and fatal hemorrhage occurs in 0.1%–1%. The risk of hemorrhage is greater if heparin is administered intermittently or is given to elderly or severely hypertensive patients.

2. **PE recurs** despite anticoagulation therapy in 1%–8% of patients.

3. **Heparin-induced thrombocytopenia** occurs in up to 5% of patients on heparin and may be related to the development of heparin-induced antibodies directed toward platelets. This response is not dose related and is usually seen 5–10 days after heparin is started. The main source of morbidity is due to small vessel thrombosis. All heparin infusions must be discontinued if thrombocytopenia occurs. Anticoagulation is continued using lepirudin or argatroban, which are direct thrombin inhibitors.

III   LYMPHATIC SYSTEM

A **Lymphedema** is a condition characterized by swelling of one or more extremities because of lymphatic insufficiency.

1. **Types.** Lymphedema may be idiopathic (**primary lymphedema**) or may be caused by acquired insufficiency due to infections, obstructions, or surgical destruction of the lymphatics (**secondary lymphedema**).

    a. **Primary lymphedema.** Three types of primary lymphedema are distinguished by age of onset.

       (1) **Congenital lymphedema** is present at birth or occurs early in infancy.

          (a) It accounts for fewer than 10% of primary lymphedema cases.

          (b) Lymphedema that is both congenital and hereditary is known as **Milroy's disease.**

       (2) **Lymphedema praecox** occurs at any time from puberty until the end of the third decade.

          (a) Most cases of primary lymphedema are of this type.

          (b) It is three times more common in women than in men.

       (3) **Lymphedema tarda** occurs after age 30.

    b. **Secondary lymphedema** is due to obstruction from a variety of causes, including infection (see III C), parasites, mechanical injury (including surgery), postphlebitic syndrome, and neoplasms.

       (1) In developed countries, the most common causes are obstruction by malignancies, postsurgical lymphedema (e.g., after mastectomy), and lymphatic destruction from therapeutic radiation.

       (2) In less well-developed countries, parasitic obstruction (elephantiasis) is a common cause. *Wuchereria bancrofti* is the most common offending parasite.

2. **Diagnosis** of lymphedema is usually made clinically.

    a. **The history** characteristically includes edema, which begins at the foot and ankle and progresses proximally. Progression is slow, usually over the course of several months.

    b. **Physical examination.** Lymphedema has no dark brawny edema or ulceration of the skin. Whereas the swelling secondary to venous disease usually starts at the ankle, lymphedema usually involves the dorsum of the foot.

    c. **Laboratory tests.** The diagnosis can be proven by lymphangiography, but this test is not done routinely because it is difficult and hazardous.

3. **Treatment**

    a. Simple measures are the first line of treatment.

       (1) Elevation of the affected limb, weight reduction, and salt restriction may be helpful.

       (2) Compressive stockings may be of benefit if worn properly.

       (3) It is extremely important to avoid trauma and infection because either will greatly exacerbate the condition.

       (4) Pneumatic compression boots may help to "squeeze" the edema from the swollen extremity in severe cases.

    b. Surgery is indicated only infrequently for advanced and severely debilitating disease.

Study Questions for Part III

Directions: Each of the numbered items in this section is followed by several possible answers. Select the ONE lettered answer that is BEST in each case.

1. A 65-year-old woman with a long history of atrial fibrillation presents to the emergency department with a history of sudden onset of severe, constant abdominal pain. After the onset of pain, she vomited once and had a large bowel movement. No flatus has been passed since that time. Physical examination reveals a mildly distended abdomen, which is diffusely tender, although peritoneal signs are absent. Ten years ago, she underwent an abdominal hysterectomy. What is the most likely diagnosis in this patient?

- [A] Acute cholecystitis
- [B] Perforated duodenal ulcer
- [C] Acute diverticulitis
- [D] Acute embolic mesenteric ischemia
- [E] Small bowel obstruction secondary to adhesions

2. A 60-year-old woman develops weakness in her right arm and leg, and she has some difficulty speaking. This condition resolves after 5 minutes, and she has no residual symptoms. Her physician does not hear a carotid bruit, and her electrocardiogram is normal. A carotid duplex ultrasound shows a 75% stenosis of the left carotid artery and an 80% stenosis of the right carotid artery; both are confirmed by a carotid arteriogram. What should be the next step in the management of this patient?

- [A] Right carotid endarterectomy
- [B] Left carotid endarterectomy
- [C] Superficial temporal artery to middle cerebral artery bypass
- [D] Percutaneous transluminal angioplasty of the left carotid artery
- [E] Bilateral carotid endarterectomy

QUESTIONS 3–4

A 70-year-old man who is a new patient presents with a history of insulin-dependent diabetes mellitus; renal insufficiency (serum creatinine, 2.5); chronic obstructive pulmonary disease; and two myocardial infarctions, the most recent being 1 year ago. His ejection fraction is 35%, and he has a right below-the-knee amputation, which he says was secondary to "peripheral vascular disease." Now, the patient has a large pulsatile nontender abdominal mass.

3. All of the following studies would be appropriate *except*

- [A] Computed tomography (CT) scan of the abdomen
- [B] Pulmonary function tests
- [C] Arteriogram
- [D] Colonoscopy
- [E] Persantine thallium scan

His workup demonstrates a 6.0-cm infrarenal abdominal aortic aneurysm with a 4-cm left common iliac artery aneurysm and normal renal arteries. He has normal external iliac arteries bilaterally, with relatively normal femoral vessels. Pulmonary function tests indicate a forced expiratory volume in 1 second (FEV_1) to be 75% of the predicted value. The Persantine thallium scan shows an old scar but no reperfusion defect.

4. What is the next step in this patient's management?

- [A] Letting the patient live with the aneurysm because he is too high a surgical risk for elective surgery
- [B] Checking the size of the aneurysm with ultrasound every year until it starts to enlarge
- [C] Not performing surgery until he develops back pain because he is currently asymptomatic

D Performing an aorto-bi-iliac bypass

E Repairing the abdominal aortic aneurysm with a tube graft

5. A 67-year-old woman notices a swollen right leg following a 6-hour plane flight. Which of the following would be a reasonable next step for the treating physician?

A Prescribe compression stockings and leg elevation

B Start 6 months of warfarin anticoagulation

C Prescribe one baby aspirin per day

D Order a venous duplex evaluation

E Order a pelvic CT scan to look for lymphadenopathy

QUESTIONS 6–9

A 59-year-old patient undergoes a craniotomy for a benign meningioma. On the tenth postoperative day, he is noted to have a swollen left calf and thigh.

6. What is the *least* accurate method to diagnose the cause of the swollen leg?

A Physical examination

B Left leg venogram

C ^{125}I Fibrinogen scan

D Impedance plethysmography

E Duplex ultrasonography

7. If deep venous thrombosis is documented, initial treatment should include which of the following?

A Subcutaneous unfractionated heparin therapy

B Intravenous heparin therapy

C Thrombolytic therapy with urokinase

D Aspirin therapy

E Warfarin treatment

8. After recovery from the acute illness, the patient returns in 6 months, complaining of persistent leg swelling. Which of the following would be the optimal long-term management as initial treatment?

A Chronic diuretic therapy

B Venous thrombectomy

C Venous bypass using an autologous vein

D Venous bypass using a prosthetic graft

E Support hose

9. This complication may have been prevented by all of the following measures *except*

A Early mobilization after surgery

B Routine use of support hose

C Routine use of pneumatic sequential compression devices on both lower legs

D Daily administration of a single dose of subcutaneous unfractionated heparin starting 12 hours after the completion of surgery

E Daily administration of low molecular weight heparin starting in the preoperative holding area

Answers and Explanations

1. The answer is D (Chapter 7, V A 1 a). The triad of a cardiac arrhythmia, the sudden onset of severe abdominal pain, and gut emptying is a classic indicator of embolic mesenteric ischemia. This combination constitutes a surgical emergency, and the patient should be treated promptly with vigorous rehydration followed by arteriography to confirm the diagnosis. Rapid embolectomy of the superior mesenteric artery could save this patient, provided that no delay occurs in her definitive surgical treatment.

Cholecystitis usually presents with right upper quadrant pain and diverticulitis with left lower quadrant pain. A perforated ulcer will have associated diffuse abdominal tenderness but also wil have signs of peritoneal irritation (guarding and rebound). A small bowel obstruction usually presents with colic or intermittent pain.

2. The answer is B (Chapter 7, VIII E 2 a–e). The symptomatic artery is usually repaired first because it carries the highest risk of stroke. Percutaneous transluminal angioplasty of the carotid artery is presently under investigation as an alternative to carotid endarterectomy, but it is not considered to be the standard of care at this point. Percutaneous transluminal angioplasty is sometimes used for smooth, regular lesions associated with fibromuscular dysplasia. The superficial temporal artery to middle cerebral artery bypass has not been shown to be effective for this patient's disease. Bilateral carotid endarterectomy is usually not performed because of the risk of recurrent laryngeal nerve trauma, which, if bilateral, could result in a tracheostomy.

3–4. The answers are 3-D (Chapter 7, VIII A), **4-D** (Chapter 7, VIII A 3). Colonoscopy is not indicated if the patient's stool is heme negative. Computed tomography (CT) can help to evaluate the proximal extent of the aneurysm. Pulmonary function tests can help to assess risk and to help plan perioperative care. An arteriogram acts as a road map, showing the renal arteries in relation to the aneurysm and the extent of occlusive disease in the iliac and femoral arteries. A Persantine thallium scan helps to define perioperative cardiac risk.

Elective repair of an abdominal aortic aneurysm (AAA) can be performed with a mortality rate lower than 5%. The leading cause of death in these patients with AAA is rupture. A 6-cm AAA has a 35% rupture rate, and surgery should be recommended unless the patient has a life expectancy of less than 1 year. Rate of enlargement is not a safe predictor of risk of rupture. Patients with symptomatic or rupturing AAA have a 75% mortality rate when operated on as an emergency. An aorto-bi-iliac graft is the appropriate procedure in this patient, rather than a tube graft, to repair the associated iliac aneurysm. With no iliac occlusive disease, an aortoiliac bypass avoids groin incisions.

5. The answer is D (Chapter 8, I B 3). A swollen leg following a period of immobilization is a typical history leading to a deep venous thrombosis (DVT). While lymphedema or other causes can also lead to leg swelling, a pelvic CT scan would not be the next step for this patient. Physical examination is reliable only 50% of the time for DVT, so an accurate diagnostic study such as a venous duplex ultrasound is needed before starting long-term anticoagulation. If no other reason for the swelling can be found, a pelvic CT scan may be reasonable. Leg elevation is helpful to reduce swelling, but compression stockings are not recommended in the acute phase for fear of dislodging the clot. Aspirin is of no proven benefit in treating DVT.

6–9. The answers are 6-A [Chapter 8, I B 3 c (1)–(4)], **7-B** [Chapter 8, I B 3 d (1)], **8-E** [Chapter 8, I B 3 f (1)]. Physical examination is the least likely method to diagnose the cause of acute leg swelling. Currently, such a patient would undergo duplex ultrasonography or venography to confirm the presumed diagnosis of DVT. Impedance plethysmography can detect increased resistance to venous flow but does not identify the cause. [125]I Fibrinogen scanning can identify ongoing thrombosis, but the scan takes 24 hours to complete and is therefore not useful in acute situations.

Intravenous heparin therapy is the most appropriate initial treatment. Subcutaneous unfractionated heparin therapy in its current form is not acceptable treatment for DVT. Thrombolytic therapy would be contraindicated in a patient with a recent craniotomy because it would increase the risk of hemorrhage.

Aspirin therapy has no role in the treatment of DVT. Warfarin can be used once the patient is discharged but not as the initial treatment. Transition from intravenous heparin to warfarin therapy should occur on the fourth or fifth day of heparin administration.

Support hose is the mainstay of treatment for patients with chronic postphlebitic syndrome. Thrombectomies have been unsuccessful, and the efficacy of venous bypass has yet to be established. There is interest in transplanting venous valves and segments of a vein to replace short-segment thromboses, but this area is still experimental. Prosthetic grafts have no role in venous reconstruction. Chronic diuretic therapy may be useful for short-term therapy but is certainly not optimal long-term management for this problem.

9. The answer is D (Chapter 8, I B 3 e). The risk of DVT can be reduced by simple measures such as leg elevation, early mobilization, support hose, and sequential compression devices. Unfractionated heparin administered subcutaneously either two or three times a day or low molecular weight heparin can both reduce the risk of DVT, but either should be started prior to surgical procedures.

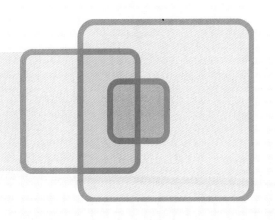

PART **IV**

Gastrointestinal Disorders

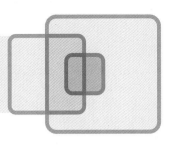

chapter 9

Common Life-threatening Disorders

VINCENT T. ARMENTI · BRUCE E. JARRELL

I ACUTE ABDOMEN

A **Definition**   Acute abdomen is the term used for an episode of severe abdominal pain with an acute onset (<8 hours) that lasts for several hours or longer and requires medical attention. Prompt diagnosis is important because an acute abdomen is caused by an intra-abdominal emergency in most patients.

B **Symptoms**   The history obtained from the patient should elicit both specific symptoms typical of a disease process and nonspecific symptoms.

1. **Nonspecific symptoms** should be elicited first.
   a. **Pain**
      (1) **Gradual periumbilical pain** indicates visceral peritoneal irritation, such as appendicitis, diverticulitis, or other inflammatory conditions. The pain may become more specifically localized as the disease process progresses.
      (2) **Severe, explosive pain** indicates a process that immediately soils the parietal peritoneum, such as perforation of a hollow viscus. The pain may be either localized or generalized.
      (3) **Progressive, severe pain** suggests a worsening intra-abdominal condition, such as that which occurs with ischemic necrosis of the bowel or other organs.
      (4) **Localized pain that recurs as a generalized pain** suggests that the inflamed organ has been perforated. For example, acute appendicitis causes right lower quadrant pain, which then becomes generalized if perforation occurs.
      (5) **Crampy pain** indicates an obstruction in the gastrointestinal (GI) tract. This type of pain has a crescendo component, building up to intense pain, followed by a decrescendo component; the patient may then have an interval with no pain.
         (a) Distinguishing between crampy pain versus constant or other types of pain is very important because crampy pain is associated with bowel obstruction.
         (b) If crampy pain develops into constant severe pain, it suggests that the involved bowel segment is now ischemic or gangrenous.
   b. **Anorexia, nausea, and vomiting** are common accompanying symptoms in acute inflammatory abdominal processes. Although they are reliably present when a problem is surgical, they also accompany nonsurgical diseases, in which case they often precede the pain (as in gastroenteritis).
   c. **Changes in bowel habits** are so common that they are seldom helpful unless very specific changes occur. For example:
      (1) Bloody diarrhea suggests colitis, *Salmonella* infestation, or colonic ischemia.
      (2) Patients with intestinal obstruction usually pass no flatus or bowel movement by rectum for 1–2 days prior to seeking medical attention.
   d. **Symptoms of sepsis,** such as **chills** and **fever,** may be nonspecific, although certain patterns are typical of certain diseases. For example:
      (1) The fever of uncomplicated appendicitis rarely exceeds 101°F, whereas that of perforation often exceeds 101°F.
      (2) Cholangitis with choledocholithiasis is often accompanied by a shaking chill.

2. **Specific symptoms** should be elicited as clues to specific diseases.
   a. **Previous surgery.** A history of previous surgery yields important information.
      (1) Adhesions may have formed within the peritoneal cavity, leading to intestinal obstruction.
      (2) If the surgery was for malignant disease, the malignancy may have recurred, causing pain, sepsis, intestinal obstruction, and other symptoms.
      (3) Previous removal of any organ (most likely the appendix, the gallbladder, or the uterus, ovaries, and fallopian tubes) eliminates that organ from consideration.
      (4) Previous surgery may point to a specific problem; e.g., suppurative cholangitis in a patient with previous choledocholithiasis and retained common duct stone.
   b. **Previous episodes of similar pain** warrant questions about the subsequent disease course and the results of any diagnostic studies that were performed.
   c. **Characteristic maneuvers** in certain diseases that provide temporary relief of pain must be sought.
      (1) A patient with acute peritonitis will lie very still; any movement results in excruciating pain.
      (2) A patient with a common duct stone or a kidney stone will pace the floor, unable to find a comfortable position.
      (3) The pain of an acute peptic ulcer may be relieved by food or antacids, whereas pain from acute cholecystitis or pancreatitis may be exacerbated by food.
   d. **Previous illnesses.** A history of disease in other body systems may be very useful.
      (1) **Urinary tract.** Symptoms such as dysuria, hematuria, or changes in urinary habits should be sought.
      (2) **Reproductive tract in the female patient.** The patient should be asked about past or present vaginal discharge, dysmenorrhea, a history of pelvic inflammatory disease, time of last menstrual period, and so forth.
      (3) **Cardiovascular system.** Atrial fibrillation of recent onset or digitalis therapy might suggest intestinal ischemia.
      (4) **Diabetes mellitus** is associated with sepsis. Poorly controlled blood sugars in a previously well-controlled diabetic may indicate infection.

C **Physical examination** of the patient with acute abdominal pain should yield new information that reinforces impressions obtained from the history. As with the history, there are both specific and nonspecific findings.

1. **Complete physical examination** must be performed so that an important related or unrelated extra-abdominal diagnosis will not be missed. Points requiring particular attention include the following:
   a. Changes in vital signs, particularly fever, tachypnea, hypotension, or cardiac rhythm irregularities
   b. Inspection for jaundice, dehydration, feculent breath, pneumonia, or mental disorientation or obtundation
   c. Examination of the extremities for loss of pulses

2. **Abdominal examination**
   a. **Overall inspection**
      (1) A distended abdomen with visible peristalsis suggests small bowel obstruction.
      (2) In a thin and muscular patient, prominent muscle guarding or rigidity may be visible, particularly if localized to one area of the abdomen.
      (3) A scaphoid abdomen may suggest herniation of the abdominal contents through the diaphragm and into the thoracic cavity, especially after blunt abdominal trauma.
      (4) Hernias are frequently visible, particularly when the patient is standing.
   b. **Palpation of the abdomen** should be done gently and should begin away from the area of maximum tenderness.
      (1) The inguinal area should be examined for hernias or inflammatory conditions.
      (2) The abdomen should be examined to determine the points of maximum tenderness or the presence of referred tenderness. **Rebound tenderness** is tenderness that occurs when the examining hand is quickly removed from the abdominal wall. It is indicative of acute peritoneal irritation.

(3) **Spasm** is determined by gently depressing the abdominal wall muscles.

  (a) Comparing two areas simultaneously allows the examiner to distinguish an abnormal area from a normal one.

  (b) A spasm is **voluntary** if the patient is tensing the muscle in response to pain and **involuntary** if the muscle is taut secondary to the underlying inflammatory process.

(4) **Palpation for abdominal masses** should be done systematically. A mass in a particular abdominal quadrant suggests a specific diagnosis.

  (a) **Right upper quadrant:** Acute cholecystitis or a complication of this diagnosis, such as subhepatic or intrahepatic abscess

  (b) **Left lower quadrant:** Acute diverticulitis or peridiverticular abscess

  (c) **Right lower quadrant:** Acute appendicitis or appendiceal abscess

  (d) **Left upper quadrant** (uncommon in the acute abdomen): Complication of gastric or colonic malignancy, subphrenic abscess, or some acute inflammatory process related to the spleen, such as infarction

  (e) **Midabdominal area:** Pancreatic malignancy or abscess, complication of a perforated ulcer, or leaking abdominal aortic aneurysm

  c. Percussion of the abdomen

  (1) Percussion is useful because it confirms areas of maximum tenderness and the presence of rebound tenderness.

  (2) On rare occasions, the hollow sound of **tympany** indicates free intraperitoneal air, but it usually is present because of air in the intestine.

  (3) A large area of tympany in the left upper quadrant suggests acute gastric dilation, a condition that can cause reflex hypotension through vagal pathways.

  d. Auscultation is useful in many acute abdominal problems.

  (1) **A silent abdomen** indicates the absence of peristalsis, suggesting diffuse peritonitis, which occurs with major abdominal sepsis, intestinal ischemia or gangrene, or prolonged (longer than 3 days) mechanical obstruction with marked distention of the bowel. Absent peristalsis may also indicate an ileus resulting from some other process, such as pneumonia, a renal stone, or trauma.

  (2) **Intermittent peristaltic rushes** that have a crescendo followed by silence suggest an intestinal obstruction. This sign is particularly useful when the peristaltic rush coincides with the onset of episodic abdominal pain. Certain nonsurgical inflammatory conditions, such as gastroenteritis, produce **high-pitched intermittent peristaltic rushes.** The pain pattern is usually not synchronous with the rushes.

3. Rectal examination should be performed routinely in patients with acute abdominal pain.

  a. Rectal palpation may localize the tenderness. In **acute appendicitis,** if the patient's appendix is located in the pelvis, the only physical finding may be a right pelvic tenderness found on rectal examination.

  b. The presence of **blood in the stool** suggests either a malignancy, hemorrhoids, or an acute inflammatory GI process, such as an ulcer or colitis.

  c. A **mass** palpable on rectal examination may be a pelvic abscess secondary to a perforated viscus, a sign of pelvic inflammatory disease, or a metastatic malignancy.

  d. Acute prostatitis in men is diagnosed rectally even though it may present with vague abdominal pain. Rectal examination reveals a tender, sometimes warm prostate gland.

4. Gynecologic examination should be performed in all women and girls with abdominal pain. (The patient's bladder should be empty.)

  a. Cervical or parauterine tenderness suggests pelvic inflammatory disease.

  b. A uterine, ovarian, or pelvic mass suggests:

  (1) Intrauterine pregnancy

  (2) Ectopic pregnancy with rupture and hemorrhage

  (3) Pelvic, ovarian, or tubal inflammatory disease with or without abscess formation

  (4) Pelvic or gynecologic malignancy

  c. Cervical discharge should be examined microscopically for gonococci.

5. Examination of the genitalia should be performed in all men and boys. Torsion of the testicle, a urologic emergency, may present as sudden onset of lower quadrant or scrotal tenderness.

6. **Special signs** are useful in diagnosing acute abdominal pain.
   a. **Tenderness to percussion over the liver or kidney** suggests acute hepatitis or pyelonephritis.
   b. **Iliopsoas sign** is pain in the lower abdomen and psoas region that is elicited when the thigh is flexed against resistance. It suggests that an inflammatory process, such as appendicitis or perinephric abscess, is in contact with the psoas muscle. Patients may also limp while walking and may lie with the ipsilateral hip flexed to minimize psoas muscle use.
   c. **Obturator sign** is pain elicited when the thigh is flexed and then rotated internally and externally. It suggests an inflammatory process in the region of the obturator muscle, such as an obturator hernia.
   d. **Murphy's sign** is elicited by palpating the right upper quadrant during inspiration: As the gallbladder descends during inspiration, acute pain is elicited, and inspiration halts. It suggests acute cholecystitis.
   e. **Cough tenderness** occurs in the area of maximum tenderness when the patient coughs. The tenderness may also be elicited by shaking the patient or by any other sudden jarring movement.
   f. **Ecchymosis** in the flank, periumbilical region, or back suggests a retroperitoneal hemorrhage. Possible causes include trauma, acute hemorrhagic pancreatitis, a leaking abdominal aortic aneurysm, and intestinal gangrene.
   g. **Subcutaneous, subfascial,** or **pelvic crepitus** suggests a rapidly spreading gas-forming infection. These infections must be rapidly diagnosed and explored surgically if they are to be cured.

D **Medical illnesses that can cause an acute abdomen**

1. Life-threatening medical illness, such as lower lobe pneumonias, acute myocardial infarction, diabetic ketoacidosis, and acute hepatitis, should be sought.

2. Acute polyserositis (occurring with collagen vascular diseases), rheumatic fever, porphyria, and chronic lead intoxication are uncommon causes of acute abdominal pain that can be exceedingly difficult to diagnose preoperatively. A careful history and physical examination may, however, raise them as possibilities.

3. Musculoskeletal problems, particularly vertebral compression of abdominal wall nerves, can also mimic acute general surgical conditions.

4. A high index of suspicion is necessary for acute abdominal emergencies in immunosuppressed patients (i.e., transplantation or steroid-dependent patients), whose symptoms and findings may be minimal.

E **Laboratory tests provide important information in many diseases.**

1. **Complete blood count**
   a. A **red cell count** may reveal anemia or suggest hemoconcentration secondary to dehydration.
   b. A **white cell differential count** is usually shifted to the left.
      (1) Leukocytosis in the 20,000–40,000 range suggests a major septic process in need of rapid surgical intervention. However, the white cell count may be misleading. For example, a normal white cell count in an elderly or diabetic patient may in fact accompany a major septic episode because advanced age can bring on an inability to generate a leukocytosis.
      (2) Profound leukopenia, particularly with a lymphocytic predominance, suggests a viral illness.
      (3) Other conditions, such as leukemia or lead intoxication, may also be diagnosed from the complete blood count.

2. **Urine examination** generally rules out urinary tract infection or kidney stone disease. Pelvic inflammatory processes in contact with the ureter or bladder may produce a few white cells and red cells in the urine. If there is doubt, intravenous pyelography or computed tomography should be performed prior to surgery.

3. **Serum amylase** should be measured in all patients with acute abdominal pain. In general, if the level is high, it usually indicates acute pancreatitis, although other surgical illnesses, such as mesenteric thrombosis and perforated ulcer, should not be overlooked.

4. **Arterial blood gases** may be very helpful in identifying a profound metabolic acidosis. This suggests either septic shock or severely ischemic or necrotic tissue, which indicates the necessity for surgery if no other obvious cause, such as diabetic ketoacidosis, can be found.

5. **Serum electrolytes, serum creatinine, coagulation profile, and liver function tests** are other studies that are often obtained.

6. **A urine or serum beta-HCG should be sent in all women of child-bearing potential.**

F **Radiographic studies**

1. **Upright chest radiograph and flat and upright radiograph of the abdomen** should be obtained in most cases of acute abdominal pain. A chest radiograph is essential to rule out other diseases, such as pneumonia, that can mimic conditions associated with an acute abdomen. Additionally, a chest radiograph is superior to an abdominal radiograph in showing intraperitoneal free air below the diaphragm. A CT scan is sensitive for free air and also provides additional information if the diagnosis is in doubt.

   a. **Bony structure abnormalities,** such as fractures or metastatic lesions, may provide important diagnostic information in trauma or malignant disease.

   b. **GI gas pattern.** Air is commonly present in the stomach and colon. However, air in the small intestine is abnormal and suggests an intra-abdominal process.

      (1) **Paralytic ileus** (see II B)

         (a) Air that is **evenly distributed** throughout the small and large intestine usually signifies paralysis of the bowel secondary to a process that is not primarily surgical.

         (b) Ileus may be **localized** to a specific area, such as the **"sentinel" loop,** an area of localized duodenal ileus adjacent to the pancreas in acute pancreatitis.

      (2) **Acute gastric dilation** is indicated by a **markedly dilated gastric bubble.** (This condition can result in severe abdominal pain and vasovagal hypotension but is easily treated by nasogastric tube decompression.)

      (3) **Mechanical obstruction of the intestine** (see II A) is revealed by the presence of **distended air- and fluid-filled loops of bowel proximal** to the obstruction and **decompressed intestine distally.** This air may be absent in the distal tract, particularly the rectum, unless air has been introduced by an enema given in the past 24 hours.

         (a) Mechanical bowel obstruction is an important diagnosis because it may be associated with strangulation of the bowel with resultant ischemia and necrosis. When both ends of a loop of bowel are obstructed, such as occurs with a volvulus, this is termed a *closed loop obstruction* and represents a surgical emergency due to the high risk of rupture and generalized peritonitis.

         (b) Postoperative adhesions, carcinoma of the colon, and inguinal hernias are the three most common **causes of bowel obstruction.** Specific causes may be diagnosed by the intestinal gas pattern.

            (i) **Hernias** may result in intestinal air located in a nonanatomic location. For example, an inguinal hernia may show gas-filled intestine extended below the inguinal ligament.

            (ii) **Volvulus** is a segment of bowel that has twisted upon itself, resulting in both mechanical obstruction and vascular compromise. It may appear on the plain film as an isolated distended loop of bowel with tapered ("bird-beak") margins. A sigmoid volvulus is treated by sigmoidoscopy and decompression. Other types of volvulus are treated operatively.

            (iii) An **ischemic** or **gangrenous bowel** may produce few radiologic findings. If the colon is affected, however, the mucosal edema may be seen as "thumbprinting" on the wall of a dilated colon.

            (iv) Isolated **distention of the colon by large amounts of air** may be seen on radiograph. It may be due to any of the acute processes, such as **distal colonic obstruction,** which may be secondary to malignancy, profound constipation, stricture, or volvulus; **"toxic megacolon,"** a massive colonic dilation that is associated with acute colitis; and **colonic ileus,** a condition of obscure etiology that results in marked distention of the cecum. If the cecum enlarges past 10–12 cm in diameter, there is a significant risk of perforation.

   c. Abnormal air collections outside the intestinal lumen

     (1) Free air within the peritoneal cavity signals a perforation of a hollow viscus and indicates a surgical emergency.

       (a) It is present in about 80% of gastroduodenal perforations but in fewer than 25% of colonic perforations.

       (b) Free peritoneal air is rarely secondary to other causes. However, it may be present in patients undergoing peritoneal dialysis and for up to 1 week after a laparotomy.

     (2) Air collections within the wall of the colon, a condition termed **pneumatosis cystoides intestinalis,** generally indicate an isolated, walled-off intestinal perforation.

     (3) Air stippling within soft tissue structures may indicate the dissection of air into the tissues from a thoracic source, such as a pneumothorax. It may, however, be due to a rapidly progressive, catastrophic gas-forming infection (see Chapter 2, V), which is a true surgical emergency.

     (4) Air-fluid level outside the intestinal tract is associated with a subphrenic or subhepatic abscess.

     (5) Air within the biliary tree indicates an abnormal communication between the biliary tree and the intestinal tract. Causes include:

       (a) A surgical connection created to provide biliary drainage (e.g., choledochoduodenostomy)

       (b) A gas-forming infection within the biliary tree (**cholangitis**). Cholangitis is associated with biliary obstruction and should be treated with antibiotics followed closely by endoscopic retrograde cholangiopancreatography (ERCP) and sphincterotomy to drain the biliary tract.

       (c) Large gallstones, particularly in the elderly, which can erode into the adjacent intestine (usually the duodenum), allowing air to enter the biliary tract and the gallstone to enter the bowel. Usually, this produces transient symptoms initially, until several days later when the gallstone impacts upon and obstructs the distal ileum, producing small bowel obstruction (gallstone ileus).

     (6) Air within the portal vein is seen when a gas-forming infection affects the portal system (**pylephlebitis**). The infection usually derives from necrotic tissue, particularly from the small intestine, appendix, or left colon.

   d. Abnormal calcifications

     (1) Renal stones are calcified in up to 85% of cases and appear along the path of the ureter.

     (2) Fecaliths (calcified material within the appendix) are strong evidence for acute appendicitis in patients with abdominal pain.

     (3) Pancreatic calcification suggests chronic pancreatitis.

     (4) Gallstones are calcified in 15% of cases.

     (5) Heavily calcified vessels may be present in mesenteric ischemia.

     (6) Masses, such as teratomas or malignant neoplasms, may calcify.

   e. Soft tissue shadows

     (1) Peritoneal fat lines and **psoas muscle shadows** may be lost in rapidly spreading infections, hematomas, or abscesses.

     (2) Margins of solid organs (liver, kidney, or spleen) may be displaced from their normal locations by an abnormal mass.

     (3) A **distended bladder** may be visible and may be responsible for marked abdominal pain.

2. Contrast roentgenography can be highly useful in patients with an acute abdominal process that remains undiagnosed after other studies.

   a. Intravenous pyelogram (IVP) should be obtained if a renal stone is suspected. It is also useful in identifying acute pyelonephritis, perinephric abscess, or renal infarction. When a patient suspected of having appendicitis has microscopic hematuria, the IVP is particularly useful for verifying that the hematuria is due to the periappendiceal inflammation rather than to a renal stone.

   b. Barium swallow is helpful if it is suspected that the patient's esophagus has ruptured during a violent episode of vomiting. Known as **Boerhaave's syndrome,** this unusual accident may result in a left pleural effusion, which communicates with the esophageal rent, as demonstrated by the barium swallow.

    c. Upper GI series, using diatrizoate meglumine (Gastrografin), a water-soluble radiopaque dye, should be performed if a perforation of the stomach or duodenum is suspected but cannot be proven because free air is not visible on the plain film.

    d. Placing contrast materials into the colon and rectum should be done very cautiously when an inflammatory condition or a perforation is suspected because even a small increase in pressure could easily convert friable tissue into a frank perforation.

      (1) This procedure is best used when the diagnosis of colon perforation is suspected and especially in a patient taking anti-inflammatory or immunosuppressive drugs, particularly corticosteroids.

      (2) In such cases, diatrizoate meglumine should be used because barium sulfate, when it mixes with stool and detritus from an infection, becomes firmly attached to the peritoneal cavity. Extensive abscess formation results, even after the surgeon attempts to irrigate the area thoroughly.

    e. Small bowel follow-through contrast study tracks the barium through the small intestine after an upper GI series. It is useful in identifying a point of small bowel obstruction when either the history, the physical examination, or plain radiography fails to verify the diagnosis of small bowel obstruction.

G Abdominal ultrasonography is usually of little diagnostic value in the patient with abdominal distention and severe pain, but it can be helpful when acute cholecystitis, cholelithiasis, biliary obstruction, or an abscess is suspected. **Computed tomography** may also be helpful, but is generally reserved for the patient whose condition remains undiagnosed after other studies have been exhausted. Some have advocated its use to assist in the diagnosis of acute appendicitis.

H General principles used in the approach to the patient with acute abdominal pain are discussed below.

    1. A careful and systematic evaluation of the patient should be routinely performed. Most patients will have a well-documented diagnosis if this principle is followed.

    2. Statistically speaking, certain diagnoses are very common, such as appendicitis and gastroenteritis, whereas **other diagnoses are quite rare,** such as pylephlebitis. The physician should not search for an occult diagnosis when a common diagnosis is more likely to be correct.

    3. When the diagnosis is not initially clear, continued observation and repeated blood studies (complete blood count, arterial blood gases, amylase, and electrolytes) may lead to the correct diagnosis as the disease process evolves.

    a. Although this practice might be desirable in a patient with gastroenteritis, **delay can be catastrophic** in acute appendicitis, ischemic bowel, small bowel obstruction, volvulus, or incarcerated hernia.

    b. If the diagnosis is not certain but the patient may have a potentially lethal condition that could be cured by an early operation, then an early operation should be performed—i.e., a small percentage of negative laparotomies are justified in patients with acute abdomen. This premise is best illustrated by the case of a patient with acute appendicitis. Here, a policy of watchful waiting may convert a simple appendicitis into a perforated appendicitis with generalized peritonitis and septic shock. The risk of death from this complication is many times higher than the risk from a small right lower quadrant incision in a patient who proves to have a normal appendix and mesenteric adenitis.

    4. Analgesics, particularly narcotics, should be withheld from the patient until the diagnosis is established or until the decision to proceed to surgery has been made. Serial physical examinations will be totally useless if the patient has been given narcotics.

    5. Antibiotics should also be withheld until a diagnosis has been made and the antibiotic therapy is needed. The only exception to this is the patient who presents in septic shock from an unknown cause. In that situation, broad-spectrum antibiotics should be part of the patient's resuscitation.

    6. Fluid deficits and electrolyte imbalances should be corrected before surgery. The few **exceptions** are:

    a. Conditions that threaten immediate exsanguination, such as a ruptured abdominal aortic aneurysm

    b. Conditions in which the fluid or electrolyte abnormality cannot be corrected in a reasonable amount of time—i.e., conditions that cause profound acidosis, such as necrotic bowel, where the acidosis cannot be corrected until the bowel is surgically removed

  7. Nasogastric tubes should be placed before the induction of anesthesia to empty the stomach, thus minimizing the risk of pulmonary aspiration.

II   INTESTINAL OBSTRUCTION

The normal flow of intestinal contents can be blocked by a mechanical obstruction or by a functional obstruction that occurs because of impaired intestinal motility. An acute abdomen often ensues.

A **Mechanical obstructions** are common and have various benign and malignant causes. If not treated expeditiously (usually by surgical removal of the cause), mechanical obstructions can rapidly become lethal. **Acute obstruction** occurs over hours to days and has a rapidly evolving course, whereas **chronic obstruction** may have a slow course with malnutrition, constipation, and other signs of chronic illness.

  1. Types

    a. Simple obstruction. There are no complicating factors, such as ischemia or perforation.

    b. Strangulating obstruction. The blood supply to the involved segment of bowel is significantly impaired. The ischemia may result from a twisting of the intestinal blood supply upon itself (**volvulus**) or from a constriction of the blood flow by a tight band or hernial opening.

    c. Closed loop obstruction. Both limbs of the bowel are obstructed; therefore, gas and liquid cannot pass in either direction.

    d. Intussusception. The bowel invaginates itself, causing a narrowing of the lumen and subsequent obstruction. It may result from either viral infections or intraluminal polypoid tumors.

    e. Perforating obstruction. The bowel proximal to the obstruction overdistends and perforates. The most common area of perforation when the colon is obstructed is the cecum.

  2. Causes (Table 9-1)

    a. Intestinal adhesions are the most common cause of obstruction.

      (1) They may result from a previous surgical exploration, particularly when talc was used to lubricate the surgeon's gloves, or their etiology may be obscure.

      (2) They may be diffuse, involving all peritoneal structures, or solitary, blocking only one area of the intestine.

    b. Hernias (see Chapter 2 III and Chapter 29 II) are a second very common cause of intestinal obstruction. A segment of intestine migrates through a defect in the abdominal wall (**external hernia**) or through a mesenteric or omental defect (**internal hernia**) and becomes blocked by the narrow ring that is present at the peritoneal communication of the hernia.

TABLE 9-1 Causes of Bowel Obstruction	
Type of Obstruction	**Examples**
Mechanical	Impaction
Lesions	
Extrinsic	
Adhesions	Previous surgery
Hernia	Incarcerated femoral hernia
Intrinsic	
Congenital	Meckel's diverticulum
Inflammatory	Diverticulitis
Malignant	Sigmoid cancer
Masses	Ovarian cancer
Volvulus	Sigmoid or cecal
Radiation injury	Previous gynecologic malignancy

    c. Intestinal tumors are the third most common cause of obstruction. The most common obstructing tumor is an adenocarcinoma of the colon or rectum. Benign lesions of the small bowel and colon, such as lipomas, can become the leading point of an intussusception. Other malignant tumors, such as carcinoid or lymphoma, can obstruct the intestinal lumen.

    d. Other intrinsic lesions within the bowel wall or the lumen can cause acute obstruction.

        (1) Congenital lesions: webs, malrotations, and atresias

        (2) Inflammatory lesions: Crohn's disease, diverticulitis, ulcerative colitis, and infections such as tuberculosis

        (3) Luminal foreign bodies: bezoars, parasites, and gallstones

        (4) Radiation injury, other **trauma,** or **endometriosis**

    e. Other extrinsic lesions, such as large intra-abdominal tumors or abscesses, can compress the intestinal lumen.

  3. Treatment

    a. Intestinal adhesions are treated by surgical lysis of the obstructing bands if the obstruction does not resolve in several days.

    b. Hernias are treated by a reduction of the contents of the hernia and subsequent repair. The bowel must always be examined for necrosis.

    c. Intestinal tumors are treated by surgical removal.

    d. Treatment of intrinsic and extrinsic lesions depend on the lesion.

B **Functional obstructions** are blockages in the intestinal flow that result from impaired motility (**paralytic** or **adynamic ileus**). These are usually **treated** by observation and by fluid and nutritional support until the causal agent resolves. Possible **causes** include:

  1. Direct irritation of the intestine, such as generalized peritonitis. Irritation may also be a factor in the postoperative adynamic ileus that can last for 3–7 days following surgery.

  2. Extraperitoneal causes, such as retroperitoneal hematoma or nerve root compression. Retroperitoneal dissections, such as a nephrectomy or sympathectomy, can cause a prolonged ileus.

III   UPPER GASTROINTESTINAL HEMORRHAGE

A **Causes** of massive upper GI hemorrhage as shown by endoscopy are given in Table 9-2.

B **Types of bleeding**   The diagnosis of hemorrhage is generally obvious, but **locating the site of bleeding** may be difficult. The **type of GI bleeding** may give a clue to its source.

  1. Hematemesis is the vomiting of blood that is either bright red or resembling coffee grounds in appearance. Hematemesis usually indicates a bleeding source proximal to the ligament of Treitz. **Coffee-grounds hematemesis** indicates that the blood has been in contact with gastric acid long enough to become converted from hemoglobin to methemoglobin.

  2. Hematochezia is the passage of bright red blood by rectum. Although it indicates GI bleeding, it does not specify the level within the GI tract.

  3. Melena is the passage of black, usually tarry, stools. Although melena signifies a longer time within the GI tract than bright red blood, it does not guarantee that the bleeding is from the upper tract.

TABLE 9-2   Causes of Upper Gastrointestinal Hemorrhage

Duodenal ulcer
Gastric ulcer
Diffuse erosive gastritis
Esophageal or gastric varices
Mallory-Weiss tear of the gastroesophageal junction
Gastric carcinoma
Arteriovenous malformations

4. Blood mixed with stool and mucus can produce a characteristic jellylike or "currant-jelly" stool. This may originate from a Meckel's diverticulum, particularly in children.

C **History**   The history should include information about previous episodes of GI bleeding, current medications (e.g., aspirin or warfarin use), and related diseases (e.g., hematologic disorders, alcoholism, peptic ulcer disease, and recent episodes of vomiting).

D **Physical examination** should specifically include a search for evidence of nasopharyngeal bleeding, portal hypertension, weight loss, malignancy, or systemic diseases such as chronic hepatic or renal failure.

E **Diagnosis**   The cause and the location of the bleeding must be confirmed unless imminent exsanguination calls for immediate measures (see Chapter 21, I D 3 e [3] [f]). In less urgent circumstances, once the patient has been stabilized, one may continue with diagnostic procedures.

1. **Fiberoptic endoscopy** of the upper GI tract has become the optimal diagnostic procedure because it allows direct visualization of the lesion in over 80% of cases.
   a. Endoscopy allows:
      (1) Determination of the size and number of lesions in most cases (lesions are multiple in 15% of cases)
      (2) Assessment of which site is actively bleeding
      (3) Assessment of the rate of bleeding. For example, if an arterial vessel is visibly bleeding in the base of a large duodenal ulcer, then there is a good chance that it will not stop bleeding.
      (4) Distinction between an ulcer, varices, gastritis, and a tear in the esophagus (Mallory-Weiss syndrome) that follows forceful vomiting
      (5) Determination of whether a lesion is benign or malignant
   b. Endoscopy is only safe if the patient's vital signs are relatively stable. Sedation is dangerous because it increases the risk of vomiting followed by aspiration of the gastric contents into the pulmonary bed.

2. **Upper GI series** helps to define anatomy or pathology more completely, but unfortunately, it sheds little light on the relationship of a particular lesion to the hemorrhage.

3. **Passage of a nasogastric tube** aids considerably in determining that the source of bleeding is proximal to the ligament of Treitz.

4. **Angiography and radionuclide scanning** may occasionally help to locate the site of bleeding, but both procedures are more useful in lower GI hemorrhage.

F **Treatment**   If treated expeditiously in a systematic fashion, the patient with upper GI hemorrhage has an excellent chance for recovery. Treatment is aimed at supporting the patient's vital signs as well as stopping the hemorrhage. **Resuscitation** measures should begin immediately when the patient is first seen.

1. **Medical treatment** of aggravating factors can then begin.
   a. **A nasogastric tube** is inserted, and the residual thrombus in the stomach is removed with an iced saline solution.
   b. **Clotting factors.** Any clotting abnormalities are corrected with appropriate factors (see Chapter 1, III C 2).
      (1) Fresh frozen plasma if the prothrombin time is abnormal
      (2) Platelets if thrombocytopenia is present
      (3) Vitamin K if bleeding is from esophageal varices
   c. **Histamine$_2$ (H$_2$) antagonists, proton pump inhibitors (PPI), and antacids.** An aggressive regimen is begun. H$_2$ antagonists given as a continuous infusion are commonly used in this setting. Oral antacids with gastric pH monitoring also have been used.
   d. **Vasopressin,** a powerful vasoconstrictor, may be useful.
      (1) It can be infused through a peripheral vein at a rate of up to 1 U/minute, or it can be infused directly into the bleeding vessel by means of angiography.
      (2) Vasopressin temporarily controls bleeding in 75% of patients; by contrast, bleeding was stopped in 30% of patients treated conventionally without vasopressin. However,

vasopressin is contraindicated in patients with significant coronary artery disease because of coronary vasoconstriction.

  e. **Fiberoptic endoscopy,** in addition to being a diagnostic procedure, may also be useful when esophageal varices are to be sclerosed (see Chapter 14, II E) or small bleeding sites are to be coagulated.

  f. **Angiography** similarly may be a therapeutic aid. It allows bleeding from small vessels to be controlled either by embolization of the bleeding vessel or by intra-arterial administration of vasopressin.

  g. **Balloon tamponade** (see Chapter 14, II E 3 d) can be important in controlling bleeding from varices.

2. **Surgical treatment.** The type of surgery performed is discussed in Chapter 11.

  a. The patient's cardiovascular status, as well as the amount and duration of bleeding, is particularly important. For example, a patient with heart disease may tolerate continued bleeding poorly and thus may need early surgery.

  b. Only about 10% of patients will require surgery.

  c. **Indications for surgery** are as follows:

    (1) **Exsanguinating hemorrhage.** A patient with uncontrollable hemorrhage who is losing blood faster than it can be replaced must be sent to the operating room immediately for control of the site of bleeding.

    (2) **Profuse bleeding,** especially in association with **hypotension.** Patients should be treated surgically:

      (a) If more than 4 U of blood are required for initial resuscitation

      (b) If bleeding continues at a rate of more than 1 U every 8 hours

      (c) If a brief hypotensive episode could have catastrophic results, as in patients with coronary artery disease or cerebrovascular disease or in patients older than 60 years of age

    (3) **Continued hemorrhage** despite resuscitation and other treatment

      (a) The mortality rate of upper GI bleeding is low among patients who need less than 6–7 U of blood.

      (b) The rate increases dramatically with requirements above 7 U. Thus, surgery should be undertaken before the blood loss reaches that point.

    (4) **Recurrent bleeding** after its initial cessation. About one fourth of patients rebleed, and the mortality rate for these patients is as high as 30%, in contrast to a mortality rate of approximately 3% among patients who do not rebleed.

    (5) **Pathologic features** of the bleeding site that **increase the risk** of recurrent bleeding include:

      (a) A posterior duodenal ulcer with the gastroduodenal artery visible in its base

      (b) A giant gastric ulcer

3. **Special situations** may call for a modification of the usual routines of management.

  a. A **patient with a rare or hard-to-find blood type** should be operated on while blood is still available.

  b. A **patient who refuses blood transfusion** for any reason should undergo surgical exploration early.

  c. A **patient with a coagulopathy** should have the disorder corrected, if possible, prior to surgical exploration.

G **Prognosis**   The prognosis for patients who are bleeding from a source other than esophageal varices is as follows:

1. Some 25%–50% will have a recurrence of bleeding during the next 5 years, and about 20% will require surgery.

2. The mortality rate is low (about 3%) if the bleeding stops spontaneously.

IV   **LOWER GASTROINTESTINAL HEMORRHAGE**

A **Overview**   Acute lower GI hemorrhage is managed initially in much the same way as upper GI hemorrhage.

1. **Resuscitation** with blood and intravenous fluids is begun immediately.
2. The **history** is taken, and a **physical examination** is performed.
3. **Diagnostic studies** are begun to identify the site and cause of the bleeding.
4. **Vasopressin** may be used as in upper GI bleeding (see III F 1 d).

B **Initial studies**

1. **Anorectal examination** is performed to determine if the source of bleeding is a hemorrhoid, anal fissure, anal carcinoma, or other anorectal lesion.
2. **A bleeding site in the upper GI tract must be ruled out.**
   a. A **nasogastric tube** is passed to ascertain that no bleeding is present in the gastroduodenal region. On occasion, however, duodenal bleeding will not reflux into the stomach because of a closed pyloric sphincter. If bile is present, duodenal bleeding is unlikely.
   b. **Endoscopy** (see III E 1) is therefore required to rule out upper GI bleeding with absolute certainty. Most physicians will withhold endoscopy when a highly probable source of the bleeding is found in the lower GI tract. However, if surgery is anticipated, particularly when one is not sure of the diagnosis, endoscopy of the upper GI tract should be performed to exclude any bleeding site there.
3. **A bleeding site in the lower GI tract must be located.** Once the upper tract has been eliminated as a source of bleeding, the lower tract should be investigated, including the distal small bowel, colon, and anorectal area (Table 9-3).
   a. **Colonoscopy** should be performed.
      (1) The presence of a mass lesion, such as rectal carcinoma, is visualized in about 3% of patients with massive lower GI bleeding.
      (2) Discrete bleeding sites from ulcers or hemorrhoids may be seen.
      (3) A diffusely hemorrhagic mucosa suggests colitis, a platelet deficiency, or a hematologic disorder.
      (4) Even if no lesion is visualized, it is important to make certain that the lower 15 cm of the rectum is normal because this region is inaccessible intraperitoneally if laparotomy is necessary. Additionally, if it is normal, it gives presumptive evidence that the bleeding is coming from a more proximal site.
   b. **Anoscopy** is frequently overlooked but should be routinely performed because bleeding lesions in the anal canal may be missed on sigmoidoscopy.

C **Subsequent diagnostic tests** will depend on whether the bleeding stops or continues. About 75% of the patients will spontaneously stop bleeding without further intervention.

1. **If bleeding stops,** the following steps are taken.
   a. A **barium enema,** a **colonoscopy,** or both procedures should be performed:
      (1) To identify or rule out diverticulosis or colon carcinoma
      (2) To provide indirect evidence for colonic mucosal ischemia
   b. The patient should be monitored thereafter.
2. **If bleeding continues,** further diagnostic studies should be done to identify the source more precisely in preparation for surgery, if it becomes necessary.

TABLE 9-3 **Causes of Lower Gastrointestinal Bleeding**	
Adults	**Children**
Anorectal disease	Meckel's diverticulum
Diverticular disease	Intussusception
Angiodysplasia	
Polyps	
Malignancy	
Inflammatory bowel disease	
Ischemic colitis	

    a. If bleeding continues, a barium enema should not be performed. The residual barium in the colon may make subsequent angiography difficult or impossible.

    b. Angiography and **radionuclide scanning** are useful.

      (1) Selective mesenteric angiogram will identify the bleeding site (or sites) in up to 80% of patients when the rate of bleeding exceeds 0.5 mL/minute. Angiography is also highly useful for identifying angiodysplastic lesions of the colon.

      (2) Radionuclide scan, which uses red blood cells labeled with technetium-99m (^{99m}Tc), is sensitive enough to detect a bleeding site when the rate is as low as 0.10 mL/minute.

    c. Colonoscopy is unsatisfactory and may be dangerous when lower GI bleeding is rapid: Visualization is poor, and there is a risk of colon perforation.

D **Indication for surgery** is persistent bleeding.

1. The patient's cardiovascular status and amount and duration of bleeding are taken into consideration, as for upper GI hemorrhage (see III F 1, 2).

2. The surgical procedure is aimed at removing the underlying cause of the bleeding.

3. On occasion, the precise point of bleeding cannot be established.

    a. In these instances, the stomach, duodenum, and small intestine should be carefully examined. Meckel's diverticulum, Crohn's disease, and other inflammatory or malignant lesions should not be overlooked.

    b. A "blind" total colectomy may be necessary if no other source of the bleeding is found.

    c. Intraoperative endoscopy of the colon, upper GI tract, and small bowel may be very useful in this setting.

4. The **mortality rate** for lower GI bleeding is currently about 10%.

chapter 10

Esophagus

WILLIAM R. ALEX · D. BRUCE PANASUK · RICHARD N. EDIE

I INTRODUCTION

A Anatomy

1. **Location.** The esophagus is approximately 24 cm in length. It extends from the C6 vertebral level to the T11 level.
   a. It originates at the **upper esophageal sphincter,** which is essentially made up of the cricopharyngeal muscle, then courses behind the arch of the aorta, and descends into the thorax on the right.
   b. It deviates anteriorly and enters the abdomen via the **esophageal hiatus,** which is formed by the right crus of the diaphragm.
   c. The tubular esophagus meets the saccular stomach at the **gastroesophageal junction,** where the esophagus is anchored by the phrenoesophageal ligament. The gastroesophageal junction is approximately 40 cm from the incisors.

2. **Histology**
   a. The esophageal mucosa consists of squamous cell epithelium except for the distal 1–2 cm, which is columnar epithelium.
   b. There are two layers of muscle throughout the esophagus, an inner circular and outer longitudinal layer. The upper one third is striated muscle, whereas smooth muscle predominates in the lower two thirds.
   c. The esophagus, unlike the rest of the gastrointestinal tract, lacks a serosal covering.

B Vasculature

1. **Arterial supply** to the esophagus is from branches of the inferior thyroid; the bronchial, intercostal, inferior phrenic, left gastric arteries; and direct esophageal branches from the aorta.

2. **Venous return** is more complicated.
   a. An extensive subepithelial venous plexus empties superiorly into the hypopharyngeal veins and inferiorly into the gastric veins. The left gastric vein is also known as the coronary vein. Segmental drainage occurs also via the azygous and hemiazygous systems.

3. **Lymphatic drainage** is to the nearest lymph nodes. Lymphatics of the upper esophagus drain into the cervical or mediastinal nodes, whereas drainage of the distal lymphatics is more often to the celiac nodes.

C Innervation
The esophagus is supplied by the sympathetic and parasympathetic system via the pharyngeal plexus, the vagus, upper and lower cervical sympathetic, and splanchnic nerves. Meissner and Auerbach's plexuses are present in the normal esophagus.

D Physiology

1. **The upper esophageal sphincter** is a high-pressure zone at the upper border of the esophagus. It is 3–5 cm in length, and it relaxes during swallowing and contracts thereafter.

2. **Peristalsis** in the central portion of the esophagus consists of wavelike movements that pass down the body of the esophagus and become stronger toward the lower portion. Esophageal peristaltic pressures range from 25–80 mm Hg.

3. **The lower esophageal sphincter (LES)** is a high-pressure zone at the lower portion of the esophagus. It is 3–5 cm in length and functions to prevent gastroesophageal reflux. LES pressure is influenced by several factors and substances.

   a. **LES pressure is increased** by a protein meal, alkalinization of the stomach, gastrin, vasopressin, and cholinergic drugs.

   b. **LES pressure is decreased** by secretin, nitroglycerine, glucagon, chocolate, fatty meals, and gastric acidification.

II   DISORDERS OF ESOPHAGEAL MOTILITY

A   Cricopharyngeal dysfunction and Zenker's diverticulum

1. **Pathophysiology**

   a. Cricopharyngeal dysfunction is caused by a failure of the upper esophageal sphincter to relax properly.

   b. The problem may be an incoordination between relaxation in the upper esophageal sphincter and simultaneous contraction of the pharynx, which results in a **pharyngoesophageal (Zenker's) diverticulum.** This is a false diverticulum that consists only of mucosa that herniate posteriorly between the fibers of the cricopharyngeal muscle.

   c. Cricopharyngeal dysfunction and Zenker's diverticulum is often associated with **hiatal hernia** and **gastroesophageal reflux.**

2. **Symptoms of Zenker's diverticulum** include dysphagia, halitosis, regurgitation of undigested food, nocturnal aspiration, and recurrent aspiration pneumonia.

3. **Diagnosis**

   a. The **history and physical examination** are usually adequate to diagnose cricopharyngeal dysfunction.

   b. **Radiographs,** which include a barium swallow, are helpful in delineating a diverticulum.

   c. Endoscopy is *contraindicated* when Zenker's diverticulum has been documented by barium swallow because the risk of perforation is high. If a diverticulum is *not* seen on contrast studies, then endoscopy is indicated to rule out other esophageal disorders, including gastroesophageal reflux or neoplasm.

4. **Treatment**

   a. **Cricopharyngeal myotomy** is the treatment of choice for cricopharyngeal dysfunction.

   b. Resection or suspension of the diverticulum is combined with the myotomy.

B   Achalasia

1. **Pathophysiology**

   a. Achalasia is an esophageal disease of unknown etiology, although it may be secondary to ganglionic dysfunction, which causes:

      (1) High resting LES pressure

      (2) Failure of the LES to relax during swallowing

      (3) Absence of coordinated peristalsis in the body of the esophagus

   b. The body of the esophagus becomes dilated, and the muscle hypertrophies in an attempt to force material through the dysfunctional LES. A similar symptom complex can be caused by **Chagas disease,** which is caused by the organism *Trypanosoma cruzi.*

   c. Carcinoma of the esophagus is 10 times more common in patients with achalasia than in the general population.

2. **Symptoms** of achalasia include dysphagia, followed by regurgitation and weight loss. Frequently, respiratory symptoms caused by aspiration are present.

3. **Diagnosis**

   a. **Radiographic studies** reveal a dilated esophagus with a bird's beaklike extension into the lower narrowed segment at the LES.

   b. **Esophageal manometry** reveals the high resting LES pressure, failure of relaxation during swallowing, higher than normal resting pressure in the body of the esophagus, and absence of peristalsis.

    c. Esophagoscopy is required to rule out neoplasia and to document the extent of esophagitis.

  4. Treatment for achalasia is palliative because LES function can never be restored to normal.

    a. Nonsurgical treatment consists of forced pneumatic dilatation of the spastic lower esophageal sphincter, which is just above the gastroesophageal junction.

    b. Surgical treatment is **esophagomyotomy** by the **modified Heller procedure,** via laparotomy/laparoscopy, or occasionally left thoracotomy. Care is taken not to disturb the vagus nerve attachments to the esophagus to prevent reflux. The myotomy is confined to the lower portion of the esophagus, usually 6–8 cm in length.

      (1) Surgical results with the Heller procedure are generally better than with pneumatic dilatation for relief of dysphagia.

      (2) Esophagomyotomy can be combined with an antireflux procedure if indicated.

C **Diffuse esophageal spasm**

  1. Pathophysiology

    a. Diffuse esophageal spasm is a disorder of esophageal motility that consists of **strong nonperistaltic contractions.**

    b. Unlike achalasia, this condition has normal sphincteric relaxation and may be associated with gastroesophageal reflux.

  2. Symptoms consist of chest pain, which can radiate to the back, neck, ears, jaw, or arms and may be confused with typical angina pectoris. The pain usually occurs spontaneously, and many patients are considered to have a psychoneurosis.

  3. Diagnosis

    a. Manometry reveals high-amplitude repetitive contractions with a normal sphincteric response to swallowing.

    b. Radiographs are normal in one half of the cases but may reveal diverticula, segmental spasm, and a corkscrew appearance of the esophagus.

  4. Treatment

    a. Surgery is moderately effective with good results obtained in over two thirds of the patients. The best results are obtained in emotionally stable patients with severe disease and without associated lower gastrointestinal problems.

      (1) Surgery consists of a long esophagomyotomy that extends from the arch of the aorta to just above the LES.

      (2) Care is taken to preserve LES function, which is usually normal in these patients.

      (3) If significant gastroesophageal reflux is present, an antireflux procedure is performed.

    b. Medical treatment. Calcium channel blockers and smooth muscle relaxants, such as nitrates, may ameliorate symptoms.

D **Esophageal reflux**

  1. Etiology. Esophageal reflux is a common condition that may affect up to 80% of the population in varying degrees. Gastroesophageal reflux disease remains a multifactorial disease.

    a. LES is a physiologic sphincter that is normally in an intra-abdominal position. Loss of LES pressure results in gastric reflux.

    b. Esophageal motility, in the normal esophagus, causes refluxed secretions to be cleared by esophageal peristalsis.

    c. Gastric secretions, gastric acid, pepsin, and bile reflux have been shown to produce severe esophagitis.

  2. Symptoms of esophageal reflux are substernal pain, heartburn, and regurgitation, all of which may increase with bending and lying down.

  3. Diagnosis is made by:

    a. Manometry, which reveals decreased LES pressure

    b. Esophagoscopy, which reveals varying degrees of esophagitis

    c. Twenty-four hour pH measurements in the lower esophageal area, which demonstrate increased acidity

4. **Treatment**
   a. **Medical treatment**
      (1) Proton pump inhibitors and H_2-receptor antagonists to reduce acidity
      (2) Cisapride and metoclopramide, which increase both LES pressure and gastric motility, thus increasing the rate of gastric emptying
      (3) Antacids
      (4) Weight reduction
      (5) Abstinence from smoking and alcohol
      (6) Elevation of the head of the bed at night
   b. **Surgical treatment**
      (1) **Indications for surgery** include:
         (a) Symptoms refractory to medical treatment
         (b) Additional problems, such as esophageal webs (see VII B) or severe esophagitis, stricture formation, or **Barrett's esophagus** with severe dysplasia (i.e., replacement of the normal epithelial lining with columnar epithelium in the lower esophagus secondary to esophagitis)
      (2) **Antireflux operations** are designed to increase LES tone. All of the operations involve wrapping the lower esophagus with gastric fundus and restoring the distal esophagus to its original intra-abdominal position with the gastroesophageal junction below the diaphragm. The three most commonly used operations are:
         (a) The **Nissen fundoplication,** which is a 360-degree wrap of the stomach around the esophagus performed through the abdomen. The procedure may now be successfully performed laparoscopically with minimal pain and a shorter recovery time.
         (b) **Belsey Mark IV operation,** which is a 270-degree wrap performed through a left thoracotomy
         (c) The **Hill repair,** or posterior gastropexy, which uses the arcuate ligament to re-establish the intra-abdominal position of the distal esophagus.

III ESOPHAGEAL STRICTURES

A Caustic stricture

1. **Etiology.** Caustic stricture is caused by the ingestion of caustic agents, such as lye, drain openers, and oven cleaners.

2. **Diagnosis**
   a. **The diagnosis may be made by the history of caustic ingestion** and the **presenting symptoms,** which may be mild or very severe. Shock may ensue from severe burning or perforation of the esophagus. It is important to identify airway compromise early.
   b. **Endoscopy** is indicated within 24 hours to determine the extent of damage.

3. **Treatment**
   a. Broad-spectrum antibiotics are administered.
   b. Corticosteroids are no longer indicated.
   c. Radiographs of the esophagus are performed at 10–14 days to determine if **strictures** are developing.
      (1) Strictures occur in 5%–10% of patients who have ingested lye.
      (2) If strictures have formed, a program of dilatation, using esophageal dilators, is begun 3–4 weeks after ingestion.
   d. Esophageal replacement with stomach or colon may be necessary.

B Strictures secondary to esophagitis and reflux

1. **Pathophysiology.** These strictures are caused by a recurrent alternating pattern of mucosal destruction secondary to gastric acid reflux and subsequent healing.
   a. The strictures most often occur at the gastroesophageal junction.
   b. In severe cases, a long stricture may result.

2. **Diagnosis**
   a. A **history** of reflux symptoms and dysphagia is suggestive of strictures.

   b. **Radiograph** of the esophagus confirms the diagnosis.
   c. **Esophagoscopy** is important to determine the extent of the disease and to rule out malignancy.

3. **Treatment**
   a. Dilatation of the esophagus is attempted first, then an antireflux operation is performed.
   b. If dilatation and an antireflux operation do not relieve the esophageal obstruction, a reconstructive procedure, using either the stomach or colon for esophageal replacement, may be necessary to restore adequate swallowing function.

IV   TUMORS OF THE ESOPHAGUS

A **Benign tumors**

1. **Leiomyomas** are intramural smooth muscle tumors that account for two thirds of all benign neoplasms of the esophagus.
   a. **Symptoms.** Dysphagia occurs when leiomyomas exceed a diameter of 5 cm as they grow within the muscular wall, leaving the overlying mucosa intact.
   b. **Diagnosis**
      (1) A **history** of dysphagia is typical.
      (2) A **barium swallow** reveals a localized smooth filling defect in the esophageal wall.
      (3) **Esophagoscopy** is performed to confirm the diagnosis.
      (4) **Biopsy** of the lesion is contraindicated because it violates the mucosa, making subsequent surgical therapy difficult.
      (5) **Endoscopic ultrasound (EUS)** is very helpful in confirming the intramural location of the lesion.
   c. **Surgical treatment**
      (1) In symptomatic patients, the **tumor is enucleated** from the esophageal wall without violating the mucosa.
      (2) A limited esophageal resection is indicated if the tumor lies in the lower esophagus and cannot be enucleated.

2. **Benign intraluminal tumors** are usually **mucosal polyps, lipomas, fibrolipomas,** or **myxofibromas.**
   a. **Symptoms** are dysphagia, occasional regurgitation, and weight loss.
   b. **Diagnosis**
      (1) **Radiographs** of the esophagus suggest the diagnosis.
      (2) **Esophagoscopy** is performed to confirm the diagnosis and to rule out malignancy.
   c. **Surgical treatment**
      (1) Esophagotomy, removal of the tumor, and repair of the esophagotomy comprise the surgical treatment.
      (2) Endoscopy should not be used to remove these tumors because of the possibility of esophageal perforation.

B **Malignant tumors**

1. **Incidence.** In the United States, the incidence of esophageal carcinoma ranges from 3.5 in 1 million for whites to 13.5 in 100,000 for blacks. The highest incidence of esophageal carcinoma is noted in the Hunan Chinese population, with as many as 130 in 100,000 individuals affected.

2. **Etiology.** The exact cause is unknown. Associated factors are tobacco use, excessive alcohol ingestion, nitrosamines, poor dental hygiene, and hot beverages. Certain pre-existing conditions also increase the likelihood of developing esophageal cancer, including achalasia and Barrett's esophagus.

3. **Pathology**
   a. **Type**
      (1) **Squamous cell carcinoma** is the most common form.
      (2) **Adenocarcinoma,** the next commonest, is the type that occurs in patients with Barrett's esophagus.

(3) Rare tumors of the esophagus include **mucoepidermoid carcinoma** and **adenoid cystic carcinoma.**

b. **Tumor spread.** Esophageal malignancies metastasize through both the lymphatic system and the bloodstream, with metastases occurring in liver, bone, and brain.

4. **Diagnosis**
   a. A **history** of dysphagia and weight loss is almost always present.
   b. **Contrast study** of the esophagus demonstrates the location and extent of the tumor.
   c. **Computed tomography (CT) scan** of the chest and abdomen is done to evaluate local lymphatic spread, and a thorough search is made for distant metastases.
   d. **Esophagoscopy** is essential for tissue diagnosis and determination of the extent of the tumor.
   e. **EUS** is done to assess the depth of the invasion and staging.
   f. **Bronchoscopy** is performed in patients with proximal esophageal lesions to assess the possibility of invasion of the tracheobronchial tree.

5. **Treatment**
   a. Overall, surgical therapy is associated with less than a 5% mortality rate. Several procedures are described for resection of the esophagus.
      (1) Transhiatal esophagectomy through a laparotomy and cervical incisions. A complete thoracic esophagectomy is performed bluntly with reconstruction of gastrointestinal continuity with the stomach or, rarely, the colon.
      (2) Ivor Lewis esophagectomy through a right thoracotomy and laparotomy. Reconstruction is also accomplished with the stomach or, rarely, the colon.
   b. **Radiotherapy and chemotherapy** are currently being investigated as adjuncts to surgery or as primary treatment modalities.
      (1) Neoadjuvant platinum-based chemotherapy in combination with X-Ray Therapy (XRT) given before surgical resection appears to shrink the tumor mass. Several studies have shown an impact on long-term survival. Clinical phase II and III studies are now under way.
      (2) Combination chemotherapy with cisplatin have shown up to a 50% response rate. However, a significant long-term survival has not been demonstrated.
      (3) Radiotherapy alone for carcinoma of the esophagus results in a 5-year survival of less than 10%.
      (4) In patients who have advanced disease with either invasion of the tracheobronchial tree or advanced metastases, palliative effects may be obtained by utilizing endoscopically placed metallic stents to allow swallowing of saliva and soft foods.

V **PERFORATION OF THE ESOPHAGUS**

A **Etiology**

1. **Perforations** of the esophagus have two basic **causes:**
   a. **Iatrogenic causes** instrumentation (e.g., esophagoscopy or dilatation) account for 50% of all esophageal perforations.
   b. **Trauma,** blunt or penetrating, 20%
   c. **Boerhaave's syndrome** (postemetic rupture of the esophagus), 15%

2. **Rupture of the esophagus** results in acute mediastinitis, which if not corrected is almost always fatal.

B **Diagnosis**

1. **History.** Patients give a recent history of instrumentation of the esophagus or severe vomiting. All patients complain of severe chest pain, which is usually most prominent in the area of the rupture.

2. **Physical examination**
   a. Crepitation in the neck results from mediastinal air.
   b. Occasionally, a crunching sound can be heard over the heart (Hamman's sign), which is caused by air in the mediastinum behind the heart.
   c. Septic shock can also occur.

3. **Chest radiograph** reveals air in the mediastinum and, possibly, a widened mediastinum.
   a. If the perforation is in the lower esophagus, air may be present under the diaphragm within the abdomen.
   b. If the pleura has been violated, a hydropneumothorax may be present.
4. A **barium swallow** should be performed if perforation is suspected. This study is preferred over esophagoscopy for identifying a perforation.
5. **CT scan** is also a very useful diagnostic modality.

C **Treatment** is to perform primary repair with tissue buttress reinforcement, combined with wide mediastinal and pleural drainage.

1. If mediastinal inflammation is severe and tissue integrity markedly is compromised, then esophageal resection with cervical esophagostomy and placement of a gastrostomy tube are performed. Esophageal reconstruction is performed at a later date when the patient has sufficiently recovered.

VI MALLORY-WEISS SYNDROME

A **Pathophysiology** This condition presents as acute upper gastrointestinal hemorrhage. The bleeding occurs in the lower esophagus, usually near the gastroesophageal junction, and is secondary to a partial-thickness tear in the lower esophagus, which follows a prolonged period of severe vomiting and retching. The tear usually extends into the stomach and may involve the greater curvature of the cardia.

B **Diagnosis** is made by endoscopy, which is performed to locate the tear and to rule out other causes of bleeding.

C **Treatment** is by supportive measures, such as blood volume replacement, antacids, and gastric lavage.

1. In most cases, the bleeding subsides spontaneously.
2. Exploratory laparotomy is performed with gastrotomy and suture of the tear of the esophagus from within the stomach if the bleeding persists. The lacerations are closed using continuous nonabsorbable sutures. A recurrence is rare.

VII ESOPHAGEAL WEBS

A Upper esophageal webs are part of the **Plummer-Vinson syndrome,** which presents in middle-age, edentulous women with atrophic oral mucosa, anemia, and dysphagia. The web occurs just below the esophageal introitus. **Treatment** is usually by esophageal dilatation.

B Lower esophageal webs, or **Schatzki's rings,** commonly occur in patients with reflux. Patients have dysphagia. **Treatment** consists of esophageal dilatation and an antireflux procedure.

chapter 11

Stomach and Duodenum

ERNEST L. ROSATO • FRANCIS E. ROSATO JR.

I STOMACH

A The **functions** of the stomach are **storage; emulsification; initial digestion** by acidification and salivary amylase; and **transmission of food** to the duodenum.

B **Embryology**

1. The stomach and duodenum are derived from a dilatation of the foregut during the fifth week of development.

2. The rate of growth of the left wall outpaces the right, thus forming the greater and lesser curvatures. Rotation of the stomach causes the left vagus to lie in the anterior position and the right vagus to lie in the posterior position.

3. The ventral and dorsal mesenteries of the foregut become the lesser and greater omentums, respectively, in adult life.

4. The stomach usually is situated between vertebral bodies T10 and L3 and is fixed at both the gastroesophageal junction and the proximal duodenum.

C **Anatomy** (Fig. 11-1). The stomach has four parts and two sphincteric mechanisms.

1. **Portions of the stomach**
    a. The **cardia** is the most proximal portion of the stomach, where it attaches to the esophagus. Immediately rostral to this area is the **gastroesophageal (GE) junction.** This transition zone is found 2–3 cm below the diaphragmatic esophageal hiatus and contains the lower esophageal sphincter mechanism.
    b. The **fundus** is the most superior extension of the stomach, bounded by the diaphragm superiorly and the spleen laterally. The angle created by the fundus and the left lateral border of the esophagus is referred to as the *angle of His.*
    c. The **body,** also referred to as the *corpus,* is the largest portion of the stomach. It consists of the lesser and greater curves. The *incisura angularis* creates an abrupt angle along the lesser curvature and marks the beginning of the antrum.
    d. The **antrum** is the distal 25% of the stomach. It begins at the incisura angularis and ends at the pylorus.

2. **Sphincters of the stomach**
    a. The **lower esophageal sphincter (LES)** is a **physiologic sphincter.** It is a **high-pressure zone of muscular activity in the distal esophagus.**
        (1) Relaxation with swallowing allows entry of food into the stomach.
        (2) Contraction prevents reflux of food from the stomach into the esophagus.
    b. The **pylorus** is an **anatomic sphincter muscle.** It controls the flow of food from the stomach into the duodenum.

3. **Arterial supply.** The stomach has an extremely rich blood supply (Fig. 11-2), provided by the following vessels:
    a. The **left gastric artery** (branch of celiac axis) supplies the lesser curvature (proximal).
    b. The **right gastric artery** (branch of common hepatic artery) supplies the lesser curvature (distal).
    c. The **left gastroepiploic artery** (branch of the splenic artery) supplies the greater curvature (proximal).

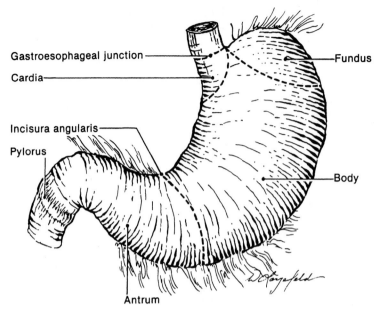

Gastroesophageal junction

Cardia

Fundus

Incisura angularis

Pylorus

Body

Antrum

FIGURE 11-1   Anatomy of the stomach.

    d. The **right gastroepiploic artery** (branch of gastroduodenal artery) supplies the greater curvature (distal).

    e. The **vasa brevia** (short gastric arteries arising from the splenic artery) supply the fundus and body.

4. Venous drainage of the stomach in general parallels the arterial supply but has some portal drainage.

    a. The **right gastric** and **left gastric** (*coronary*) veins drain into the portal vein, while the right gastroepiploic vein drains into the superior mesenteric vein, and the left gastroepiploic vein drains into the splenic vein.

    b. The **left gastric vein** (coronary vein) has multiple anastomoses with the lower esophageal venous plexus. These drain systemically into the azygous vein.

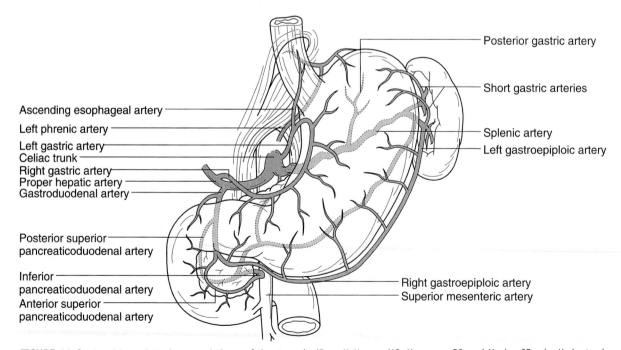

Posterior gastric artery

Short gastric arteries

Ascending esophageal artery

Left phrenic artery

Left gastric artery
Celiac trunk
Right gastric artery
Proper hepatic artery
Gastroduodenal artery

Splenic artery
Left gastroepiploic artery

Posterior superior
pancreaticoduodenal artery

Inferior
pancreaticoduodenal artery
Anterior superior
pancreaticoduodenal artery

Right gastroepiploic artery
Superior mesenteric artery

FIGURE 11-2   Arterial supply and venous drainage of the stomach. (From McKenney MG, Mangonon PC, and Moylan JP, eds. *Understanding Surgical Disease.* Philadelphia: Lippincott–Raven Publishers; 1998:118. Used by permission of Lippincott Williams & Wilkins.)

5. The **nervous innervation** of the stomach is via parasympathetic and sympathetic fibers.
   a. The **vagus (parasympathetic) nerves** stimulate parietal cell secretion, gastrin release, and gastric motility. Acetylcholine is the primary neurotransmitter used by the efferent fibers.
      (1) The **left vagus nerve** lies anterior to and left of the esophagus. It supplies branches to the anterior portion of the stomach and a hepatic branch to the liver, gallbladder, and biliary tree.
      (2) The **right vagus nerve** lies posterior to and right of the esophagus. It supplies branches to the posterior stomach and a celiac branch to the pancreas, small bowel, and right colon. Its first branch is called the *criminal nerve of Grassi* and is recognized as a cause of recurrent ulcer when left undivided.
      (3) The vagus nerves become the anterior and posterior nerves of **Laterjet,** which terminate at the pylorus as the "**crow's foot.**"
   b. **Sympathetic innervation** is via the **greater splanchnic nerves** derived from spinal segments T5 through T10. These fibers terminate in the **celiac ganglion,** and **postganglionic fibers** follow the gastric arteries to the stomach. The **afferent fibers** are the pathway for perception of visceral pain.

6. **Lymphatic drainage** of the stomach is extensive but can be divided into four general zones. It is important to note that cancer anywhere in the stomach can spread equally to any zone.
   a. **Superior gastric nodes** drain the upper lesser curve and cardia region.
   b. **Pancreaticolienal nodes** drain the upper great curve and splenic nodes.
   c. **Suprapyloric nodes** drain the antral segment of the stomach.
   d. **Inferior gastric/subpyloric nodes** drain along the right gastroepiploic vessels.

7. The **four layers of the stomach wall** are the **serosa, muscularis, muscularis mucosa,** and **mucosa.**
   a. The layers of muscle fibers found in the muscularis are the inner **oblique,** middle **circular,** and outer **longitudinal.**
   b. The mucosal morphology is composed of distinctly different types of glands unique to the **cardia, fundus/body,** and **pylorus/antrum.**
      (1) **Cardiac glands** occupy a narrow zone up to 4 cm long adjacent to the LES. These glands function mainly in producing mucus.
      (2) The fundus and body contain gastric glands with specialized cell types.
         (a) **Mucous cells** provide an alkaline coating for the epithelium. This coating facilitates food passage and provides some mucosal protection.
         (b) **Chief cells** are found deep in the fundic glands. They secrete **pepsinogen,** which is the precursor to **pepsin.** Pepsin is active in protein digestion. Chief cells are stimulated by cholinergic impulses, gastrin, and secretin.
         (c) **Oxyntic** or **parietal cells** are found exclusively in the fundus and body of the stomach. They are stimulated by gastrin to produce **hydrochloric acid** as well as **intrinsic factor.**
      (3) The **pyloroantral mucosa** is found in the antrum of the stomach.
         (a) Parietal and chief cells are absent here.
         (b) **G cells,** which secrete gastrin, are found in this area. They are part of the amine precursor uptake and decarboxylase system of endocrine cells. Gastrin stimulates hydrochloric acid and pepsinogen secretion and gastric motility.

II   DUODENUM

A **Anatomy**   (Fig. 11-3). The duodenum is divided into four sections. The first portion (duodenal cap) is 5 cm long, the second (descending) portion is 7 cm long, the third (transverse) portion is 12 cm long, and the fourth portion is 2.5 cm long.

B **Vasculature**

1. **Arterial supply** of the duodenum is via the **superior pancreaticoduodenal artery,** which is a branch of the gastroduodenal artery, and the **inferior pancreaticoduodenal artery,** which is a branch of the superior mesenteric artery.

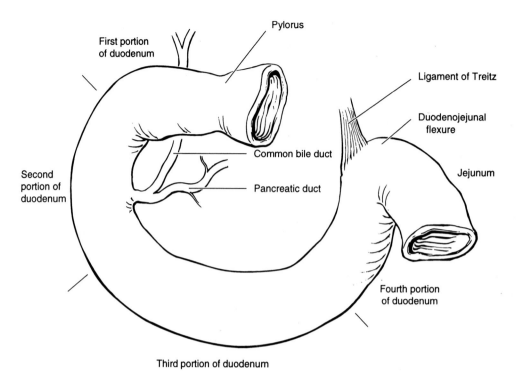

FIGURE 11-3 Anatomy of the duodenum. The *first portion* is partially retroperitoneal at its distal margin. The *common bile duct* and the *pancreatic duct* empty into the *second portion* of the duodenum. The *third portion* runs horizontally to the left and ends to the left of the third lumbar vertebra. At the terminal portion of the *fourth portion*, the *duodenojejunal flexure* changes direction sharply and becomes the *jejunum*. This area of the duodenum is fixed in position by the *ligament of Treitz*.

2. **Venous drainage** is via **anterior and posterior pancreaticoduodenal venous arcades.** These drain into portal and superior mesenteric veins.

C The layers of the duodenum are the **serosa (only on the anterior wall),** the **muscular layer,** the **muscularis mucosae,** and the **mucosa.**

1. The **muscular layer** contains inner **longitudinal** and outer circular muscle fibers.

2. The **mucosa** of the proximal duodenum contains Brunner's glands, which secrete a protective alkaline mucus.

III   GASTRIC AND DUODENAL DIGESTION

A Gastric acid secretion is mediated by a complex interplay of neuronal and hormonal influences. The **secretory response during eating** is divided into three **phases.**

1. The **cephalic phase** is initiated by sight, smell, and thought of food.
   a. Vagal stimulation causes parietal cells to secrete acid.
   b. Vagal stimulation also causes release of gastrin from the antrum. **Gastrin** is the most potent stimulator of gastric acid secretion.

2. The **gastric phase** is initiated by mechanical distention of the antrum. This stimulates additional gastrin release.

3. The **intestinal phase** of secretion is not well understood. Intestinal factors, such as **cholecystokinin,** are mild stimulators of acid production.

B **Negative acid feedback mechanisms** include a decline in vagal stimulation, increased acid content, and duodenal negative feedback. An antral pH of 2 inhibits gastrin release. Acid chyme in the duodenum stimulates secretin release, which further inhibits gastrin secretion.

IV ULCER DISEASE

A Gastric ulcers

1. **Etiology.** The etiology of gastric ulcers is multifactorial and not completely delineated. **Damage to the gastric mucosal barrier** appears to be the most important factor.
   a. **Reflux of bile** into the stomach changes the mucosal barrier, allowing gastric acid to enter the mucosa and injure it.
   b. **Drugs** alter the mucosal barrier to hydrogen ion. **Nonsteroidal anti-inflammatory drugs (NSAID), salicylates, steroids, ethanol,** and the **combination of smoking and salicylate ingestion** are causative agents.
   c. **Acid secretion** is necessary for ulcer formation, but persons with gastric ulcers tend to have **lower than normal** rates of acid secretion, both basal and stimulated. Their serum gastrin levels, however, are approximately twice the normal levels.
   d. *Helicobacter Pylori* infection is present in more than 80% of patients with gastric ulcers. *H. pylori* weakens the protective gastric mucous barrier, increases the basal and stimulated concentrations of gastrin, and impedes gastric healing after injury, resulting in gastric ulcer formation.

2. **Incidence.** Gastric ulcers are more common in men, the elderly, and lower socioeconomic groups. Duodenal ulcers are twice as common as gastric ulcers.

3. **Location/Type**
   a. **Type 1** gastric ulcers occur within the body of the stomach, most often along the lesser curve at the **incisura angularis** along the **locus minoris resistentiae.** This term refers to the histologic transition zone between the parietal cells of the body and the gastrin-secreting cells of the antrum.
   b. **Type 2** gastric ulcers occur in the body of the stomach in combination with duodenal ulcers. These ulcers are associated with acid oversecretion.
   c. **Type 3** gastric ulcers develop in the pyloric channel within 3 cm of the pylorus. These ulcers are associated with acid oversecretion.
   d. **Type 4** gastric ulcers are located high in the stomach adjacent to the esophagus.
   e. **Type 5** gastric ulcers are secondary to chronic NSAID and aspirin use and can occur throughout the stomach.

4. **Diagnosis**
   a. **History of burning midepigastric pain** that is stimulated by or follows eating is a common presentation of gastric ulcers.
   b. **Upper gastrointestinal (UGI) radiographs** will show barium in an ulcer crater.
   c. **Endoscopy** detects 90% of ulcers and allows multiple biopsy samples to be taken to rule out cancer or control bleeding.
   d. *H. plyori* can be confirmed by urease breath test, tissue biopsy, or antibody titer measurement.

5. **Gastric ulcers and malignancy**
   a. A gastric ulcer does not degenerate into carcinoma.
   b. Gastric cancer will ulcerate in 25% of cases. **It is, therefore, mandatory to prove that the ulcer is not carcinoma; 10% of gastric ulcers are malignancies with ulceration.**

6. **Treatment**
   a. **Medical treatment** of gastric ulcers is indicated initially. Most gastric ulcers will heal in 8–12 weeks.
      (1) **Avoidance of ethanol, tobacco, and drugs** that irritate the gastric mucosa is important.
      (2) **Histamine (H$_2$) blockers** are effective in healing gastric ulcers. Gastric ulcers associated with NSAID use may not respond as well to H$_2$ blockers.
      (3) **Proton pump inhibitors** block the enzyme involved in the parietal cell secretion of acid.
      (4) **Antacid therapy** in high doses has been demonstrated to be superior to placebo.
      (5) **Sucralfate** is a sulfated sucrose that binds to the ulcer crater and protects for 6 hours.
      (6) *H. pylori* treatment reduces the recurrence rates for gastric ulcer. Treatment requires antisecretory agents (omeprazole, etc.), antibiotics (amoxicillin or clarithromycin and metronidazole) and/or bismuth. Ninety-percent cure rates are reported with dual antibiotic and omeprazole treatment.

   b. Surgical treatment is indicated in the following situations.

   (1) **Intractability.** The ulcer fails to heal after 8–12 weeks of medical therapy or recurs despite adequate medical therapy.

   (2) **Bleeding** not controlled by endoscopy or medical therapy

   (3) **Perforation**

   (4) **Gastric outlet obstruction**

   (5) **Malignancy** cannot be excluded

7. **Operative procedures** (Fig. 11-4). The operative procedure is determined by the type of ulcer, location, and condition of the patient at the time of surgery.

   a. Type 1 ulcer

   Hemigastrectomy (excision of the distal 50% of the stomach with excision of the ulcer) is historically the procedure of choice.

   (1) **Gastroduodenal anastomosis (Billroth I gastrectomy)** is used for reconstruction **if the duodenum can be mobilized** (Fig. 11-4A).

   (2) **Gastrojejunal anastomosis (Billroth II gastrectomy)** is used for reconstruction **if the duodenum cannot be mobilized** (Fig. 11-4B).

   b. Types 2 and 3 ulcers

   Vagotomy with antrectomy with extension to include excision of the ulcer. Vagotomy is necessary for pyloric channel ulcers or gastric ulcers occurring with duodenal ulcers in order to reduce acid secretion.

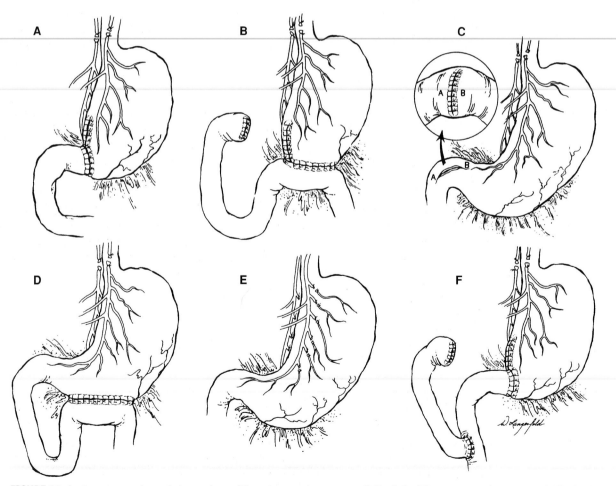

FIGURE 11-4 Common gastric surgical procedures: **(A)** vagotomy and antrectomy (Billroth I); **(B)** vagotomy and antrectomy (Billroth II); **(C)** vagotomy and pyloroplasty; **(D)** vagotomy and gastrojejunostomy; **(E)** parietal cell vagotomy; and **(F)** Roux-en-Y gastrojejunostomy.

    c. Type 4 ulcer
      (1) Antrectomy with extension of resection to include the ulcer
      (2) Antrectomy with wedge excision of the ulcer
    d. Type 5 ulcer

Surgical intervention for chemical-induced ulcers is reserved for emergency situations (**perforation and hemorrhage**). Primary closure, omental patch, or wedge excision combined with cessation of non-steroidal anti-inflammatory drugs and acetylsaliclyic acid (ASA) are standard treatments.

B Duodenal ulcers

1. **Etiology.** Peptic ulceration occurs when an imbalance develops between mucosal integrity and acid production.
   a. Most, although not all, duodenal ulcer patients experience **acid hypersecretion.** This condition may be related to an increased mass of acid-secreting cells. The parietal cells in duodenal ulcer patients are more sensitive to gastrin secretion. The feedback inhibition of gastrin release by acid may be impaired in these patients.
   b. **Mucosal resistance** may be altered by bacteria (*H. pylori*). This gram-negative rod is found in the antrum of 95% of duodenal ulcer patients, and eradication of this organism in patients with ulcers may be therapeutic. Many patients without ulcer disease may have *H. pylori*.

2. **Location**
   a. Most duodenal ulcers are located in the first portion of the duodenum. Ulcers on the posterior wall may bleed from the gastroduodenal artery. Ulcers on the anterior wall may perforate freely into the abdominal cavity.
   b. About 5% of duodenal ulcers are postbulbar, located in the more distal duodenum.
   c. **Pyloric channel ulcers** occur in the gastric antrum within 3 cm of the pylorus and are treated like duodenal ulcers. They frequently do not respond to medical therapy and often require surgery, largely because of the development of gastric outlet obstruction. This results from scarring, inflammation, and stricture formation.

3. **Diagnosis**
   a. **History of epigastric pain** radiating to the back is the usual presentation. The pain is relieved by food; however, the period of relief becomes shorter as symptoms progress. The pain typically wakes the patient at night.
   b. **Studies. Esophagoduodenoscopy** is the major diagnostic tool. **UGI radiographs** may also be used.
   c. **Gastric pH analysis** may be used to provide data on acid output in planning for surgery.
   d. **Serum gastrin level measurements** are obtained in patients with recurrent ulceration after surgery, ulcers that fail to respond to medical management, suspected endocrine disorders (MEN I), and Zollinger-Ellison syndrome. Normal serum gastrin levels are less than 200 pg/mL.
   e. *H. pylori* can be confirmed by urease breath test, tissue biopsy, or antibody titer measurement.

4. **Medical treatment** of uncomplicated duodenal ulcer disease is usually successful.
   a. **Avoidance of aspirin, caffeine, alcohol, and tobacco** is recommended.
   b. **Stress reduction** may be beneficial.
   c. Eradication of *H. pylori*
   d. **Pharmacologic therapy** is the mainstay of treatment of peptic ulcer disease. H_2-receptor antagonists and proton pump inhibitors are used most commonly for initial treatment and then are decreased to a single bedtime dose for maintenance therapy. Most duodenal ulcers heal in 6–8 weeks with such therapy. Maintenance therapy is recommended because ulcer recurrence after discontinuing medical therapy occurs in 50%–80% of patients (Table 11-1).

5. **Surgical treatment** of duodenal ulcer is reserved for patients who have ulcers that fail to respond to medical therapy or who have complications, such as perforation or bleeding. There are a number of surgical options. The goal of each is to reduce acid secretion; therefore, most approaches concentrate on interrupting vagal stimulation, antral gastrin secretion, or both.
   a. **Vagotomy with antrectomy** (Fig. 11-4B) is the procedure associated with the lowest recurrence rate.

TABLE 11-1   Drug Therapy of Peptic Ulcer Disease

Agent	Effect	Advantages and Disadvantages
Decrease Gastric Acidity		
Antacids	Neutralize gastric acid; also may increase mucosal resistance	Inexpensive; readily available
H_2-receptor antagonists (e.g., cimetidine)	Inhibit histamine receptor on parietal cell, which decreases acid output dosing for maintenance therapy	Excellent results; mainstay therapy; once daily evening
Proton-pump inhibitors (e.g., omeprazole)	Inhibit ATP-ase proton pump, which is final step in acid secretion from parietal cell	Quicker healing, but more expensive than preceding agents
Increase Mucosal Defense		
Cytoprotective topical agent (e.g., sucralfate)	Binds to proteins in ulcer to form protective mucosal barrier	Not proven for gastric ulcers
Antibiotics (e.g., amoxicillin)	Eradicate *H. pylori*	Inexpensive; important in preventing recurrences in patients with *H. pylori*

ATP, adenosine triphosphate.

    b. Vagotomy with drainage is associated with a recurrence rate of 6%–7%. After vagotomy, the motility of the stomach and pylorus is impaired, creating a functional obstruction. For this reason, a drainage procedure, such as a **pyloroplasty** (Fig. 11-4C) or **gastrojejunostomy** (Fig. 11-4D), is required.

    c. Parietal cell vagotomy (Fig. 11-4E), also known as highly selective vagotomy, is gaining in popularity, especially when the indication for surgical intervention is intractable pain. Only the gastric branches of the vagus nerve are divided. Because innervation of the pylorus is maintained, a drainage procedure is not necessary. Recurrence rates with this procedure are somewhat higher (approximately 10%), but the morbidity is less as compared with truncal vagotomy with antrectomy. This procedure is often performed laparoscopically, further decreasing its morbidity.

  6. Complications of ulcers include perforation, hemorrhage, and obstruction.

    a. Perforations occur most commonly with ulcers on the anterior surface of the duodenum. Gastric perforations are less common. Occasionally, gastric ulcers can perforate posteriorly into the lesser sac.

      (1) Signs and symptoms

        (a) Typical symptoms of perforation include sudden onset of severe abdominal pain, radiation of pain to the shoulder, nausea, and vomiting.

        (b) Signs include a rigid, boardlike abdomen and shock. An upright chest radiograph frequently demonstrates free air under the diaphragm.

      (2) Treatment

        (a) Occasionally, **observation** may be used if the patient is hemodynamically stable and the initial event occurred several hours previously. A monitored setting, antibiotics, and intravenous fluids are required.

        (b) Simple operative closure of the perforated ulcer, often with a patch of omentum (Graham patch), is the usual treatment.

        (c) Definitive treatment of the ulcer (e.g., by vagotomy with antrectomy) may be indicated in low-risk patients with minimal soilage of the peritoneal cavity, especially if they give a long history (more than 3 months) of ulcer symptoms—or proven failure of the medical treatment.

    b. Hemorrhage occurs in approximately 15%–20% of patients with ulcers. Medical management controls the hemorrhage in most cases.

        (1) Endoscopy is necessary to evaluate the site of the hemorrhage. A "visible vessel" in the ulcer crater is an ominous sign and is associated with a higher risk of rebleeding and a need for surgical intervention.

        (2) Thermal techniques performed through the endoscope may be effective. These techniques include electrocoagulation, laser, or heater probe.

        (3) Injection of sclerosing or vasoconstrictive agents may also be used.

        (4) Surgery. Surgical intervention is usually needed to control **massive hemorrhage,** defined as blood loss that requires transfusion of more than 1500 mL of blood products without stabilization of vital signs or continued blood loss requiring more than 6 units of transfused blood in a 24-hour period.

            (a) Techniques

                (i) Oversewing of the bleeding point is done via a longitudinal opening through the pylorus.

                (ii) If this fails to control the vessel, it is necessary to isolate and ligate the gastroduodenal artery.

                (iii) The incision through the pylorus is then closed transversely, which is known as a **pyloroplasty,** or **widening of the pylorus.**

            (b) A **truncal vagotomy** (division of the two main vagal trunks) is also done to reduce acid stimulation (Fig. 11-4C).

            (c) Vagotomy with antrectomy is another option in low-risk patients.

  c. Gastric outlet obstruction can be caused by **prepyloric ulcers** and by **chronic scarring of the pyloric channel.**

        (1) Symptoms. Obstruction causes symptoms of crampy abdominal pain, nausea, and vomiting. The stomach is usually markedly dilated. Prolonged vomiting due to obstruction can lead to electrolyte disorders, particularly hypokalemic metabolic alkalosis from the large hydrochloric acid losses.

        (2) Initial treatment consists of several days of nasogastric suction to allow the stomach to decompress.

        (3) Surgery. Vagotomy with antrectomy or **vagotomy with drainage** is the standard procedure.

V   GASTRITIS

A Uncomplicated acute gastritis

  1. Etiology. Acute diffuse gastritis can be due to a number of irritating agents, particularly aspirin and ethanol.

  2. Hemorrhage can occur and be massive.

  3. Treatment. Removal of the inciting agent and antacid therapy usually result in prompt healing.

B Stress ulceration (acute hemorrhage gastritis) is another form of acute gastritis. Ischemia of the gastric mucosa is the inciting event. The injury is compounded by the effect of the intraluminal acid. Although stress ulceration is common in critically ill patients, only 5% develop significant gastric bleeding.

  1. Location. Stress ulcers are characteristically shallow mucosal lesions that start in the fundus. They then spread distally and can involve the entire stomach.

  2. Clinical presentation. Affected patients frequently have sepsis, multiple organ system failure, severe trauma, or a complicated postoperative course or are on assisted ventilation. Stress ulceration that occurs in burn patients is known as **Curling's ulcer,** and stress ulceration occurring in patients with head injury is known as **Cushing's ulcer.**

  3. Treatment

    a. Prophylaxis against stress ulceration can be achieved with antacids given as needed to keep the gastric pH above 5. H_2-receptor antagonists and proton pump inhibitors are equally effective at maintaining an adequate gastric pH.

b. **Medical treatment** involves correcting the underlying problems (e.g., sepsis) and vigorous use of antacids. Cimetidine is not helpful once bleeding has occurred.

c. **Surgical treatment** is rarely necessary and is associated with a high mortality. In the case of uncontrollable bleeding, near total gastrectomy is usually the best option.

d. **Radiographic embolization** can be performed to identify the main artery bleeding and stop blood flow.

VI GASTRIC CANCER

A **Gastric tumors** Approximately 90%–95% of gastric tumors are malignant, and of the malignancies, 95% are adenocarcinomas. Other histologic types include squamous cell, carcinoid, gastrointestinal stromal tumor (GIST), and lymphoma.

B **Gastric adenocarcinoma**

1. The **incidence** of gastric adenocarcinoma has been decreasing for many years and is now stabilized. Gastric adenocarcinoma is the tenth most common cancer, with an estimated annual incidence of 22,000 cases and 13,000 deaths. The **trend is increasing toward lesions more proximally located** in the stomach.

2. **Risk factors** for gastric cancer include:
   a. Age >70 years
   b. Diet high in salt, smoked foods, low protein, low vitamins A and C
   c. *H. pylori* infection
   d. Previous gastric resection
   e. Chronic gastritis and pernicious anemia
   f. Blood group A
   g. Radiation exposure
   h. Tobacco use
   i. **Male gender**
   j. Low socioeconomic status
   k. Adenomatous polyps

3. **Symptoms** include epigastric pain, anorexia, fatigue, vomiting, and weight loss. Proximal tumors can present with dysphagia, while more distal tumors may present as gastric outlet obstruction. Symptoms tend to occur late in the course of the disease. Physical signs can include palpable supraclavicular (Virchow's) or periumbilical (Sister Mary Joseph's) lymph nodes.

4. **Diagnosis** is suggested on UGI radiographs and is confirmed by upper endoscopy with biopsy.

5. **Preoperative evaluation** may include computed tomography (CT) scan to look for local extension, ascites, and distant metastases. Endoscopic ultrasound has been shown to be useful in determining the depth of penetration and in detecting nodal metastases. Staging laparoscopy may detect small peritoneal metastases and is required before most neoadjuvant protocols.

6. **Involvement beyond the stomach** may include direct spread to adjacent organs (e.g., spleen, diaphragm, omentum, colon); "drop metastases" to the ovary (Krukenberg's tumor) or the pelvis (Blumer's shelf tumor); or distant disease (e.g., to liver, lung).

7. **Classification.** Gastric carcinoma is classified according to its gross characteristics.
   a. **Intestinal type** is a well-differentiated, glandular tumor found most commonly in the distal stomach.
   b. **Diffuse type** is a poorly differentiated, small cell infiltrating tumor found most commonly in the proximal stomach.

8. **Surgical treatment** depends on nodal disease and distant metastases.
   a. **Potentially curable lesions**
      (1) Potentially curable lesions are treated with subtotal or total gastrectomy, depending on tumor location.
      (2) Wide margins (>6 cm) on the stomach are necessary because extensive submucosal tumor spread can occur. Lesions of the fundus and cardia may require resection of the spleen, pancreas, or transverse colon to completely remove the cancer.

(3) The role of lymphadenectomy is controversial, but for favorable lesions, there is some advantage to removing the local draining nodes. Removal of the omentum and its nodes is included. Radical lymphadenectomy that includes distant nodal basins has not been shown to improve survival and may increase morbidity. It is recommended that a least 15 regional lymph nodes be sampled to ensure adequate staging of the tumor.

    b. Palliative resections are indicated in the presence of obstructing or bleeding gastric cancers. Treatment may include resection, bypass alone, or either one in conjunction with endoscopic or radiotherapeutic techniques.

9. Adjuvant chemotherapy (5-fluorouracil/leucovorin and radiation therapy) after potentially curative resection improves median survival and is the current standard of care. Neoadjuvant chemoradiation is being studied in several clinical trials but remains unproven at this time. Unresectable tumors may show some response to chemotherapy. The addition of radiation therapy may improve results and can control bleeding symptoms.

10. Prognosis depends largely on the depth of invasion of the gastric wall, involvement of regional nodes, and presence of distant metastases but still remains poor. Overall 5-year survival after the diagnosis of gastric cancer is 10%–20%. Tumors not penetrating the serosa and not involving regional nodes are associated with a 5-year survival rate of approximately 70%. This number decreases dramatically if the tumor is through the serosa or into regional nodes. Recurrence rates after gastric resection are high, ranging from 40%–80%. Potentially curative surgical resection does offer a better 5-year prognosis; however, only 40% of patients have potentially curable disease at the time of diagnosis.

C **Gastric lymphoma**   The stomach is the most common site of **primary intestinal lymphoma;** however, gastric lymphoma is relatively uncommon, accounting for only 15% of all gastric malignancies and only 2% of lymphomas.

1. Symptoms are usually vague, namely abdominal pain, early satiety, and fatigue. Rarely ever do patients present with constitutional symptoms (i.e. "B" classification of lymphoma). Patients at risk for developing lymphomas are those who are immunocompromised or are harboring an *H. pylori* infection.

2. Diagnosis consists of endoscopy with biopsy and endoscopic ultrasound for staging. As with all lymphomas, assessment of distant disease should include bone marrow biopsy; CT of chest, abdomen, and pelvis; as well as an upper airway exam. Testing for *H. pylori* should also be performed.

3. Treatment consists of a multimodality regimen, with the role of gastric resection remaining highly controversial.

    a. Medical treatment combining chemotherapy and radiation is now the most accepted first-line therapy for treating gastric lymphoma. The most common chemotherapy combination is cyclophosphamide, hydroxydaunomycin, Oncovin, and prednisone (CHOP). Some variants of lymphoma may also be treated effectively by the eradication of *H. pylori* infection alone.

    b. Surgical treatment is now used mostly for the complications of bleeding and perforation that arise from locally advanced disease. The treatment involves the removal of all gross disease via partial gastrectomy.

4. Prognosis is good, with a 5-year survival greater than 95% when disease is localized to the stomach and 75% when local lymph nodes are involved.

D **Gastric sarcomas** arise from the mesenchymal cells of the gastric wall and constitute 3% of all gastric cancers. Gastrointestinal stromal tumors (GIST) are the most common and are found predominately in the stomach.

1. Gastrointestinal stromal tumors (GIST) arise from mesenchymal cells of the GI tract, usually the pacemaker cell of **Cajal.**

2. Histologic diagnosis is confirmed by immunohistochemical staining for **CD 117,** a cell surface antigen.

3. Presentation varies from incidental asymptomatic endoscopy or CT findings to symptomatic large tumors causing obstruction, pain, bleeding, or metastases.

4. Treatment is complete surgical removal. Clinical behavior and malignant potential are based on several factors, including mitotic count >5 per 50 high-power fields; size >5 cm; and cellular atypia, necrosis, or local invasion. **Tumor recurrence or unresectable disease** can be treated by **imatinib mesylate (Gleevec),** which inhibits the **c-KIT gene**–associated tyrosine kinase receptor responsible for tumor growth. Overall 5-year survival is 50%.

VII BENIGN LESIONS OF THE STOMACH

A **Gastric polyps** are usually found incidentally. They often can be excised via endoscopy.

1. **Hyperplastic polyps** are the most common and arise most often in the setting of chronic atrophic gastritis. These polyps are non-neoplastic, and treatment consists of polypectomy.

2. **Adenomatous polyps** are associated with a 20% risk of malignancy, especially in those greater than 1.5 cm. Treatment consists of endoscopic polypectomy. Surgery is required for evidence of invasion on polypectomy specimen, for sessile lesions >2 cm, and polyps with symptoms of bleeding or pain.

B **Ectopic pancreas** occurs during development and is rare. The majority of cases are found in the stomach, duodenum, and jejunum. The most common presenting symptoms are abdominal pain, nausea and vomiting, and bleeding. Surgical excision is the recommended treatment.

C **Ménétrier's disease** (hypoproteinemic hypertrophic gastropathy) is a premaliganant abnormality of the gastric mucosa with an unknown etiology.

1. **Characteristics** include the following:
   a. A **hypertrophic gastric mucosa** is seen by radiographic or endoscopic evaluation.
      (1) Giant rugae are characteristic.
      (2) Mucous cells are increased in number.
      (3) Parietal and chief cells are decreased in number.
   b. There is gastric hypersecretion of mucus as well as excessive protein loss and hypochlorhydra.

2. **Treatment** consists of anticholinergics, acid suppression, octreotide, and *H. pylori* eradication. Total gastrectomy is required in patients with severe hypoproteinemia despite maximal medical therapy.

D **Mallory-Weiss tears** are linear mucosal lesions found at the gastroesophageal junction and are related to repeated forceful vomiting. These tears account for 15% of all upper GI bleeds. Massive hemorrhage is rare but is greater in those with pre-existing portal hypertension. Most cases of bleeding can be controlled by endoscopic interventions, intra-arterial infusions, or transcatheter embolization. Only 10% of patients require surgery to stop the bleeding, which consists of oversewing the mucosal tear (see Chapter 10, VI).

E **Dieulafoy's gastric lesion** is caused by an abnormally large tortuous artery located in the submucosa. The classic presentation is a sudden onset of massive upper GI bleeding with associated hypotension. Endoscopy is both diagnostic and therapeutic. Surgery is rarely needed.

F **Gastric volvulus** is an uncommon entity. The volvulus may be intermittent. It is caused by laxity of the ligaments supporting the stomach and is frequently associated with congenital diaphragmatic defects, traumatic injuries to the diaphragm, and paraesophageal hernias.

1. **Types**
   a. **Organoaxial volvulus** is a rotation around the cardiopyloric line, a line drawn along the length of the stomach between the cardia and pylorus (most common).
   b. **Mesentericoaxial volvulus** occurs around a line perpendicular to the cardiopyloric line.
   c. Volvulus may also occur as a combination of these two types.

2. The sudden onset of constant, severe abdominal pain, wretching without vomitus, and the inability to pass a nasogastric tube constitutes Borchardt's triad.

3. **Surgical treatment** includes reducing the torsion and fixation of the stomach.

G **Bezoars** are agglutinated masses of hair (**trichobezoars** occur most commonly in young, neurotic women), vegetable matter (**phytobezoars** are seen after a partial gastric resection and tend to be more common in older men), or a combination of the two that form within the stomach.

1. **Symptoms** of a bezoar include nausea, vomiting, weight loss, and abdominal pain. **Complications** include obstruction and ulceration.

2. **Treatment** generally requires endoscopic or surgical removal, although enzymatic dissolution of some bezoars has been successful.

VIII DUODENAL TUMORS

A **Malignant tumors** are usually adenocarcinomas. Treatment of resectable lesions is pancreaticoduodenectomy (Whipple's procedure). Other tumors include carcinoids, GISTs, gastrinomas, and parcomas.

B **Benign tumors** include lipomas, benign GISTs, hamartomas, and adenomas. Surgical resection is the treatment of choice.

IX MISCELLANEOUS DISORDERS OF THE STOMACH AND DUODENUM

A **Gastric outlet obstruction** (see IV B 6 c)

B **Superior mesenteric artery syndrome** Especially in young, thin women, the third portion of the duodenum can be obstructed by the superior mesenteric artery, which takes a sharp angle from the aorta and courses over the duodenum. This anatomic configuration is combined with **predisposing factors,** such as a lack of the retroperitoneal fat cushion, prolonged immobilization, and pressure (e.g., from a body cast). The syndrome is also known as **cast syndrome** because of its association with patients in body casts.

1. **Symptoms** include vomiting and postprandial pain.

2. **Treatment**
   a. **Medical treatment** consists of eliminating all contributing factors, such as casts, girdles, and lying in the supine position. Weight gain may alleviate symptoms. Increasing oral intake, enteral feeding beyond the ligament of Treitz, and parenteral supplementation may be tried.
   b. **Surgical treatment** includes either releasing the ligament of Treitz, which moves the duodenum out from beneath the superior mesenteric artery, or bypassing the obstruction.

C **Duodenal (pulsion) diverticula** are frequently asymptomatic. The most common location is opposite the ampulla of Vater. Severe hemorrhage or perforation can occur; but in the absence of such complications, no treatment is indicated.

X POSTGASTRECTOMY SYNDROMES

These symptom complexes can be disabling.

A **Alkaline reflux gastritis** is the most common problem after a gastrectomy, occurring in about 25% of all patients.

1. **Symptoms** are postprandial epigastric pain, nausea, vomiting, and weight loss.

2. **Diagnosis. Endoscopy** demonstrates the gastritis and a free reflux of bile.

3. **Treatment** is conversion of the Billroth I or II gastrectomy (Fig. 11-4A,B) to a Roux-en-Y anastomosis (Fig. 11-4F).

B **Afferent loop syndrome** is caused by intermittent mechanical obstruction of the afferent loop of a gastrojejunostomy.

1. **Symptoms** include early postprandial distention, pain, and nausea, which are relieved by vomiting of bilious material not mixed with food.

2. **Treatment** consists of providing good drainage of the afferent loop, usually by conversion to a Roux-en-Y anastomosis.

C **Dumping syndrome** affects most postgastrectomy patients but is a significant problem in only a few. It exists in either an early or late form with the former occurring more frequently.

1. **Early dumping syndrome** occurs within 20–30 minutes following ingestion of a meal. It is more common after partial gastrectomy with Billroth II reconstruction. It results from the rapid movement of a hypertonic food bolus into the small intestine. Rapid fluid shifts into the small bowel cause distention and a subsequent autonomic response along with the release of several humoral agents.

2. **Late dumping syndrome** occurs 2–3 hours after a meal and is far less common. The large carbohydrate load passed into the small intestine causes on over-release of insulin resulting in profound hypoglycemia. This stimulates the adrenal gland to release a large amount of catecholamines producing confusion tachycardia, lightheadedness and tremulousness.

3. **Signs and symptoms** may include epigastric fullness or pain, nausea, palpitations, dizziness, diarrhea, tachycardia, and elevated blood pressure.

4. **Treatment**
   a. **Conservative nonsurgical measures** include octreotide to control symptoms. Patients are advised to avoid a high-carbohydrate diet and not to drink fluids with meals.
   b. **Surgical treatment** is used to delay gastric emptying, including interposition of an antiperistaltic jejunal loop between the stomach and small bowel or conversion to a long limb Roux-en-Y reconstruction.

D **Postvagotomy diarrhea** is common in its mild form but seldom is a disabling problem. Symptoms usually improve during the first year after surgery.

chapter 12

Small Intestine

KAREN A. CHOJNACKI • DAVID J. MARON

I — INTRODUCTION

A — Anatomy

1. **External structure.** The small intestine is the length of bowel that extends from the pylorus to the cecum.
   a. The **duodenum,** which is retroperitoneal, extends from the pylorus to the ligament of Treitz.
   b. The **jejunum** (proximal 40%) and **ileum** (distal 60%), which are intraperitoneal, make up the remainder of the small intestine.
   c. The total length of small bowel is approximately 3 m (the duodenum measures 30 cm; the jejunum is 110 cm; and the ileum is 160 cm).

2. **Vasculature.** The **arterial supply** to the small intestine is primarily from the jejunal and ileal branches of the superior mesenteric artery (except the duodenum, which is also supplied by the branches of the celiac axis).
   a. Jejunal mesenteric arteries have only one or two arcades and a long vasa recta (the small arteries directly adjacent to the bowel wall).
   b. Ileal arteries have multiple arcades that extend closer to the bowel and have short vasa recta.

3. **Layers of the wall of the small intestine**
   a. The **mucosa** consists mostly of absorptive columnar epithelium and mucous-producing goblet cells. The absorption of nutrients takes place through the epithelial cells that cover the intestinal villi and have a total surface area of approximately 500 m^2. Mucosal cells proliferate rapidly and have a life span of 5 days.
   b. The **submucosa** is the strongest layer and provides strength to an intestinal anastomosis. It contains nerves, Meissner's plexus, blood vessels, lymphoid tissue (Peyer patches), and fibrous and elastic tissue.
   c. The **muscularis**—the muscle layer—consists of an outer longitudinal layer and an inner circular layer with Auerbach's myenteric plexus of ganglion cells in between.
   d. The serosa is the outermost layer and derives embryologically from the peritoneum.

4. **Internal structure**
   a. Spiral folds of mucosa and submucosa, also known as plicae circulares or valvulae conniventes, are more prominent proximally.
   b. The jejunum is larger in diameter, thicker walled, has more prominent plicae circulares, and has less mesenteric fat than the ileum.
   c. The lymphoid tissue (Peyer patches) becomes more prominent distally in the ileum.

B — Physiology
The **primary functions** of the small intestine are **digestion** and **absorption.** All ingested food and fluid, plus secretions from the stomach, liver, and pancreas, reach the small intestine. The total volume may reach 9 L/day, and all except 1–2 L will be absorbed.

1. **Motility**
   a. Two types of contractions **occur after a meal.**
      (1) **To-and-fro motion** mixes chyme with digestive juices and provides prolonged exposure to the absorptive mucosa.
      (2) **Peristaltic contractions** move food distally.

b. In the fasting state, a strong contraction begins in the duodenum and occurs every 2 hours (migrating motor complex). This completes the emptying of residual food from previous meals.

c. Parasympathetic stimulation promotes contractions, whereas sympathetic stimulation inhibits them.

2. Absorption. Vitamins, fat, protein, carbohydrates, water, and electrolytes are all absorbed in the small intestine.

a. Water is absorbed throughout the small intestine, although most water is absorbed in the jejunum. Passive absorption is the mechanism.

b. Electrolytes

  (1) Potassium is absorbed by passive diffusion through intercellular pores in the jejunum.

  (2) Sodium is actively transported, and once a gradient is established, **chloride** follows passively.

  (3) Calcium is actively transported in the jejunum (enhanced by vitamin D and parathyroid hormone).

  (4) Iron is absorbed as the ferrous (reduced) ion Fe^{2+}. Conversion of the ferric to the ferrous ion is enhanced by an acid milieu and the presence of reducing substances in the diet, such as vitamin C (ascorbic acid). Absorption is via active transport in the duodenum and jejunum, and 10%–26% (maximally) of dietary iron is absorbed.

c. Fat absorption occurs mainly in the jejunum. Fat is digested by pancreatic lipase and becomes emulsified in bile salt micelles. The micelles release fatty acids and monoglycerides to the epithelial cells. After absorption, the epithelial cells resynthesize triglycerides, which are assembled into chylomicrons and transported into the lymphatics. (All other absorbed nutrients are transported directly into the portal venous system.)

d. Carbohydrates are digested by salivary and pancreatic amylase. Enzymes of the mucosal cell surface further reduce sugars to the monosaccharides galactose and glucose, which are absorbed by active transport, and fructose, which is absorbed by diffusion.

e. Protein digestion begins in the stomach (by pepsin) and continues in the small bowel by pancreatic proteases. The process is completed at the brush border, yielding tripeptides, dipeptides, and amino acids. All are absorbed by active transport.

f. The **fat-soluble vitamins** A, D, E, and K are absorbed from micelles by the mucosa. Vitamin B_{12} is complexed with intrinsic factor and absorbed in the distal ileum. Vitamin C, thiamine, and folic acid are actively transported. The remaining water-soluble vitamins are absorbed by passive diffusion.

II ▪ SMALL BOWEL DISEASES

A Small bowel obstruction (SBO)

1. Causes

  a. Adhesions **account for more than half of SBO cases.** Adhesions from lower abdominal procedures carry a higher risk of causing obstruction.

  b. Hernias of all types can cause obstruction. Femoral hernias are particularly prone to incarceration and bowel necrosis.

  c. Obstruction can be caused by malignancy, most commonly adenocarcinoma or lymphoma.

  d. Other less likely causes include gallstone ileus (which is caused by obstruction of the ileocecal valve by a gallstone), Crohn's disease (see II C 5 a), intussuception, and volvulus.

2. Symptoms include crampy abdominal **pain,** nausea and **vomiting,** and abdominal **distention.** Patients with complete bowel obstruction typically do not pass any flatus or bowel movements.

3. Diagnosis

Abdominal x-rays show dliated loops of small bowel on flat plate and air-fluid levels on upright films. Air in the colon may represent early complete or incomplete obstruction.

Small bowel follow-through and computed tomography (CT) scan can also be used to localize the point of obstruction and to determine the nature of the lesion.

4. Treatment includes resuscitation with intravenous (IV) fluids, nasogastric tube decompression, and placement of a urinary catheter to monitor urine output. Abdominal exploration is performed in patients with peritoneal signs, leukocytosis, fever, or failure of resolution of obstructive symptoms.

B **Tumors of the small intestine**

1. **Benign neoplasms** are usually asymptomatic. They are ten times more common than are malignant tumors (autopsy data). Surgery is indicated for bleeding, obstruction, or intussusception.
   a. **Adenomas** are **rare** in the small intestine.
      (1) Duodenum is the most common site of small bowel adenomas.
      (2) There are three types of small bowel adenomas: **tubular, villous,** and **Brunner's gland.**
      (3) **Villous adenomas** have the highest malignancy potential.
      (4) Adenomas are usually discovered **incidentally** or as a source of gastrointestinal (GI) **bleeding, obstruction,** or **intussusception.**
      (5) Adenomas are treated by endoscopic or surgical resection.
   b. **Hamartomatous polyps** are found in patients with Peutz-Jeghers syndrome (mucocutaneous pigmentation accompanied by widespread intestinal polyposis). There is little malignant potential in this syndrome.
   c. **Juvenile (retention) polyps** are benign hamartomas and not true neoplasms. They are more common in the rectum and usually autoamputate.
   d. **Gastrointestinal stromal tumors (GIST)** are mesenchymal neoplasms of the small bowel formerly called *leiomyomas.*
      (1) These tumors are most commonly benign and present with bleeding, obstruction, or intussusception.
      (2) Their origin is the **cells of Cajal.** They stain positive for **CD 117** on immunohistochemical analysis.
      (3) The most common site is the **ileum.**
      (4) Ten to 30% of GIST tumors are malignant. Malignancy is based on tumor size greater than 5–10 cm, >10 mitotic figures per 50 high-power fields, necrosis, and/or the presence of metastases.
      (5) Treatment is wide surgical resection. Metastases should be debulked, if possible, for palliation. **Imatinib mesylate,** a tyrosine kinase inhibitor, has recently been shown to effective for patients with unresectable or metastatic GIST.
   e. Other benign small bowel tumors **include lipomas, hemangiomas, fibromas,** and **neurofibromas.**

2. **Malignant neoplasms**
   a. Overview
      (1) **Incidence.** The most common tumors are adenocarcinoma (40%), carcinoid (30%), lymphoma (20%), and sarcoma. Metastases from other intraabdominal malignancies are common, especially with peritoneal carcinomatosis. Metastases from extra-abdominal malignancies are rare except for the tendency of malignant melanoma to metastasize to the small bowel.
      (2) **Symptoms. Malignant tumors constitute 75% of symptomatic small bowel tumors** and usually present with bleeding, diarrhea, perforation, or obstruction (which may be caused by intussusception).
      (3) **Diagnosis** is frequently made late in the course of disease because symptoms are often subtle and insidious in onset.
      (4) **Treatment** involves segmental resection, including adequate margins proximally and distally and as much mesentery as possible without compromising the blood supply to the remaining small intestine.
   b. **Adenocarcinoma** is most common in the duodenum and proximal jejunum.
      (1) Adenocarcinomas of the first and second portions of the duodenum are best managed by Whipple pancreaticoduodenectomy. Unresectable tumors at this location should be palliated by gastrojejeunostomy or stents.
      (2) Tumors of the distal duodenum and small bowel should be managed by wide local resection of the bowel and intervening mesentary.
      (3) Metastases are often found at the time of presentation.

(4) For patients with node-negative disease, 5-year survival may be as high as 80%. For those with node-positive disease, 5-year survival is only 10%–15%.

c. Carcinoid tumors are derived from enterochromaffin cells. These cells are part of the amine precursor uptake and decarboxylation system (APUD cells) and secrete various vasoactive amines. **Carcinoid tumors** are most common in the **appendix,** followed by the **small bowel (usually the ileum)** and the **rectum.** Other sites are uncommon.

(1) The **prognosis** is related to the presence of metastases at diagnosis, which is strongly associated with the size of the tumor. Both carcinoid tumors and metastases grow slowly, and prolonged survival is common.

(a) Tumors less than 1 cm in diameter (75% of total) have a 2% incidence of metastases.

(b) Tumors larger than 1 cm (20% of total) have a 50% rate of metastases.

(c) Tumors larger than 2 cm (5% of total) have an 80%–90% rate of metastases.

(2) Only small bowel carcinoids tend to be multicentric (30%).

(3) Carcinoid syndrome—flushing, diarrhea, bronchoconstriction, and tricuspid and pulmonary valvular disease—is caused by serotonin and other vasoactive substances secreted by the tumor.

(a) These substances are cleared by the liver, thus the syndrome can only occur in patients with liver metastases (which drain into the systemic veins) or primary extraintestinal carcinoids (e.g., bronchial carcinoids). Approximately 10% of patients with small bowel carcinoids develop the syndrome.

(b) Diagnosis is confirmed by finding elevated urinary levels of 5-hydroxyindoleacetic acid (5-HIAA), which is the breakdown product of serotonin.

(c) Treatment includes resection of the primary tumor and resection or "debulking" of metastases. Liver metastases can be resected (when solitary) but usually require palliative local therapies (e.g., intra-arterial chemotherapy, hepatic arterial chemoembolization, or local destruction) (Chapter 14, I E).

(d) Prognosis. The overall 5-year survival rate for patients with small bowel carcinoids is 70%. If liver metastases are present at diagnosis, the 5-year survival rate is 20%.

d. Small bowel lymphomas may present as primary neoplasms or as part of a disseminated lymphoma. Small bowel lymphomas usually arise in the ileum.

(1) Most primary lesions are non-Hodgkins B-cell lymphomas.

(2) There is an increased incidence of small bowel lymphomas in patients who are immunosuppressed or have inflammatory conditions such as Crohn's disease.

(3) The most common symptoms are abdominal pain, fatigue, and weight loss. Diffuse adenopathy is uncommon.

(4) Complications include bowel perforation, hemorrhage, obstruction, and intussusception.

(5) Treatment is wide local resection. Liver biopsy and distant nodal biopsies are done for accurate staging.

(6) Chemotherapy and local radiation are used for patients with disseminated disease.

(7) Overall 5-year survival rates are 20%–40%.

e. Leiomyosarcoma is the most common of the small bowel sarcomas.

C Crohn's disease (regional enteritis; granulomatous ileitis) is a chronic, transmural granulomatous inflammatory disease that can involve any area of the GI tract. Its cause is unknown.

1. Distribution. The small bowel alone is involved in 25% of patients, both the small and the large bowel in 50%, and the colon alone in almost 25%. The distal ileum (the most common site) is involved in 70% of all cases, which accounts for the older name, **terminal ileitis.**

2. Diagnosis

a. The **peak age of onset** is between the second and fourth decades.

b. Symptoms include abdominal pain, diarrhea (usually not bloody), lethargy, fever, weight loss, and anorectal disease. Anal fissures, fistulas, ulcers, or perirectal abscesses are seen in 50% of patients with colonic involvement and in 20% of patients with small bowel disease.

c. Signs include an abdominal mass, anemia, and malnutrition. Extraintestinal manifestations include inflammatory ocular (uveitis, iritis), joint (arthralgias, arthritis), skin (erythema nodosum, pyoderma gangrenosum), and biliary (primary sclerosing cholangitis) conditions.

    d. Radiographic findings on contrast study characteristically include segmental areas of stricture separated by "skip areas" of uninvolved bowel (string sign), cobblestone appearance of the mucosa, and fistulas.

    e. Gross appearance includes thickened, shortened mesentery, grayish-pink to purple discoloration of the bowel, and fat wrapping (circumferential growth of mesenteric fat around the bowel wall).

    f. Pathologically, there is mucosal ulceration that progresses to transmural inflammation, and noncaseating granulomas are found in the bowel wall and regional lymph nodes.

3. Differential diagnosis includes ulcerative colitis, lymphoma, and infectious enteritides (tuberculosis; amebiasis; and *Yersinia*, *Campylobacter*, and *Salmonella* infections).

4. Medical treatment includes a low-residue diet, aminosalicylates, prednisone, oral antibiotics (sulfasalazine, metronidazole), sedatives, antispasmodics, and, when necessary, total parenteral nutrition (TPN). Although antibiotics and steroids are helpful in acute active disease, their effectiveness in preventing relapses has not been established.

    a. Infliximab, a chimeric IgG_1 monoclonal antibody that binds to tumor necrosis factor-alpha, helps enterocutaneous fistulas close and results in improvement in 80% of chronic refractory patients, almost half of whom achieve short-term remission (8–12 weeks).

5. Surgical treatment is reserved for **complications** of the disease and ultimately becomes necessary in 70% of cases. Surgical therapy is conservative—resecting as little bowel as necessary. Margins of resection need only be to grossly uninvolved bowel. If resection is hazardous, bypass or exclusion of the involved segment may be necessary.

    a. Intestinal obstruction, which is usually caused by stricture and inflammation, is the most common indication for surgery. Short strictures can be repaired by a stricturoplasty, thus avoiding resection.

    b. Abscesses and fistulas are also common. Abscesses may be intra- or retroperitoneal. Fistulas (see Chapter 2, VII) form from bowel to skin, bladder, vagina, urethra, or other loops of bowel.

    c. Perianal disease is best treated with oral metronidazole therapy.

        (1) Perirectal abscesses require drainage. Anal fistulas and fissures may need surgery if they are multiple or severe.

        (2) In general, surgery for perianal disease should be as limited as is practical, because wound healing in these patients is poor and recurrence is common.

    d. Perforation, hemorrhage, intractable symptoms, cancer, and growth retardation (in children) are less common indications for surgery.

6. The **prognosis** is only fair. Approximately 50% of patients who require surgery will require it again within 5 years. The likelihood of a recurrence after each reoperation is again approximately 50%.

7. There is an increased risk of small bowel and colon adenocarcinoma associated with the severity and chronicity of inflammation.

D Diverticular disease

1. Duodenal diverticula are common (seen on 10%–20% of upper GI radiographs), but more than 90% are asymptomatic.

    a. Approximately 70% of duodenal diverticula are in the periampullary region.

    b. Periampullary diverticula can impair the emptying of bile through the ampulla, resulting in cholangitis, pancreatitis, and common bile duct stones.

2. Jejunoileal diverticula are rare.

    a. They may cause obstruction (from intussusception), bleeding, or perforation.

    b. They may also cause malabsorption owing to bacterial overgrowth within the diverticulum.

3. Meckel's diverticulum is the most common diverticulum of the GI tract (**incidence 2%**). It is located approximately **2 ft** from the ileocecal valve. The male:female ratio is **2:1**. Over a lifetime, approximately 95% of Meckel's diverticula will remain asymptomatic.

    a. Meckel's diverticula are true diverticula.

b. Most symptomatic Meckel's diverticula occur in children younger than age 2 and usually cause bleeding. Bleeding is due to heterotopic gastric mucosa in the diverticulum, which causes "peptic" ulceration in adjacent ileal mucosa. Heterotopic pancreatic mucosa may also be found within a Meckel's diverticulum.

c. Problems in adults include bowel obstruction (from intussusception), bleeding, and acute diverticulitis, which may be indistinguishable from appendicitis.

d. Management of asymptomatic Meckel's divericulum is controversial. Relative indications for resection include patient age <40, diverticulum >2 cm in length, fibrous bands between the diverticulum and the umbilicus, or mesentery.

E **Small bowel fistulas** (see Chapter 2, VII)

F **Short bowel syndrome** is a complication of extensive small bowel resection.

1. **Symptoms.** It is characterized by malabsorption with diarrhea and excessive loss of fat and protein in the stool. Inadequate absorption of water, electrolytes, minerals, and vitamins also invariably occurs. The length of bowel necessary to avoid the syndrome is variable, but patients with less than 100 cm (3.5 ft) of small bowel are most susceptible. An intact ileocecal valve, colon, or both decreases the amount of residual small bowel needed.

2. **TPN** (see Chapter 1, II E 2) is essential postoperatively. The small bowel will hypertrophy with time, and most patients can be weaned from TPN gradually. For refractory cases, long-term parenteral nutrition (**home TPN**) is available.

3. **Oral nutrition.** In order to ensure that oral nutrition is adequate, attention should be paid to several points.

   a. The total calories ingested must increase to compensate for the portion that is not absorbed.

   b. A low-residue or elemental diet is needed. An elemental diet contains only components that are directly absorbed by the intestinal mucosa without any enzymatic digestion (medium- and short-chain triglycerides, monosaccharides and disaccharides, monopeptides and dipeptides), plus vitamins and minerals.

   c. Antiperistaltic agents and histamine$_2$ (H$_2$)-receptor antagonists or proton pump inhibitors should be given.

   d. Fat and water soluble vitamin supplementation is needed.

   e. Parenteral vitamin B$_{12}$ is needed if the distal ileum has been resected.

   f. Calcium and magnesium supplementation should be given.

   g. Medium-chain triglycerides should replace dietary fats because they do not require micelles for absorption.

4. **Surgical therapy** is available, consisting of reversal of a short segment of distal small bowel to slow the intestinal transit time if adequate oral nutrition cannot be attained.

G **Radiation injury to the small bowel** occurs in two phases.

1. **Acute-phase injury** is caused by mucosal injury. Symptoms, which include nausea, vomiting, and diarrhea, are transient. Rarely, bleeding or perforation occurs and requires surgery.

2. **Chronic effects** appear months to years later and are caused by an obliterative vasculitis. The symptoms and signs are similar to those associated with a recurrent malignancy and, indeed, this possibility must always be fully evaluated.

   a. **Minor symptoms**—abdominal pain, malabsorption, and diarrhea—require symptomatic therapy only.

   b. **Major complications** that require surgery include bowel obstruction (unrelieved by decompression with a nasogastric or long tube), perforation, abscess, fistula, and hemorrhage. Hemorrhage may be caused by mucosal erosion or by an enteroarterial fistula.

   c. Surgery is technically difficult owing to fibrosis and scarring. With resection or bypass, unirradiated bowel must be used for any anastomosis. Even so, the anastomosis or surgical wound is likely to break down with subsequent fistula formation or other complications.

chapter 13

Colon, Rectum, and Anus

SCOTT D. GOLDSTEIN • PAUL A. MANCUSO

I INTRODUCTION

A Anatomy

1. **Colon.** The colon, or large intestine, is approximately 3–5 ft in length and is divided into several parts: the **cecum, ascending colon, transverse colon, descending colon,** and **sigmoid colon.**
   a. **Arterial blood supply** (Fig. 13-1)
      (1) Branches from the **superior mesenteric artery** supply the cecum, ascending colon, and proximal transverse colon.
      (2) Branches of the **inferior mesenteric artery** supply the distal transverse, descending, and sigmoid colon.
   b. **Venous drainage**
      (1) The **inferior mesenteric vein** carries blood from the left side of the colon to the splenic vein.
      (2) The **superior mesenteric vein** drains the right side of the colon, joining the splenic vein to form the portal vein.
   c. **Lymphatic drainage**
      (1) Lymph channels generally follow the arterial blood vessels.
      (2) Metastases from colon cancers generally spread through lymphatic paths in progressive fashion. The nodes closest to the cancer are involved first, and more distant nodes become involved as the disease advances.
   d. **Bowel wall**
      (1) Layers consist of **mucosa, submucosa, muscularis,** and **visceral peritoneum (serosa).**
      (2) There are no villi in the colonic mucosa; the **crypts of Lieberkühn** are the distinguishing histologic feature of the colonic mucosa.
      (3) The outer longitudinal muscle of the colon is incomplete; it forms three distinct bands, the **tenia coli.**
      (4) **Haustra** are the outpouchings of the colonic wall between the tenia coli.

2. **Rectum.** The rectum extends from the sigmoid colon to the anus and is approximately 15 cm in length.
   a. **Arterial blood supply** (Fig. 13-1)
      (1) The **superior rectal artery,** which is the terminal branch of the inferior mesenteric artery, supplies the upper and middle rectum.
      (2) The lower portion of the rectum is supplied with arterial branches from the internal iliac artery: the **middle rectal arteries** and **inferior rectal arteries.**
   b. **Venous drainage**
      (1) The **superior rectal veins** drain the upper and middle rectum, communicating with the portal vein via the inferior mesenteric vein.
      (2) The **middle rectal veins** drain the lower rectum and anal canal, emptying into the vena cava via the internal iliac veins.
      (3) Note that tumors in the rectum may metastasize into venous channels that enter either the portal system (portal vein) or the systemic system (vena cava).
   c. **Lymphatic drainage**
      (1) Lymph from the upper and middle rectum flows in channels that parallel the arterial supply and is filtered by the **inferior mesenteric nodes.**

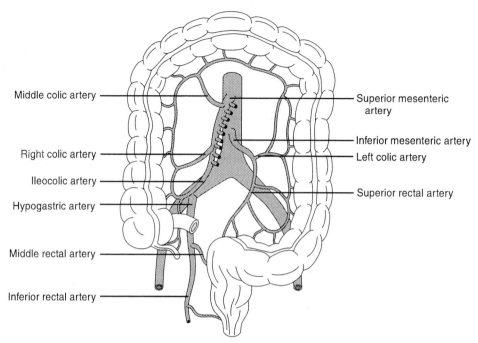

FIGURE 13-1 Arterial supply of right (ascending) colon via branches of superior mesenteric artery; left (descending) colon and rectum via branches of inferior mesenteric artery. Distal rectum supplied by branches from hypogastric artery.

    (2) Lymph from the distal rectum flows into channels adjacent to the middle and inferior rectal arteries. These channels drain to **iliac nodes.**

d. Bowel wall

    (1) In contrast to the colon, the rectum is lined by *complete* layers of inner circular and outer longitudinal muscle.

    (2) The proximal third of the rectum is covered with peritoneum, but the rectum descends beyond the peritoneal cavity, and the lower third has no peritoneal covering.

    (3) The **valves of Houston, usually three in number,** are mucosal folds that project into the lumen of the rectum.

3. Anus. The anus is the terminal portion of the intestinal tract. It is surrounded by two muscular tubes, which are involved in the mechanism of continence. The anus is also enveloped by the **puborectalis,** which is palpable by digital examination of the anus as the **anorectal ring.**

  a. The anal canal is lined by **anoderm,** a specialized epithelium that is devoid of hair follicles, sebaceous glands, or sweat glands but has a rich nerve supply. The junction between the anoderm and perianal skin is the **anal verge.**

  b. The colonic mucosa joins the anoderm at the **dentate line,** located approximately 1.5 cm above the anal verge.

  c. A **transitional zone** of 6–12 mm in length resides above the dentate line. In this zone, squamous epithelium gradually changes to cuboidal epithelium and then to columnar epithelium.

  d. The **columns of Morgagni** are longitudinal mucosal folds located just above the dentate line, where they meet to form the **anal crypts.**

  e. Small **anal glands** are present beneath the anoderm; these glands are located between the internal and external sphincters and communicate with the anal crypts via **anal ducts.**

  f. The **anal canal** is surrounded by two muscular sphincters, which provide continence.

    (1) The **internal sphincter**—a continuation of the inner circular muscle of the rectum—is a smooth muscle with involuntary control and autonomic innervation.

    (2) The **external sphincter** is a striated muscle under voluntary control with somatic innervation.

B **Physiology**

1. **Absorption of water and electrolytes**
   a. The colon receives from 900–1,500 mL of ileal chyme each day, of which all but 100–200 mL are absorbed. **Sodium** is actively absorbed across the colonic mucosa, whereas **potassium** moves into the colonic mucosa by passive diffusion.
   b. Water is absorbed passively, accompanying sodium molecules across the mucosa.

2. **Bacterial fermentation** of undigested carbohydrates in the colon produces **short-chain fatty acids,** which provide energy for sodium transport across the colonic mucosa.

3. **Storage of feces**
   a. Nondigestible waste is stored in the colon until voluntary evacuation occurs.
   b. Approximately one third of the dry weight of feces consists of bacteria. Each gram of feces contains 10^{11} to 10^{12} bacteria, with anaerobes being 100 to 10,000 times more prevalent than aerobes.
      (1) *Bacteroides*, an anaerobic bacterium, is the most common colonic organism.
      (2) *Escherichia coli* is the most common colonic aerobe.

4. **Colonic gas** can come from three sources: swallowed air, intraluminal production, and diffusion from the blood. Five gases constitute 98% of colonic gas: **nitrogen, oxygen, carbon dioxide, hydrogen,** and **methane.**

II **EVALUATION OF THE COLON, RECTUM, AND ANUS**

A **History**   The history provides very important information in the evaluation. A properly taken history most often establishes the diagnosis or at least suggests it. Inquiries should include the following:

1. **Bleeding:** passage of bright red blood (**hematochezia**) or dark, tarry stools (**melena**)
2. **Pain,** either abdominal or anal
3. Presence of an **anal or perianal mass**
4. **Rectal discharge**
5. **Change in bowel habit**
6. **Incontinence**
7. **History of cancer,** both personal and family
8. **History of colorectal polyps** or **inflammatory bowel disease,** both personal and family

B **Physical examination**

1. Pertinent aspects of the physical examination should be directed by the patient's complaints. Abdominal complaints require a standard, thorough abdominal examination. The examination for anorectal problems may require modification, depending on the patient's symptoms. For example, the patient with severe anal pain may not be able to tolerate examination with an anoscope or proctosigmoidoscope. If the cause of the pain is revealed by simple inspection (e.g., a thrombosed hemorrhoid), further methods of examination may not be necessary.

2. **Anorectal examination** is usually performed with the patient in the left lateral position and includes **four basic steps:**
   a. **Inspection.** Skin abnormalities, masses, protrusions, and drainage sites should be noted.
   b. **Palpation.** The perineum, anal canal, and lower rectum should be gently palpated with a gloved, well-lubricated index finger. Sphincter tone, areas of tenderness, and any masses should be noted.
   c. **Anoscopy** with a small anoscope provides the best method to evaluate fissures, hemorrhoids, anal papillae, or other anal canal lesions.
   d. **Proctosigmoidoscopy.** The rigid 20-cm proctosigmoidoscope remains a valuable instrument for studying the rectum. Often, the examination can be accomplished without preparation. A single enema may occasionally be required. The rectal mucosa should be inspected for any abnormalities such as ulceration, granularity, or tumors.

C **Radiographic studies**

1. **Barium enema** remains the most cost-effective method of identifying colon pathology. Unfortunately, it cannot reliably detect small tumors and thus is not effective for screening patients for cancer.

2. **Water-soluble contrast enema.** If colonic perforation is suspected, barium enema is contraindicated; extravasation of barium and feces can cause a severe peritonitis with a high mortality rate. The water-soluble material, although safer, is quickly diluted, giving these studies lesser diagnostic quality than barium studies.

3. **Computed tomography (CT) scan** is an excellent method of evaluating the patient suspected of having diverticulitis (contrast enemas may worsen the inflammation in such situations). Pericolic inflammation may be revealed, as well as abscesses, which may be drained under CT scan guidance. The CT scan is also useful for detecting metastases in patients with known colorectal cancer.

4. **Magnetic resonance imaging (MRI)** appears to offer little advantage over CT scans for evaluation of colorectal disease, with the possible exception of distinguishing between recurrent cancer and fibrosis in postoperative situations.

5. **Defecography** is a dynamic radiologic study by which the distal colon and rectum are imaged as the patient eliminates barium. It is useful in studying disorders of defecation.

D **Flexible endoscopy** permits a more extensive evaluation of the bowel than is possible with short, rigid instruments. Smaller lesions as well as mucosal irregularities can be evaluated more accurately with a flexible endoscope than with a barium enema.

1. **Flexible sigmoidoscopy** permits examination of the rectum and sigmoid colon (and occasionally the descending colon) with a flexible instrument that is 65 cm in length.

2. **Colonoscopy** enables evaluation of the entire colonic mucosal surface in more than 90% of patients. The flexible instrument used is 160 or 185 cm in length. Lesions can be biopsied and polyps removed with this instrument. **Indications** for its use include:
   a. Evaluation of **abnormalities noted on barium enema**
   b. Evaluation and surveillance of **inflammatory bowel disease**
   c. Differential diagnosis between **diverticular disease** and **cancer**
   d. Presence of a **polyp** (or history of previous polyp)
   e. **Gastrointestinal symptoms** (e.g., bleeding, abdominal pain, iron deficiency anemia) not clarified by contrast studies
   f. **Follow-up** of patients with prior colon cancer
   g. **Acute lower gastrointestinal bleeding**
   h. Reduction of **sigmoid volvulus**
   i. Evaluation of the entire colon in a patient with known **colorectal cancer** to evaluate for synchronous lesions

E **Fecal occult blood determination**   Stool is placed on guaiac-impregnated paper. If hemoglobin is present, a blue color appears when a peroxide-containing developer is added.

1. A daily loss of approximately 20 mL of blood into the gastrointestinal tract is required to consistently produce a positive result on a fecal occult blood test.

2. Red meat, turnips, radishes, tomatoes, aspirin, nonsteroidal anti-inflammatory drugs, and iron may cause false-positive results.

3. Vitamin C (ascorbic acid) can cause false-negative results.

4. A properly performed, positive fecal occult blood test requires adequate investigation of the gastrointestinal tract to determine the cause.

F **Anorectal physiologic studies**   The exact role of anorectal physiologic studies in the clinical setting has yet to be determined. Often, a thorough history and physical examination are adequate to determine the diagnosis and the treatment. However, further studies are sometimes required to define a problem.

1. **Anorectal manometry** provides information concerning anal sphincteric tone and the ability of the sphincter to contract. It can also document the presence of the normal **rectosphincteric reflex,** which is absent in Hirschsprung's disease.

2. **Electromyography** (pudendal nerve conduction velocity) may provide evidence of injury to the pudendal nerves that supply the anal sphincter.

G **Endorectal ultrasound** may provide information in certain anorectal disorders, including:

1. The depth of invasion into the bowel wall by **rectal cancer**

2. The site of **anal sphincter injury** in the incontinent patient

3. The path of **complicated anal fistulas**

III **BOWEL PREPARATION**

The colon must be adequately cleansed before surgical resection or before studies such as barium enema and colonoscopy. Feces must be removed from the bowel lumen; and, for surgery, the bacterial population must be reduced to minimize the risk of infection. Many methods are available to accomplish these goals, but almost all use a combination of cathartics, enemas, and antibiotics. The type of preparation depends somewhat on specific requirements (e.g., only mechanical cleansing is necessary for barium enema).

A **Diet**   Solid food should be avoided for at least 24 hours and preferably 48 hours before the anticipated procedure.

1. **Clear liquids** should be ingested to maintain adequate hydration.

2. **Intravenous fluids** are occasionally required for patients with cardiac or renal disease.

B **Cathartics** or **laxatives** are almost always required. Preferences are quite variable.

1. **Mannitol,** a nonabsorbable sugar, is an osmotic agent that attracts water into the bowel lumen and thus purges the gut. It is pleasant tasting but has disadvantages.
   a. Colonic bacteria metabolize the sugar and produce **hydrogen** and **methane,** which are gases that may explode if electrocautery is used.
   b. **Wound infections** are increased in patients prepared with mannitol. Apparently, mannitol promotes growth of *E. coli.*

2. **Polyethylene glycol (PEG)** is an isotonic lavage solution that acts as an osmotic purgative but is not fermented by bacteria. Approximately 4 L of PEG must be ingested within 4 hours for adequate cleansing.

3. **Castor oil** (2 oz) and **magnesium citrate** (10 oz) ingested 24 hours before the planned procedure have equivalent efficacy.

4. **Bisacodyl tablets** are often used as an element of the bowel preparation. They are taken 36 hours before the anticipated procedure.

C **Enemas** are at least as important as laxatives and cathartics to cleanse the colon. Either **saline enemas** or commercial **phosphasoda enemas** should be administered the night before the procedure until returns are clear.

D **Antibiotics** are important to reduce concentrations of colonic bacteria, with the goal of preventing postoperative infections.

1. Antibiotics must be given **preoperatively.** Postoperative antibiotics have no effect in the reduction of postoperative infections.

2. Oral antibiotics often recommended before surgery are **neomycin** and **erythromycin base.** These antibiotics achieve high concentrations in the colonic lumen and are administered the day before surgery, along with the purgative.

3. A broad-spectrum **intravenous antibiotic** is usually administered immediately before the start of a surgical procedure and is given again in the immediate postoperative period. Prophylactic antibiotics should not be continued after the day of operation.

IV **BENIGN AND MALIGNANT COLORECTAL TUMORS**

A **Polyps**   A polyp may be defined as any projection from the surface of the intestinal mucosa.

1. **Gross appearance**
   a. **Pedunculated polyps** are attached to the bowel wall by a stalk.
   b. **Sessile polyps** are flat growths with no stalk.

2. **Histologic types**
   a. **Hyperplastic polyps** are small (usually 5 mm) lesions of thickened mucosa without cellular atypia. They are present in 50% of adults, which makes them the most common type of polyp. There is no malignant potential, and treatment is usually unnecessary.
   b. **Hamartomatous polyps** are non-neoplastic growths that consist of an abnormal mixture of normal tissue. **Juvenile polyps** are hamartomas that occur most frequently in children and may cause gastrointestinal bleeding or intussusception.
   c. **Inflammatory polyps** are growths resulting from tissue reaction to inflammation, such as **pseudopolyps** in ulcerative colitis (UC) or benign **lymphoid polyps.** They have no neoplastic potential.
   d. **Neoplastic polyps** are by definition benign, but they have the potential to develop into cancer. These polyps are classified by histology into three types:
      (1) **Tubular adenomas** (75% of adenomas) have a smooth, firm surface and are often on a stalk.
      (2) **Villous adenomas** (10% of adenomas) are soft, sessile lesions with frondlike projections. Large villous adenomas may cause watery diarrhea and potassium loss.
      (3) **Tubulovillous adenomas** (15% of adenomas) have elements of both tubular and villous adenomas.

3. **The adenoma-carcinoma sequence.** Cumulative evidence suggests a progression from benign neoplasia to malignancy in colorectal polyps. Supporting observations include:
   a. Patients with colorectal cancer often have **synchronous adenomatous polyps.**
   b. **Histopathologic studies** have shown a transition from adenoma to carcinoma in polyps. The **peak incidence** for discovery of colon polyps is 50 years of age; the peak incidence for development of cancer is 60 years of age. This fact suggests a 10-year span for adenomas to transform to cancer.
   c. Patients with **familial adenomatous polyposis (FAP)** invariably develop colon cancer if not treated.
   d. **Polypectomy** has been shown to reduce the risk of colorectal cancer.
   e. **Molecular genetic studies** have detected four main genetic alterations in colorectal adenomas and carcinomas (*ras* **mutations** and deletions from chromosomes 5, 17, and 18).

4. **Malignant potential.** Probably more than 95% of colorectal cancers arise from neoplastic polyps. At least three characteristics of polyps are associated with malignancy:
   a. **Size**
      (1) Polyps <1 cm: 1% malignant
      (2) Polyps 1–2 cm in size: 10% malignant
      (3) Polyps >2 cm in size: 50% malignant
   b. **Histologic type**
      (1) Tubular: 5% malignant
      (2) Tubulovillous: 20% malignant
      (3) Villous: 40% malignant
   c. **Grade of atypia**
      (1) Mild: 5% malignant
      (2) Moderate: 20% malignant
      (3) Severe: 35% malignant

5. **Treatment of polyps.** Neoplastic polyps should be removed because of their malignant potential.
   a. **Endoscopic polypectomy** (excision with a colonoscope or sigmoidoscope) is ideal for pedunculated polyps. Small, superficial, sessile polyps are often amenable to piecemeal removal by this technique.
   b. **Transanal polypectomy.** Rectal polyps may be removed surgically through the anus.

    c. Segmental colectomy is required both for sessile polyps that cannot be excised with an endoscope and for most polyps that are malignant. Removal of the polyp through a **colotomy,** or a surgically made opening in the colon, is a historical procedure that has no place in treatment of polyp disease.

    d. A **malignant polyp** may be treated by endoscopic polypectomy if all of these characteristics are present:

      (1) The polyp is pedunculated.

      (2) The cancer is confined to the head (i.e., does not invade the stalk).

      (3) There is no venous or lymphatic invasion.

      (4) The polyp is moderately differentiated or well differentiated histologically.

B **Polyposis syndromes**

  1. Peutz-Jeghers syndrome is an autosomal dominant disorder characterized by **hyperpigmented spots** on the lips, buccal mucosa, face, and digits and **hamartomas** throughout the gastrointestinal tract.

    a. Complications. The polyps may cause gastrointestinal bleeding and intussusception.

    b. Cancer risk. There is an increased risk of malignancy of the intestine and other organ systems.

    c. Treatment. Symptomatic polyps should be removed, with a goal of preservation of intestine.

  2. Diffuse juvenile polyposis is an autosomal dominant disease characterized by a heterogeneous population of polyps, both **hamartomas** and **adenomas.**

    a. Complications. Intussusception, diarrhea, and protein loss may occur.

    b. Cancer risk. There is at least a 10% risk of developing colon cancer.

    c. Treatment is most commonly subtotal colectomy and ileorectal anastomosis.

      (1) Proctoscopy of the remaining rectum should be done every 6 months, and any new rectal polyps should be excised.

      (2) If there are **diffuse rectal polyps,** total protocolectomy with either an ileostomy or preferably an ileal pouch—anal anastomosis is indicated.

  3. Cowden's syndrome is an autosomal dominant disorder characterized by **hamartomas** throughout the gastrointestinal tract; **mucocutaneous abnormalities** (e.g., facial and oral papules, keratotic growths on the hands and feet); and **breast, thyroid,** or **uterine cancer. Treatment** is not usually required for the polyps but is directed toward the extraintestinal malignancies.

  4. Cronkhite-Canada syndrome is a noninherited syndrome characterized by generalized intestinal **hamartomas** in association with **alopecia, cutaneous pigmentation,** and **atrophy of the fingernails and toenails.**

    a. Symptoms include **vomiting, diarrhea, malabsorption,** and **protein-losing enteropathy.**

    b. The cause is unclear. **Mortality** is usual; most patients die within a short time after diagnosis, but there have been reports of **spontaneous remission.**

    c. Treatment is reserved for complications such as intestinal obstruction.

  5. FAP is characterized by more than 100 adenomatous polyps throughout the colon and rectum. If untreated, almost 100% of patients develop colon cancer by the fifth decade of life.

    a. Genetic transmission

      (1) FAP is an **autosomal dominant syndrome** with high penetrance. Fifty percent of offspring of affected patients develop the disease.

      (2) Almost all cases caused by germline mutations of adenomatous polyposis coli (APC) gene located on **chromosome 5.**

      (3) One third of patients with FAP have no family history of the disease: They represent **spontaneous mutations.**

    b. Clinical presentation. Although the disease is inherited, polyps are not present at birth, and they rarely appear before puberty. Fifty percent of FAP patients develop adenomas by age 15 and 95% by age 35.

      (1) Complications. The polyps may cause **bleeding** or, rarely, **intussusception.**

      (2) Extraintestinal expressions are common and include:

        (a) Epidermoid cysts

        (b) Osteomas

(c) Cutaneous fibromas

(d) Desmoid tumors of the abdomen and mesentery

(e) Gastrointestinal polyps

(f) Retinal pigmentation

(g) Periampullary carcinoma

(h) Thyroid carcinoma

c. **Screening.** First-degree relatives of FAP patients should undergo screening for FAP at age 10–12 years. Screening test of choice is testing for mutation of the APC gene. If genetic testing cannot be done, patients are advised to pursue yearly endoscopy beginning at age 12.

d. **Diagnosis** is made by confirming the numerous polyps by endoscopy and obtaining a biopsy to ensure the adenomatous nature of the polyps.

e. **Treatment:** If untreated, virtually all patients will develop colon cancer with the average age of onset between 34 and 43 years. Treatment is aimed at colectomy and includes:

(1) **Total proctocolectomy with ileostomy.** This procedure removes all colorectal mucosa, and the patient must wear an appliance.

(2) **Total proctocolectomy and continent ileostomy.** A reservoir is fashioned from the ileum to prevent outflow; the ileostomy must be intubated several times a day for elimination. The patient does not have to wear an appliance, but the operation is technically difficult and has a high incidence of complications.

(3) **Colectomy with ileorectal anastomosis.** The colon is excised, and the ileum is anastomosed to the rectum, which leaves only 15 cm of bowel at risk for cancer.

(a) Patients must be examined by **proctoscopy every 6 months,** and all rectal polyps are destroyed when they appear.

(b) **Celecoxib,** a selective cyclooxygenase-2 inhibitor, has been reported to cause regression of polyps in some patients with FAP. This feature may be advantageous for patients treated by this operation.

(4) **Total protocolectomy with ileal pouch–anal anastomosis.** This operation is especially attractive for patients with "carpeting" of the rectum by polyps too numerous to remove.

(a) **Advantages**

(i) Removes all colorectal mucosa at risk for cancer

(ii) Frequent proctoscopic examinations not required

(b) **Disadvantages**

(i) Some complications, including **sepsis, impotence,** and **fistula** are more likely with this procedure.

(ii) More frequent stools

(iii) Higher incidence of **anal incontinence** and **nocturnal seepage**

6. **Gardner's syndrome** is **FAP** with **osteomatosis, epidermoid cysts,** and **skin fibromas.**

7. **Turcot's syndrome** is **FAP** associated with **central nervous system malignancies** (e.g., medulloblastoma of the spinal cord, glioblastoma of the cerebrum).

C Carcinoma of the colon and rectum

1. **Incidence.** Colorectal cancer is the most common malignancy of the gastrointestinal tract.

a. It is the third most lethal cancer in women (after lung and breast).

b. It is the third most lethal cancer in men (after lung and prostate).

c. An American has approximately a **5% probability** of developing colorectal cancer during a 70-year life span.

d. Most cancers are detected after the age of 50; **incidence rises with age.**

2. **Site.** During the past 50 years, there has been a shift in the location of carcinomas from the rectum and left colon toward the right colon. This fact suggests that methods for detecting early large bowel cancer should be directed at the entire colon, rather than the rectosigmoid.

3. **Etiology.** Neither the cause nor the pathogenesis is well understood. A number of factors are considered important in the development of colorectal cancer.

a. The **polyp–cancer sequence** has been discussed previously (Chapter 13, IV B).

b. **Inflammatory bowel disease**

(1) Patients with **UC** have an increased risk of colorectal cancer, estimated to be more than 40% at 25 years after the onset of pancolitis.

(2) Patients with **Crohn's colitis** have a lower risk of cancer than those with UC but a higher risk than the general population.

c. Genetics. The importance of genetic causes of colon cancer is becoming increasingly obvious.

(1) There is an increased incidence of first-degree relatives of patients with colorectal cancer.

(2) The genetic transmission in FAP was described previously (Chapter 13, IV B).

(3) **Hereditary nonpolyposis colorectal carcinoma (HNPCC).** HNPCC, unlike FAP, cancer arises from a single colorectal lesion in the absence of polyposis.

(a) Characteristics include:

(i) Accounts for 3%–5% of all colorectal cancers

(ii) Autosomal dominant inheritance

(iii) Predominance of proximal colon cancers

(iv) Increased synchronous colon cancers

(v) Early age of onset (average age is 44 years)

(vi) Increased risk of metachronous cancers

vii) Increased incidence of mucinous or poorly differentiated carcinomas

(viii) Improved survival stage for stage compared with those who have sporadic tumors

(b) Increased incidence of **extracolonic malignancies,** including endometrium, ovary, breast, stomach, hematopoietic, small bowel, and skin.

(c) **HNPCC is caused by a single mutation of a DNA mismatch repair gene.** These genes are responsible for maintaining the fidelity of DNA during replication. Alterations in these genes lead to microsatellite instability (MSI), a phenomenon characterized by expansion or deletion of repeated units of DNA. Mismatch repair genes include: **hMSH2, hMLH1,** hPMS1, hPMS2, hMSH6.

(d) **Diagnosis of HNPCC is based the Amsterdam criteria,** which includes the following:

(i) Three or more relatives with histologically verified colorectal cancer, one of whom is a first-degree relative of the other two.

(ii) Colorectal cancer involving at least two generations.

(iii) One or more colorectal cancer cases diagnosed before the age of 50.

(e) **Recommendations for screening in HNPCC:**

(i) In the absence of genetic testing, first-degree relatives of affected individuals should undergo colonoscopy every 1–2 years beginning at age 20 and yearly past the age of 40.

(ii) In known germline mutation individuals, it is recommended that colonoscopy begins either at age 25 or when the age is 5 years younger than the first diagnosed family member, whichever comes first, and should continue annually.

d. Risk factors for colon and rectal cancer: Researchers have identified several risk factors that increase a person's chance of developing colorectal cancer:

(1) **A family history of colorectal cancer.** If there is a first-degree relative (parent, sibling, or offspring) who has had colorectal cancer, the risk for developing this disease is increased.

(a) People who have two or more close relatives with colorectal cancer make up about 20% of all people with colorectal cancer.

(b) **FAP and HNPCC,** discussed previously (Chapter 13, IV B), accounts for 5%–10% of patients with colorectal cancer.

(2) **Ethnic background.** Jews of Eastern European descent (Ashkenazi Jews) are thought to have a higher rate of colorectal cancer.

(3) A **personal history of colorectal cancer,** even though it has been completely removed, increases likelihood of developing new cancers in other areas of the colon and rectum.

(4) A **personal history of colorectal polyps** is associated with an increased risk for colorectal cancer. This is especially true if the polyps are numerous or large.

(5) A **personal history of chronic inflammatory bowel disease** including UC and Crohn's disease (CD) increases the risk of developing colorectal cancer (see Chapter 13, VII B 1 and VII C 5).

(6) **Age.** Chances of developing colorectal cancer increase markedly after age 50. Greater than 90% of people found to have colorectal cancer are older than 50.

(7) **Diet**

(a) Diets high in **fat,** especially from animal sources, can increase the risk of colorectal cancer. It is recommended to eat foods from plant sources and to limit the intake of high-fat foods such as those from animal sources.

(b) **Fruits and vegetables** contain substances that interfere with the process of cancer formation, and their consumption is believed to lower the risk for development of colorectal cancers.

(c) **Fiber.** Eating a diet high in fiber has traditionally been thought to decrease the risk of colorectal cancer. However, recent evidence suggests that fiber may not be as beneficial as previously assumed.

(d) **Calcium.** It has been observed that increased dietary calcium decreases the incidence of colorectal cancer.

(8) **Activity.** Physically inactive individuals are at increased risk of developing colorectal cancer.

(9) **Obesity.** Risk of dying of colorectal cancer is increased overweight people.

(10) **Diabetes** increases the chance of developing colorectal cancer by 30%–40%. Diabetics also tend to have a higher death rate after diagnosis.

(11) **Smoking.** Smokers are 30%–40% more likely than nonsmokers to die from colorectal cancer. Smoking may be responsible for causing about 12% of fatal colorectal cancers.

(12) **Alcohol intake.** Colorectal cancer has been linked to the heavy use of alcohol.

4. **Clinical presentation** depends on the location, size, and extent of the tumor.

a. **Right-sided cancer**

(1) Melanotic stools

(2) Iron deficiency anemia

(3) Right-sided abdominal mass

b. **Left-sided cancer**

(1) Change in bowel habits

(2) Passage of red blood via rectum

(3) Cramping abdominal pain (caused by partial obstruction)

5. **Patient evaluation** includes the following:

a. **Abdominal examination**

b. **Rectal examination**

(1) **Digital examination** is useful to assess the location, size, and extent of invasion of a tumor in the distal rectum.

(a) Hard areas in a tumor suggest carcinoma, whereas soft polyps are more likely to be benign.

(b) If a tumor feels fixed or "tethered" to the adjacent pararectal tissues, malignant invasion of the bowel wall is likely.

(2) **Rigid proctosigmoidoscopy** is useful to determine the exact location of a rectal tumor in relation to the anal verge.

(3) **Endorectal ultrasound** provides information concerning the depth of invasion into the bowel wall by a rectal tumor and involvement of lymph nodes.

c. **Colonoscopy** with biopsy of the lesion and inspection of the remaining colon is necessary to exclude synchronous lesions. A **barium enema** is often not required if the colonoscopic examination is satisfactory. If the colonoscope does not reach the cecum, a barium enema should be obtained to evaluate the entire colon.

d. **Chest radiograph**

e. **Laboratory studies** include carcinoembryonic antigen (CEA); liver enzymes; and hemoglobin, hematocrit, or both.

f. **CT scan** is used to evaluate the liver and abdomen for metastases and both kidneys for ureteral obstruction.

6. **Treatment. Surgical resection** is the preferred treatment for most cases of colorectal cancer. Important aspects of surgery include:
   a. Proper preparation of the patient, including **bowel preparation**
   b. **Thorough exploration** of the abdomen to search for metastases and other intra-abdominal disease
   c. **Removal** of the segment of colon containing the tumor and the lymphovascular pedicle, which contains the lymph nodes that drain the cancer
   d. **Anastomosis without tension** between segments of bowel with **satisfactory blood supply**
   e. Operations for **rectal cancer** require special considerations.
      (1) **Upper-third lesions** (10–15 cm above the anus) can be treated by resection through the abdomen with anastomosis between the left colon and the remaining rectum (**low anterior resection**).
      (2) **Middle-third lesions** (5–10 cm above the anus) are usually amenable to low anterior resection, using circular stapling instruments to fashion the anastomosis.
      (3) **Lower-third lesions.** Several options may be considered.
         (a) Resection of the rectum, anus, and anal sphincters by a combined abdominal and perineal approach requires construction of a colostomy (**abdominoperineal resection,** also called **Miles procedure).**
         (b) Resection of the distal rectum using a transanal approach, resection of the proximal rectum using an abdominal approach, or anastomosis between the colon and distal rectum through the anus can be performed. There are several modifications of these technically difficult operations, and they may be referred to as **pull-through operations.** In almost all patients, a temporary colostomy is fashioned to allow the anastomosis to heal without the danger of anastomotic leak and sepsis. The colostomy may be closed 10–12 weeks after the initial operation.
         (c) **Local excision, fulguration, and contact radiotherapy** may be used for select, very favorable rectal cancers in which the chance of metastases is small, for example:
            (i) **Superficial lesions,** freely moveable by digital examination
            (ii) Those that are **not poorly differentiated** histologically
            (iii) Those that are **confined to the rectal wall,** as detected by endorectal ultrasound
            (iv) Those in which there are no palpable retrorectal lymph nodes
            (v) Nonulcerated, exophytic lesions
   f. **Adjuvant therapy**
      (1) **Chemotherapy,** as combinations of **5-fluorouracil (5-FU), leucovorin,** and more recently **oxaliplatin** are currently recommended for patients with positive lymph nodes or metastatic disease.
      (2) **Radiation therapy** given preoperatively to patients with advanced rectal cancer has been shown to shrink the cancer and reduce local recurrence.
      (3) Combinations of adjuvant radiation therapy and chemotherapy for advanced rectal cancers are also being employed.

7. **Staging.** The American College of Surgeons' Commission on Cancer has urged adoption of the **TNM staging system.** This system identifies the depth of invasion of the tumor (**T**), the regional lymph node status (**N**), and the presence of distant metastases (**M**) (Tables 13-1 and 13-2).

8. **Prognosis,** determined by 5-year survival, is clearly related to the stage of disease, as demonstrated in Table 13-3.

9. **Follow-up**
   a. **Physical examination** seldom reveals early tumor recurrences.
   b. **Colonoscopy** should be performed 1 year after surgery to detect any new polyps.
      (1) If polyps are found and removed, the colonoscopy should be repeated annually until there are no polyps.
      (2) After a negative colonoscopy, the examination should be repeated every 3–5 years to detect any new polyps.
   c. **CEA** is the most sensitive indicator of recurrent colorectal cancer. CEA is a glycoprotein that is secreted by colorectal tumors. It cannot usually be detected if the tumor has not penetrated

TABLE 13-1 TNM Classification of Colorectal Cancer

TNM Classification	Abbreviation	Definition
Primary tumor (T)	TX	Primary tumor that cannot be assessed
	T0	No evidence of primary tumor
	Tis	Carcinoma in situ
	T1	Tumor that invades submucosa
	T2	Tumor that invades muscularis propria
	T3	Tumor that invades the muscularis propria into the subserosa or into nonperitonealized periocolic or perirectal tissues
	T4	Tumor that perforates the visceral peritoneum or directly invades other organs
Regional lymph nodes (N)	NX	Regional lymph nodes that cannot be assessed
	N0	No regional lymph node metastasis
	N1	Metastasis in one to three pericolic or perirectal lymph nodes
	N2	Metastasis in four or more pericolic or perirectal lymph nodes
	N3	Metastasis in any node along the course of a named vascular trunk
Distant metastasis (M)	MX	Presence of distant metastases not able to be assessed
	M1	No distant metastases
	M2	Distant metastases

the bowel wall, and it is often increased if there are metastases. CEA may be elevated in patients with cirrhosis, pancreatitis, renal failure, UC, and other types of cancer and can also be influenced by smoking; thus, measuring the CEA level is a nonspecific test. Most surgeons recommend obtaining CEA levels:

(1) Every 3 months during the first two postoperative years

(2) Every 6 months during the third, fourth, and fifth postoperative years

    d. A **rising CEA level** is an indication for a **chest radiograph** and an **abdominal CT scan.**

    e. There is sufficient reason to attempt to detect an early recurrence.

        (1) **Isolated hepatic metastases** may be resected with a 25% 5-year survival.

        (2) **Solitary pulmonary metastases** may be resected with a 20% 5-year survival.

    f. **Chemotherapy** and **radiation therapy** are palliative for recurrent nonresectable colorectal cancer.

D **Carcinoid tumors** arise from neuroectodermal cells. They have the ability to incorporate and store amine precursor (5-hydroxytryptophan) and to decarboxylate this substrate, which produces several biologically active amines (i.e., amine precursor uptake and decarboxylation [**APUD**] **tumors**). The gastrointestinal tract is the most common site, and (in decreasing order of frequency) carcinoids arise in the appendix, ileum, rectum, stomach, and colon. The tumors are usually small, submucosal nodules.

1. **Colon carcinoids** account for less than 2% of gastrointestinal carcinoids; they may be multicentric, and they may cause the **carcinoid syndrome** from liver metastases.

2. **Rectal carcinoids** account for 15% of gastrointestinal carcinoids. They are usually solitary, and they do not cause the carcinoid syndrome.

3. **Treatment** is related to size of the tumor.
   a. Tumors smaller than 2 cm seldom metastasize and can be locally excised.
   b. Tumors larger than 2 cm are usually malignant and should be treated by radical resection.

TABLE 13-2 Dukes Classification of Colorectal Cancer

Class	Description
A	Tumor is confined to the bowel wall.
B	Tumor penetrates the bowel wall into serosa or perirectal fat.
C	Lymph node metastasis is present.
D	Distant metastasis is present.

TABLE 13-3 Stage and Prognosis of Colorectal Cancer

Stage	Dukes Classification	T Level	N Level	M Level	Cure Rate
0	—	Tis	N0	M0	100%
I	A	T1 or T2	N0	M0	90%
II	B	T3 or T4	N0	M0	80%
III	C	Any T	N1, N2, or N3	M0	60%
IV	D	Any T	Any N	M1	5%

T, tumor; N, regional lymph nodes; M, distant metastases.

E **Other neoplasms** may arise from normal colorectal tissues but are rare, including:

1. Lymphoid tissue (lymphoma and lymphosarcoma)
2. Adipose tissue (lipoma and liposarcoma)
3. Muscle tissue (leiomyoma and leiomyosarcoma)

V DIVERTICULAR DISEASE

A Terminology

1. **Diverticulum:** abnormal sac or pouch protruding from the wall of a hollow organ (e.g., the colon)
2. **True diverticulum:** diverticulum composed of all layers of bowel wall (rare in the colon)
3. **False diverticulum:** diverticulum lacking a portion of the bowel wall (common)
4. **Diverticula:** more than one diverticulum
5. **Diverticulosis:** the presence of diverticula
6. **Diverticulitis:** infection associated with diverticula

B Epidemiology and etiology

1. **Diverticulosis is a disease of modern times.**
   a. It was not recognized until after the Industrial Revolution (1880).
   b. Its appearance seems to be related to processing wheat flour in a roller mill and reducing fiber in the diet.
2. It is common in Western societies and rare in unindustrialized nations.
3. Populations who eat high-fiber, low-sugar foods (e.g., sub-Saharan Africans) have a low incidence of diverticulosis.
4. The incidence of this acquired disorder increases with age.
   a. Diverticulosis is rare in persons younger than 30 years of age.
   b. It is present in 75% of people older than 80 years.

C Pathogenesis

1. **Diverticula** are herniations of mucosa through the colonic wall.
   a. They occur at sites where arterioles traverse the wall.
   b. These herniations lack a muscular layer: They are **false diverticula.**
2. The **sigmoid colon** is the most common site for diverticula.
   a. Diverticula occur with decreasing frequency in the descending, transverse, and ascending colon.
   b. It is rare for diverticula to occur in the rectum.
3. **Increased intraluminal pressure** in the colon, which is thought to be associated with a low-fiber diet, has been proposed as the cause of mucosal herniation.
   a. **Segmentation** of isolated areas of colon can produce high pressures.

    b. By **Laplace's law, P = T/R,** the highest pressure across the colon wall occurs in the sigmoid colon, which has the smallest radius in the colon.

  4. Muscular hypertrophy of the colon wall often accompanies diverticula and is especially common in the involved sigmoid colon.

  5. The diverticula are in close proximity to arterioles that traverse the colon wall.

D **Diverticulitis** is caused by a perforation of one or more diverticula.

  1. The perforation occurs in the **sigmoid colon** in more than 90% of cases.

  2. Extravasation of colonic bacteria results in a **pericolic infection.**

  3. A wide spectrum of disease is possible, ranging from:
    a. Localized cellulitis, which is a **pericolic phlegmon**
    b. An intra-abdominal **abscess**
    c. Generalized purulent peritonitis (from ruptured abscess)
    d. Feculent peritonitis (persistent leakage of feces from the perforation)
    e. Fistula formation, including fistulas from the colon to the **bladder, vagina, skin,** or other sites

  4. Clinical presentation is variable, depending on the location of the perforation and the extent of the infection.
    a. Left lower abdominal pain is the most common symptom. Pain may radiate to the **suprapubic area, groin,** or **back.**
    b. Abdominal or **pelvic mass** may be caused by a phlegmon or abscess.
    c. Fever and **leukocytosis** are common.
    d. Associated **ileus** may cause small bowel distention and vomiting.
    e. Generalized peritonitis may be present in severe cases.
    f. Pneumaturia, dysuria, pyuria, or **fecaluria** may be caused by colovesical fistula. Similarly, colovaginal fistula may be accompanied by vaginal drainage of pus or stool.

  5. Initial evaluation
    a. A **CT scan of the abdomen and pelvis** is the most helpful test to confirm the suspected diagnosis of diverticulitis.
      (1) If intravenous contrast is given before the CT scan, the kidneys and ureters can be evaluated simultaneously, and intravenous pyelography (IVP) is not usually necessary.
      (2) If an abscess is revealed, it may be amenable to **CT-guided percutaneous** drainage.
      (3) Air in the bladder is highly suggestive of **colovesical fistula.**
      (4) Contrast enema should generally be avoided if diverticulitis is suspected; hydrostatic pressure can worsen the situation by causing extravasation of contrast and feces through the perforation.
    b. Chest radiography. Subdiaphragmatic air is detected in fewer than 3% of cases of diverticulitis.
    c. The **leukocyte count** should be obtained initially as a baseline and serially to evaluate the response to treatment.
    d. Frequent abdominal examinations are necessary to determine the activity of the disease.

  6. Subsequent evaluation. After the patient's condition has stabilized and signs of sepsis have subsided, further evaluation may be necessary.
    a. Colonoscopy may be indicated to exclude a **sigmoid cancer.**
    b. Barium enema is less useful than colonoscopy because small tumors may be masked by diverticula and may not be detected by barium enema.
    c. Cystoscopy should be done if a colovesical fistula is suspected to determine the probable site of the fistula.

  7. Treatment depends on the severity of the disease, the number of previous attacks, the presence of complications, and the overall condition of the patient.
    a. Initial treatment for a **phlegmon of the sigmoid colon** includes:
      (1) Intravenous fluids
      (2) Nothing orally (a nasogastric tube is placed if ileus is present)
      (3) Broad-spectrum intravenous antibiotics

b. Treatment if an **intra-abdominal abscess** is present
  (1) Intravenous fluids
  (2) Nothing orally (a nasogastric tube is placed if ileus is present)
  (3) Broad-spectrum intravenous antibiotics
  (4) Drainage of the abscess, preferably by percutaneous drainage using CT guidance
c. Treatment for **purulent** or **feculent peritonitis**
  (1) Administration of fluid and antibiotics
  (2) Resection of the diseased segment of bowel (if possible)
  (3) Closure of rectal stump and construction of colostomy (**Hartmann's operation**)
    (a) It is not safe to make an anastomosis in the presence of severe infection.
    (b) The colostomy can be taken down, and the colon can be anastomosed to the rectum after the patient has recovered from the illness and surgery, which is usually at least 10 weeks later.
d. Treatment for **recurrent attacks of diverticulitis**
  (1) Sigmoidectomy and primary colorectal anastomosis
  (2) Considerable clinical judgment is required to determine indications.
    (a) Young patients with a single severe attack may warrant elective surgery to prevent another attack, because this group of patients has a very high incidence of complicated diverticulitis.
    (b) Elderly patients should probably not have surgery unless more than one episode of diverticulitis has occurred.
    (c) The chance of recurrent episodes of diverticulitis after a single, uncomplicated episode is approximately 10%.
    (d) The chance of recurrent episodes after a complicated episode of diverticulitis (with abscess formation) is probably higher than 30%.
    (e) The risk of complications increases with subsequent episodes of diverticulitis.
e. Treatment for **fistulas caused by diverticulitis**
  (1) Treat initially with antibiotics to allow acute inflammation to resolve.
  (2) Sigmoidectomy and primary colorectal anastomosis
    (a) Excising the diseased sigmoid colon with anastomosis is usually possible if acute inflammation has resolved.
    (b) If considerable inflammation persists, **Hartmann's operation** is indicated. The colostomy can be closed at a later date, as discussed previously (Chapter 13, V D 7 c).

8. Surgical treatment of diverticulitis
  a. Abscesses should be drained by percutaneous, transvaginal, or transrectal route, if possible.
    (1) Laparotomy for abscess drainage risks spreading infection throughout the peritoneal cavity, and a colostomy almost always is required in such cases.
    (2) If the abscess can be successfully drained, the patient usually recovers sufficiently to permit a single-stage sigmoidectomy with colorectal anastomosis.
  b. If there is significant pelvic inflammation, **ureteral catheters** may be placed prior to surgery to assist intraoperative location of the left ureter.
  c. All hypertrophied muscular colon should be removed.
  d. The **anastomosis** should be made at the level of the rectum.
    (1) The distal sigmoid colon almost always has a hypertrophied muscular wall, which should not be incorporated into the anastomosis (this is thought to be a cause of recurrence).
    (2) The rectum is almost never involved in diverticular disease.
  e. It is not necessary to remove all segments of colon containing diverticula; only the hypertrophied muscular segment (which is usually confined to the sigmoid) must be removed.

E **Hemorrhage** is the other major complication of diverticular disease.
  1. An arteriole adjacent to a diverticulum may disrupt, causing massive bleeding. Such bleeding is most frequent in elderly patients.

  2. Presentation. Abdominal pain is rare; patients usually pass large amounts of bright-red blood via the rectum. Rapid blood loss may result in shock.

3. Diagnostic tests that accompany resuscitation

    a. Preparation. A crystalloid solution is administered intravenously. Blood is transfused, if required, for hemodynamic stabilization. A nasogastric tube is passed to rule out gastroduodenal hemorrhage.

    b. Proctoscopy is done to rule out anorectal hemorrhage (from hemorrhoids or rectal varices).

    c. Coagulation studies (e.g., prothrombin time [PT], partial thromboplastin time [PTT], platelets) are obtained, and clotting factors are corrected if they are abnormal.

    d. A **nuclear scan** (labeled red blood cell scan) is obtained if the patient's condition permits.

    e. A **mesenteric arteriogram** is indicated if the nuclear scan indicates the site of bleeding.

        (1) If the mesenteric arteriogram shows the site of bleeding, **vasopressin** can be infused through the mesenteric catheter to constrict the mesenteric artery and lower portal pressure. This infusion stops 90% of diverticular hemorrhages.

        (2) If bleeding persists and the mesenteric arteriography has shown the site of hemorrhage, a **segmental colectomy** is indicated.

        (3) If bleeding persists and the site cannot be detected by arteriography, a **total abdominal colectomy with ileostomy** is indicated.

VI   ANGIODYSPLASIA

A   This **acquired vascular lesion** joins diverticulosis as a major cause of colonic hemorrhage. Other names for this entity include angiectasis, arteriovenous malformation, and vascular ectasis.

1. These acquired vascular lesions occur most commonly in the right colon.

2. They rarely occur in persons before 40 years of age, and they increase in frequency with age.

3. It has been suggested that the lesions are the result of chronic, intermittent obstruction of the submucosal veins.

    a. This chronic obstruction results eventually in incompetence of the precapillary sphincters, which in turn causes small arteriovenous communications within the bowel wall.

    b. These lesions are probably present in most people older than 70 years of age. The reason why some lesions bleed, whereas most do not, remains unknown.

4. Hemorrhage from angiodysplasia tends to be slower than that from diverticulosis. Stools may be melanotic or bright red, depending on the rate of hemorrhage.

B   **Evaluation and treatment** are similar to those for a patient with bleeding diverticulosis. However, angiodysplasia tends to bleed intermittently, whereas diverticular bleeding is caused by an arteriolar disruption with massive bleeding that does not usually recur after it ceases.

1. Some angiodysplastic lesions can be detected by **colonoscopy** as **"cherry-red spots"** on the mucosa. These lesions may be eradicated by endoscopic electrocoagulation.

2. If the bleeding persists or recurs and can be isolated to a colonic segment by nuclear scans, arteriography, or colonoscopy, segmental colectomy is indicated.

3. If the bleeding persists and the site cannot be identified, total abdominal colectomy with ileostomy may be required as a lifesaving measure.

VII   INFLAMMATORY BOWEL DISEASE

A   **General considerations**   Two major types of idiopathic inflammatory bowel disease (IBD) may cause colitis of the large bowel: **CD** and **UC**.

1. Presentation. There is considerable overlap in the presentation of these diseases (Table 13-4). In approximately 15% of patients with idiopathic colitis, a distinction between the two cannot be made on pathologic or clinical grounds. In such situations, the disease is called **indeterminate colitis**.

2. Etiology of both diseases remains unknown.

    a. Genetic, environmental, infectious, and autoimmune mechanisms have been suggested, but a clearly defined cause has not been identified.

    b. Both diseases can occur at any age, but they tend to be diseases of young adults.

TABLE 13-4 Inflammatory Disease of the Colon

Characteristics	Ulcerative Colitis	Crohn's Colitis
Usual location	Rectum, left colon	Any segment of colon; ileocolic disease most common
Rectal bleeding	Common, continuous	Less common, intermittent
Rectal involvement	Almost always	Approximately 50%
Fistulas	Rare	Common
Ulcers	Shaggy, irregular, continuous distribution	Linear with transverse fissures ("cobblestone")
Bowel stricture	Rare; should raise suspicion of cancer	Common
Carcinoma	Increased incidence	Increased incidence but less than with UC

c. It is helpful to distinguish between the two types of colitis, because the medical and surgical treatments are slightly different for each.

3. **Serologic markers** can be a useful tool for the confirmation of IBD. Perinuclear antineutrophil cytoplasmic antibody (**pANCA**) and anti–*Saccharomyces cerevisiae* antibodies (**ASCA**) are two antibodies frequently detected in the serum of IBD patients. pANCA has been observed in 60%–70% of patients with UC but only in 5%–10% of CD patients and in 2%–3% of the general population. Conversely, positivity for ASCA is typically seen in 60%–70% of CD patients, in 10%–15% of those with UC, and in 5% of the general population.

B **Ulcerative colitis**

1. **Important features**
   a. **Inflammation. Mucosal inflammation** (as opposed to transmural inflammation) occurs, as does **rectal inflammation.** The rectum is virtually always involved, with inflammation extending proximally for variable distances. Inflammation is **continuous;** that is, there are no skipped areas of normal mucosa between inflamed segments.
   b. **Involvement.** There is usually **no anal** or **perianal disease** in patients with UC. Anal abscesses, fistulas, and fissures are rare. There is **no involvement of the small bowel.**
   c. **Histology. Crypt abscesses** may be present but not granulomas. **Pseudopolyps** may be present.
   d. **Extraintestinal manifestations** of the disease may be present, including:
      (1) Ankylosing spondylitis and sacroileitis
      (2) Peripheral arthritis
      (3) Erythema nodosum and pyoderma gangrenosum
      (4) Aphthous stomatitis
      (5) Iritis and episcleritis
      (6) Sclerosing cholangitis
   e. **Risk for colon cancer** occurs in patients with chronic disease.
      (1) The risk is minimal until after 10 years of onset, and then it increases by approximately 2% each year thereafter.
      (2) The risk is minimal in patients with disease limited to the rectum and is highest in patients with pancolitis.
      (3) **Dysplasia** of the mucosa is associated with an increased risk of cancer.
      (4) Patients who have had UC for longer than 10 years should have an annual **surveillance colonoscopy** with multiple mucosal biopsies to search for dysplasia.
      (5) Cancers in patients with UC are flat, invasive lesions and are not readily identified by barium enema.

2. **Clinical presentation**
   a. **Bloody diarrhea** is the most common symptom. Rarely, bleeding may be massive and life threatening.
   b. **Mucus** and **pus** may accompany the passage of loose stools.

   c. Cramping abdominal pain often occurs.

   d. Malaise, fever, weight loss, and **anemia** are common.

   e. Severity of disease ranges from occasional episodes of diarrhea to **fulminant colitis with toxic megacolon,** which is characterized by:

     (1) Dilatation of the transverse colon

     (2) Abdominal pain, tenderness, and distention

     (3) Fever, leukocytosis, and hypoalbuminemia

     (4) Significant risk of colonic perforation

3. Evaluation depends on the severity of the disease. Mild cases can be evaluated on an outpatient basis, whereas fulminant colitis with toxic megacolon is a life-threatening situation requiring hospitalization, intensive medical treatment, and emergency surgery if medical treatment fails.

   a. Proctoscopy is the most valuable test to establish the diagnosis.

     (1) Mucosal inflammation beginning at the level of the dentate line is highly suggestive of UC.

     (2) In the presence of fulminant colitis, colonoscopy and barium enema should be avoided because these tests may worsen the condition and lead to toxic megacolon.

     (3) Mucosal biopsies should be taken to confirm the diagnosis. Such biopsies are also helpful in distinguishing UC from Crohn's colitis and infectious colitis.

   b. Abdominal radiographs should be obtained if abdominal tenderness is present and symptoms are severe to rule out colonic dilatation.

   c. Stool samples should be cultured for pathogens and examined for ova and parasites.

   d. Serologic markers for IBD, mainly pANCA (see Chapter 13, VII A 3)

   e. If symptoms are mild, the entire colon should be evaluated by **colonoscopy** and **barium enema.**

   f. Small bowel contrast studies should be obtained to rule out small bowel involvement, which would indicate CD.

4. Medical treatment

   a. Steroids are effective for short-term treatment, but side effects prevent their long-term use.

   b. Sulfasalazine remains the main therapeutic agent. It is recommended even if disease is in remission because it decreases the incidence and severity of a recurrence.

   c. Aminosalicylates (5-aminosalicylic acid [5-ASA]) are beneficial to patients who are allergic to sulfasalazine.

   d. Immunosuppressive agents include:

     (1) 6-Mercaptopurine

     (2) Azathioprine

     (3) Methotrexate

     (4) Intravenous cyclosporine

   e. Broad-spectrum antibiotics are indicated for patients with fulminant colitis and toxic megacolon.

   f. TPN may be required for patients with severe debilitating disease, usually to prepare the patient for surgery.

5. Surgical treatment

   a. Indications

     (1) Hemorrhage

     (2) Fulminant colitis or toxic megacolon that is not responsive to intensive medical treatment

     (3) Debilitating disease that is not refractory to medical treatment

     (4) Colonic stricture (at least 30% incidence of cancer)

     (5) Dysplasia or cancer

   b. Procedures

     (1) Total proctocolectomy with a permanent ileostomy

     (2) Proctocolectomy with anal sphincter preservation and ileal pouch anal anastomosis (restorative proctocolectomy)

       (a) This operation is the most common for UC. It is usually accompanied by a temporary ileostomy, which is closed 10 weeks after the initial operation.

(b) This operation is **contraindicated for patients with CD** because of the high incidence of recurrent diseases in the ileal pouch.

(3) **Abdominal colectomy with closure of the rectal stump**

(a) This procedure is indicated for patients with fulminant colitis.

(b) This procedure is helpful in patients with indeterminate colitis, because it allows examination of the entire colon to distinguish between CD and UC.

(c) Restorative proctectomy with an ileal pouch anal anastomosis can be performed at a later time.

(4) **Ileostomy and blowhole colostomy.** This operation is rarely used. The indication is life-threatening toxic megacolon when the colonic wall is too thin and friable to permit resection without rupture. In such situations, the colon is decompressed with a skin-level transverse colostomy, and an ileostomy diverts feces from the colon. After the patient has recovered from the fulminating illness, the standard operations for UC may be performed.

(5) **Total proctocolectomy and continent (Kock) ileostomy.** The main indication for this procedure is a patient who has already had a total proctocolectomy and is allergic to the ileostomy appliance.

(a) In this procedure, an ileal pouch is fashioned with a nipple valve that is attached to the abdominal wall and requires intubation to evacuate the ileum several times daily.

(b) This operation is associated with a high incidence of complications, usually associated with the nipple valve.

C **Crohn's (granulomatous) colitis**

1. **Important features**

    a. **Inflammation**

    (1) **Transmural inflammation.** The full thickness of the bowel wall is inflamed.

    (2) **Noncontinuous inflammation.** "Skip areas" of normal bowel may separate inflamed regions (another term for this disease is **segmental colitis**).

    b. **Involvement. Rectal sparing** may be present. Disease does not always involve the rectum. The **small bowel is frequently involved** (especially terminal ileum). **Anal** or **perianal disease** (e.g., fistulas, abscesses, fissures) may be present.

    (1) Approximately one third of all patients with CD develop anal disease.

    (2) Anal disease is more common in patients with colon disease (50%) than in patients with small bowel disease (25%).

    c. **Histology. Granulomas** are present in 30%–50% of cases. Linear ulcers may join transverse fissures to give a "cobblestone" appearance to the mucosa.

    d. **Extraintestinal manifestations** are generally the same as for UC, except that sclerosing cholangitis is less common than with UC.

    e. Risk for cancer in the diseased segments is increased but less than with UC.

2. **Clinical presentation**

    a. **Diarrhea** (with diffuse colonic disease) is common.

    b. **Cramping abdominal pain** and **right lower quadrant tenderness** (with ileocolic disease) are common.

    c. **Malaise, fever, weight loss,** and **leukocytosis** are common.

    d. **Abdominal abscess** (usually right lower quadrant) may occur.

    e. **Fistulas** may occur between the involved bowel and the bladder, vagina, skin, or other segments of intestine.

    f. **Anal abscess** or **fistula** is a presenting symptom in 5% of cases.

    g. **Fulminant colitis** may be as severe as UC (see VII B 2 e).

    (1) The colon usually does not dilate ("megacolon") with fulminant CD, which is thought to be due to the transmural inflammation with thickening of the wall.

    (2) Patients with fulminant colitis must be treated as vigorously as patients with UC and megacolon. Risk of perforation is the same as in those conditions.

3. **Evaluation.** As with UC, evaluation depends on the severity of the disease.

    a. **Abdominal examination** is important to evaluate areas of tenderness or mass.

    b. **Anorectal examination** should detect abscesses, fissures, or fistulas.

    c. Proctoscopy is important. If rectal mucosa is not involved, UC is essentially excluded as a diagnostic possibility.

    d. Serologic markers for IBD, mainly ASCA (see VII A 3).

    e. Stool samples should be cultured and examined for ova and parasites.

    f. Barium studies of the small bowel and colon are indicated to determine the extent of disease.

    g. Colonoscopy is helpful to evaluate the extent of colonic involvement.

    h. A **CT scan** is helpful if abdominal or pelvic abscess is suspected.

4. Medical treatment

    a. Steroids are helpful for acute disease. Budesonide, a rapidly metabolized glucocorticoid with high topical activity and poor systemic absorption, has been shown to be effective in inducing remissions in patients with CD, with less adrenal suppression than traditional steroids.

    b. Immunosuppressive agents appear to provide clinical improvement, steroid sparing, and fistula healing in patients with active CD:

        (1) 6-Mercaptopurine

        (2) Azathioprine

        (3) Methotrexate

        (4) Intravenous cyclosporine

    c. Infliximab therapy, monoclonal antibodies to the proinflammatory cytokine tumor necrosis factor **(TNF),** is indicated for reducing signs and symptoms and inducing and maintaining clinical remission in patients with moderately to severely active CD and for reducing the number of draining enterocutaneous and rectovaginal fistulas and maintaining fistula closure in patients with fistulizing CD.

    d. TPN permits bowel rest and induces remission in some patients with significant CD. This remission rate is much higher than the rate for patients with severe UC treated by TPN.

    e. Broad-spectrum antibiotics are beneficial to decrease luminal bacterial concentrations, tissue invasion and cellulitis, and bacterial translocation.

    f. Metronidazole and **ciprofloxacin** appear to be beneficial for treatment of anal disease.

5. Surgical treatment

    a. Indications

        (1) Intestinal obstruction

        (2) Anorectal abscesses or **fistulas** that require special considerations (pus should be drained, but large incisions are avoided to prevent sphincter injury)

        (3) Abdominal abscesses, which are preferably drained percutaneously with CT guidance

        (4) Fistulas between the intestine and bladder, skin, bowel, or vagina (there have been reports of such fistulas closing after treatment by immunosuppressive agents)

        (5) Debilitating disease that is not refractory to medical treatment

        (6) Fulminant colitis

        (7) Hemorrhage (rare)

        (8) Cancer (much less common than with UC)

    b. Surgical considerations

        (1) A **high recurrence rate** (50% within 5 years) follows intestinal resection. The most likely site of recurrence is at the anastomosis from the previous operation.

        (2) A **goal of surgery is to conserve bowel.**

            (a) Wide margins of normal bowel are not required; only grossly involved bowel should be resected.

            (b) To conserve bowel, **strictureplasty** may sometimes be indicated to relieve obstruction (rather than intestinal resection).

        (3) Abdominal abscesses should be drained percutaneously prior to laparotomy.

        (4) Total proctocolectomy with ileostomy is required for severe rectal disease. **Ileal pouch anal anastomosis is contraindicated** because of the high incidence of anal disease and recurrent bowel disease in the pouch.

        (5) TPN and bowel rest for 7–10 days preoperatively will promote resolution of intra-abdominal inflammation and will reduce the risk of injury to adjacent, secondarily inflamed bowel.

(6) In most cases, the plan of surgery should be to resect the involved bowel and to fashion a primary anastomosis.

VIII PSEUDOMEMBRANOUS COLITIS (ANTIBIOTIC-ASSOCIATED COLITIS)

A Epidemiology and clinical presentation

1. **Acute diarrhea associated with the use of antibiotics**
   a. **Clindamycin** and **ampicillin** most often are implicated, but almost every antibiotic has been reported to be associated with this syndrome.
   b. In 25% of cases, the antibiotic has been discontinued before the development of diarrhea.
2. This syndrome is **common in hospitals and nursing homes.**
   a. Epidemics of the disease have been reported in these institutions.
   b. This syndrome may occur after intestinal operations, especially after antibiotic bowel preparation.
3. *Clostridium difficile* has been shown to be the causative organism.
   a. *C. difficile* elaborates two exotoxins.
   b. Colonic inflammation is probably caused by the exotoxins.
   c. Yellow plaques, or **pseudomembranes,** may cover the mucosa.
      (1) Pseudomembranes are composed of fibrin and cellular debris.
      (2) The absence of pseudomembranes does not rule out this syndrome.

B Pathogenesis

1. Antibiotics alter the normal colonic bacterial population.
2. *C. difficile,* an organism that is normally suppressed by colonic bacteria, emerges as a pathogen and causes mild diarrhea to severe life-threatening colitis.

C Diagnosis

1. A history of diarrhea after treatment with an antibiotic is suspicious.
2. **Proctoscopy** or **colonoscopy** may reveal pseudomembranes, which are virtually diagnostic if present.
3. A stool sample should be sent for ***C. difficile* toxin titer.**

D Treatment

1. The causative antibiotic should be stopped.
2. **Metronidazole** is the treatment of choice and may be given orally or intravenously. Oral **vancomycin** is also effective but is reserved for refractory or persistent cases. The daily cost for metronidazole treatment is less than $1 but is $200 for vancomycin.
3. Constipating agents (e.g., loperamide) should be avoided.
4. **Cholestyramine** may be administered to bind the toxin, but it may also inhibit the therapeutic antibiotic and therefore is seldom indicated.
5. **Recurrence** is common (25%) and requires retreatment. Metronidazole is again the agent of choice if the patient initially responded to it.
6. **Abdominal colectomy with ileostomy** has been required for rare cases of fulminant pseudomembranous colitis.

IX ISCHEMIC COLITIS

A Etiology

1. Points of communication between collateral arteries are theoretically at increased risk for ischemia. These points include the **splenic flexure** and the **midsigmoid colon.** However, any segment of the colon may be involved (rectal involvement is very rare).
2. Predisposing factors include:
   a. Surgery, especially ligation of the inferior mesenteric artery during aortic surgery
   b. Atherosclerosis, vasculitis, collagen vascular diseases

   c. Polycythemia vera
   d. Congestive heart failure
   e. Digitalis, oral contraceptives, antihypertensive medications, and vasopressors
   f. Low-flow states (myocardial infarction, sepsis)

3. **Three phases of ischemic colitis** may be recognized.
   a. Transient ischemia (mucosal involvement)
      (1) Symptoms are usually mild abdominal pain and passage of maroon-colored stool.
      (2) Barium enema may reveal "thumbprinting" (mucosal hemorrhage).
      (3) Colonoscopy reveals dusky, hemorrhagic mucosa.
   b. Partial-thickness ischemia with late stricture. Symptoms are more severe and include abdominal tenderness, fever, and leukocytosis.
   c. Gangrenous ischemia. Symptoms of an acute abdomen are present with abdominal pain, peritonitis, and signs of sepsis.

B **Treatment**

1. **Transient ischemia** is treated symptomatically.
   a. Hospitalization and observation are indicated until the severity of disease is determined.
   b. Any causative factors should be corrected, if possible.

2. **Partial-thickness ischemia**
   a. Close observation, intravenous fluids, and broad-spectrum antibiotics are usually required.
   b. If a stricture develops and is asymptomatic, no treatment is required. Symptomatic strictures require resection.

3. **Gangrenous ischemia**
   a. Emergency resection of nonviable bowel is required.
   b. Anastomosis is not usually safe in such circumstances, thus a colostomy is required.

X VOLVULUS

A **Overview**

1. Volvulus is a twist or torsion of an organ on a pedicle.

2. **Symptoms** are produced by occluding the bowel lumen (**obstruction**) or occluding the blood supply (**ischemia**).

3. The **incidence** is low in the United States.
   a. Diverticulitis and cancer are more common causes of colon obstruction.
   b. Volvulus is the most common cause of colon obstruction in Africa.

B **Sigmoid volvulus** accounts for more than 80% of cases of colonic volvulus. Patients with this condition are often from **nursing homes** or **mental institutions.** Sigmoid volvulus is most common in **men,** and it occurs more often in blacks. The average age of a patient with this condition is **60 years.**

1. **Etiology.** Several predisposing conditions are required:
   a. A long, freely movable sigmoid colon
   b. An ample, freely mobile sigmoid mesentery
   c. A point of fixation about which the colon can twist (a loop of bowel with the limbs lying close together)

2. **Pathogenesis.** The sigmoid colon usually twists counterclockwise around the axis of the mesentery. This torsion about the mesentery is accompanied by an axial torsion of the bowel wall. The combined torsions of the mesentery and bowel cause obstruction of the colon lumen.

3. **Diagnosis**
   a. History usually indicates increasing **abdominal distention, discomfort,** and **obstipation.**
   b. Physical examination reveals **abdominal distention** and **tympany.**
   c. Abdominal radiographs usually show a massively distended loop of bowel, with both ends in the pelvis and the bow near the diaphragm (i.e., bent inner tube sign).

d. Barium enema reveals the pathognomonic obstructing twist (i.e., ace of spades or bird's beak deformity).

4. Treatment

a. Sigmoidoscopic decompression is indicated for nonstrangulated sigmoid volvulus. This procedure should be terminated if necrotic mucosa is observed or if the volvulus cannot be reduced by gently inserting a rubber tube through the sigmoidoscope past the point of torsion. If the tube successfully reduces the volvulus, it should be left in the sigmoid and taped to the skin of the thigh to prevent immediate recurrence.

b. Sigmoidectomy with colostomy (Hartmann's operation) is indicated if decompression cannot be achieved or if there is gangrenous bowel.

c. Elective sigmoidectomy with colorectal anastomosis is recommended after the bowel has been decompressed and prepared as usual for colonic resection.

C **Cecal volvulus** occurs much less frequently than sigmoid volvulus. It occurs most commonly in **women,** and patients are often **younger than 40 years.**

1. Etiology. A **congenital anatomic anomaly** is required for cecal volvulus.

a. Incomplete peritoneal fixation of the right colon is required for the cecum and right colon to have the mobility to form a volvulus.

b. Other contributing factors may include:

(1) Cancer of the distal colon

(2) Midgut nonrotation

(3) Adhesions from previous surgery

2. Pathogenesis. The cecum and ascending colon usually twist clockwise. Bowel and vascular obstruction occur in a manner similar to that described for sigmoid volvulus.

3. Diagnosis

a. History usually indicates increasing abdominal pain. Diarrhea may have occurred initially. Obstipation follows.

b. Physical examination reveals **abdominal distention** and **tympany. Rebound tenderness** suggests gangrenous bowel.

c. Abdominal radiographs reveal a **large, distended cecum** that may occupy the left upper quadrant.

d. Barium enema reveals the **ace of spades** or **bird's beak deformity.**

4. Treatment

a. Right colectomy with ileotransverse colonic anastomosis is generally indicated if the bowel is viable.

b. Colonoscopic decompression has been successfully performed, but right colectomy is still indicated to prevent recurrence.

c. Cecopexy is an alternative to right colectomy, but recurrence rates have been high in some reports.

XI   DYSFUNCTION OF THE ANORECTUM

A **Incontinence** is the inability to control elimination of rectal contents.

1. Etiology

a. Mechanical defects of the anal sphincter

(1) Episiotomy injuries

(2) Previous anal fistulotomies

(3) Anorectal trauma (impalement injuries)

b. Neurogenic causes

(1) Pudendal nerve injury due to prolonged labor

(2) Pudendal nerve injury due to perineal descent

(3) Systemic neurologic disease (multiple sclerosis)

c. Systemic disease

(1) Scleroderma

(2) Diabetes

     d. Causes unrelated to the anal sphincter
       (1) Severe diarrhea
       (2) Severe proctitis with decreased rectal capacity
       (3) Fecal impaction with overflow incontinence
       (4) Large rectal tumors

2. Evaluation. History and **anorectal examination** often suffice to establish the diagnosis.

  a. Anterior sphincter defect and **patulous anus** after midline episiotomy may be confirmed by a thorough examination and, if necessary, endorectal ultrasound of the anal musculature.

  b. Physiologic evaluation may be helpful if the cause of incontinence is not obvious.

    (1) **Anal manometry** can document the resting pressure, squeeze pressure, sphincter length, and minimal sensory volume of the rectum.

    (2) **Pudendal nerve terminal motor latency** can be tested to determine if the cause of incontinence is neurogenic in nature.

3. Surgical treatment

  a. Sphincter defects, such as those caused by obstetric injuries, may be corrected by **anal sphincter repair** with excellent results.

  b. More extensive loss of the anal sphincter may be treated by **gracilis muscle transposition,** which mobilizes the gracilis muscle to encircle the anus or by implantation of an **artificial anal sphincter** device.

  c. Colostomy may be required for severe sphincter injuries or for neurogenic or systemic causes of incontinence.

B **Obstructed defecation (pelvic floor–outlet obstruction)**

1. Anal stenosis may be caused by circumferential hemorrhoidectomy (Whitehead deformity), trauma, or radiation. It may result in the inability to evacuate formed stool, with resultant abdominal bloating, intestinal dilatation, and discomfort. **Treatment** generally entails repeated dilation or advancing full-thickness pedicles of skin to the anal canal.

2. Nonrelaxation of the puborectalis is a functional disorder characterized by the inability to relax the puborectalis muscle at the time of defecation.

  a. Symptoms include the need for digital maneuvers to eliminate stool, pelvic pain, a sense of incomplete evacuation, and severe straining during defecation.

  b. The syndrome occurs in women nine times more often than in men.

  c. Normal function of the colon is demonstrated by **colonic transit time,** which is measured by following radiopaque markers through the colon.

  d. Diagnosis may be confirmed by defecography, which demonstrates the failure of the muscle to relax appropriately. Another simple diagnostic test reveals the inability of the patient to expel an air-filled balloon from the rectum.

  e. Treatment is nonsurgical. Biofeedback to develop cognitive aspects of defecation is the treatment of choice.

3. Internal intussusception (internal prolapse of the rectum). This condition is characterized by the distal bowel telescoping into itself to cause partial obstruction to defecation. Patients complain of an urgency to defecate, a feeling of rectal fullness, and pelvic pain.

  a. A **solitary rectal ulcer** is now recognized as the cause of this syndrome.

    (1) The ulcer is usually located in the anterior rectal wall. Biopsies reveal a bland, non-neoplastic ulcer.

    (2) **Colitis cystica profunda,** which is characterized by glandular tissue beneath the mucosa, may accompany this condition. It is important to distinguish this benign lesion from cancer (for which it may be confused by histologic appearance).

  b. Internal intussusception is accompanied by **abnormal rectal fixation,** which permits the rectum to descend toward the perineum.

  c. Medical treatment suffices for most patients and consists of:

    (1) Increased dietary fiber
    (2) Stool softeners
    (3) Glycerine suppositories or small enemas

  d. Indications for surgical treatment include:

   (1) **Debilitating symptoms** despite maximum medical therapy and psychological counseling

   (2) **Impending anal incontinence** due to stretch injury to the pudendal nerves caused by constant straining (and subsequent perineal descent)

   (3) **Chronic bleeding** from a solitary rectal ulcer

  e. Surgical treatment is low anterior resection of the sigmoid and proximal rectum, with colorectal anastomosis and rectal fixation.

4. Rectal prolapse is the protrusion of the **full thickness** of the rectum (and occasionally the sigmoid colon) through the anus. This condition should be distinguished from **mucosal prolapse,** which is the protrusion of only the rectal mucosa through the anal orifice. Full-thickness prolapse has concentric mucosal folds. Mucosal prolapse has radial folds in prolapsing mucosa.

  a. Etiology and epidemiology

   (1) Rectal prolapse may be the result of long-term internal intussusception.

   (2) There is an **increased incidence** in:

    (a) Patients in mental institutions

    (b) Women who have had a hysterectomy

    (c) Elderly women

   (3) There is no increased incidence in women who have had multiple deliveries.

  b. Symptoms include:

   (1) Mucosa-lined bowel protruding through the anus

   (2) Bleeding

   (3) Anal pain

   (4) Mucous discharge

   (5) Anal incontinence of varying degrees, caused by stretch of the anal sphincters or by stretch injury to the pudendal nerves (from perineal descent that is associated with the prolapse)

  c. Treatment is surgical. The prolapse may become incarcerated and strangulated if not reduced.

   (1) Patients in satisfactory health and with satisfactory anal continence should be treated by **low anterior resection with rectopexy.**

   (2) An alternative treatment is to fix the rectum to the sacrum with a synthetic sling (**Ripstein's procedure).** This operation may increase the difficulty of evacuation.

   (3) Patients who are poor surgical risks may be treated by **perineal proctectomy with low colorectal (or coloanal) anastomosis.** An abdominal incision is avoided, but recurrence is higher.

   (4) **Anal encircling procedures** are at times advocated for poor-risk patients. A band of synthetic material (wire or mesh) is placed subcutaneously around the anus. Encircling procedures are often complicated by infection, and results are generally unsatisfactory.

   (5) Patients with total incontinence may require treatment by **anterior resection of the rectum and colostomy (low Hartmann's procedure).**

XII BENIGN ANORECTAL DISEASE

A **Hemorrhoids**

1. Etiology

  a. Anal cushions are complexes of vascular and connective tissue normally located in the right anterolateral and posterolateral positions and the left lateral position in the anal canal. This normal tissue protects the sphincter during defecation and permits complete closure of the anus during rest.

  b. Engorgement of the vascular tissue in the anal cushions causes these complexes to enlarge and form hemorrhoids.

  c. Prolonged straining during defecation and increased abdominal pressure are thought to contribute to formation of hemorrhoids.

2. Classification

  a. Internal hemorrhoids are located above the dentate line and are covered by rectal mucosa.

   (1) **First-degree hemorrhoids** bleed but do not prolapse.

   (2) **Second-degree hemorrhoids** bleed and prolapse through the anus but reduce spontaneously.

(3) **Third-degree hemorrhoids** bleed and prolapse and must be manually reduced.

(4) **Fourth-degree hemorrhoids** protrude through the anus and cannot be manually reduced.

b. **External hemorrhoids** reside below the anal verge and are lined by squamous epithelium. A thrombosis within an external hemorrhoid may cause acute swelling and anal pain.

3. **Symptoms**

a. **Bleeding, mucous discharge, prolapse,** and **pruritus** are symptoms of internal hemorrhoids.

b. Internal hemorrhoids seldom cause pain unless acutely prolapsed and incarcerated. **Anal pain should not be attributed to thrombosed internal hemorrhoids.** Another source must be sought to explain the pain.

4. **Treatment** of hemorrhoids depends on the symptoms.

a. **Medical therapy** consists of the addition of dietary fiber and stool softeners and education of the patient to avoid prolonged straining.

b. **Rubber band ligation** can provide satisfactory treatment for first- and second-degree hemorrhoids and selected cases of third- and fourth-degree hemorrhoids.

(1) The rubber bands must be placed above the dentate line, or severe pain will be associated with the procedure.

(2) External hemorrhoids are not amenable to this form of treatment.

c. **Sclerotherapy** (submucosal injection of phenol in oil or sodium morrhuate) may be used for first- and second-degree hemorrhoids.

d. **Infrared photocoagulation** is accomplished by placing an infrared probe proximal to the internal hemorrhoids and delivering therapy in three pulses of 1.5 seconds each. This treatment has been successful for first and second-degree hemorrhoids.

e. **Hemorrhoidectomy,** which may be required to relieve the symptoms of third- and fourth-degree hemorrhoids may be performed by:

(1) **Surgical excision** of all hemorrhoidal tissue, leaving the mucosa open or sutured closed.

(2) **Stapled hemorrhoidectomy,** which removes a ring of anal rectal tissue above the hemorrhoids, severing the blood supply and lifting and flattening the hemorrhoids in the anal canal.

f. **Thrombosed hemorrhoids** may require excision for relief of pain. However, most cases resolve within 2 weeks without any specific therapy. The most intense pain is within the first 48 hours after thrombosis; thereafter, pain usually subsides rapidly.

B **Anal fissure** is a tear in the anoderm, which is usually caused by constipation and, less often, repeated episodes of diarrhea. This leads to excessive tension in the internal anal sphincter and sesequent ischemia of the muscle with overlying anoderm breakdown. The fissure is located near the posterior midline of the anus 98% of the time in men and 90% of the time in women. Otherwise, the fissure is near the anterior midline.

1. **Symptoms** are **anal pain** and **bleeding** associated with defecation.

2. **Physical findings** may include the following:

a. Fissure or ulcer distal to the dentate line

b. **Sentinel skin tag** at the anal verge adjacent to the distal edge of fissure

c. **Hypertrophied anal papilla** at the proximal edge of the fissure

d. **Spasm of the internal sphincter** (in chronic cases)

3. **Treatment**

a. **Medical** (most fissures will heal with medical treatment)

(1) Stool softeners, increased dietary fiber, and warm sitz baths are beneficial.

(2) Suppositories are usually not beneficial.

(3) Topical application of 0.2% **nitroglycerin ointment** has been shown to be effective treatment in some patients by increasing blood flow to the ischemic internal sphincter muscle.

(4) **Botulinum toxin** injection into the internal sphincter muscle. This causes temporary paralysis of the muscle, allowing the fissure to heal.

b. **Surgical** (indications are persistent symptoms despite medical treatment)

(1) **Lateral internal sphincterotomy.** This procedure may be done by either an open or a closed technique and is highly curative.

(2) Anal sphincter stretch. This procedure is done under local anesthesia and is also effective. This approach may be associated with a slightly higher risk of incontinence than the risk with lateral sphincterotomy.

C **Anorectal abscess and fistula**

1. **Pathogenesis**
   a. These infections are **cryptoglandular** in origin: They begin in the anal glands that empty into the anal crypts.
   b. An **abscess** is the acute stage, and a **fistula** is the chronic stage of the same disease process.
   c. Most abscesses originate between the internal and external sphincters and are thus called **intersphincteric abscesses.**
      (1) Downward extension results in **perianal abscess.**
      (2) Lateral extension through the low external sphincter results in an **ischiorectal fossa abscess.**
      (3) Upward extension (rare) results in **supralevator abscess.**

2. **Signs and symptoms**
   a. **Anorectal pain** is constant but is not associated with defecation.
   b. **Swelling and fluctuance** are late signs.
   c. **Drainage of pus and blood** signifies spontaneous rupture of the abscess and is usually associated with pain relief.
   d. **Fever and leukocytosis** may be present.

3. **Treatment** is **incision and drainage** and should be done when the diagnosis is made. Treatment with antibiotics is inappropriate.
   a. The ischiorectal fossa may contain a large volume of pus before fluctuance is obvious.
   b. Antibiotics are not required unless immune status is compromised (e.g., diabetes, leukemia).
   c. Incision and drainage are curative 50% of the time; the other 50% of patients will develop anorectal fistula.

4. **Anorectal fistula** is a communication between an anal crypt (internal opening) and the perianal skin (external opening).
   a. The **internal opening must be identified** to allow proper treatment.
      (1) The most common site of the internal opening is the posterior anal crypt.
      (2) Anterior abscesses may originate from anterior anal crypts.
      (3) **Goodsall's rule** states that external openings posterior to a transverse line that bisects the anus will connect to the posterior midline crypt; external openings anterior to this line will communicate to an anterior crypt by a short, direct tract.
      (4) **Exception to Goodsall's rule.** An anterior external opening greater than 3 cm from the anal margin usually communicates with the posterior midline crypt.
   b. **Treatment** of simple anal fistula is to identify both openings and open the tract by **fistulotomy.**
   c. A complicated fistula that tracks above the external sphincter may require a procedure that eradicates the internal opening.
      (1) A fistulotomy can cause incontinence.
      (2) A flap of rectal mucosa is used to close the internal opening in these rare cases.

D **Pilonidal disease**

1. **Pathophysiology.** Pilonidal disease is characterized by hair from the skin of the postsacral superior gluteal cleft that drills below the skin level, causing foreign body reaction and localized infection.

2. **Treatment**
   a. **Incision and drainage** of acute abscesses
   b. **Excision with closure by secondary intention** of chronic sinus tracts
      (1) Healing may be promoted by marsupialization of the sinus.
      (2) Excision and primary closure of the sinus are accompanied by a high incidence of recurrence.

E **Hidradenitis suppurativa** is an infection of the apocrine sweat glands. The infected glands form subcutaneous sinus tracts that can spread to the perineum, scrotum, or labia.

1. **Pathophysiology.** The disease should be distinguished from cryptoglandular disease.
   a. Hidradenitis suppurativa does not involve the anal canal because there are no apocrine glands in anoderm.
   b. Cryptoglandular disease originates in the anal canal.
2. **Clinical presentation** is numerous, often complicated fistulas and sinus tracts around the anus.
3. **Treatment** is excision of involved skin, with healing by contracture. Recurrence is common and should be treated by prompt excision.

F **Condyloma acuminatum** (genital warts)

1. **Etiology.** The causative agent is the **human papillomavirus (HPV).**
   a. Transmission is usually sexual, with increased incidence in patients who practice receptive anal intercourse.
   b. There is an increased incidence in male homosexuals.
   c. Certain viral strains (HPV-16 and HPV-18) found in condyloma are associated with an **increased risk of anal cancer.**
2. **Clinical presentation.** The lesions vary from tiny excrescences to cauliflowerlike masses. They may be sessile or pedunculated, and they are usually located on the perianal skin, penis, vulva, vagina, or cervix or in the anal canal. Pruritus, anal wetness, discomfort, and the presence of a mass are the usual symptoms.
3. **Treatment**
   a. Bichloroacetic acid is applied topically to lesions every 7 days.
   b. Local excision and electrocoagulation with local anesthesia may also be performed and offers the best chance of cure.
   c. Interferon has been suggested for refractory warts.
   d. Patients should be followed closely because of the risk of associated cancer if carcinogenic viral strains are identified.

XIII **PERIANAL AND ANAL CANAL NEOPLASMS**

A **Anal margin** (below the dentate line) neoplasms include the following (Table 13-5):

1. Squamous cell carcinoma
2. Basal cell carcinoma
3. Bowen's disease
4. Perianal Paget's disease

B **Anal canal** (above the dentate line) neoplasms include:

1. **Epidermoid carcinoma** includes squamous cell, basaloid, cloacogenic, and mucoepidermoid carcinoma.
   a. **Clinical presentation** may be bleeding, pain, or anal mass.
   b. **Diagnosis and evaluation**
      (1) **Physical examination**
          (a) Assess tumor size, depth of invasion, and ulceration.
          (b) Examine for retrorectal and inguinal lymph nodes.
      (2) Anoscopy, proctoscopy, and biopsy
      (3) Endorectal ultrasound
      (4) CT scan of the pelvis and liver
      (5) Chest radiograph
   c. **Treatment**
      (1) Combined modality therapy consists of 5-FU, mitomycin C, and external beam radiation.
      (2) Abdominal perineal resection is performed for treatment failures.
   d. **Prognosis**
      (1) The effectiveness of combined modality therapy depends on the size of the primary lesion. Tumors larger than 6 cm seldom respond completely.

TABLE 13-5 Anal Margin Neoplasms

Tumor Type	Presentation	Treatment
Squamous cell carcinoma	Polypoid, fungating, or ulcerated abdominal mass	Local excision or radiation; perineal resection for advanced lesions
Basal cell carcinoma	Central ulceration with irregular, raised edges	Local excision for most lesions; radiation or abdominal perineal resection for rare, advanced lesions
Bowen's disease	Carcinoma in situ (erythematous, crusty, scaly plaques), itching, burning, bleeding; 10% develop squamous cell carcinoma	Wide local excision
Perianal Paget's disease	Erythematous, eczematous rash; intractable pruritus; intraepithelial adenocarcinoma; high incidence of visceral carcinoma	Wide local excision; if underlying cancer, abdominal perineal resection

(**2**) Overall, combined treatment has a response rate of 90% and a 5-year survival rate higher than 80%.

2. **Adenocarcinoma** is most commonly an extension from cancer in the distal rectum.
   a. Cancer arises from anal glands and ducts. It may arise from outside the lumen of the anal canal and may present as an anal fistula that does not respond to fistulotomy.
   b. **Treatment** is, generally, similar to that for rectal cancer, using preoperative radiation therapy followed by abdominal resection.

3. **Melanoma**
   a. **Characteristics.** The anal canal is the third most common site (after skin and eyes). Not all anal melanomas are darkly pigmented (i.e., some are amelanotic).
   b. **Symptoms and presentation.** Anal mass, pain, and bleeding are the most common symptoms. Regional lymphatic and distant metastases are common at the time of diagnosis.
   c. **Treatment.** Abdominal perineal resection is recommended if no metastases are detected. Abdominal perineal resection is no more effective than wide local excision for local control. The 5-year survival rate is less than 15%.

chapter 14

Liver, Portal Hypertension, and Biliary Tract

BENJAMIN PHILOSOPHE · DAVID D. NEAL · MICHAEL J. MORITZ ·
BRUCE E. JARRELL

I   LIVER

A **Anatomy**   The liver is the largest, heaviest intra-abdominal organ, weighing about 2% of total body weight.

1. **Segmentation.** The liver is composed of two lobes (left and right), and each lobe has two segments (Fig. 14-1).
   a. These lobes are divided by the **interlobar fissure,** an invisible line between the gallbladder fossa anteriorly and the inferior vena cava posteriorly.
   b. The **falciform ligament,** the only externally visible boundary, marks the **segmental fissure** between the median and lateral segments of the left lobe.
   c. The right lobe segmental fissure has no external landmarks.

2. **Vascular supply (hepatic arterial and portal venous).** The segmental anatomy of the liver is determined by the vascular supply and biliary tree.
   a. **Arterial supply** is from the common **hepatic artery,** a branch of the celiac axis.
      (1) The hepatic artery carries fully oxygenated blood and comprises 25% of the liver blood flow.
      (2) The common hepatic artery enters the porta hepatis medially to the common bile duct, gives off the gastroduodenal artery to become the proper hepatic artery, and bifurcates into right and left hepatic arteries.
      (3) The **cystic artery** usually arises from the right hepatic artery.
      (4) In 20% of the population, the left hepatic artery arises from the left gastric artery. In approximately 20%, the right hepatic artery arises as a branch of the superior mesenteric artery.
   b. **Venous supply and return**
      (1) The **portal vein** carries partially oxygenated blood as it drains the entire splanchnic circulation (all structures that receive blood from the celiac, superior mesenteric, and inferior mesenteric arteries) and comprises 75% of the liver blood flow.
         (a) It is formed by the confluence of the superior mesenteric, splenic, inferior mesenteric, and coronary veins (Fig. 14-2).
         (b) It enters the liver hilum, where it divides to form **right** and **left branches,** which supply the right and left hepatic lobes.
         (c) It lies posteriorly in the porta hepatis.
      (2) Blood leaves the liver via the hepatic veins.
         (a) The hepatic veins course **between segments** (rather than into segments like the segmental vascular supply). For example, the middle hepatic vein lies between the right and left hepatic lobes and is exposed when opening the interlobar fissure (Fig. 14-3).
         (b) The hepatic veins drain directly into the inferior vena cava just inferior to the diaphragm.

3. **The biliary tree** follows the segmental divisions of the hepatic artery and portal vein intrahepatically. The bile ducts lie anterolaterally in the porta hepatis.

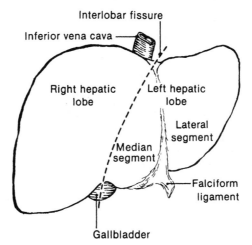

FIGURE 14-1   Surgical anatomy of the liver: left and right lobes.

4. **Hepatic resections** are based on the segmental anatomy. The surgeon divides the vascular-biliary supply to the portion to be removed and preserves the vascular-biliary structures to the portion to be retained.
   a. **Right hepatic lobectomy** transects the liver through the interlobar fissure between the gallbladder fossa and the inferior vena cava (Fig. 14-3).
   b. **Left hepatic lobectomy** uses the same guidelines.
   c. **Trisegmentectomy** removes the entire right lobe and the median segment of the left lobe across the anatomic division of the falciform ligament (leaving only the left lateral segment).
   d. **Left lateral segmentectomy** removes the segment of liver to the left of the falciform ligament.
   e. **Wedge resections** are performed for small lesions near the liver surface that do not require a full lobectomy. These resections do not adhere to anatomic boundaries but are safe because a limited amount of tissue is transected.

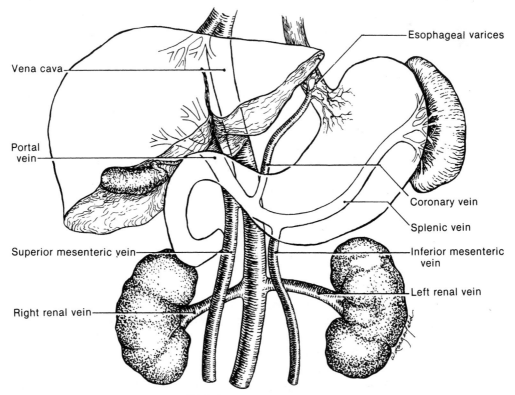

FIGURE 14-2   Portal circulation.

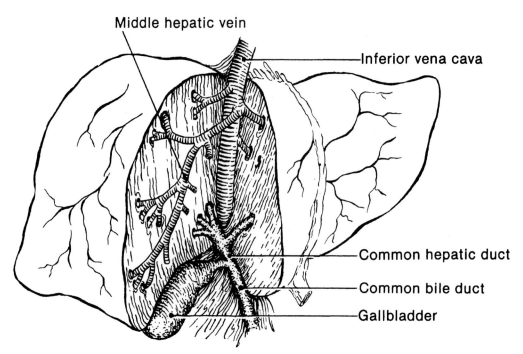

Middle hepatic vein

Inferior vena cava

Common hepatic duct

Common bile duct

Gallbladder

FIGURE 14-3   Plane of resection for right and left hepatic lobectomy.

B **Studies of the liver**

1. **Liver function tests** are blood tests of a few of the myriad functions that the liver performs.
   a. **Synthetic function** of hepatocytes is reflected by:
      (1) Serum proteins, such as albumin or fibrinogen
      (2) Clotting factors, as measured by coagulation tests (see Chapter 1, III)
      (3) Cholesterol
      (4) Blood glucose
   b. **Clearance function** of hepatocytes is estimated by:
      (1) Ammonia
      (2) Indirect bilirubin, which is taken up from the blood by hepatocytes
   c. **Excretory function** of hepatocytes and patency of the biliary tree is reflected by:
      (1) Direct bilirubin
      (2) Enzyme levels, such as alkaline phosphatase and gamma glutamyl transferase
   d. **Extent of injury** to the hepatocytes is reflected by the serum levels of the enzymes, aspartate transaminase, also called *glutamic-oxaloacetic transaminase*, and alanine transaminase, also called *glutamic-pyruvic transaminase.*

2. **Imaging of the liver** is used to define parenchymal lesions and plan liver resections when appropriate.
   a. The sulfur-colloid **liver-spleen scan,** which visualizes the reticuloendothelial system, is rarely used because more accurate studies are now available. However, it still remains useful in delineating an adenoma from focal nodular hyperplasia.
   b. **Ultrasound** is excellent for detecting the texture of the parenchyma and any lesions within the parenchyma. It is especially useful in assessing hepatic vascular flow and characterizing cystic lesions.
   c. **Computed tomography (CT)** and **magnetic resonance imaging (MRI)** visualize the parenchyma and adjacent tissues with great clarity. The availability of higher resolution technology and three-dimensional (3D) reconstruction with the use of intravenous contrast have made CT and MRI the procedures of choice to distinguish parenchymal or biliary pathology.
   d. **Arteriography** is used to determine the arterial supply and can detect large parenchymal lesions.
   e. **Angioportography** combines CT scanning with contrast infusion through a catheter placed in the superior mesenteric artery. It is especially useful in assessing the portal vein.

    f. Hepatobiliary scanning is a nuclear medicine scan used to visualize the liver and biliary tree (see III B 4).

3. Needle biopsy (either percutaneous or at surgery) provides liver tissue for histologic study.

C **Benign tumors of the liver** In women, oral contraceptive use has increased the incidence of benign primary liver tumors.

1. Hemangioma, the most common benign hepatic tumor, is usually asymptomatic. Usually, it is discovered as an incidental finding (i.e., calcification on abdominal radiograph or a characteristic mass on ultrasound) and is managed by observation.

    a. Clinical presentation. Hemangiomas can produce symptoms by compressing adjacent structures or by stretching the liver capsule.

    b. Pathology. Grossly, there may be single or multiple masses, and microscopically, there are vascular lacunae lined with normal endothelial cells.

    c. Treatment. Only symptomatic hemangiomas should be resected.

2. Hepatocellular adenoma is an uncommon benign tumor usually seen in women that is strongly associated with oral contraceptive use. It is also found in men and women who take anabolic (androgenic) steroids.

    a. Clinical presentation. There may be no symptoms or physical findings.

        (1) Approximately 25% of patients have a palpable abdominal mass or abdominal pain.

        (2) Up to 30% of patients present with spontaneous rupture and hemorrhage into the peritoneal cavity. The mortality rate for rupture is about 9%.

    b. Pathology. Adenomas are soft tumors with sharply circumscribed edges but no true capsule. Histologically, only normal hepatocytes are present, and there is no evidence of malignancy.

    c. Diagnosis

        (1) The tumor is usually suspected when a mass is seen on ultrasound or other scan of the liver.

        (2) MRI with gadolinium enhancement is the diagnostic procedure of choice because it can often differentiate adenomas from focal nodular hyperplasia or malignant lesions.

        (3) Arteriograms are rarely used anymore.

        (4) Liver function studies are generally normal.

        (5) Biopsy is needed to exclude malignancy.

    d. Treatment

        (1) Oral contraceptives, anabolic steroids, and pregnancy should be avoided, as in the absence of these, the tumor can regress. If the diagnosis is confirmed and the lesion is small, intrahepatic, and associated with oral contraceptive use, it may be safely observed.

        (2) Occasionally, the tumor is exophytic on a narrow pedicle and can be easily excised.

        (3) If the tumor is large and superficial or if a woman anticipates pregnancy in the near future, it should be resected because of the risk of spontaneous rupture and hemorrhage.

        (4) In cases of **spontaneous rupture with hemorrhage** into the peritoneal cavity, the patient should initially be resuscitated. If it is recognized that this patient has a ruptured adenoma and is hemodynamically stable, the bleeding can be successfully managed by identifying the bleeding vessel with angiography and embolizing it with thrombus. If angiography is not immediately available, if the patient remains unstable, or if a hepatic adenoma or other hepatic tumor is not suspected, the patient should be taken to the operating room.

           (a) The recommended procedure is hepatic artery ligation. This frequently controls the bleeding and is associated with only minor aberrations in liver function when the liver is not cirrhotic.

           (b) Hepatic resection in the presence of acute rupture has a high mortality rate. Elective resection should, however, be performed at a later date.

           (c) If the patient is very unstable after rupture despite major resuscitative efforts, open packing or angiographic embolization of the hepatic artery may control the hemorrhage.

        (5) Although the risk of carcinoma developing in this adenoma is low, there are several case reports of this progression. If not excised, adenomas should be followed indefinitely for significant growth or other changes.

3. **Focal nodular hyperplasia (FNH)** is the third most common benign liver tumor. It occurs most often in women and has a weak association with oral contraceptive use.
   a. **Clinical presentation.** Symptoms and physical findings, when they occur, are similar to those seen with hepatocellular adenoma; however, FNH is usually asymptomatic and discovered as an incidental finding. Spontaneous rupture is rare.
   b. **Pathology.** Single or multiple lesions with a nodular appearance externally and a central scar with radiating septa on cut section are seen.
   c. **Histology.** The tumors contain all hepatic elements and are composed of hyperplastic hepatocytes with inflammatory (Kupfer) cells. Bile duct epithelium is a prominent finding in contrast to hepatocellular adenoma. Overall, the lesions resemble regenerating nodules of cirrhosis.
   d. **Diagnosis and treatment** are similar to those for hepatocellular adenoma. The Kupfer cells in FNH take up the sulfur colloid in the sulfur-colloid scan, and the lesion appears indistinguishable from normal liver parenchyma. In contrast, adenomas contain no Kupfer cells and would appear as a filling defect. For this reason, the sulfur colloid scan can be a valuable adjunct to differentiate these two lesions that commonly present in the same patient population.

4. **Infantile hemangioendothelioma** is a benign liver tumor of children that has malignant potential.
   a. **Clinical presentation.** It may present as hepatomegaly and high-output cardiac failure in an infant with a large arteriovenous fistula.
   b. **Pathology.** Grossly, it is a nodular lesion, and microscopically, it shows dilated vascular spaces lined by endothelium.
   c. **Treatment** is by excision or hepatic artery ligation.

D **Primary malignant tumors of the liver** account for 0.7% of all cancers. In men, 90% of primary liver tumors are malignant; in women, only about 40% are malignant.

1. **Hepatocellular carcinoma (hepatoma)** is the most common primary malignant liver tumor.
   a. **Incidence** of hepatocellular carcinoma varies geographically, being highest in Africa and Asia and lowest in the Western world.
      (1) Men are affected twice as often as women.
      (2) The average age of affected individuals is 50 years, but hepatocellular carcinoma can occur at any age.
   b. **Associations.** The tumor shows an association with a number of pre-existing diseases and environmental substances, such as:
      (1) Chronic hepatitis B virus (HBV) infection (present in as many as 80% of cases worldwide). The risk of developing hepatocellular carcinoma is increased 200-fold for chronic HBV carriers. The risk in male carriers is as high as 50%. Hepatocellular carcinoma is associated with chronic hepatitis C infection.
      (2) Cirrhosis, regardless of etiology (present in approximately 60%–90% of patients), especially macronodular cirrhosis
      (3) Hemochromatosis with iron overload and cirrhosis
      (4) Schistosomiasis and other parasitic infestations
      (5) Environmental carcinogens
         (a) Industrial substances, including polychlorinated biphenyls; chlorinated hydrocarbon solvents, such as carbon tetrachloride; nitrosamines; vinyl chloride and polyvinyl chloride; and organochloride pesticides
         (b) Organic materials, including aflatoxins (produced by *Aspergillus flavus* or *A. fumigatus* and found on foods, such as peanuts)
         (c) Thorotrast, an intravenous contrast agent that is no longer used
   c. **Clinical presentation**
      (1) Smaller hepatocellular carcinomas are usually asymptomatic. Larger and more advanced tumors often present as a dull, aching pain in the right upper quadrant; malaise, fever, and jaundice may also be present.
      (2) Physical examination reveals hepatomegaly (present in 88% of cases), weight loss (in 85%), a tender abdominal mass (in 50%), or findings associated with cirrhosis (60%).

(3) About 10%–15% of patients present with acute hemorrhage into the peritoneal cavity with resultant shock.

(4) Paraneoplastic syndromes also may occur in which tumor cells secrete hormonelike substances that cause unusual syndromes, such as Cushing's syndrome.

d. **Diagnosis.** Liver function test results are usually abnormal, but there is no particular diagnostic pattern.

(1) Alpha-fetoprotein, a protein made by embryonal hepatocytes, is elevated in 70% of cases.

(2) Hepatic ultrasound, CT scan, and MRI are the most reliable and commonly used studies for determining the presence and operability of the lesions. These studies are positive in up to 90% of cases. Smaller lesions require CT or MRI with intravenous contrast enhancement because they will only be evident in the arterial phase. Ultrasound is not an adequate modality to assess lesions <2 cm.

e. **Pathology.** Hepatocellular carcinoma occurs as a solitary mass or as multiple masses. Local invasion, especially into the diaphragm, is common, as are distant metastases with the lung being most commonly involved (in up to 45% of cases).

f. **Surgical treatment** includes resection and transplantation. To catch tumors early and increase the potential for cure, high-risk individuals (e.g., those with chronic HBV or those with cirrhosis) should be screened every 6 months with imaging studies and measurement of alpha-fetoprotein.

(1) If lesions are resectable, the average survival is 3–4 years, and 5-year survival rate can now be achieved in 40% of patients.

(2) The operative mortality rate is approximately 5% but is significantly higher in patients with coexistent cirrhosis.

(3) If lesions are unresectable, and transplantation is not an option, patients have a mean survival time of 4 months.

(4) Attempts to induce tumor necrosis by hepatic artery ligation have shown poor results.

g. **Chemotherapy** has been ineffective when given systemically, but administration of drugs into the hepatic artery has given some promising preliminary results.

h. Combination therapy using chemoembolization and local ablation may be palliative for patients with unresectable lesions. Chemoembolization is the technique of embolizing the arterial supply of the tumor with chemotherapeutic agents mixed with thrombus. Ablative therapies include instillation of absolute ethanol into the lesion or insertion of a probe and delivery of radio frequency energy into the lesion. Both chemoembolization and local ablation cause local necrosis of the tumor, and the combination may improve survival.

2. **Hepatoblastoma**

a. **Clinical presentation.** Hepatoblastoma is the most common primary malignant liver tumor in children and presents with abdominal distention, failure to thrive, and other symptoms of liver failure. Alpha-fetoprotein is frequently positive.

b. **Pathology.** Approximately 80% are solitary liver masses that microscopically show nests and cords of primitive cells, resembling embryonic hepatocytes.

c. **Treatment** is surgical excision. Inoperable tumors are treated with irradiation or chemotherapy but with poor results.

3. **Cholangiocarcinoma** is a tumor that arises from the bile duct epithelium; it represents 5%–30% of all primary hepatic malignancies.

a. **Clinical presentation.** Signs and symptoms include right upper quadrant pain, jaundice, hepatomegaly, and occasionally a palpable mass. Patients are usually 60–70 years of age.

b. **Pathology.** A hard grayish mass is found that microscopically shows adenocarcinoma of the biliary epithelium. Metastasis occurs initially to the regional lymph nodes or to the liver.

c. **Etiology.** Associated conditions include parasitic infections (e.g., *Clonorchis sinensis*), primary sclerosing cholangitis, or Thorotrast exposure.

d. **Treatment** of intrahepatic tumors is resection when feasible. Overall survival is poor.

4. **Angiosarcoma, or malignant hemangioendothelioma,** is a highly malignant liver tumor composed of irregular spindle cells lining the lumina of hepatic vascular spaces.

a. **Etiology.** Most cases (85%) occur in men, and there is a high association with chemical agents, especially vinyl chloride, Thorotrast, arsenicals, and organochloride pesticides.

      b. Clinical presentation. The tumor commonly spreads locally to the spleen (80% of cases) and distantly to the lungs (60% of cases).

      c. Treatment is resection when feasible, but patients rarely survive 1 year.

    5. Sarcomas other than angiosarcoma are rare but are highly malignant and frequently not curable.

E **Metastatic tumors of the liver** are much more common than primary tumors (ratio 20:1).

    1. Overview. The liver is the second most common site of metastasis (exceeded only by regional lymph nodes) for all primary cancers of the abdominal viscera. Over two thirds of all colorectal cancers ultimately involve the liver, and up to 50% of cancers outside the abdomen metastasize to the liver. Fully one third of all cancers ultimately spread to the liver, which is the most common site of hematogenous spread.

    2. Diagnosis may be difficult because liver metastases are often asymptomatic.

      a. Laboratory studies. In a recent National Cancer Institute study, no single laboratory blood test could predict liver metastases in more than 65% of patients with subclinical disease. This percentage can only be increased by using imaging techniques.

        (1) Liver function studies (e.g., aspartate transaminase or alkaline phosphatase) detect only 50%–65% of subclinical metastases.

        (2) Testing for carcinoembryonic antigen has been valuable for predicting the presence of liver metastasis in colorectal cancer because it is positive in over 85% of patients with proven disease. Unfortunately, this test lacks specificity.

      b. Imaging techniques are expensive screening tests but are currently the most reliable nonsurgical method of finding liver metastases.

        (1) CT scans and MRIs are the most accurate imaging techniques but are expensive screening tests.

        (2) Ultrasonography is almost as reliable as CT and MRI, and it provides a reasonable screening test.

    3. Treatment for metastatic disease to the liver depends on the type of primary tumor. Because colorectal cancer has generated the most reliable statistics, those figures are cited here.

      a. Chemotherapy for liver metastasis from colorectal cancer has been disappointing.

        (1) Systemic 5-fluorouracil therapy has resulted in a response rate of 9%–33% and a median survival of 30–60 weeks. (A response is defined as a 50% decrease in the size of an existing tumor and the development of no new lesion for a period of 1–2 months.)

        (2) Hepatic arterial infusion of floxuridine has shown an increase in response rate but little or no improvement in patient survival.

      b. Radiation therapy is poorly tolerated by the liver but may be palliative for painful liver metastases.

      c. Hepatic artery ligation may cause a dramatic shrinkage in tumor size, but this is only transient. (Although most splanchnic primary cancers metastasize via the portal vein, they quickly become vascularized by the hepatic artery.)

      d. Cryoablation, or local freezing of the metastasis, may palliate the symptoms and slow the progression of disease in unresectable metastases.

      e. Surgical resection is the most effective mode of therapy but is limited to the few patients who have unilobar liver lesions and no evidence of extrahepatic disease.

        (1) The incidence of liver metastasis at the time of surgery for primary colorectal cancer is 8%–25%, and approximately one fourth of these lesions are solitary and resectable, so only about 5% of patients are potential resection candidates.

        (2) The 5-year survival rate approaches 40% in patients with these criteria. The operative mortality rate is less than 5%, an acceptable risk.

F **Hepatic abscesses and cysts**

    1. Nonviral liver infections (i.e., bacterial, protozoal, or parasitic) generally localize as abscesses or cysts. Mortality without prompt, appropriate treatment is high.

      a. Etiology is dependent on environmental factors, particularly geographic location and the presence of endemic parasites.

b. Clinical presentation. Abscesses and cysts produce few localizing symptoms (i.e., chiefly pain and a mass in the right upper quadrant), while causing major systemic effects (i.e., fever, malnutrition, sepsis, or anemia).

c. Diagnosis. Diagnostic tests used are similar to those used for tumors of the liver (see I B 2).

2. **Bacterial abscesses** are the most common hepatic abscesses in the Western world.
   a. Etiology
      (1) These are most commonly secondary to infectious processes in the abdomen, particularly cholangitis, appendicitis, or diverticulitis.
      (2) They may also result from seeding from a distant infectious source, such as endocarditis.
      (3) In 10%–50% of cases, no source can be identified.
      (4) The **infecting organism** is related to the primary source.
         (a) When the source is abdominal, the most common organisms are gram-negative rods (especially *Escherichia coli*), anaerobes (typically a *Bacteroides* species), and anaerobic streptococci (*Enterococci*).
         (b) When the source is extra-abdominal, gram-positive organisms predominate.
   b. Clinical presentation includes sepsis, fever and chills, leukocytosis, and anemia.
      (1) Liver function studies show elevated enzyme levels, particularly alkaline phosphatase.
      (2) The patient may have right upper quadrant pain, and the liver may be tender or enlarged.
      (3) On occasion, sepsis may be overwhelming.
      (4) Hemobilia may also occur due to erosion of the abscess into the biliary tree.
   c. Treatment
      (1) The standard surgical treatment for hepatic abscess is operative surgical drainage and antibiotic therapy, which have good results.
      (2) Hepatic abscesses also are well managed by percutaneous drainage, using catheter aspiration guided by ultrasonic or CT imaging. This closed procedure may be curative, particularly for abscesses with minimal accompanying necrotic debris. Periodic sinograms of the abscess cavity are used to monitor healing and the adequacy of drainage.
      (3) Multiple abscesses are difficult to manage and rely heavily on appropriate antibiotic coverage. Percutaneous drainage with multiple drains can be curative. It is important to determine the antibiotic sensitivity of the infecting organisms and to administer a full course of antibiotics to reduce the risk of recurrent or persistent infection.
   d. Mortality rate for hepatic abscess may be as high as 40% in difficult cases. This high rate is related principally to three factors.
      (1) Delay in diagnosis. The possibility of an abscess is often overlooked in the critically ill patient. The use of CT scans and ultrasonography should improve this situation.
      (2) Multiple abscesses. These are more difficult to drain properly, and therefore, the patient may continue to be septic.
      (3) Malnutrition. Patients with sepsis are very catabolic. Caloric supplementation, either orally or parenterally, is critical for the patient's well-being, wound healing, and immunocompetence.

3. **Amebic abscess** is the second most common hepatic abscess in the Western world and is more common than bacterial abscesses in third world countries.
   a. Etiology. Amebic abscess is due to infection with the protozoan *Entamoeba histolytica*, which typically reaches the portal vein from intestinal amebiasis.
   b. Clinical presentation includes fever, leukocytosis, hepatomegaly, and right upper quadrant pain. Occasionally, liver enzyme levels are elevated.
      (1) The abscess is usually solitary and affects the right lobe of the liver in 90% of patients.
      (2) Indirect hemagglutination titers for *Entamoeba* are elevated in up to 85% of patients with intestinal infestation and in 98% of patients with hepatic abscess.
      (3) The pus within the abscess is usually sterile and has the appearance of anchovy paste. Trophozoites are occasionally present in the periphery of the abscess.
   c. Treatment of choice is parenteral antibiotics, particularly metronidazole. The abscess is aspirated if it is large or adjacent to important structures, but surgical drainage is not usually necessary. Complications include secondary bacterial infection of the cavity and rupture into adjacent structures, such as the pleural, pericardial, or peritoneal spaces.

4. Hydatid cysts of the liver

    a. Etiology. Hydatid cysts result from infection with the parasite *Echinococcus granulosus*. Dogs are the definitive host, shedding ova in the feces, which infect intermediate hosts, such as man, sheep, and cattle. This infection is endemic in southern Europe, the Middle East, Australia, and South America—all areas where sheep are raised.

    b. Clinical presentation

        (1) Hydatid cysts can develop anywhere in the body, but two thirds occur in the liver.

            (a) The cyst and cyst lining contain parasites fully capable of spreading the infection.

            (b) The adjacent compressed liver tissue and scar form the ectocyst, which is not infective and should be retained when evacuating the cyst.

        (2) Hydatid cysts undergo progressive enlargement and may rupture.

            (a) Approximately 50% rupture within the hepatic parenchyma to form daughter cysts.

            (b) Cysts may rupture into bile ducts, where the debris can cause biliary obstruction.

            (c) Cysts may rupture into the free peritoneal cavity, resulting in urticaria, eosinophilia, or anaphylactic shock and implantation into other viscera.

            (d) About 30% of patients develop cysts in the lungs or other extrahepatic organs.

        (3) Symptoms include liver enlargement and right upper quadrant pain in a patient with a history of exposure to an endemic area. Eosinophilia is present in 40% of patients, and serum tests for the parasite antigen are diagnostic.

            (a) All symptomatic cysts require surgery.

            (b) Small cysts deep within the parenchyma should be followed up (for months to years) until they are sufficiently superficial to be removed.

            (c) When pericystic calcification is visible on an abdominal radiograph, it signifies the death of a parasite, a condition that requires no further treatment.

    c. Treatment

        (1) Because the cyst is quite fragile and easily ruptured, a hydatid cyst can rarely be removed intact. If the scolices spill into the peritoneal cavity, the parasite will multiply and form new cysts.

        (2) The current method of treatment is controlled rupture of the cyst, followed by its removal.

            (a) This is accomplished by careful isolation of the operative field to prevent spillage, followed by aspiration of the cyst.

            (b) Once decompressed, the cyst and its contents are peeled off the ectocyst lining and removed, thus removing all living cyst elements.

            (c) The residual space is then sterilized with fresh 0.5% silver nitrate solution or hypertonic saline, which are potent scolicide agents and relatively nontoxic. (There is no systemic scolicidal agent currently in use.)

            (d) The residual cavity is carefully inspected for bile leakage from cyst-biliary communications, and these are sutured closed.

            (e) If the cyst ruptured into a major bile duct, common bile duct exploration is done to remove all debris.

            (f) The cyst is closed. No drains are used.

G **Trauma**   Due to its large size, the liver is frequently injured by both blunt and penetrating trauma.

    1. Mortality. Due to its high blood flow, proximity to the inferior vena cava, nearby vital structures, and propensity to develop infections, the overall mortality of liver trauma remains about 10%–20%. Injury to the hepatic veins and retrohepatic inferior vena cava has a mortality of over 50%, regardless of the method used to obtain control of the bleeding.

    2. Diagnosis is usually related to intraperitoneal bleeding. Ongoing bleeding mandates surgery.

    3. Nonsurgical management. In a hemodynamically stable patient, some trauma centers angiographically visualize the liver and occlude disrupted arteries with thrombus in an attempt to control hemorrhage and avoid surgery. The safety of this approach is being evaluated, but the approach seems to be safe in many patients.

    4. Surgical management. At surgery, hemostasis is usually obtained via **packing** and the **Pringle maneuver** (control and compression of the porta hepatis). Further exposure and ligation of individual parenchymal bleeders is not typically necessary. Less common methods to control bleeding include:

    a. Tractotomy or opening of a missile tract or fracture to expose bleeding parenchyma

    b. Resectional debridement, the removal of nonviable parenchyma without an anatomic (i.e., segmental or lobar) resection

    c. Anatomic resection has a high mortality (about 50%) when done as an emergency procedure.

    d. Hepatic artery ligation may control arterial bleeding but is associated with infectious complications in the compromised parenchyma.

    e. Definitive packing can be useful when other methods are unavailable or fail. Ideally, it provides time (24–48 hours) to restore normothermia and clotting factors.

  5. Late complications are common.

    a. Subcapsular and intrahepatic hematomas can be carefully observed, but many ultimately require drainage.

    b. Perihepatic collections, whether of blood or bile, usually become infected and must be drained.

    c. Biliary fistulas may track to the skin or into the chest (biliary-pleural, bronchobiliary fistula). Treatment is similar to the treatment for gastrointestinal fistulas (see Chapter 2, VII).

    d. Traumatic arteriovenous fistulas may result from penetrating trauma. Large fistulas are best treated by arterial embolization.

    e. Hemobilia is due to arteriobiliary fistula formation.

      (1) Patients present late (more than 1 month after injury) with gastrointestinal bleeding (hematemesis or melena), jaundice, biliary colic, or fever.

      (2) Diagnosis and treatment are via arteriography and embolization.

II   PORTAL HYPERTENSION

A **Anatomy**   (see I A 2 b; Fig. 14-2)

B **Pathophysiology**   Portal hypertension is an abnormal elevation in portal venous pressure (normal is 5–6 mm Hg).

  1. The increase in pressure stimulates the development of venous collaterals, which attempt to decompress the portal system into the systemic venous system.

  2. The collateral veins are very fragile. They form portosystemic connections between the portal system and the inferior vena cava or the superior vena cava via the azygos system.

  3. When portal pressure exceeds 20 mm Hg, **dilated veins** or **varices** are likely to develop. When the varices form in a submucosal location, such as at the gastroesophageal junction, they are subject to rupture and hemorrhage.

C **Etiology**

  1. Intrahepatic causes are most common.

    a. Cirrhosis causes 85% of portal hypertension in the United States. The most common etiology of cirrhosis is alcohol abuse, followed by hepatitis C.

      (1) Pathologically, cirrhosis produces:

        (a) Progressive narrowing of sinusoidal and postsinusoidal vessels due to centrilobular collagen deposition

        (b) Distortion of the sinusoidal anatomy by cirrhotic regenerative nodules

      (2) The resultant sinusoidal block increases resistance to portal blood flow through the liver and increases portal pressure.

    b. Schistosomiasis is a common cause worldwide. Portal hypertension develops when parasitic ova in small portal venules cause a presinusoidal block.

    c. Wilson's disease, hepatic fibrosis, and **hemochromatosis** are occasional causes of portal hypertension.

  2. Prehepatic causes of portal hypertension are rare but are more common in children. Examples of prehepatic causes are portal vein obstruction due to either thrombosis, congenital atresia, or stenosis caused by extrinsic compression, such as occurs with tumors.

3. **Posthepatic causes** of portal hypertension are also rare.
   a. **Budd-Chiari syndrome** is characterized by hepatic vein thrombosis, which causes a postsinusoidal block with resultant hepatomegaly and ascites. This syndrome may be idiopathic or due to a hypercoagulable state as occurs with tumors, hematologic disorders, oral contraceptive use, and trauma. In Asia, inferior vena caval webs are the most common cause of hepatic vein obstruction. Oddly, this syndrome is not uncommon after bone marrow transplantation.
   b. **Constrictive pericarditis** produces a markedly elevated inferior vena cava pressure, resulting in resistance to hepatic venous outflow. It should be suspected when calcification of the pericardium is present.

4. **Increased portal venous flow** may result in portal hypertension. This is due to primary splenic disease and splenic arteriovenous fistulas or shunts.

5. **Splenic vein thrombosis** may cause left-sided portal hypertension, resulting in varices confined to the gastric fundus. This is usually due to pancreatitis or a pancreatic tumor (see II K 2 c).

D **Clinical presentation**   The following are common findings in portal hypertension:

1. **Encephalopathy**
   a. This is secondary to portosystemic collaterals (with shunting of portal blood around the liver) and hepatic insufficiency.
   b. It may be related to elevated serum levels of ammonia in some patients, but the correlation is unreliable.

2. **Gastrointestinal hemorrhage,** frequently from gastroesophageal varices and complicated by impaired coagulation

3. **Malnutrition,** particularly in alcoholic cirrhosis

4. **Ascites** (see II L) secondary to hepatic sinusoidal hypertension, hypoalbuminemia, and hyperaldosteronism

5. Other manifestations of **collateral venous development,** such as a periumbilical caput medusae or hemorrhoids

6. **Splenomegaly,** which may be associated with hypersplenism (see II K)

E **Medical management of acute variceal hemorrhage**   Variceal hemorrhage is life threatening and is the principal complication of portal hypertension that requires emergency intervention.

1. The management of acute upper gastrointestinal (UGI) hemorrhage is described in Chapter 9, III F.

2. Gastroesophagoscopy should be performed as soon as possible to find the site of bleeding and determine the presence of varices.
   a. The cause of an UGI hemorrhage in cirrhotic patients is varices in 20%–50%, erosive gastritis in 20%–60%, peptic ulcer disease in 6%–19%, and esophageal tears (Mallory-Weiss syndrome) in 5%–18%.
   b. Up to 8% of patients have two bleeding sites.

3. **Measures for controlling acute variceal bleeding** (Fig. 14-4) include the following:
   a. **Variceal banding** with small rubber bands is the treatment of choice for bleeding varices. This procedure is performed endoscopically. It is at least as effective as sclerotherapy and is safer (Fig. 14-5).
   b. **Injection sclerotherapy**
      (1) Injection of a sclerosing agent is currently the preferred method of managing acute variceal bleeding. The injection into a varix results in thrombosis of the vein.
      (2) The procedure is done endoscopically and controls bleeding temporarily in 80%–90% of patients; it is associated with a mortality rate of 1%–2%.
      (3) Injection sclerotherapy has a complication rate of approximately 20%–40%, which includes esophageal perforation, worsening of hemorrhage, and more minor complications such as esophageal ulceration, fever, retrosternal chest pain, and pleural effusions.
   c. **Pharmacotherapy**

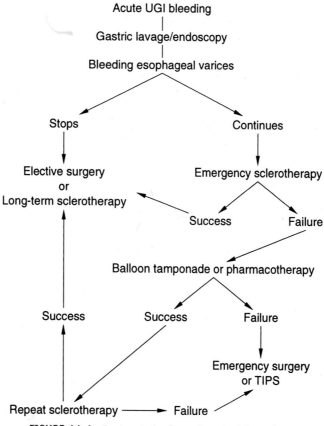

FIGURE 14-4 Treatment plan for acute variceal hemorrhage.

(1) Vasopressin and nitroglycerin

    (a) Vasopressin, a potent vasoconstrictor, lowers portal pressure by splanchnic vasoconstriction, which results in diminished mesenteric blood flow. Vasopressin is useful only for short-term hemorrhage control; it does not improve patient survival rates.

    (b) Nitroglycerin lowers portal pressure independently and helps to counteract some of the systemic side effects of vasopressin (e.g., myocardial ischemia, limb ischemia, and bowel necrosis).

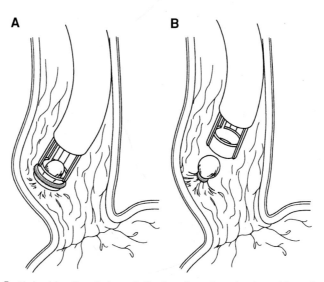

FIGURE 14-5 Variceal banding. Endoscopic ligation of esophageal varices with small rubber bands.

(2) **Somatostatin** causes splanchnic vasoconstriction and decreases portal pressure with fewer side effects than vasopressin.

(3) **Metoclopramide and pentagastrin** constrict the lower esophageal sphincter, which may help to control bleeding.

d. **Balloon tamponade.** The Sengstaken-Blakemore tube is a nasogastric tube with esophageal and gastric balloons for tamponade of varices.

(1) These tubes control bleeding in up to 80% of patients, but bleeding may resume in approximately 20%–50% of patients when the balloon is deflated.

(2) Pneumonia, due to the inability to clear salivary secretions, is common unless a proximal suction tube is placed above the esophageal balloon.

(3) Esophageal rupture may result from mechanical disruption or ischemia of the esophagus.

(4) To minimize these complications, this tube should be used for a limited time, such as 48 hours.

e. **Transjugular intrahepatic portosystemic shunt (TIPS)** is now the preferred procedure for controlling variceal bleeding (Fig. 14-6).

(1) Using angiographic techniques, the physician creates an 8- to 12-mm shunt between one of the hepatic veins and a branch of the portal vein and inserts a stent to maintain patency.

(2) The rate of postoperative encephalopathy is approximately the same as the surgical shunts—10%–30%.

(3) Complications include early rebleeding, shunt stenosis, and thrombosis.

(4) TIPS is very helpful in acute hemorrhage in patients with portal hypertension, particularly in those awaiting liver transplantation.

F **Surgical management of acute massive bleeding** Acute massive bleeding that fails to respond to nonsurgical maneuvers requires emergency surgery, especially if hypotension is present. The possibility of bleeding from sources other than varices should be eliminated before any surgical procedure. TIPS has significantly reduced the number of patients requiring surgical shunts emergently.

1. **The decision to proceed with surgery** is made if bleeding continues despite transfusion of five units or more of blood, especially within 24 hours. The risk of death rises dramatically after ten units of blood have been transfused, due to both sepsis and the worsening of cirrhotic coagulopathy from the use of banked blood.

2. Surgery is not advisable in the presence of pneumonia, moderate or severe encephalopathy, severe coagulopathy, alcoholic hepatitis (see II G 1 b), or severe liver failure.

3. **Type of surgery** performed may be either surgery to decompress the portal venous system or surgery to directly ligate the bleeding varices.

a. **Emergency portacaval shunting,** although very effective in controlling hemorrhage (over 95% of patients stop bleeding), has a high operative mortality related to the Child's classification of the patient (Table 14-1).

(1) The usual procedure performed is an end-to-side portacaval shunt or a mesocaval shunt (see II H).

(2) The acute reduction of portal blood flow to the liver after shunting may lead to hepatic failure, accounting for two thirds of the perioperative deaths. Pneumonia, renal failure, and delirium tremens are lethal contributing factors.

b. **Ligation of varices** (see Figure 14-12), either directly or by esophageal transection using a stapling device, usually stops the bleeding.

(1) Ligation is associated with an operative mortality rate of up to 30%.

(2) Bleeding recurs within several months in up to 80% of survivors.

(3) In most patients, ligation probably offers no advantage over shunt procedures.

G **Elective management of esophageal varices** is used when patients are not actively bleeding. The goal of this type of surgery is to prevent rebleeding with its concomitant risk of death.

1. **Preoperative evaluation** includes the following:

a. Endoscopy is used to prove that the esophageal varices bled.

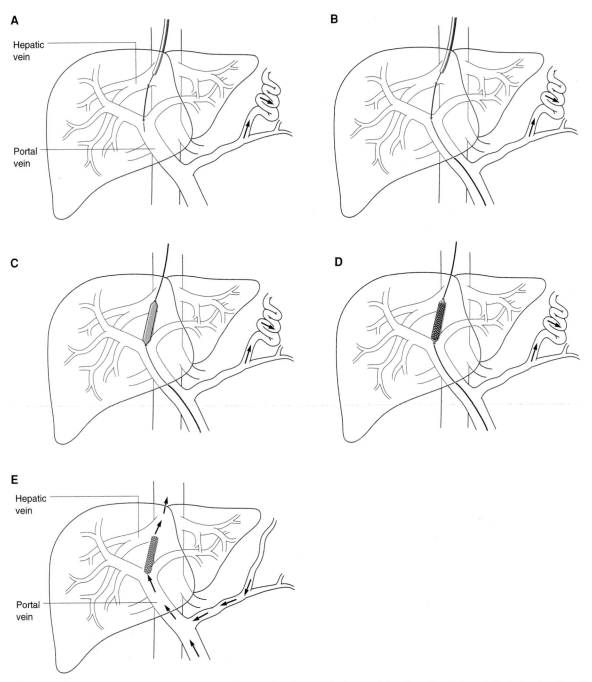

FIGURE 14-6 Transjugular intrahepatic portosystemic shunt (TIPS). **A,** a wire is placed from hepatic vein to portal vein in a transhepatic path; **B,** a balloon catheter is passed over the wire and inserted into the portal vein; **C,** the balloon is inflated to dilate the path; **D,** a stent is expanded to maintain patency of the transhepatic path; and **E,** once established, portal blood may flow freely into the hepatic vein and IVC.

TABLE 14-1 The Child's Classification for Determining the Operative Risk of a Shunting Procedure in a Patient with Portal Hypertension

	Child Group		
	A	B	C
Serum bilirubin (mg/dL)	<2	2–3	>3
Serum albumin (g/dL)	>3.5	3–3.5	<3
Presence of ascites	Absent	Easily controlled	Refractory
Presence of encephalopathy	Absent	Minimal	Severe
Presence of malnutrition	Absent	Mild	Severe
Operative mortality rate	2%	10%	50%

    b. Acute alcoholic hepatitis must be excluded.
        (1) This syndrome presents as liver failure with a diffusely tender liver.
        (2) Histologically, hepatocyte necrosis is seen with discrete hyaline bodies (Mallory's bodies) in hepatic cells.
        (3) Liver enzyme levels and liver function improve if the patient survives the acute episode.
        (4) A liver biopsy should be performed if the diagnosis is in question because the operative mortality rate exceeds 50% when surgery is performed in the presence of alcoholic hepatitis.
    c. The **Child's classification** (Table 14-1) is used to evaluate the operative risk.
    d. The patient's portal venous anatomy is determined, verifying the presence of a patent portal vein by the following.
        (1) Splenic and superior mesenteric arteriography followed by delayed venous-phase imaging is the most accurate method.
        (2) Doppler ultrasound examination to identify the portal vein and its tributaries and ascertain patency and direction of flow is simple and noninvasive.
        (3) Splenoportography, the injection of radiopaque dye into the spleen followed by imaging of the portal system, is reserved for specific visualization of the splenic vein.
    e. The portal venous pressure can be measured indirectly by measuring the wedged hepatic venous pressure.

  2. Type of nonoperative management depends on the surgeon's preference and on the patient's pathologic and physiologic status. The choices are as follows:
    a. TIPS (see II E 3 e)
    b. Direct occlusion of varices
        (1) Endoscopic variceal banding or sclerosis (sclerotherapy) is initially effective in up to 80%–90% of patients and has become the principal initial method of management for esophageal varices.
        (2) Many patients require resclerosis procedures because nothing has been done to lower the portal pressure.
        (3) A major risk of chronic therapy is esophageal stricture.

H **Shunting procedures** are designed to lower the portal venous pressure, thereby decompressing esophageal varices and diminishing their propensity to bleed. **Portosystemic shunts** may be prophylactic or therapeutic and may be nonselective or selective.

  1. Prophylactic shunts are performed on patients with proven varices but prior to any episodes of esophageal variceal bleeding.
    a. Only 30%–40% of these patients ultimately bleed from their varices, making 60% of the procedures unnecessary.
    b. Nonselective shunts decrease hepatic portal venous flow, increasing the risk of hepatic decompensation.
    c. In randomized trials, prophylactic shunts have not improved survival rates. They are currently not recommended.

  2. Therapeutic shunts are performed on patients who have had a variceal hemorrhage. Patient survival is principally a function of the Child's classification (Table 14-1) prior to surgery. Long-term survival in the alcoholic patient is principally determined by whether or not the patient continues to abuse alcohol.

  3. Nonselective portosystemic shunts decompress the entire portal venous system into the inferior vena cava, lowering portal pressure. The type of shunt used depends partly on surgeon preference and whether the patient is likely to be a candidate for a liver transplant.
    a. The end-to-side portacaval shunt (Fig. 14-7) is the shunt procedure most commonly performed.
        (1) The hepatic end of the portal vein is ligated, and the inferior end of the portal vein is sutured to the inferior vena cava, which results in dramatic lowering of portal pressure and decompression of varices.
        (2) The rebleeding rate is <5%, but the major problem is that portal flow into the liver is reduced to zero, which increases the risk of encephalopathy and hepatic failure.

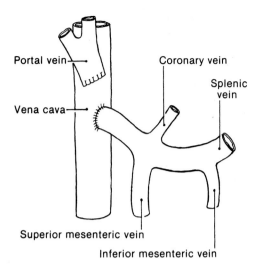

FIGURE 14-7 End-to-side portacaval shunt.

b. The **mesocaval shunt** is constructed with a large-diameter (16–18 mm) prosthetic vascular graft to connect the superior mesenteric vein to the inferior vena cava (Fig. 14-8). It is the preferred shunt in potential liver transplant recipients.

(1) With this shunt and the side-to-side portacaval shunt, the effect on portal blood flow into the liver is unpredictable; as portal pressure falls, portal flow into the liver falls. In fact, blood may flow out of the liver via the portal vein, thereby stealing hepatic arterial flow. Thus, the risk of hepatic failure may be higher than for end-to-side portacaval shunts.

(2) The advantage of this shunt is the relative ease of exposing the mesenteric vein and the avoidance of any dissection in the porta hepatis, hence facilitating future transplantation.

(3) There are two disadvantages:

(a) This shunt uses prosthetic material, which has the potential for infection.

(b) There is a somewhat lower long-term patency rate as compared with shunts without prosthetic material.

(4) As with all shunts, **thrombosis of the shunt returns the patient to a high risk of variceal hemorrhage.**

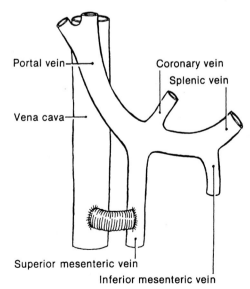

FIGURE 14-8 Inferior vena cava–superior mesenteric vein (mesocaval) shunt.

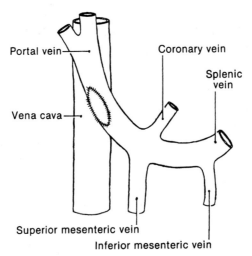

FIGURE 14-9 Side-to-side portacaval shunt.

    c. The side-to-side portacaval shunt is technically more difficult because a longer length of both veins must be prepared (Fig. 14-9). Its use is reserved for situations in which it is necessary to decompress the liver.

      (1) In the Budd-Chiari syndrome, this shunt or a mesocaval shunt converts the portal vein into an outflow vessel, replacing the thrombosed hepatic veins.

      (2) With refractory ascites and variceal hemorrhage, this shunt decompresses the liver and decreases ascites (see II L 1 b).

  4. Selective portosystemic shunts decrease the pressure in the gastroesophageal bed only and reduce the risk of gastroesophageal varices by shunting only gastroesophageal venous blood into the systemic circulation. Prospective trials have shown a significant decrease in the incidence of postoperative encephalopathy with the selective shunt as compared with the nonselective shunts. The **distal splenorenal (Warren) shunt** is most commonly performed (Fig. 14-10).

    a. In this procedure, the distal end of the splenic vein (i.e., the portion coming directly from the splenic hilum) is anastomosed to the left renal vein, a low-pressure vein. The proximal splenic vein is ligated.

    b. The coronary vein, the right gastroepiploic vein, and other collaterals between the portal system and the gastric, pancreatic, and splenic region are ligated.

    c. As can be seen from Figure 14-10, portal venous flow into the liver is maintained, thus minimizing the problem of hepatic insufficiency and consequent encephalopathy.

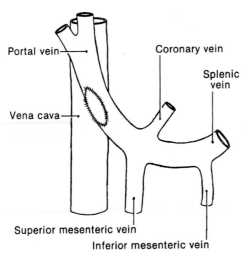

FIGURE 14-10 Distal splenorenal (Warren) shunt.

   d. Because portal sinusoidal pressure remains high, ascites is common after this procedure.
   e. Chylous ascites may also occur as a result of surgical dissection in the retroperitoneum adjacent to the major lymphatic channels.

I **Nonshunt surgical procedures**

   1. Paraesophageal devascularization combined with esophageal transection and reanastomosis (Sugiura procedure) has, in some series, been highly effective in preventing bleeding and has shown a low operative mortality rate.
   a. The procedure consists of transthoracic esophageal devascularization, transabdominal proximal gastric devascularization, splenectomy, selective vagotomy, and pyloroplasty (Figs. 14-11 and 14-12).
   b. The operative mortality rate has been as low as 5% and the rebleeding rate as low as 4% in the Japanese series. These excellent results have not been duplicated for European or American individuals with cirrhosis.

   2. Liver transplantation is the only therapy that addresses the underlying liver disease and restores the patient's hepatic functional reserve to normal. It is generally reserved for patients who have poor hepatic reserve and are otherwise good candidates for transplantation (i.e., other organic systems are healthy, and the psychosocial status of the patient is acceptable).

J **Prognosis**   Ultimately, in alcoholic patients with cirrhosis, regardless of the treatment, the potential for hepatic failure and death depends on whether the patient continues to consume alcohol. The prognosis for other causes of cirrhosis is not quite as poor, although the trends are the same. The overall statistics for alcoholic cirrhotic patients are as follows:

1. Approximately 15% of alcoholics develop cirrhosis, and 30% of these individuals die within a year of the diagnosis.

2. Approximately 40% (i.e., 13%–70%) of cirrhotic individuals develop bleeding varices, and without definitive treatment, 66% of these individuals die within a year.

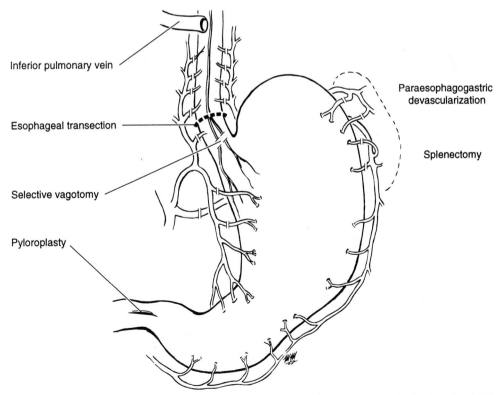

FIGURE 14-11 Sugiura procedure: esophageal transection and paraesophagogastric devascularization. (Reprinted with permission from Sugiura M, Futagawa S. Further evaluation of the Sugiura procedure in the treatment of esophageal varices. *Arch Surg.* 1977;112:1317–1321.)

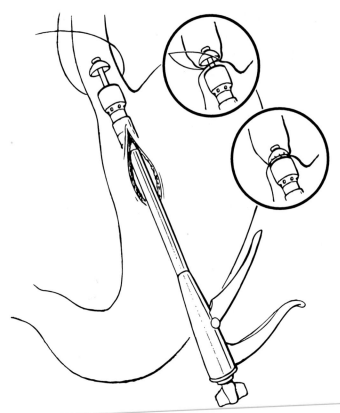

FIGURE 14-12 End-to-end anastomosis (EEA). The EEA stapler is introduced, and the esophagus is securely tied over the center rod 2 cm above the gastric junction. The instrument gap is closed, and the trigger is fired, which completes the simultaneous transection and reanastomosis. (Reprinted with permission from Wexler MJ. Treatment of bleeding esophageal varices by transabdominal esophageal transection with the EEA stapling instrument. *Surgery.* 1980;88:410.)

    a. Approximately 50%–80% of patients die from their first variceal hemorrhage without definitive treatment.

    b. Of those patients who survive the initial hemorrhage to bleed a second time, the same proportion will die from their second hemorrhage.

K **Hypersplenism** is common in patients with portal hypertension.

  1. It should be treated conservatively (i.e., nonoperatively). Approximately half of patients who undergo shunting show improvement of the hypersplenism.

  2. Splenectomy should be performed rarely for portal hypertension and variceal hemorrhage.

    a. It is associated with a variceal hemorrhage recurrence rate as high as 90%.

    b. Sepsis and death may follow splenectomy, especially in children.

    c. Indication for splenectomy in a patient with variceal bleeding is radiographic proof of **splenic vein thrombosis.**

      (1) This occurs as a result of an obstruction in the vein due to a pancreatic disorder, such as pancreatitis or a neoplasm.

      (2) The varices are generally limited to the stomach (gastric varices) and therefore are **curable** by splenectomy.

L **Ascites** is a complication of hepatic disease.

  1. Etiology. It results from sinusoidal hypertension, hypoalbuminemia, abnormal hepatic and abdominal lymph production, and abnormal salt and water retention by the kidneys.

    a. Salt and water retention are due to **hyperaldosteronism,** which is related to decreased breakdown of aldosterone by the liver.

    b. Ascites may be worsened by portosystemic shunts with exception of side-to-side portacaval and mesocaval shunts (see II H 3 b, c).

2. **Medical management** of ascites is efficacious and involves salt and water restriction and diuretics, especially the aldosterone antagonists.

3. **Peritoneal-jugular shunting** may be used to treat ascites that is refractory to medical management. Its efficacy in either controlling ascites or improving survival has not yet been definitely demonstrated.

   a. A plastic tube is implanted surgically, originating in the peritoneal cavity and terminating in the jugular vein. A valve in the tubing controls the direction of flow out of the peritoneal cavity.

   b. Diuretics should be continued for optimal shunt results.

   c. Peritoneal-jugular shunts may result in bleeding due to the presence of factors in ascitic fluid that stimulate the development of disseminated intravascular coagulation.

4. **TIPS** (see II E 3 e) has also been found effective in controlling refractory ascites.

III GALLBLADDER AND EXTRAHEPATIC BILIARY TREE

A Overview

1. **Embryology**
   a. **Development** of the liver and biliary structures begins during the fourth week of fetal life.
   b. The **hepatic diverticulum** forms as an outpouching of the foregut.
      (1) The **cranial portion** forms the liver, the larger branches of the intrahepatic ducts, and the proximal extrahepatic biliary tree.
      (2) The **caudal portion** forms the gallbladder, cystic duct, and common bile duct.

2. **Anatomy** (Fig. 14-13)
   a. **Extrahepatic biliary tree**
      (1) **Structure**
         (a) The **left** and **right hepatic ducts** join together after leaving the liver. This confluence forms the **common hepatic duct** (3–4 cm in length).
         (b) The common hepatic duct is joined at an acute angle by the cystic duct to form the common bile duct (10 cm in length; 3–10 mm in diameter).

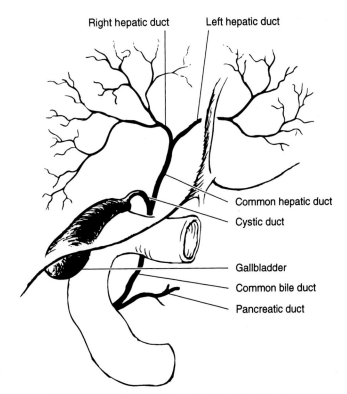

FIGURE 14-13 Gallbladder and extrahepatic biliary tree.

        (c) The **common bile duct** is lateral to the common hepatic artery and anterior to the portal vein. The distal one third of the common bile duct passes behind the pancreas to the **ampulla of Vater,** also called the *papilla.*

        (d) The common bile duct joins the **pancreatic duct** in one of three ways.

           (i) Most commonly, the ducts unite outside the duodenum and traverse the duodenal wall and papilla as a single duct.

          (ii) They may join within the duodenal wall and have a short common channel.

         (iii) Least commonly, they enter the duodenum independently.

    (2) The **sphincter of Oddi** surrounds the common bile duct as it traverses the ampulla of Vater and controls bile flow.

    (3) **Blood supply to the ducts**

        (a) The **hilar ducts** within the liver parenchyma are supplied primarily from the hepatic arteries.

        (b) The blood supply to the **supraduodenal common bile duct** is variable, but generally blood flows superiorly. The most important vessels (the **"three o'clock"** and **"nine o'clock"** arteries) run along the sides of the duct, as their names imply.

  b. The **gallbladder** is located on the inferior aspect of the liver and marks the division of the liver into its right and left lobes.

    (1) **Anatomic portions**

        (a) **Fundus** (most anterior)

        (b) **Body,** which serves as the storage area

        (c) **Infundibulum (Hartmann's pouch),** located between the neck and the body (most posterior)

        (d) **Neck,** which connects with the cystic duct

    (2) The **wall of the gallbladder** is composed of smooth muscle and fibrous tissue; the lumen is lined with high columnar epithelium.

    (3) **Vasculature**

        (a) **Arterial supply.** The gallbladder is supplied by the **cystic artery,** which is usually (95% of the time) a branch of the right hepatic artery that passes behind the cystic duct.

        (b) **Venous return** is via cystic veins to the portal vein and small veins that drain directly into the liver.

        (c) **Lymphatic drainage** from the gallbladder goes both to the liver and to hilar nodes.

    (4) **Innervation** is from the **celiac plexus.**

        (a) **Motor innervation** travels via vagal postganglionic fibers from the celiac ganglia. The preganglionic sympathetic level is T_8–T_9.

        (b) **Sensory innervation** travels from sympathetic fibers coursing to the celiac plexus through the right posterior root ganglion at levels T_8–T_9.

    (5) The **valves of Heister** are mucosal folds in the cystic duct. Despite their name, they have no valvular function.

  c. Anomalies of the arterial and biliary systems are common. Because "normal" anatomy occurs in fewer than 50% of individuals, the surgeon must have a thorough knowledge of both normal and anomalous anatomy.

3. Physiology. Bile is produced by the liver and is transported via the extrahepatic ducts to the gallbladder, where it is concentrated and released in response to humoral and neural control.

  a. Hepatic production of bile is under neural and humoral control. Vagal and splanchnic stimulation, secretin, theophylline, phenobarbital, and steroids all increase bile flow. Approximately 600 mL of bile are produced daily (normal range: 250–1,000 mL/day).

  b. Composition of bile. Because the electrolyte concentration of bile approximates that of plasma, **lactated Ringer's solution** is a good replacement fluid for biliary losses. Bile is composed of:

    (1) Electrolytes and water

    (2) Bile pigments

    (3) Protein

    (4) Lipids

        (a) Phospholipids, primarily lecithin

        (b) Cholesterol

        (c) Bile acids (bile salts); chenodeoxycholic acid and cholic acid conjugated with taurine and glycine

   c. Functions of the gallbladder include:

      (1) Storage of bile

      (2) Concentration of bile

         (a) The absorption of water and electrolytes by the gallbladder mucosa results in a 10-fold increased concentration of lipids, bile salts, and bile pigments compared with hepatic bile.

         (b) The **secretion of mucus** protects the gallbladder mucosa from the irritant effects of bile and facilitates the passage of bile through the cystic duct. This mucus secretion represents the **"white bile"** seen with **hydrops of the gallbladder,** which results from cystic duct obstruction.

      (3) Release of bile

         (a) The coordinated release of bile requires simultaneous contraction of the gallbladder and relaxation of the sphincter of Oddi.

         (b) This process is predominantly under humoral control (via cholecystokinin [**CCK**]), but vagal and splanchnic nerves also play a role.

B **Radiologic diagnosis of biliary tract disease**

   1. Plain abdominal films demonstrate the 15% of gallstones that are radiopaque.

   2. Real-time ultrasonography has a 90%–95% accuracy in identifying calculi. It is also useful in determining the presence of biliary ductal dilation, gallbladder wall thickening, and the presence of pericholecystic fluid.

      a. Ultrasonography can be performed in a jaundiced patient.

      b. It is usually the initial test obtained in the workup of a patient with biliary tract disease.

   3. Oral cholecystography (OCG) is an alternative method for demonstrating biliary calculi in patients with an equivocal gallbladder sonogram. It is rarely used today.

      a. This technique identifies abnormalities (visualization of stones or nonvisualization of the gallbladder) with a 95%–98% accuracy.

      b. The patient must ingest iopanoic acid tablets on the evening before the study. The chief disadvantages lie in its reliance on:

         (1) Absorption of contrast medium from the gastrointestinal tract

         (2) Uptake and excretion of contrast medium from the hepatocytes

         (3) Concentration of contrast medium in the gallbladder

         (4) Patency of hepatic and cystic ducts

      c. Cholecystokinin stimulation is used to diagnose gallbladder disease in symptomatic patients with a normal OCG. A positive study is presented by either of the following:

         (1) Failure of the gallbladder to contract more than 40% at 20 minutes after CCK injection

         (2) Reproduction of the patient's pain after CCK injection

   4. Hepatobiliary iminodiacetic acid (HIDA) scan (cholescintigraphy) makes use of a gamma-ray–emitting radioisotope (i.e., ^{99m}Tc) attached to a variety of lidocaine analogs bound to iminodiacetic acid, which is excreted in the bile.

      a. A HIDA scan provides images of the liver, the biliary tree, and the intestinal transit of bile.

      b. The HIDA scan is useful in the diagnosis of acute cholecystitis, choledochal cyst, bile leak (after laparoscopic cholecystectomy), and common bile duct obstruction.

      c. A **HIDA scan in conjunction with a CCK injection** and subsequent ejection fraction calculation (normal is >35%) may be of value in diagnosing biliary dyskinesia and calculous and acalculous cholecystitis. In acute cholecystitis, the gallbladder cannot be visualized due to obstruction of the cystic duct. In common duct obstruction, the nuclide fails to enter the duodenum.

   5. Endoscopic retrograde cholangiopancreatography (ERCP) is also useful in evaluating a patient with biliary tract disease. The procedure is both diagnostic and therapeutic.

      a. This procedure permits evaluation of the stomach, duodenum, ampulla of Vater, pancreatic duct, and common bile duct.

      b. If stones are present within the common bile duct, endoscopic papillotomy can be performed along with extraction of the stones. This procedure has a 90%–95% success rate.

    c. If a stricture is present, a stent can be inserted.

    d. Complications include pancreatitis, bleeding, and duodenal perforation. The complication rate is approximately 10%, with a mortality rate of 1%.

6. **Percutaneous transhepatic cholangiography (PTHC)** is useful in evaluating a jaundiced patient. It can localize the site of the obstruction and also allows the placement of biliary drainage catheters. PTHC is usually performed when ERCP cannot be performed or when ERCP cannot visualize the proximal biliary systems because of a near-complete obstruction secondary to tumor, stone, or stricture.

7. **CT** and **MRI** are expensive, but they delineate dilated ducts as well as retroperitoneal lymphadenopathy and lesions of the pancreas and liver.

8. **Intravenous cholangiography** is no longer performed.

C **Cholelithiasis (gallstones)**

1. **Types and mode of formation.** Gallstones form as a result of biliary solids precipitating out of the solution. Most stones (70%) are made up of cholesterol, bilirubin, and calcium, with cholesterol as the major component.

    a. Cholesterol stones are large and smooth.

        (1) The solubility of cholesterol in bile depends on the concentration of bile salts, lecithin, and cholesterol. Lecithin and cholesterol are insoluble in aqueous solution but dissolve in bile salt–lecithin micelles.

        (2) Failure of the liver to maintain a micellar liquid can be caused by an increase in the concentration of cholesterol or a decrease in the concentration of bile salts or lecithin; either can result in cholesterol stone formation.

        (3) Conversely, increasing the biliary concentration of lecithin and bile salts should hinder cholesterol stone formation.

            (a) This theory has been investigated by treating patients with cholesterol stones with oral bile salts.

            (b) In the National Cooperative Gallstone Study, patients with cholesterol gallstones were treated with chenodeoxycholic acid over a 2-year period. Complete resolution of stones was found in 13% of the patients, and partial dissolution in 41%. The recurrence rate is 50% at 5 years.

    b. Pure pigment (bilirubin) stones are smooth and are green or black in color; they are associated with hemolytic disorders, such as sickle cell anemia or spherocytosis.

    c. Calcium bilirubinate stones are associated with infection or inflammation of the biliary tree.

        (1) Infection results in an increase in biliary calcium as well as an increase in β-glucuronidase (which converts conjugated bilirubin to the unconjugated form).

        (2) The calcium binds to the unconjugated bilirubin and precipitates to form calcium bilirubinate stones.

        (3) Normal bile contains glucaro-1,4-lactone, which inhibits the conversion of conjugated to unconjugated bilirubin, and thus deters calcium bilirubinate stone formation.

2. **Clinical presentation** of cholelithiasis varies. It can present as (in increasing order of severity):

    a. Asymptomatic cholelithiasis

    b. Chronic cholecystitis

    c. Acute cholecystitis

    d. Complications of cholecystitis

    e. Choledocholithiasis (common bile duct stones)

3. **Asymptomatic cholelithiasis.** The treatment of asymptomatic cholelithiasis is somewhat controversial.

    a. Each year, approximately 1%–4% of patients with asymptomatic gallstones develop symptoms or complications of their disease. Most patients do develop symptoms before developing a severe complication of cholelithiasis.

    b. There is little evidence that prophylactic treatment is justified in the management of cholelithiasis, with the exception of calcified or porcelain gallbladder, which should be removed because the risk of malignancy exceeds 25%.

   c. The National Institutes of Health Consensus Conference on Gallstone and Laparoscopic Cholecystectomy, held in September 1992, does not recommend cholecystectomy for asymptomatic diabetic patients with gallstones. The opposite was widely practiced until recently.

D **Cholecystitis** is inflammation of the gallbladder. In 85%–90% of patients, cholecystitis is caused by calculi, bile stasis, and bacteria; pancreatic juice irritation may play a lesser role.

   1. **Chronic cholecystitis**
      a. **Clinical presentation.** The patient complains of moderate intermittent pain in the right upper quadrant and epigastric region, nausea, and vomiting. The pain may radiate to the back or right scapular region. Symptoms may be associated with eating fatty foods.
      b. **Diagnosis.** Laboratory studies are generally normal. With an OCG, the gallbladder fails to appear or shows filling defects. Ultrasonography reveals stones.
      c. **Treatment** is elective cholecystectomy. Approximately 95% of patients receiving surgery for cholecystitis secondary to cholelithiasis are completely relieved of their symptoms. Approximately 5% of patients retain mild symptoms that presumably are unrelated to the biliary tree.
      d. **Nonoperative treatment** (e.g., oral bile salts, lithotripsy) may be appropriate for patients with small stones and functioning gallbladders (determined by OCG) who are not operative candidates or who refuse surgery.

   2. **Acute cholecystitis**
      a. **Pathophysiology**
         (1) Most cases are due to an impacted stone in the gallbladder neck or the cystic duct with resultant obstruction. Direct pressure from the stone on the mucosa or duct obstruction causes ischemia, ulceration, edema, and impaired venous return, all of which lead to extensive inflammation in and around the gallbladder.
         (2) In 75% of cases, bacterial infection of the bile and gallbladder wall occurs.
         (3) Unchecked, these changes can lead to complications of acute cholecystitis.
      b. **Clinical presentation**
         (1) The greatest incidence of acute cholecystitis is in adults 30–80 years old; women are affected more often than men.
         (2) Most patients give a history consistent with prior chronic cholecystitis, except this episode is worse or lasts longer.
         (3) Fever, nausea, and vomiting; right upper quadrant tenderness with or without rebound tenderness; and Murphy's sign are common. The gallbladder may be palpable.
      c. The **differential diagnosis** includes:
         (1) Perforated or penetrating peptic ulcer
         (2) Myocardial infarction
         (3) Pancreatitis
         (4) Hiatal hernia
         (5) Right lower lobe pneumonia
         (6) Appendicitis
         (7) Hepatitis
         (8) Herpes zoster
      d. **Diagnosis**
         (1) Gallbladder ultrasound is the diagnostic study of choice. If acute cholecystitis needs to be documented further, a HIDA may be performed.
         (2) Other mandatory studies include a complete blood count; measurement of serum amylase, serum bilirubin, and liver enzymes; an electrocardiogram; and chest radiograph.
         (3) Levels of the following may be elevated in patients with acute cholecystitis:
            (a) Serum alkaline phosphatase in 23%
            (b) Bilirubin in 45%
            (c) Aspartate transaminase in 40%
            (d) Amylase in 13%
         (4) Ultrasonography may show stones and a thick-walled edematous gallbladder wall.
         (5) Cholescintigraphy will show any existing failure of the gallbladder.

e. Treatment

(1) Cholecystitis should be treated with cholecystectomy. As the bile is usually infected, perioperative antibiotics are needed. There are two approaches to the timing of surgery.

(a) Immediate surgery; that is, within 72 hours of the onset of symptoms

(b) Delayed surgery; that is, after recovery from the acute attack with intravenous fluids and antibiotics. Surgery should be performed approximately 6 weeks after the acute inflammation has resolved.

(2) Most surgeons now advocate **early surgical intervention** in the treatment of acute cholecystitis. This is due to the improved safety of current techniques, the effectiveness of perioperative antibiotics, and the high risk (at least 50%) of recurrent acute cholecystitis if surgery is delayed. Our **approach** is as follows.

(a) If symptoms began within 72 hours of the time of presentation, laparoscopic cholecystectomy is performed.

(b) If symptoms began more than 72 hours before the time of presentation and the patient is responding to medical management (i.e., a nasogastric tube, intravenous fluids, nothing by mouth, and antibiotics), then surgery is delayed for 4–6 weeks.

(c) Deterioration or failure to improve on medical management is an indication for surgery.

3. Acalculous cholecystitis is acute or chronic **cholecystitis in the absence of stones.** The acute form occurs as a complication of burns, sepsis, trauma, or collagen vascular disease. The chronic condition may also be referred to as *biliary dyskinesia.*

a. Etiology. Possible causes include:

(1) Kinking or fibrosis of the gallbladder

(2) Thrombosis of the cystic artery

(3) Sphincter spasm with obstruction of the biliary and pancreatic ducts

(4) Prolonged fasting

(5) Dehydration

(6) Systemic disease, such as the multiorgan failure associated with trauma

(7) Generalized sepsis

b. Diagnosis. Diagnostic tests used and their results are similar to those for calculous cholecystitis, except that no stones are seen. The cholescintigram is especially accurate for cholecystitis when it fails to visualize the gallbladder.

c. Treatment is cholecystectomy or cholecystostomy if the patient is too ill to tolerate cholecystectomy.

4. Complications of cholecystitis (and cholelithiasis) require urgent surgery.

a. Emphysematous cholecystitis is an acute, usually gangrenous cholecystitis complicated by secondary invasion of the gallbladder wall by gas-forming organisms.

(1) Unlike acute cholecystitis, emphysematous cholecystitis is three times more prevalent in men than women and may occur without cholelithiasis.

(2) Radiologically, the gallbladder is filled with gas in the absence of any communication between the gallbladder and the gastrointestinal tract.

(3) Treatment is urgent cholecystectomy. Antibiotics effective against *Clostridia* and coliform organisms are given.

b. Gangrenous cholecystitis results when extensive inflammation causes thrombosis of the cystic artery and resultant necrosis of the gallbladder. Bile cultures and appropriate antibiotics are essential.

c. Perforated cholecystitis results from necrosis of the gallbladder wall and leakage of bile into the peritoneal cavity. Peritonitis or, more commonly, subhepatic abscess may result.

d. Biliary-enteric fistula and gallstone ileus are complications of cholelithiasis, cystic duct obstruction, recurrent cholecystitis, adhesions to the surrounding viscera, perforation, fistula formation, and passage of the stone into the bowel.

(1) The **site of fistula** with the gallbladder is most commonly the duodenum, but the colon or any other intra-abdominal viscera may be involved.

(2) Site of bowel obstruction

(a) As the stone travels in the gastrointestinal lumen, the terminal ileum is the most common site of obstruction because this is the narrowest portion of the small bowel. Stones smaller than 2–3 cm are usually passed per rectum.

(b) If a stone is passed free into the peritoneal cavity, extraluminal obstruction secondary to inflammation and adhesions can occur anywhere.

(3) **Clinical presentation**

(a) Bowel obstruction is a disease of the elderly, and concomitant multisystem disease is common.

(b) The patient presents with symptoms of small bowel obstruction (i.e., nausea, vomiting, obstipation, pain, and distention).

(c) About 25% of patients have symptoms of acute cholecystitis immediately preceding the episode of obstruction. About 70% of the patients have a history of cholelithiasis.

(4) **Diagnosis**

(a) The correct diagnosis is made preoperatively in fewer than 25% of cases.

(b) The diagnosis is suggested by the history and by plain films of the abdomen. These may show small bowel obstruction accompanied by air in the biliary tree or a radiopaque stone in the right lower quadrant (seen in only 15% of cases).

(5) **Treatment**

(a) Because these patients are often extremely ill, emergency laparotomy may permit only localization of the stone, proximal enterotomy, stone extraction, and closure of the enterotomy.

(b) The whole small bowel, common bile duct, and gallbladder must be palpated for stones, as recurrent gallstone ileus (due to other stones) develops in 5%–9% of patients.

(c) Cholecystectomy and closure of the biliary fistula can be performed either concomitantly or after an interval, depending on the patient's condition.

5. **Treatment of cholecystitis. Cholecystectomy** is designed to remove the gallbladder without damage to structures in the porta hepatis.

a. Either an **open** cholecystectomy or a **laparoscopic** cholecystectomy can be performed.

(1) An **open cholecystectomy** involves making a right subcostal incision and placing mechanical abdominal wall retractors. The gallbladder is moved off the liver, usually starting at the top. The cystic duct and artery are ligated and divided during the course of the operation.

(2) **Laparoscopic cholecystectomy** involves placing 10-mm and 5-mm ports through the abdominal wall and filling the peritoneal cavity with CO_2 gas. Using the laparoscope with an attached video camera and long instruments, the gallbladder is removed, starting from the bottom, after the cystic duct and artery are clipped and divided. This topic is discussed further in Chapter 30. Advantages and contraindications are shown in Table 14-2.

b. A **common bile duct cholangiogram** via the cystic duct (operative cholangiogram) is performed by filling the ducts with radiopaque dye and taking a radiograph. Operative cholangiography is done whenever there is suspicion of common bile duct stones or the biliary tract anatomy is unclear. This procedure can be performed during open or laparoscopic cholecystectomy.

TABLE 14-2   Advantages and Contraindications of Laparoscopic Cholecystectomy

Advantages	Relative Contraindications
Cosmetic	Coagulopathy
Shorter hospital stay	Cirrhosis, portal hypertension
Rapid return to activity	Pregnancy
	Generalized peritonitis
	Prior surgery (adhesions)
	Severe cardiopulmonary disease
	Hypotension, especially secondary to hypovolemia

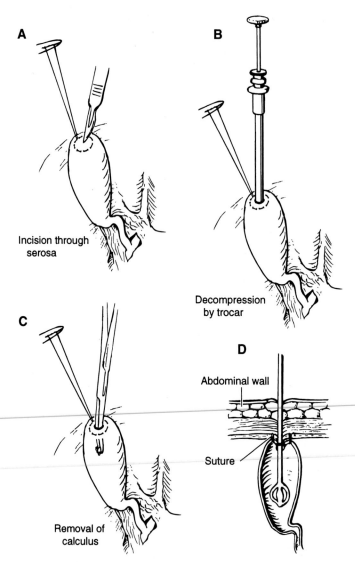

A: Incision through serosa

B: Decompression by trocar

C: Removal of calculus

D: Abdominal wall / Suture

FIGURE 14-14 Cholecystostomy. **A:** Placement of purse-string suture in fundus of gallbladder and incision through serosa; **(B)** trochar decompression; **(C)** removal of calculus from ampulla; **(D)** sagittal section demonstrating two concentric purse-string sutures, intraluminal catheter, and suturing of serosa of gallbladder to peritoneum. (Reprinted with permission from Schwartz S, Shires G. Tom, Spencer Frank C. *Principles of Surgery*, 5th ed. New York: McGraw-Hill; 1989:1405.)

    c. Cholecystostomy is an alternative procedure when extensive inflammation makes cholecystectomy too dangerous or a patient is too ill to undergo cholecystectomy. In this procedure, the gallbladder fundus is opened, bile and stones are removed, and a tube is placed in the gallbladder for external drainage. This procedure can be done operatively or percutaneously (Fig. 14-14).

E **Postcholecystectomy syndrome** is the term given to symptoms that develop after or persist despite cholecystectomy.

    1. In patients who have undergone cholecystectomy for chronic cholecystitis and cholelithiasis, postcholecystectomy symptoms are usually **extrabiliary** in origin and caused by:
        a. Hiatal hernia
        b. Peptic ulcer
        c. Pancreatitis
        d. Irritable bowel
        e. Food intolerance

2. Symptoms may be **biliary** in origin and caused by:
   a. A stone in the common bile duct
   b. A stone in the stump of the cystic duct
   c. Stenosis of the sphincter of Oddi
   d. Biliary stricture

3. Evaluation should be directed toward identifying these extrabiliary and biliary etiologies and may include ERCP, esophagogastroduodenoscopy, UGI radiograph, ultrasound, and CT scan.

F **Bile duct disorders**

1. Choledocholithiasis (stones in the common bile duct) can be single or multiple and are found in 10%–20% of patients who undergo cholecystectomy. Most stones are formed in the gallbladder and pass into the duct. However, **primary common duct stones** can form in the absence of a gallbladder.

   a. Clinical presentation. Some patients are asymptomatic. Most patients present with right upper quadrant pain that radiates to the back and right shoulder, intermittent obstructive jaundice, acholic stools, or bilirubinuria.

   b. Diagnosis
   (1) In contrast to neoplastic obstruction of the common bile duct, the gallbladder is not palpable.
   (2) Diagnostic studies include ultrasonography, ERCP, and, less commonly, transhepatic cholangiography or a radionuclide scan.
   (3) Liver function test results are consistent with obstructive jaundice and include elevations in bilirubin and alkaline phosphatase.

   c. Surgical treatment involves cholecystectomy, choledochotomy (opening the common duct), common bile duct exploration, stone removal, T tube placement, and T tube operative cholangiography (Fig. 14-15).
   (1) Operative cholangiography has decreased the need for common bile duct exploration but has increased the proportion of positive explorations, that is, explorations in which stones are found.
   (2) The only absolute indication for common bile duct exploration is a palpable stone in the common bile duct.
   (3) When any of the following are present, operative cholangiography is performed, although these were at one time considered to be indications for duct exploration:
      (a) Increased size of the common bile duct
      (b) History of jaundice
      (c) Small stones in the gallbladder with a large cystic duct
      (d) A history of cholangitis or pancreatitis
   (4) Common bile duct exploration is not necessary if the operative cholangiogram is of good quality and demonstrates both:
      (a) No filling defects
      (b) Free flow of contrast medium into the duodenum
   (5) Common bile duct exploration is indicated if the operative cholangiogram shows either:
      (a) Filling defects within the intrahepatic or extrahepatic biliary tree
      (b) Obstruction of the flow of bile into the duodenum

   d. Complications. Stones that remain after surgery complicate up to 5%–10% of common bile duct explorations.
   (1) No treatment is necessary for **small stones,** as they usually pass spontaneously.
   (2) Treatment options for **large stones** are:
      (a) Chemical dissolution by intraductal administration of methyl-tert-butyl ether or mono-octanoin
      (b) Mechanical extraction under fluoroscopic guidance
   (3) Primary or recurrent common bile duct stones can be treated surgically with a biliary-enteric connection to allow stones to pass out of the biliary tree. The two most common methods are choledochoduodenostomy or choledochojejunostomy; transduodenal sphincteroplasty or endoscopic sphincterotomy are also acceptable options.

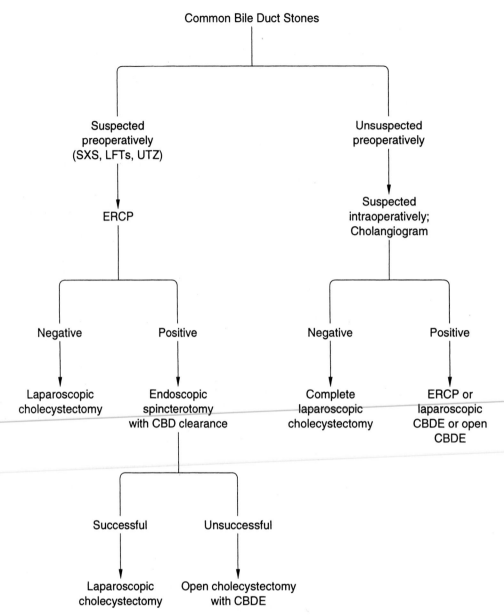

FIGURE 14-15 Algorithm for treatment of common bile duct stones. SXS, symptoms; LFTs, liver function tests; UTZ, ultrasound; ERCP, endoscopic retrograde cholangiopancreatography; CBD, common bile duct; CBDE, common bile duct exploration.

2. **Cholangitis,** or **infection of the bile ducts,** is a potentially life-threatening disease that results from concurrent biliary infection and obstruction. *E. coli* is the most common offending organism.
   a. **Etiology.** Benign postoperative strictures and common bile duct stones account for 60% of the cases. Neoplasms, sclerosing cholangitis, plugged biliary drainage tubes, and biliary contrast studies are other causes.
   b. **Clinical presentation. Charcot's triad** of fever, jaundice, and right upper quadrant pain is present in 70% of cases. In severe cases, hypotension may be present.
   c. **Treatment** includes antibiotics, resuscitation with fluids and electrolytes, and relief of the obstruction.
   d. **Prognosis** depends on the cause of the obstruction; from best prognosis to worst, the order is stones, benign stricture, sclerosing cholangitis, and neoplasm.

3. **Primary sclerosing cholangitis** is a disease of unknown etiology that affects the biliary tract, resulting in stenosis or obstruction of the ductal system. Progressive obstruction, if not relieved, results in biliary cirrhosis and liver failure.

a. **Clinical presentation**

   (1) Symptoms and signs include right upper quadrant pain or painless jaundice, usually without fever or chills, pruritis, fatigue, nausea, and symptoms of hepatic failure.

   (2) Other inflammatory conditions, particularly ulcerative colitis, may be present.

b. **Histology.** The bile ducts show edema and areas of inflammation and fibrosis.

c. **Diagnosis**

   (1) The diagnosis is usually made by ERCP or a transhepatic cholangiogram and occasionally by intraoperative cholangiography.

   (2) Criteria needed to fulfill the diagnosis are:

      (a) Thickening and stenosis of a major portion of the biliary ductal system

      (b) Absence of prior surgery, choledocholithiasis, malignancy, or congenital biliary anomalies

      (c) No evidence of primary liver disease, particularly primary biliary cirrhosis

d. **Treatment.** Operative management is dependent on the level of bile duct involvement and the amount of fibrosis present. Restoration of adequate and permanent biliary drainage is the goal of operative management.

   (1) **Internal biliary drainage,** via either a hepaticoenteric or choledochoenteric anastomosis, is the preferred method of management. This is successful only when the major area of involvement is the extrahepatic bile ducts.

   (2) **External biliary drainage,** using a T tube or other percutaneous stent, establishes adequate drainage initially, but inevitably it becomes contaminated, and the patient may contract bacterial cholangitis.

   (3) Cholecystectomy is performed only when gallbladder disease requires it.

e. **Postoperative treatment** is strongly dependent on the presence of preoperative sepsis and the adequacy of drainage. Steroids are not beneficial and could potentially complicate the postoperative course.

f. **Prognosis** is poorly defined at present. If the liver parenchyma has been damaged or if the intrahepatic ducts are significantly involved, only hepatic transplantation offers a real chance of longevity, and this procedure is only possible when the patient is free of sepsis.

4. **Fibrosis of the sphincter of Oddi** is a disorder of uncertain etiology that causes colicky right upper quadrant pain, nausea, vomiting, and frequently recurrent pancreatitis. Treatment is by endoscopic papillotomy of transduodenal sphincteroplasty.

[G] **Neoplasms**

1. **Benign tumors of the gallbladder** are rare. They include papilloma, adenomyoma, fibroma, lipoma, myoma, myxoma, and carcinoid.

2. **Carcinoma of the gallbladder** accounts for 4% of all carcinomas. It is the most common cancer of the biliary tract and occurs in 1% of all patients undergoing biliary tract surgery.

a. **Etiology.** Although the cause is not known, 90% of the patients have cholelithiasis. About 80% of the tumors are adenocarcinomas. Metastases occur by lymphatic spread to the pancreatic, duodenal, and choledochal nodes and by direct extension to the liver.

b. **Clinical presentation.** The most common complaint is right upper quadrant pain. This is often associated with nausea and vomiting. The diagnosis is rarely made preoperatively. Patients with calcification of the wall of the gallbladder (porcelain gallbladder) that is seen on plain radiograph of the abdomen have a carcinoma of the gallbladder in approximately one half of cases.

c. **Treatment.** The only truly curable cases are those in which the tumor is found incidentally at cholecystectomy for other reasons. If there is microscopic invasion of the gallbladder, cholecystectomy with wedge resection of the liver and regional lymphadenectomy may improve the survival.

d. **Prognosis** is poor: The 5-year survival rate ranges from 0%–10%.

3. **Common bile duct malignant tumors** are rare and difficult to cure.

a. **Clinical presentation**

   (1) The patient usually complains of pruritus, anorexia, weight loss, and an aching right upper quadrant pain. Jaundice is usually severe.

      (2) The following diseases may be associated with this malignancy:
        (a) Sclerosing cholangitis
        (b) Chronic parasitic infection of the bile ducts
        (c) Gallstones (present in 18%–65% of cases)
        (d) Prior exposure to Thorotrast

  b. Diagnosis may be made by percutaneous transhepatic cholangiography or ERCP. Both procedures are capable of biopsy for pathologic examination.

  c. Pathology. These tumors are called *cholangiocarcinoma.*

    (1) The gross pathologic finding is a mass involving a portion of the bile ducts. The microscopic appearance is that of adenocarcinoma, although the distinction from sclerosing cholangitis may be difficult.

    (2) The tumor may be located in the distal common bile duct, the common hepatic duct or cystic duct, or the right or left hepatic duct (most common location). When the confluence of the hepatic ducts is involved, the tumor is termed a **Klatskin tumor.**

    (3) The tumor initially metastasizes to the regional lymph nodes (16% of cases), spreads by direct extension into the liver (14%), or metastasizes to the liver (10%).

  d. Treatment. The management of common bile duct tumors is generally surgical, although fewer than 10% are resectable at the time of the initial diagnosis.

    (1) Tumors in the distal duct may be resected by pancreaticoduodenectomy (Whipple procedure) with biliary and gastrointestinal reconstruction. More proximal lesions can sometimes be locally resected with biliary reconstruction. The average length of survival after resection is 23 months. Postoperative radiation may improve the life expectancy.

    (2) Unresectable lesions should have rigid stents placed to provide palliation of the biliary obstructive symptoms.
      (a) Laparotomy with no bypass is associated with an average survival time of less than 6 months.
      (b) With stenting, the average survival time is 19 months.
        (i) In this procedure, either a transhepatic stent is placed percutaneously or a U tube is placed surgically.
        (ii) The U tube passes from the skin, through the liver, through the tumor, into the common bile duct, and then out through the abdominal wall (Fig. 14-16).

  e. Prognosis

    (1) Metastatic spread of the tumor is usually slow and is not responsible for death.

    (2) The usual cause of death is related to the following:
      (a) Progressive biliary cirrhosis due to inadequate biliary drainage
      (b) Persistent intrahepatic infection and abscess formation
      (c) General debility
      (d) Sepsis

H **Choledochal cysts** are congenital malformations of the pancreaticobiliary tree.

1. Classification (Fig. 14-17)
  a. Type I: fusiform dilatation of the common bile duct
  b. Type II: diverticulum of the common bile duct
  c. Type III: choledochocele involving the intraduodenal portion of the common bile duct
  d. Type IV: cystic involvement of the intrahepatic bile ducts (**Caroli's disease**)

2. The pathogenesis is not known. Pathologically, patients show cystic dilatation of the common bile duct, a normal liver parenchyma and (except in Caroli's disease) a normal intrahepatic biliary tree, and partial obstruction of the terminal common bile duct.

3. Clinical presentation. The most common presenting symptom is intermittent jaundice. The classic triad of pain, jaundice, and an abdominal mass occurs in only 30% of the patients.

4. Diagnosis. Ultrasonography is the best initial investigative study, followed by radionuclide scanning. Transhepatic cholangiography and ERCP can define the extent of the disease but are not necessary.

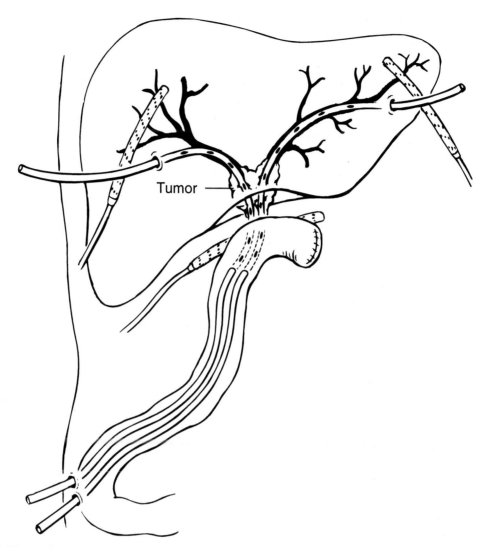

FIGURE 14-16 Transhepatic tubes after hepaticojejunostomy. (Reprinted with permission from Braasch Albert E, Braasch John W. *Atlas of Abdominal Surgery*. Burlington, MA: Lahey Clinic Medical Center; 1991.)

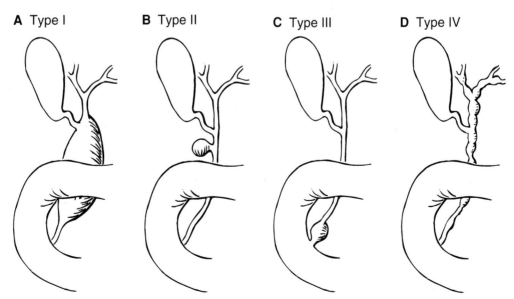

A Type I   **B** Type II   **C** Type III   **D** Type IV

FIGURE 14-17 Biliary cysts. Longmire's modification of Alonso-Lej's classification. (Reprinted with permission from Longmire W. Congenital cystic disease of the liver and biliary system. *Ann Surg*. 1971;174:721.)

5. **Treatment.** Due to the risk of malignancy, cyst excision (rather than bypass) is the cornerstone of surgery.

   a. Type I patients are treated with cholecystectomy, cyst excision, and a Roux-en-Y choledochojejunostomy.

   b. Type II patients are treated by excision of the common bile duct diverticulum.

   c. Type III patients are treated by cyst excision and choledochoduodenostomy or by transduodenal sphincteroplasty.

   d. The type IV anomaly may be fatal. Patients require liver transplantation.

I **Congenital biliary atresia** (see Chapter 29, IX B)

J **Trauma**

1. **Gallbladder injuries** are uncommon but are seen after both penetrating and nonpenetrating trauma. Associated visceral injuries are common and most frequently (72%) involve the liver.

   a. **Types of injuries** to the gallbladder include contusions, avulsion, rupture, and traumatic cholecystitis.

   b. **Clinical presentation.** Right upper quadrant pain, right chest pain, biliary leakage through a penetrating wound, and shock are the most common presenting symptoms.

   c. **Diagnosis** is most frequently made at laparotomy. A peritoneal tap may be negative.

2. **Extrahepatic bile duct injuries**

   a. **Operative injury.** Most extrahepatic bile duct injuries are iatrogenic, occurring during cholecystectomy.

      (1) **Clinical presentation.** Only 15% of intraoperative injuries are diagnosed at the time of surgery, and 85% present days to years later with progressive jaundice, cholangitis, or cirrhosis and its complications.

      (2) **Diagnosis** is by transhepatic cholangiography or ERCP.

      (3) **Treatment.** End-to-end (duct-to-duct) anastomosis may be done at the time of initial injury; otherwise, a Roux-en-Y choledochojejunostomy is necessary.

      (4) **The mortality rate** after repair of a chronic biliary stricture is 8%–10%, and death is usually secondary to liver failure.

   b. **Other extrahepatic bile duct injuries** almost always accompany other visceral injuries and result from trauma, such as gunshot wounds. Isolated bile duct injuries are rare.

      (1) **Clinical presentation** is the same as those in gallbladder injuries.

      (2) **Diagnosis** is made at laparotomy.

      (3) **Treatment,** aside from administration of antibiotics, involves meticulous exploration of the ducts. Either a primary end-to-end (duct-to-duct) anastomosis, or, more commonly, a Roux-en-Y choledochojejunostomy is appropriate. If the patient is unstable, drainage with a T tube is expedient.

   c. **Intraperitoneal extravasation of bile**

      (1) The extravasation of **sterile bile** results in chemical peritonitis.

         (a) This may be a mild peritonitis, producing ascites, or a localized collection.

         (b) Continuous outpouring of sterile bile may produce an extensive chemical peritonitis and shock.

      (2) **Infected intraperitoneal bile** induces a fulminant and frequently fatal peritonitis.

chapter 15

Pancreas

JEROME J. VERNICK • RONALD J. WEIGEL

I ANATOMY

The pancreas (Fig. 15-1) is a retroperitoneal, pistol-shaped organ. The handle of the pistol lies in the duodenal C-loop, and the barrel extends to the left upper quadrant. The average **weight** of the pancreas is 85 g, and the usual **length** is 12–15 cm.

A Relations

1. **The head of the pancreas** lies over the aorta and under the stomach and transverse colon, posteromedially to the inferior vena cava.
   a. The superior limit of the head is the **portal vein.** The anterior limit is the **gastroduodenal artery.**
   b. The **common bile duct** courses posteriorly to the head of the pancreas and partially within it.
   c. The head of the pancreas has a common blood supply with the medial wall of the **duodenal C-loop.** The serosal surface of the duodenum is intimately related to the capsule of the pancreas in that area.
2. The **uncinate process** lies posteriorly to the head of the pancreas and is that portion of the pancreas that is posterior to the portal vein.
3. The **tail of the pancreas** is in close relation to the spleen and most accessory spleens, and it contains the splenic artery (see Chapter 22, I A 3a).
4. The **neck of the pancreas** lies at the confluence of the splenic and inferior mesenteric veins. The **posterior aspect of the pancreas** lies over this confluence at the origin of the portal vein.
5. The **anterior aspect of the pancreas** lies against the posterior wall of the **stomach,** forming the posterior border of the lesser omental bursa, or lesser sac.

B Vasculature

1. The splenic artery and vein provide the **blood supply** to the pancreas. The pancreatic body and tail are related to these vessels, which run posteriorly and superiorly into the hilus of the spleen.
2. The **superior mesenteric artery** and the **superior mesenteric vein** exit below the pancreas at the junction of the body and head and are surrounded by the uncinate process.
3. A replaced right hepatic artery (incidence 25%) or a replaced common hepatic (incidence 2.5%) arising from the superior mesenteric artery can complicate pancreatic surgery and may lead to injuries to these vessels during pancreaticoduodenectomy.

C Functions
The **pancreatic ducts** drain pancreatic secretions into the duodenum. They comprise two separate systems:
1. The **duct of Wirsung,** which empties into the ampulla of Vater in conjunction with the common bile duct, is the major system.
2. The **duct of Santorini,** which empties into a minor papilla approximately 2 cm above and medial to the ampulla of Vater, is the minor system.

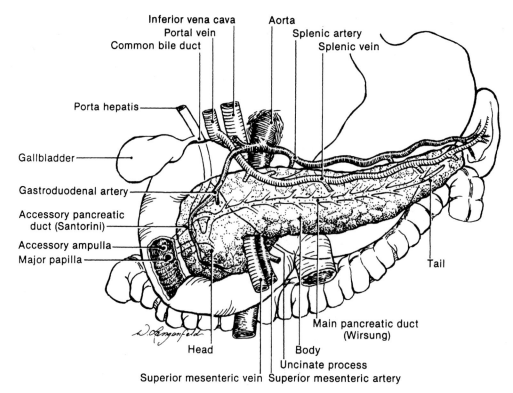

FIGURE 15-1 Anatomy of the pancreas. The normal anteroposterior thickness of the head is less than 2.5 cm; the neck, 1.5 cm; the body, 2 cm; and the tail, 2.5 cm.

II PANCREATITIS

Pancreatitis is an inflammatory process in the pancreas.

A **Classification** Pancreatitis is divided into four categories to clarify the different syndromes that are found and to improve the standardization of treatment and prognosis.

1. **Acute pancreatitis** arises in a previously asymptomatic patient and subsides with appropriate treatment. Acute pancreatitis can involve other regional tissues or remote organ systems. The International Symposium on Acute Pancreatitis produced a clinically based classification:
   a. **Severe acute pancreatitis**
   b. **Mild acute pancreatitis**
   c. **Acute fluid collection**
   d. **Pancreatic necrosis**
   e. **Acute pseudocysts**
   f. **Pancreatic abscess**

2. **Acute relapsing pancreatitis** is a series of recurrent episodes of acute pancreatitis in an otherwise asymptomatic patient. A quiescent, asymptomatic phase always precedes and follows each attack.

3. **Chronic relapsing pancreatitis** is a chronic inflammation of the pancreas with chemical evidence of pancreatitis, which fluctuates in its intensity without a period of resolution.

4. **Chronic pancreatitis** shows unrelenting symptoms that are due to inflammation and fibrosis of the pancreas; the pancreatic duct and parenchyma usually show calcification. Chronic pancreatitis is often associated with malabsorption and even with pancreatic endocrine insufficiency (diabetes).

B **Etiology** Approximately 75% of pancreatitis cases can be explained on the basis of biliary tract disease or alcohol abuse, although the exact mechanism for the production of pancreatitis remains theoretical.

1. **Gallstone pancreatitis** is thought to be induced by the inflammation that results from continued passage of stones into the common bile duct. Most often, the gallstone has passed by the time the patient is studied.
   a. The pancreatic duct and the bile duct empty into a common papilla, which is subject to trauma in a patient with biliary calculi.
   b. The entire common channel can be obstructed if a large calculus becomes impacted in the papilla, and this situation can cause reflux of bile into the pancreatic duct. Experiments have shown that such reflux can induce pancreatitis. However, it is unclear whether this reflux actually occurs in humans.

2. **Alcohol-induced pancreatitis** may be the result of various mechanisms. Alcohol has been implicated in the direct damage of acinar cells and the increase of the concentration of enzymes in pancreatic secretion. High protein concentration with calcium carbonate precipitation in the protein-filled spaces encourages the development of stones. The resultant multifocal ductal obstruction and increased intraductal pressure along with increased permeability caused by alcohol destroys parenchyma and leads to inflammation and fibrosis.

3. **Congenital abnormalities and hereditary pancreatitis.** Duct strictures, pancreas divisum, cystic fibrosis, and various metabolic disorders (e.g., hypertriglyceridemia) are implicated as contributing factors in a small percentage of cases.

4. **Iatrogenic.** Pancreatitis can be caused by instrumentation (e.g., endoscopic retrograde cholangiopancreatography [ERCP]) or certain drugs.

C Acute pancreatitis

1. **Clinical presentation** of acute pancreatitis may vary from mild abdominal discomfort to profound shock with hypotension and hypoxemia. Usually the patient presents with epigastric pain that radiates to the back and is associated with nausea and vomiting. Findings vary with the severity of the inflammatory process.
   a. Most patients have mild-to-moderate abdominal tenderness.
   b. In severe cases, a rigid abdomen with epigastric guarding, rebound tenderness, and marked abdominal pain may be present.
   c. Severe pancreatic inflammation and necrosis may cause **retroperitoneal hemorrhage,** which can lead to large third-space fluid losses, hypovolemia, hypotension, tachycardia, and shock with blood dissection (i.e., the blood extravasates and forces its way between tissue planes).
      (1) When blood dissection extends to the flank tissues, resulting in flank ecchymoses, it is known as **Turner's sign.**
      (2) When blood dissects up the falciform ligament and creates a periumbilical ecchymosis, it is known as **Cullen's sign.**

2. **History.** Often the patient mentions recent consumption of a heavy meal, many times with generous quantities of alcoholic beverages. The pain typically begins 1–4 hours after a meal and is often less severe when the patient is slumped forward.

3. **Diagnosis** of acute pancreatitis is aided by the following studies:
   a. **Serum amylase level.** This level is increased in 95% of patients with acute pancreatitis.
      (1) Approximately 5% of all amylase determinations are falsely positive, and only 75% of patients with abdominal pain and an increased amylase level have pancreatitis.
      (2) The increase in amylase level is not proportional to the severity of the pancreatitis. Some inferences, however, can be made from the degree of increase.
         (a) An amylase level higher than 1,000 Somogyi units usually indicates gallstone pancreatitis.
         (b) An amylase level between 200 and 500 Somogyi units often indicates alcoholic pancreatitis. Approximately 17% of patients with amylase levels in this range have no other evidence of pancreatitis.
      (3) The pancreas must be intact and functional to synthesize amylase and release it into the circulation. Therefore, patients with acute pancreatitis superimposed on chronic pancreatitis may not show an increase in serum amylase.
      (4) A significant amount of circulating amylase is not of pancreatic origin. The major alternative source is the salivary glands.
      (5) An elevated **lipase** is also seen in pancreatitis.

b. Amylase:creatinine clearance ratio. Amylase determinations are more sensitive identifiers when the amylase clearance rate is compared with the creatinine clearance rate and a ratio is established.

(1) An amylase:creatinine clearance ratio higher than 5 is strongly suggestive of pancreatitis.

(2) Using this ratio avoids the problem of rapid renal clearance of amylase, which tends to reduce serum levels below the point where a simple serum amylase determination would be positive.

(3) Impaired renal function affects the creatinine clearance rate sooner than the amylase clearance rate. Even in this situation, however, the amylase:creatinine clearance ratio appears to be more sensitive than the serum amylase level if urine specimens are collected for at least 1 hour.

c. Radiographic imaging

(1) **Plain films** of the upper abdomen are relatively insensitive with regard to diagnosing pancreatitis. Significant findings include the following:

(a) Calcification in the area of the lesser sac and pancreas may indicate chronic pancreatitis, which is most often found in association with alcoholism.

(b) A gas collection in the lesser sac suggests abscess formation in or around the pancreas.

(c) Blurred psoas shadows from retroperitoneal pancreatic necrosis and fluid in the retroperitoneum may be found on plain films.

(d) Soft tissue shadows and gas-containing viscera may be visibly displaced by collections and edema in the lesser sac and structures adjacent to the pancreas.

(e) An area of colonic spasm adjacent to an inflamed pancreas causes the gas in the transverse colon to end abruptly (the **"cutoff" sign**).

(f) Focal duodenal and jejunal ileus in the area of the pancreas can cause the **reversed 3, or inverted 3 sign.**

(2) **Barium studies** may show upper gastrointestinal (GI) abnormalities.

(a) The duodenal C-loop may be widened by pancreatic edema.

(b) Hypotonic duodenography may show the **"pad" sign,** a smoothing out or obliteration of the duodenal mucosal folds by the edematous pancreas and the inflammatory response on the medial aspect of the C-loop.

(3) **Angiography** is useful for delineating pancreatic and hepatic blood supply before radical surgery. Diagnostic aspects have been superseded by spiral computed tomography (CT) scan and magnetic resonance (MR) imaging.

d. Ultrasound (US) imaging of the pancreas is especially useful in the diagnosis of pancreatitis.

(1) **Changes** in the normal anatomy of the pancreas and its vascular landmarks **can be delineated.**

(a) Acute pancreatitis is suggested by swelling that is greater than the normal anteroposterior thickness and loss of tissue planes between the pancreas and the splenic vein.

(b) Other anomalies of the pancreas may also be found (e.g., a change in duct size or calcification).

(c) Chronic pancreatitis is often manifested by the presence of calcification or pseudocysts containing fluid or showing a complex cystic structure.

(d) Ascites, which is easily diagnosed by US, may or may not be present in chronic pancreatitis.

(2) Various pancreatic disorders can change the US echogenicity.

(a) Most diseases decrease the echogenicity in the pancreas because they include edema and inflammation. Tumors are also often hypoechogenic.

(b) Increased echogenicity is generally due to gas or calcification.

(3) **Fluid densities** lying within the pancreas indicate cysts, abscesses, or possibly lymphoma.

(4) **Cholelithiasis** may be identified, suggesting gallstone pancreatitis. US may also show the presence of cholecystitis or a dilated common bile duct.

(5) US has a major **limitation** in that it cannot be performed when excessive bowel gas is present, as occurs with an ileus.

e. CT scan of the pancreas is **extremely** helpful. It provides higher resolution than US, and it is not limited by the masking effect of intestinal gas. The improvements in availability, speed,

(3) Peritoneal lavage can be useful in excluding other severe intra-abdominal processes and can be therapeutic in severe pancreatitis. However, peritoneal lavage appears to improve early mortality rates but not ultimate survival rates in acute severe pancreatitis.

(a) **Catheters** can be placed percutaneously, and antibiotics can be included in the lavage solution.

(b) Peritoneal lavage can be undertaken as part of a **laparotomy** performed for diagnosis and lesser sac exploration.

(c) **Complications** include a deterioration of pulmonary function, which can be compromised by abdominal distention from the dialysis solutions. A high glucose load in the dialysis solution can induce severe hyperglycemia.

D **Relapsing pancreatitis** frequently occurs in nonalcoholic patients and results from biliary tract disease—either calculi in the ducts or inflammation and spasm of the sphincter of Oddi.

1. **Diagnosis** of relapsing pancreatitis can be made by demonstrating the presence of biliary stones or biliary sphincter dysfunction.

a. **US** (see II C 3 d) is useful for diagnosing biliary calculi.

b. **Microscopic examination of the bile** is also useful.

(1) Bile is aspirated through a suction tube placed in the duodenum.

(2) The bile is examined for white blood cells (WBC), cholesterol crystals, and microspheroliths.

(3) These signs of occult biliary disease are an indication for cholecystectomy.

c. **Provocative testing** (i.e., the **Nardi test**) can show whether narcotic-induced stimulation or spasm will reproduce the abdominal pain and amylase increase.

(1) Morphine and neostigmine are given intramuscularly, and baseline levels are obtained for glutamine-oxaloacetic transaminase and glutamic-pyruvic transaminase, γ-glutamyl transferase, amylase, and lipase.

(2) Determinations are repeated hourly for 4 hours, and a final determination is made at 8 hours.

(3) The test is positive if biliary pain is reproduced within 15–20 minutes after the injection and if the enzyme levels increase at least four times the baseline levels.

(4) In the presence of sphincteric disease, the following situations occur:

(a) Amylase levels increase whether or not the gallbladder is present.

(b) Liver-related enzymes do not increase if the gallbladder is present and can distend to relieve pressure on the hepatic ductal system.

(c) The Nardi test can, therefore, be used to infer sphincteric disease in any pancreatic or biliary ductal system without a gallbladder.

(5) Although the test is controversial, it has been accurate in the diagnosis of perisphincteric disease. The test is not in common use.

(6) At the time of surgery, the test results can be confirmed by measuring the pressure and flow in the common bile duct.

d. **US observation** of duct dilatation after secretin administration has shown promise in the diagnosis of sphincteric disease.

2. **Treatment** of relapsing pancreatitis is based on the cause.

a. In a patient with biliary calculi, the following procedures can be performed:

(1) Cholecystectomy

(2) Common bile duct exploration

(3) Biliary manometry

(4) Sphincteroplasty plus pancreaticobiliary septum resection

b. The **treatment of perisphincteric disease** is removal of the gallbladder and a wide sphincteroplasty that includes the pancreaticobiliary septum. The results have been very good in patients who have had a positive Nardi test.

c. Many patients have had a cholecystectomy, yet continue to have recurrent pancreatitis, biliary tract disease symptoms, or both.

(1) These patients often have a positive provocative test and can be treated successfully by sphincteroplasty.

(2) Patients who have had negative provocative test require further workup, including ERCP [see III A 3 b]. Alcohol abuse should be ruled out.

d. Patients with severe intrinsic pancreatic disease respond poorly to sphincteroplasty.

E **Chronic pancreatitis** is often progressive.

1. **Pathologic findings** include fibrosis and calcification throughout the gland.

   a. Early pancreatic changes may consist of plugging of the small pancreatic ducts with proteinaceous material containing eosinophils.

   b. With progression of the disease, the calcification becomes prominent, and multiple areas of ductal dilatation can result.

   c. The ductal dilatation in its end stages produces a "chain-of-lakes" appearance.

   d. Common bile duct obstruction or duodenal obstruction can occur in advanced cases of chronic pancreatitis as a result of inflammation in surrounding areas.

2. **The cause** is almost always alcohol related. However, certain congenital anomalies can produce chronic ductal obstruction and chronic pancreatitis.

3. **Clinical presentation**

   a. A history of unrelenting pain is usual in advanced cases of chronic pancreatitis. The pain is usually the major indication for surgical intervention.

   b. Pancreatic damage may be severe enough to cause pancreatic endocrine insufficiency, with impaired glucose tolerance or true diabetes.

   c. Exocrine pancreatic insufficiency results in malabsorption, with consequent weight loss and steatorrhea.

   d. Plain films may show the calcifications in the ductal system or may aid in delineating neighboring areas that are caught in the inflammatory process.

   e. Severe disease in the head of the pancreas can mimic carcinoma and cause bile duct obstruction.

   f. Chronic pancreatitis can cause **splenic vein thrombosis** that may be a cause for upper GI bleeding.

4. **Medical treatment**

   a. Analgesia

   b. Endocrine replacement as needed

   c. Exocrine replacement with pancreatic enzymes, such as pancrelipase (Viokase or Pancrease) or pancreozymin. High-dose pancreatic enzymes (i.e., 5 g four times daily) can suppress pancreatic secretion by the feedback phenomenon.

   d. General measures, such as avoidance of alcoholic beverages and correction of malnutrition

5. **Surgical treatment** of chronic pancreatitis depends on the condition of the pancreatic ducts, as determined by ERCP. If ERCP is not possible and the patient must undergo an operation, pancreatograms can be obtained.

   a. **Puestow operation** (Fig. 15-2). A dilated chain-of-lakes duct is treated by wide unroofing of the duct and dilated ductules, with drainage of the entire open pancreas into a defunctionalized jejunal loop. A side-to-side procedure may be used, or the surgeon may choose an invagination in which the pancreas is placed into the jejunal loop.

   b. **Distal pancreatectomy** is used to treat a distal ductal obstruction.

   c. **Duval operation** (Fig. 15-2). A proximal ductal obstruction can be treated by amputating the tail of the pancreas and draining the pancreas retrogradely into a defunctionalized jejunal loop. This is a simple operation and is not as effective or long lasting as lateral pancreaticojejunostomy.

   d. For a patient with severe pain and a fibrotic, nondilated duct, possible surgical procedures include:

      (1) **Child operation** (Fig. 15-2), which is a 95% pancreatectomy

      (2) **Splanchnicectomy,** either abdominal or thoracic

         (a) This procedure merely divides the splanchnic nerves and serves only to relieve the pain of pancreatitis, with no direct effect on the underlying disorder.

         (b) A splanchnicectomy also eradicates the pain from appendicitis and other intra-abdominal problems, which may lead to the delayed diagnosis of an abdominal emergency.

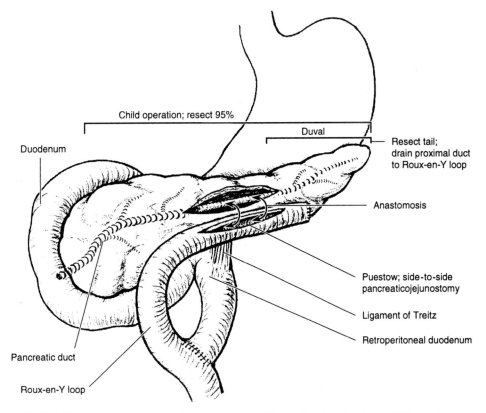

Child operation; resect 95%

Duodenum

Duval

Resect tail;
drain proximal duct
to Roux-en-Y loop

Anastomosis

Puestow; side-to-side
pancreaticojejunostomy

Ligament of Treitz

Retroperitoneal duodenum

Pancreatic duct

Roux-en-Y loop

FIGURE 15-2 Surgical treatments for chronic pancreatitis: the Puestow, Duval, and Child operations.

(3) Duodenum-sparing pancreatic head resection. This approach has become a popular option for patients who have had failed sphincteroplasties.

F **Pseudocyst** is a late complication of pancreatitis.

1. **Pathologic findings**
   a. The pseudocyst begins as a lesser sac collection and forms as a result of fibrosis, thickening, and organization of the organs bordering the collection.
   b. The pseudocyst is **not lined by epithelium** and consists only of the inflammatory response of the neighboring organs.
   c. The organs forming the walls are the stomach, duodenum, colon, and transverse mesocolon. The major organ involved is generally the stomach, which forms the anterior surface of the pseudocyst.
   d. Maturation of the pseudocyst takes 3–5 weeks. It is not truly formed until the walls are sufficiently organized to become firm anatomic structures.
   e. The natural history of the pseudocyst depends on its size. Small pseudocysts may resolve; large pseudocysts with mature organized walls generally do not resolve.

2. **Clinical presentation**
   a. During the maturation phase, the patient recovers from a bout of pancreatitis but develops a persistent increase of amylase, a low-grade fever, a minimally increased WBC count, and chronic pain.
   b. Continuous minor bleeding into the pseudocyst tends to cause a gradual decrease in hemoglobin and hematocrit. More significant bleeds are associated with acute abdominal pain or hemorrhagic shock. Bleeding into a pseudocyst is an indication for surgical intervention.
   c. Pseudocysts are usually diagnosed by US or CT scan.

3. **Treatment**
   a. The **goal** is to allow the maturation phase to continue until the walls of the pseudocyst have matured.

(1) The patient is generally treated with total parenteral nutrition (TPN) or an elemental diet for 3–4 weeks, until maturation has occurred. Prematurely starting the patient on a full diet is likely to cause an exacerbation of the pancreatitis.

(2) Maturation-phase treatment sometimes must be cut short because of sepsis or hemorrhage within the pseudocyst.

(3) Small pseudocysts may resolve with medical treatment.

b. **Surgical treatment of mature pseudocysts**

(1) **Internal drainage,** if possible

(a) The best approach is through the anterior wall of the stomach to locate the firm connection that usually exists between the posterior stomach and the pseudocyst.

(i) The first step is to **aspirate the cyst** through the wall of the stomach. After aspirating the cyst, an opening is made between the stomach and the pseudocyst, and the wall of the opening is sutured for hemostasis.

(ii) The pseudocyst then drains into the stomach and generally resolves.

(b) If the pseudocyst is not fixed to an organ that lends itself to internal drainage, a defunctionalized (Roux-en-Y) loop of jejunum may be sutured to the pseudocyst wall to establish internal drainage.

(2) **External drainage** is used if the pseudocyst is not found to be mature and if suturing of the pseudocyst wall is not safe. The external drainage results in a pancreatic fistula, which usually heals with continued TPN.

(3) **Excision** of a pseudocyst is rare; however, this removal may be indicated if the pseudocyst is small and is located distally in the tail of the pancreas.

III PANCREATIC MALIGNANCIES

A Pancreatic adenocarcinoma

1. The **incidence** of pancreatic adenocarcinoma is rapidly increasing, especially in men.

a. It is now the fourth most common cause of cancer death in the United States.

b. It accounts for approximately 30,000 fatalities annually, according to the American Cancer Society estimate for 2003. The annual death rates for pancreatic cancer is equal to the annual incidence of the disease.

c. Increased risk is associated with multiple environmental factors, including tobacco use and some dietary and occupational exposures. Hereditary factors include familial cancer and polyposis syndromes. Diabetes and chronic pancreatitis are possible increased risk factors.

d. The tumor occurs most often in people who are between 50 and 70 years of age and has increased incidence among blacks, males, and those of Jewish descent.

2. **Clinical presentation**

a. **Early symptoms** are usually vague (e.g., epigastric pain, weight loss, backache, and depression).

b. **Thrombophlebitis** may be the initial presentation. It is migratory and ultimately develops in as many as 10% of patients.

c. The **symptoms at the time of presentation** are related to the **location of the tumor** within the pancreas.

(1) The **head of the pancreas** is the most common site. Tumors here produce weight loss and obstructive jaundice in 75% of patients.

(a) The jaundice is painless, although back pain or vague abdominal discomfort may be present in up to 25% of patients at this stage.

(b) Because of the retroperitoneal location of the pancreas, tumors must be very large or metastatic to become evident on physical examination. However, an upper abdominal mass may be palpable.

(i) It represents the tumor mass in as many as 20% of patients and indicates incurability.

(ii) If the mass represents an enlarged, nontender gallbladder (**Courvoisier's gallbladder**), the cause is most commonly an obstructing pancreatic neoplasm, but the gallbladder is palpable in fewer than 50% of patients.

(2) Carcinomas of the **body or tail of the pancreas** are less common and generally present at a more advanced stage because only about 10% produce obstructive jaundice.

3. **Diagnosis.** Routine screening of asymptomatic populations is currently not feasible. Progress in serologic testing for tumor markers provides hope for the future. Definitive diagnosis requires at least a minimally invasive procedure.

   a. **Percutaneous fine-needle aspiration,** which is a highly reliable technique to diagnose a malignancy, uses US or CT scanning to direct a small-bore needle to a mass. A cytologic specimen is obtained. **This technique should not be used when lesions are potentially resectable.**

   b. **ERCP** uses a flexible duodenoscope to cannulate the pancreatic duct. Contrast medium is injected, and radiographs are taken.

      (1) Small pancreatic cancers can be found using this technique, and specimens can be collected from the pancreatic duct for cytologic examination.

      (2) Successful cannulation requires a highly skilled endoscopist. A stent is usually placed to relieve the biliary obstruction.

      (3) **Endoscopic US** can be combined with other endoscopic procedures. This provides very high resolution of small lesions and can allow transduodenal needle biopsies without the risk of peritoneal seeding.

   c. **Percutaneous transhepatic cholangiography** is useful in the evaluation of patients who have obstructive jaundice.

      (1) With the patient under local anesthesia, a long small-bore needle is inserted through the liver into a dilated hepatic duct, and contrast medium is injected to identify the site of obstruction.

      (2) Jaundice is relieved preoperatively by passing a catheter through the site of obstruction, because very high bilirubin levels can be associated with an increased risk of postoperative complications.

      (3) Potential complications of the procedure include bleeding from the needle track in the liver and sepsis.

4. **Treatment**

   a. **Pancreaticoduodenectomy (Whipple procedure)** is the standard surgical treatment for adenocarcinoma of the head of the pancreas when the lesion is curable by resection. Many patients can be deemed unresectable, as evidenced by metastatic disease identified by abdominal imaging and confirmed by percutaneous biopsy.

      (1) **Resectability** is determined at surgery from several criteria:

         (a) There are no metastases outside the abdomen.

         (b) The tumor has not involved the porta hepatis, the portal vein as it passes behind the body of the pancreas, and the superior mesenteric artery region.

         (c) The tumor has not spread to the liver or other peritoneal structures.

         (d) **Laparoscopy** is receiving increased use to rule out peritoneal seeding before proceeding with laparotomy. This is especially indicated in tumors involving the body and tail of the pancreas and in patients with a CA 19-9 level >400.

      (2) Histologic **proof of malignancy** is obtained by needle aspiration, either before or during surgery. A tru-cut biopsy can be performed through the duodenum after a Kocher maneuver.

      (3) The **Whipple procedure** (Fig. 15-3) involves removal of the head of the pancreas, duodenum, distal common bile duct, gallbladder, and distal stomach.

         (a) The GI tract is then reconstructed with creation of a gastrojejunostomy, choledochojejunostomy, and pancreaticojejunostomy.

         (b) The operative mortality rate with this extensive operation can be as high as 15% but should be 2% or lower in centers where this surgery is frequently performed. According to recent publications, the lower mortality rate is realized in institutions doing at least five pancreaticoduodenectomies per year.

         (c) The complication rate is also considerable, the most common complications being hemorrhage, abscess, and pancreatic ductal leakage.

   b. **Distal pancreatectomy,** usually with splenectomy and lymphadenectomy, is the procedure performed for carcinoma of the midbody and tail of the pancreas. Staging for this procedure

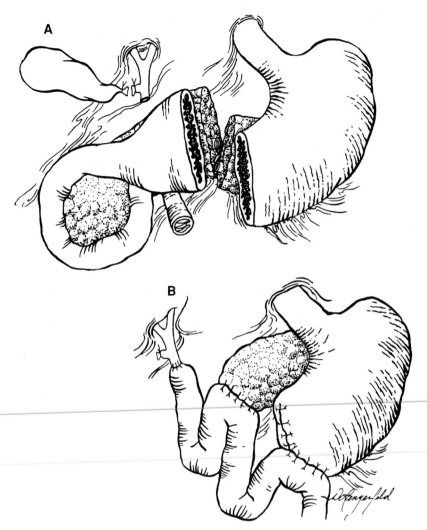

FIGURE 15-3   Whipple procedure. **A,** the head of the pancreas, distal common bile duct, gastric antrum and duodenum are removed. **B,** the GI tract, pancreatic duct and bile duct are reconstructed.

should include **laparoscopy.** Distal pancreatectomy is often performed for benign mucinous pancreatic tumors or occassionally a cystic pancreatic cancer.

  c. Total pancreatectomy has been proposed for the treatment of pancreatic cancer.
    (**1**) The procedure has two potential advantages:
      (**a**) Removal of a possible multicentric tumor (present in up to 40% of patients)
      (**b**) Avoidance of pancreatic duct anastomotic leaks
    (**2**) However, survival rates are not markedly better, and the operation has not been widely adopted.
    (**3**) In addition, it has resulted in a particularly brittle type of diabetes, making for an unpleasant postoperative life.

  d. Palliative procedures are performed more frequently than curative ones because so many of these tumors are incurable.
    (**1**) Palliative procedures attempt to relieve biliary obstruction by using either the common bile duct or the gallbladder as a conduit for decompression into the intestinal tract.
    (**2**) As many 20% of patients may require further surgery for gastric outlet obstruction if a gastric bypass procedure is not performed initially. Therefore, many centers combine a gastrojejunostomy with choledochojejunostomy as the initial procedure.
    (**3**) Percutaneous transhepatic biliary stents can sometimes be used to provide internal biliary drainage for obstructive jaundice, thereby avoiding a major operative procedure.

    e. Chemotherapy has been used in the treatment of pancreatic adenocarcinoma. Multidrug regimens that include 5-fluorouracil have produced a response (temporary tumor regression or, rarely, cure) in about 20%–25% of patients with metastases. New agents including gemcitabine have added to the palliative armamentarium.

    f. Combination treatment of pancreatic adenocarcinoma has been used experimentally to improve local control and to prevent metastases. Intraoperative radiotherapy is today's treatment. Results are encouraging, with a median survival of 9 months with unresectable disease.

5. Prognosis

    a. The prognosis for patients with pancreatic adenocarcinoma is extremely poor.

        (1) Overall, the 5-year survival rate is less than 5%, and cures are extremely rare. Most patients die in less than 1 year.

        (2) The median length of survival for patients with unresectable tumors is 6 months.

        (3) Even for those few patients with resectable tumors, results of surgery are not good. Only about 20% of patients who undergo resection will live 5 years.

    b. The poor prognosis is due in part to the difficulty in making a diagnosis while the tumor is at an early stage: Only about 10% of pancreatic adenocarcinomas are resectable at the time of diagnosis.

B **Other pancreatic malignancies** are infrequent. They include cystadenocarcinomas (which typically occur in women); nonfunctional islet cell tumors; and peptide-producing tumors, such as insulinomas and Zollinger-Ellison tumors (gastrinomas) (see Chapter 17, II A 2 b).

CRITICAL POINTS

Acute Pancreatitis

1. Suspected in patients with abdominal pain and elevated serum amylase and lipase.

2. Dynamic CT is used to confirm diagnosis and to evaluate anatomy and extent of necrosis.

3. Admit patient, keep nothing by mouth (NPO), manage fluid requirements, and assess for complications of pancreatic abscess or bleeding.

4. For gallstone pancreatitis, cholecystectomy after resolution of symptoms and amylase normal.

Chronic Pancreatitis

1. Fibrosis of gland is associated with alcoholism.

2. Medical management of pain, diabetes, and pancreatic enzymes.

3. Surgical treatment is based on duct anatomy, including Peustow (for chain of lakes), distal pancreatectomy, or Duval (distal obstruction).

4. Pseudocysts can occur (or as sequela of acute pancreatitis) and require drainage procedure for continued symptoms or bleeding.

Pancreatic Cancer

1. Very poor prognosis. Fourth leading cause of cancer death in the United States.

2. Patients who present with painless jaundice are usually the only ones considered for curative resection.

3. CT and ERCP are used to establish diagnosis and stent biliary obstruction

4. Consider pancreaticoduodenectomy (Whipple) in patients without evidence of distant spread.

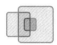

Study Questions for Part IV

Directions: *Each of the numbered items in this section is followed by several possible answers. Select the ONE lettered answer that is BEST in each case.*

1. A 15-year-old boy is admitted with a history and physical findings consistent with appendicitis. Which finding is most likely to be positive?

- [A] Pelvic crepitus
- [B] Iliopsoas sign
- [C] Murphy sign
- [D] Flank ecchymosis
- [E] Periumbilical ecchymosis

2. A 50-year-old man is admitted with massive bright red rectal bleeding. He recently had a barium enema that demonstrated no diverticular or space-occupying lesion. Nasogastric suction reveals no blood but does produce yellow bile. The patient continues to bleed. What is the next diagnostic step?

- [A] Repeat barium enema
- [B] Colonoscopy
- [C] Upper gastrointestinal series
- [D] Mesenteric angiography
- [E] Small bowel follow-through with barium

3. A 15-year-old boy awakens with sudden onset of right lower quadrant and scrotal tenderness accompanied by nausea and vomiting. Which of the following is the most appropriate diagnosis and represents a surgical emergency?

- [A] Acute prostatitis
- [B] Acute epididymitis
- [C] Torsion of the testicle
- [D] Acute appendicitis
- [E] Gastroenteritis

4. A 47-year-old woman presents with dysphagia to both solids and liquids equally. She has experienced a 10-kg weight loss over the last several months. A barium swallow reveals a birdlike narrowing in the distal esophagus. What is the underlying cause of her symptoms?

- [A] Disorganized, strong nonperistaltic contractions in the esophagus
- [B] Failure of the lower esophageal sphincter to relax
- [C] Hiatal hernia
- [D] Barrett's esophagus
- [E] Esophageal stricture secondary to untreated gastroesophageal reflux

5. A 45-year-old male executive is seen because he is vomiting bright red blood. There are no previous symptoms. The man admits to one drink a week and has no other significant history. In the hospital, he bleeds five units of blood before endoscopy. What is the most likely diagnosis?

- [A] Gastritis
- [B] Duodenal ulcer
- [C] Esophagitis
- [D] Mallory-Weiss tear
- [E] Esophageal varices

6. Massive bleeding from the lower gastrointestinal tract is occurring in a 55-year-old man who is otherwise healthy. After continued bleeding equivalent to one unit of blood, what should be the initial management?

- [A] Emergency laparotomy and total colectomy and ileoproctostomy
- [B] Emergency laparotomy and colostomy with operative endoscopy

C Arteriography to identify the bleeding site after anoscopy and sigmoidoscopy have ruled out a distal site

D Infusion of vitamin K and fresh frozen plasma

E Colonic irrigation with iced saline solution

QUESTIONS 7–8

A 45-year-old man is seen in the emergency department after vomiting bright red blood. He has no previous symptoms. He drinks one alcoholic beverage a day.

7. What is the most reliable method for locating the lesion responsible for the bleeding?

A Upper gastrointestinal series

B Exploratory laparotomy

C Upper endoscopy

D Arteriography

E Radionuclide scanning

8. After several hours in the hospital, he begins to have recurrent bleeding. He is transferred to a critical care bed and is persistently hypotensive despite trasnfusion of nine units of packed red blood cells. Which is the most appropriate next step in management of this patient?

A Upper endoscopy with attempt at cauterization of bleeding

B Transport to the interventional radiology unit to identify and embolize bleeding source

C Placement of a Blakemore tube to temporarily tamponade bleeding and to allow for stabilization of blood pressure

D Laparotomy to control bleeding

E Infusion of vasopressin and additional units of blood

9. A 45-year-old woman who has had a hysterectomy presents to the emergency department with abdominal pain and vomiting. A mechanical small bowel obstruction is seen on the abdominal radiograph. What is the most likely cause for this obstruction?

A Carcinoma of the colon

B Small bowel cancer

C Adhesions

D Incarcerated inguinal hernia

E Diverticulitis

10. A 25-year-old man is admitted with a history of sudden onset of severe midepigastric abdominal pain. Upright chest radiograph reveals free intraperitoneal air. What is the therapy for this patient?

A Upper endoscopy

B Barium swallow

C Gastrografin swallow

D Observation

E Laparotomy

11. An 80-year-old male patient is referred for dysphagia with reflux of undigested food. The patient occasionally notices a bulging in his left neck. Which of the following is the most appropriate definitive treatment?

A Barium swallow

B Upper endoscopy

C Cricopharyngeal myotomy

D Computed tomography (CT) scan of the chest

E Liquid diet

12. A 42-year-old female patient is diagnosed with gastroesophageal reflux and is started on medical therapy. Which of the following would be an indication for surgical antireflux procedure?

- [A] Development of esophageal stricture(s)
- [B] Barrett's esophagus with severe dysplasia
- [C] Esophagitis by biopsy
- [D] High lower esophageal sphincter pressure demonstrated by esophageal manometry
- [E] Slow and uncoordinated swallowing by barium study

13. A 75-year-old male patient presents to the emergency room 2 hours after developing severe chest pain with repeated episodes of vomiting. He is tachycardic and febrile. A chest radiograph demonstrates a left pleural effusion. Emergent barium swallow reveals extravasation of contrast into the left chest. Proper definitive treatment of this patient would include which of the following?

- [A] Observation
- [B] Emergent surgical intervention
- [C] Placement of left chest tube
- [D] Intravenous antibiotics and admission to the hospital
- [E] Upper endoscopy

QUESTIONS 14–15

A 65-year-old patient has been treated with pharmacologic therapy for an antral gastric ulcer for 12 weeks. A repeat upper gastrointestinal series shows approximately 50% shrinkage of the ulcer.

14. What further management should the patient undergo at this time?

- [A] Continued pharmacologic therapy with a repeat upper gastrointestinal series in 8–12 weeks
- [B] A change in pharmacologic therapy with a repeat upper gastrointestinal series in 12 weeks
- [C] An upper endoscopy with multiple biopsies
- [D] Total gastrectomy
- [E] Surgery with limited excision of the ulcer

After further diagnostic work-up, the patient is found to have a gastric adenocarcinoma. Metastatic work-up is negative.

15. Therapy with curative intent would involve which of the following?

- [A] Radiation therapy followed by chemotherapy alone
- [B] Distal gastrectomy followed by adjuvant chemoradiotherapy
- [C] Total gastrectomy
- [D] Total gastrectomy and splenectomy
- [E] Local excision of the ulcer with clear margins followed by radiotherapy

16. Which of the following statements is true about the performance of a parietal cell vagotomy?

- [A] It divides the vagus nerve at the gastroesophageal junction.
- [B] It maintains innervation of the pylorus so that a drainage procedure is not required.
- [C] The recurrence rate is less than 5%.
- [D] It cannot be performed laparoscopically.
- [E] It is contraindicated for bleeding or perforated ulcers.

17. What innerves the stomach resulting in parietal cell secretion and gastrin release?

- [A] Phrenic nerve
- [B] Vagus nerve
- [C] Greater splanchnic nerves

    ⊡ D ⊡ Celiac ganglion
    ⊡ E ⊡ T4 root

18. Which of the following is true regarding intestinal absorption of nutrients?

    ⊡ A ⊡ Bile or bile salts are essential for absorption of vitamin B_{12}.
    ⊡ B ⊡ An iron-deficient individual can absorb up to 80% of dietary iron.
    ⊡ C ⊡ Parathormone increases the intestinal absorption of dietary calcium.
    ⊡ D ⊡ Intestinal epithelial cells resynthesize triglycerides before their release into the portal circulation.
    ⊡ E ⊡ Triglycerides are absorbed intact in a bile salt micelle-dependent process.

QUESTIONS 19–20

A previously healthy 43-year-old man presents with a 6-month history of nonbloody diarrhea, fever, and 10-pound weight loss and now develops urosepsis. On evaluation, an enterovesical fistula (from the ileum to the bladder) is found. At laparotomy, findings include inflammation and "fat wrapping" of three separate segments of ileum. Each segment is approximately 20 cm in length and is separated by less than 20-cm segments of normal-appearing bowel (skip areas). The distal-most of the three segments is more severely inflamed than the others and involves the terminal ileum all the way to the cecum. This segment of ileum is densely adherent to the right superior aspect of the bladder.

19. Which of the following is true?

    ⊡ A ⊡ All of the abnormal-appearing bowel should be resected.
    ⊡ B ⊡ This patient has complications of Meckel's diverticulitis.
    ⊡ C ⊡ All of the bladder wall involved in the inflammatory process must be removed.
    ⊡ D ⊡ Extensive resection can reduce the potential for a recurrence to less than 10%.
    ⊡ E ⊡ Closure of the fistula and resection of the involved bowel are preferred.

20. The patient returns to the office 3 years later complaining of abdominal pain, abdominal distention, bloating after meals, and intermittent constipation interspersed with diarrhea. He has lost 20 pounds during the last 3 months, which he ascribes to the aforementioned abdominal symptoms. An upper gastrointestinal series with a small bowel follow-through reveals one area of tight stricture in the distal small bowel. The stricture appears to be 10 cm in length. Which of the following is true?

    ⊡ A ⊡ All strictures require resection; bypass of the involved segment is not an option.
    ⊡ B ⊡ Postoperatively, this patient's chance of another recurrence requiring surgery is 50%.
    ⊡ C ⊡ Because this patient requires surgery for the second time, his risk of cancer is extremely high, and he should have an extensive small bowel resection.
    ⊡ D ⊡ Postoperative anastomotic strictures typically cause symptoms years later.
    ⊡ E ⊡ Because of the patient's prior surgery, folate replacement is essential.

QUESTIONS 21–23

A 32-year-old male executive with long-standing Crohn's disease presents with a complete obstruction of the small bowel. At laparotomy, scarring of the distal ileum and cecum cause an obstruction. A 10-cm segment of mid small bowel shows moderate nonobstructive Crohn's disease.

21. Which operative procedure should be performed at this time?

    ⊡ A ⊡ Radical resection of the involved segment of mid small bowel, all of the ileum, the cecum, and the right colon
    ⊡ B ⊡ Resection of the distal ileum and right colon with the involved mesentery and lymph nodes

C. Bypass of the obstructing segment with a side-to-side anastomosis between the ileum and the right colon and no resection

D. Stricturoplasty of the obstruction plus resection of the short involved segment of mid small bowel

E. Resection of the distal ileum and cecum

22. Postoperatively, the patient requires an indwelling bladder catheter for 5 days to treat urinary retention. He does well until the tenth postoperative day, at which point he develops a fever of 103°F, right lower quadrant pain, and an ileus. The midline wound is not inflamed. Which of the following is most likely to have developed?

A. Blind loop syndrome
B. Pyelonephritis
C. Recurrent Crohn's disease
D. Intra-abdominal abscess
E. Pseudomembranous enterocolitis

23. After successful surgery and discharge from the hospital, which of the following is true?

A. If the diseased bowel is removed, therapy with prednisone and metronidazole can best prevent a recurrence.
B. The chance of a cure is greater than 60%.
C. The recurrence rate is higher than 50% during the next 5–10 years.
D. If the terminal ileum is removed, the risk of a recurrence is less.
E. If the terminal ileum is removed, the patient will require long-term therapy with oral iron to prevent anemia.

QUESTIONS 24–25

A 63-year-old man presents with a 3-day history of increasing cramping abdominal pain, constipation, and intermittent vomiting. He continues to pass gas. Other than the present complaints, he has been healthy. Examination reveals a distended abdomen with high-pitched bowel sounds. No localized tenderness and no rectal masses are present. The stool is heme positive.

24. Diagnostically, the first step should be to perform which of the following?

A. Total colonoscopy
B. Mesenteric angiography
C. Flat plate and erect abdominal radiographs
D. Upper gastrointestinal radiographs with small bowel follow-through
E. Barium enema

25. Therapeutically, the first step should be which of the following?

A. A Fleet enema, clear liquids by mouth, and careful observation
B. Emergency colonoscopy for colonic decompression
C. Intravenous fluids, nasogastric suction, and careful observation
D. Colonoscopic decompression with use of a rectal tube, if necessary
E. Immediate exploratory laparotomy

QUESTIONS 26–27

A 60-year-old patient who is finishing a course of antibiotic therapy for bacterial pneumonia develops cramping abdominal pain and profuse watery diarrhea. A diagnosis of pseudomembranous or antibiotic-associated colitis is suspected.

26. Which of the following is the quickest way to establish the diagnosis?

- [A] Stool culture
- [B] Barium enema
- [C] Stool titer for *Clostridium difficile* toxin
- [D] Proctoscopy
- [E] Blood culture

27. What would the initial treatment involve?

- [A] Metronidazole
- [B] Vancomycin
- [C] Imodium
- [D] Cephalexin
- [E] Total abdominal colectomy

28. During exploration for a transverse colon tumor, a surgeon incidentally notices a 2-cm diverticulum of the small bowel located 2 ft proximal to the ileocecal valve. Which of the following statements are not true?

- [A] This diverticulum should be resected when found due to an associated increased risk of malignancy
- [B] This is an example of the most common type of diverticulum of the gastrointestinal tract, present in 2% of the population
- [C] It is more commonly found in men than women
- [D] When symptomatic in children, it presents as a source of bleeding
- [E] It can cause obstruction via intussusception

29. A 55-year-old man presents with a 24-hour history of increasingly severe left lower quadrant abdominal pain. On examination, he has tenderness localized in the left lower quadrant with rebound. Fever and leukocytosis are present. The clinical suspicion of diverticulitis would best be confirmed by which of the following?

- [A] Barium enema
- [B] Colonoscopy
- [C] CT scan of the abdomen and pelvis
- [D] Magnetic resonance imaging of the abdomen and pelvis
- [E] Chest radiograph

30. A 45-year-old woman with diabetes presents with a 2-day history of acute perirectal pain. On examination, a tender fluctuant mass is present to the left of the anus. What treatment should be administered at this time?

- [A] Broad-spectrum antibiotic therapy
- [B] Abscess drainage and excision of the fistulous tract
- [C] Incision and drainage of the abscess
- [D] Continued observation
- [E] Treatment of Crohn's disease

QUESTIONS 31–32

A 34-year-old female patient in previous good health presents in the emergency department with spontaneous intraperitoneal hemorrhage. Her only medication is an oral contraceptive that she has been taking for the past 5 years. During resuscitation, a bedside ultrasound reveals a large amount of intraperitoneal blood and a 3-cm mass in the right lobe of the liver.

31. What is the likely cause of her hemorrhage?

- [A] Hepatoma
- [B] Hemangioma

C   Focal nodular hyperplasia
D   Hepatic cell adenoma
E   Metastatic neoplasm

The patient continues to bleed and requires transfusion.

32. What further treatment should be undertaken?

A   Observation in the intensive care unit
B   Right hepatic artery ligation
C   Right hepatic lobectomy
D   Angiographic embolization of hepatic artery
E   CT portogram

33. A 45-year-old man presents to the emergency room with 24 hours of left lower quadrant abdominal pain. Examination reveals fever and focal tenderness in the left lower quadrant but no generalized peritoneal signs. CT scan reveals a collection containing air and fluid. Optimal management of this patient includes which of the following?

A   Admission for intravenous antibiotics and serial abdominal exams
B   Urgent operation with resection of diseased bowel and primary anastomosis
C   Urgent operation with resection of diseased bowel and diverting colostomy
D   Colonoscopy to rule out the possibility of a perforated cancer followed by CT-guided drainage
E   CT-guided drainage followed by bowel resection once the patient has fully recovered

QUESTIONS 34–36

A 52-year-old alcoholic man with known cirrhosis presents to the emergency department with hematemesis.

34. After resuscitation and stabilization, which procedure should take place?

A   Arteriography
B   Upper gastrointestinal series
C   Endoscopy
D   Tagged red cell scan
E   Liver biopsy

Work-up reveals acutely bleeding esophageal varices.

35. What should the next treatment be?

A   Transjugular intrahepatic portosystemic shunt
B   Emergency portacaval shunt
C   Splenectomy
D   Sclerotherapy
E   Gastroesophageal devascularization

After appropriate therapy, the bleeding ceases and the patient stabilizes. He is found to be a Child's C alcoholic cirrhotic who has been abstinent for 1 year. Evaluation for an orthotopic liver transplant has begun.

36. If his variceal bleeding recurs, it could be managed by all *except* which of the following?

A   Portacaval shunt
B   Mesocaval shunt
C   Sclerotherapy

D Transjugular intrahepatic portosystemic shunt

E Selective Warren shunt

37. A 73-year-old previously healthy man presents to the emergency room with several days of jaundice followed by 12 hours of right upper quadrant pain and fever. He is mildly hypotensive. CT scan of the abdomen reveals dilatation of the biliary tree. The next step in management includes which of the following?

A Laparoscopic cholecystectomy

B Open cholecystectomy and T tube placement

C Open cholecystectomy and choledochojejunostomy

D Fluid resuscitation, antibiotics, and endoscopic retrograde cholangiopancreatography (ERCP)

E Fluid resuscitation and hepatitis serologies

QUESTIONS 38–39

A 33-year-old man with no significant past medical history presents to the emergency room with abdominal pain and nausea. He is afebrile, and laboratory studies reveal a serum amylase level of 1200 U/L.

38. Which of the following would not be part of initial management?

A Intravenous hydration

B Nasogastric decompression

C Abdominal imaging with ultrasound and/or CT scan

D ERCP to evaluate pancreatic duct anatomy

E Intravenous narcotic pain medicine

39. Ten days into his course of pancreatitis, this patient is found to have a fluid collection measuring 4 cm in diameter near the tail of his pancreas. He had a recurrence of his abdominal pain when he was restarted on a diet 2 days prior but is otherwise asymptomatic. He remains on total parenteral nutrition. Appropriate management of this collection would include which of the following?

A CT-guided aspiration to assess for infection

B Endoscopic drainage via an ultrasound-guided cystogastrostomy

C Operative debridement and external drainage

D CT-guided percutaneous drainage

E Observation alone

40. A 59-year-old patient undergoes exploration for a 4-cm mass in the head of the pancreas that has caused obstructive jaundice. The patient had a biliary stent endoscopically placed prior to the procedure with complete resolution of jaundice. At the time of surgery, two small liver metastases are noted. Which of the following is not part of appropriate management at this point?

A Transduodenal pancreatic biopsy

B Hepaticojejunostomy

C Gastrojejunostomy

D Cholecystectomy

E Celiac ganglion nerve block

41. A 65-year-old patient presents with a history significant for obstructive jaundice and weight loss. A workup reveals a 2.5-cm mass in the head of the pancreas; needle aspiration reveals adenocarcinoma. Which of the following findings on preoperative CT scan would preclude operative exploration for curative resection?

A Presence of replaced right hepatic artery

B Loss of fat plane between tumor and portal vein

C Loss of fat plane between tumor and superior mesenteric artery

D Occlusion of gastroduodenal artery

E Occlusion of superior mesenteric vein

Directions: *The group of items in this section consists of lettered options followed by a set of numbered items. For each item, select the lettered option(s) that is(are) most closely associated with it. Each lettered option may be selected once, more than once, or not at all.*

Match the portion of the stomach, duodenum, or pancreas to the appropriate arterial supply.

- A Left gastric artery
- B Right gastroepiploic artery
- C Splenic artery
- D Vasa brevia (short gastric arteries)
- E Superior mesenteric artery

42. Body and tail of pancreas

43. Duodenum and head of pancreas

44. Proximal lesser curvature of stomach

45. Distal greater curvature of stomach

46. Fundus of stomach

Answers and Explanations

1. The answer is B (Chapter 9, I C 6 b). The iliopsoas sign is pain in the lower abdomen and psoas region that is elicited when the thigh is flexed against resistance. It suggests an inflammatory process, such as appendicitis. Crepitus suggests a rapidly spreading gas-forming infection. Murphy sign is elicited by palpating the right upper quadrant during inspiration and suggests acute cholecystitis. Flank and periumbilical ecchymoses suggest retroperitoneal hemorrhage.

2. The answer is D (Chapter 9, IV C 2 b (1)). The most likely cause of massive lower gastrointestinal bleeding in the absence of diverticula is an angiodysplastic lesion of the colon, particularly the right colon. An upper gastrointestinal series and small bowel studies should be done only after an exhaustive colonic workup has failed to demonstrate the source of bleeding. Colonoscopy in the face of massive bleeding is unreliable and difficult and carries the risk of colonic perforation. In addition, it will not usually demonstrate an angiodysplastic lesion. A repeat barium enema is also unlikely to help. The most helpful study in this patient would be selective mesenteric angiography.

3. The answer is C (Chapter 9, I C 3 d (5)). The history described would be more typical for either testicular torsion or acute epididymitis, of which only torsion represents a surgical emergency. Torsion of the testicle is likely the result of an abnormal attachment of the tunica vaginalis around the cord that allows the testis to twist (bell-clapper deformity). Compromise of the blood supply causes exquisite pain and produces gangrene and atrophy of the testis unless the torsion is treated immediately. Torsion is usually seen in young males, most often occurring spontaneously and even during sleep. It is associated with an onset of severe pain and is accompanied by nausea, vomiting, and abdominal pain. Acute prostatitis may present with vague abdominal pain. A more typical presentation for appendicitis would be pain preceded by nausea or anorexia. This presentation is not typical for gastroenteritis (which is not a surgical emergency).

4. The answer is B (Chapter 10, II B). This patient is presenting with classic symptoms of achalasia. The dysphagia to both solids and liquids is classic, as is the bird-beak narrowing on radiographs. The underlying defect is failure of the lower esophageal sphincter to relax, causing increased pressure in the esophagus and dysfunctional swallowing. Disorganized, strong nonperistaltic contractions in the esophagus are characteristic of diffuse esophageal spasm. Strictures typically have dyspahgia to solids well before liquids cause symptoms.

5. The answer is B (Chapter 9, Table 9-1). Massive upper gastrointestinal bleeding is usually due to a bleeding source proximal to the ligament of Treitz. The cause is most likely to be a posterior duodenal ulcer that is eroding into the gastroduodenal artery. Gastritis, esophagitis, a Mallory-Weiss tear, and esophageal varices are less likely causes of massive upper gastrointestinal bleeding.

6. The answer is C (Chapter 9, IV B, C). Arteriography is most often used as the initial evaluation step for continued bleeding after anorectal bleeding sources have been eliminated by endoscopy. Arteriography allows identification of diverticular bleeding as well as an angiodysplastic lesion of the right colon. Surgery is generally not indicated until four to six units of blood have been shed. Coagulation products are of no use unless the patient has abnormal clotting studies. Saline lavage of the colon is not a routine procedure.

7–8. The answer are 7-C (Chapter 9, III E 1), **8-D** (Chapter 11, IV B). Upper endoscopy is the most reliable method for precisely locating the site of upper gastrointestinal bleeding. Endoscopy can almost always be used unless bleeding is massive. Patients who are unstable or have blood losses requiring more than six units of blood within a 24-hour period require surgical intervention. Unstable patients should not typically be transported to interventional radiology. A Blakemore tube is only useful for bleeding esophageal varices. This patient, who does not have a history indicative of cirrhosis, is unlikely to have bleeding from varicies.

9. The answer is C (Chapter 9, II A 3 a). Obstructing adhesive bands after abdominal surgery are the most common cause of intestinal obstruction. They may be diffuse or solitary. A partial small bowel obstruction often responds to conservative management with nasogastric decompression and hydration. Complete small bowel obstruction typically requires operative intervention.

10. The answer is E (Chapter 9, I F 1 c [1]). Free air within the peritoneal cavity signals perforation of a hollow viscus. It is present in about 80% of gastroduodenal perforations. Because free peritoneal air is rarely secondary to other causes, additional studies in this patient would not be necessary before laparotomy.

11. The answer is C (Chapter 10, II A 3–4). This patient's symptoms are consistent with a Zenker's diverticulum. A barium swallow would be diagnostic but not therapeutic. Endoscopy is contraindicated secondary to the risk of diverticular perforation by the endoscope. Surgical myotomy of the cricopharyengeous muscle with resection or suspension of the diverticulum is the treatment of choice. Computed tomography (CT) scan of the chest is not necessary. Changing the diet would not alter the underlying pathology.

12. The answer is A (Chapter 10, II D 4). Development of esophageal strictures is an indication for surgical antireflux procedures. Uncomplicated Barrett's esophagus is a controversial indication for an antireflux procedure, as available studies do not agree as to whether or not surgery reverses the mucosal changes associated with Barrett's esophagus. Confirmed severe dysplasia is an indication for esophagectomy, not antireflux surgery. Gastroesophageal reflux is associated with a lower esophageal sphincter pressure. Esophageal dysmotility is a contraindication to reflux surgery. Esophagitis should heal with appropriate medical management.

13. The answer is B (Chapter 10, V A–C). This patient's history, physical examination, and diagnostic studies are consistent with an acute esophageal perforation, and the situation represents a surgical emergency. Whenever possible, primary surgical repair is indicated regardless of the time since perforation. If sepsis and regional inflammation preclude primary repair, resection with cervical esophagostomy and gastrostomy and jejunostomy tube insertion should be performed. Restoration of alimentary continuity with stomach or colon can then be performed in 2–3 months.

14–15. The answers are 14-C (Chapter 11, IV A 4–5), **15-B** (Chapter 11, V C 2 h [1] [c]). Benign gastric ulcers should heal in 8–12 weeks with maximal medical therapy. If the ulcer does not heal completely during this time period, repeat endoscopy should be performed with biopsy. If gastric adenocarcinoma is diagnosed in this location, the optimal surgical therapy for this condition would be a distal gastrectomy with D1 (regional) lymph node dissection. More extensive surgery, such as total gastrectomy or splenectomy, would be reserved for more proximal gastric lesions. Neither radiation therapy followed by chemotherapy alone without surgery or limited surgery followed by radiotherapy is a treatment plan with curative intent.

16. The answer is B (Chapter 11, IV B 5 c). Parietal cell vagotomy, also termed *highly selective vagotomy*, maintains the nerves of Laterjet that innervate the pylorus. By dividing only the branches that innervate the parietal cells, pyloric function is preserved and outflow of the stomach is maintained. It is a technically demanding operation, in that failure to adequately sever the appropriate nerves will result in recurrences of more than 10%. However, parietal cell vagotomy can be performed for bleeding or perforated ulcers.

17. The answer is B (Chapter 11, I B 5). The vagal nerves are one of the principal stimulants of gastric acid secretion through direct stimulation of the parietal cells and via gastrin release from antral cells. Although the splanchnic and celiac ganglions are important in gastric motility and sensation, they do not stimulate acid secretion. The T4 root and phrenic nerve are not involved in gastric nervous supply.

18. The answer is C (Chapter 12, I B 2). Both parathormone and vitamin D increase intestinal absorption of dietary calcium. Bile salts are essential for absorption of fats and fat-soluble vitamins. Vitamin B_{12} is a water-soluble vitamin that complexes with intrinsic factor, which is a protein produced by the stomach, and the protein–vitamin B_{12} complex is absorbed in the terminal ileum. The range of iron absorption is only 10%–26% of dietary iron. Triglycerides are not absorbed intact but must first be broken down into free fatty acids and monoglycerides. Once absorbed, they are resynthesized into triglycerides, but they are not released into the portal circulation. Rather, the triglycerides are packaged as chylomicrons and released into the lymphatic circulation.

19. The answer is E (Chapter 12, II B). The diagnosis of Crohn's disease is supported by the enterovesical fistula, the presence of "fat wrapping" of the bowel, inflammation, and the clinical history. To prevent ongoing contamination of the urinary tract, the fistula must be closed, and resection of the involved segment of bowel would be the standard approach. Regarding the extent of resection, the 50% risk of recurrence is not decreased by more extensive resections, thus the less bowel removed the better. In this case, with three widely separated segments of ileum involved, removal of all involved bowel could result in loss of more than half of the ileum and would not be advisable. Crohn's disease does not directly involve the bladder and thus resection of the bladder wall is unnecessary except when needed to close the opening of the fistula. Meckel's diverticulum occurs proximal to the terminal ileum; it would not affect multiple bowel segments and does not cause "fat wrapping."

20. The answer is B (Chapter 12, II B). This patient presents with recurrent Crohn's disease in the form of an obstruction from stricture, which is the most common manifestation that requires surgery. After surgery, the risk of recurrent manifestations of Crohn's disease requiring reoperation is 50%, and the risk remains 50% after each surgical procedure. Strictures, unlike fistulas and perforations, can be treated via bypass of the involved segment of bowel, although resection is preferred except when the risk is too great. The risk of cancer is related to the chronicity of the disease and would almost never require extensive small bowel resection, which may leave the patient with short bowel syndrome (a difficult disorder to treat in this population). Postoperative anastomotic strictures cause symptoms very early postoperatively, not years later. If this patient had previously had a resection of the terminal ileum, he would develop a deficiency of vitamin B_{12}, not folate.

21–23. The answers are 21-E (Chapter 12, II B 5), **22-D** (Chapter 12, II B 3, 5), **23-C** (Chapter 12, I B 2 f–g; II B 4–6). When surgery is necessary to treat complications of Crohn's disease, the operations are "conservative," as defined by the length of the resection. Therefore, when an obstructive lesion is present, only a short length of bowel needs to be resected. In the case described, the distal ileum and cecum should be removed. Radical resections are not necessary, as they do not reduce the risk of recurrence and may ultimately contribute to short bowel syndrome if several resections are required over long periods. In addition, resection of mesentery and lymph nodes (e.g., for a cancer operation) is unnecessary. Bypass procedures without resection are reserved for only the most difficult cases where resection cannot be undertaken safely. A stricturoplasty is appropriate occasionally for short symptomatic strictures in the small bowel only.

The second postoperative week is the usual time for the development of serious complications, such as abdominal wound dehiscence, intestinal anastomotic breakdown, and intraperitoneal abscess. Blind loop syndrome occurs rarely; and although it does cause pain and diarrhea, it does not cause fever and ileus. Pyelonephritis usually causes flank pain and pyuria. Crohn's disease does not recur immediately or cause the signs unless complications have occurred. Pseudomembranous enterocolitis causes tenderness over the transverse colon and occasionally over the descending colon, with diarrhea. Of the choices listed, an intra-abdominal abscess is the most likely diagnosis.

The prognosis of Crohn's disease, which requires surgery, is not good because 50% of patients require additional surgical procedures within 5 years of the first operation. Therefore, the chance of cure is less than 50%. Medical therapy (including anti-inflammatory agents and antibiotic drugs) has not proved effective for preventing recurrence of the disease. Removal of the terminal ileum has no effect on disease recurrence or iron absorption; however, the absorption of vitamin B_{12} is significantly impaired.

24–25. The answers are 24-C (Chapter 13, VIII A 6; XIV B 3), **25-C** (Chapter 13, XV A 3 a). Flat plate and erect radiographs of the abdomen should be performed first. Further studies may be needed based on the results of this initial survey. As with all bowel obstructions, the initial treatment involves nasogastric suction, intravenous fluids, and resuscitation with careful attention to correcting metabolic and electrolyte abnormalities. Once a patient has been adequately resuscitated, the decision to either observe carefully or intervene operatively can be made.

26–27. The answers are 26-D (Chapter 13, VIII C 1), **27-A** (Chapter 13, VIII D 2). Crampy abdominal pain and diarrhea after a course of antibiotic therapy is highly suggestive of antibiotic-associated or pseudomembranous colitis. Diagnosis can be made either by proctoscopy, which demonstrates pseudomembranes, or by stool titer for *Clostridium difficile* toxin. Proctoscopy establishes the diagnosis immediately. Barium enema is contraindicated. The antibiotics should be stopped, and the patient should be started on metronidazole. Oral vancomycin is also effective, but it is more expensive. Colectomy is rarely required only in severe cases.

28. The answer is A (Chapter 12, II C). Meckel's diverticulum is the most common diverticulum of the gastrointestinal tract and goes by the rule of 2's: 2 ft from ileocecal valce, 2% incidence, 2 cm long, 2:1 male to female ratio. They can cause bleeding due to heterotropic gastric mucosa as well as intussusception and obstruction. An asymptomatic Meckel's diverticulum should not be resected.

29. The answer is C (Chapter 13, IV D 5 a–b). CT scan of the abdomen and pelvis is the most helpful test to confirm the suspected diagnosis of diverticulitis. Free air is detected on the chest radiograph in less than 3% of patients with diverticulitis. Contrast enema should generally be avoided in the initial stages of diverticulitis. Colonoscopy to exclude a sigmoid cancer may be of value after the condition of the patient has stabilized.

30. The answer is C (Chapter 13, XII C 1 f (1)). This patient presents with a classic history and physical findings of perirectal abscess. Antibiotic therapy will not cure an abscess. Definitive drainage is required. This therapy will be curative in approximately 50% of the patients, and the remainder will develop a fistula. However, the physician should deal with the abscess itself at the initial presentation. Attempts to definitely address any fistula tract at initial presentation is not recommended due to potential complications such as injury to the sphincter muscles and difficulties with continence.

31–32. The answers are 31-D (Chapter 14, I C 2 a, d), **32-D** (Chapter 14, I C 2 a, d). Although many liver tumors undergo spontaneous hemorrhage, this condition occurs most frequently with hepatic cell adenomas. Up to 30% of patients present with spontaneous rupture into the peritoneal cavity as their initial finding.

The patient continues to bleed. Emergency liver resection after an acute rupture would be associated with high morbidity and mortality. While hepatic artery ligation may control the bleeding, this can probably be accomplished less invasively by radiologic embolization. Once the bleeding is controlled and the patient recovers, elective resection should be undertaken to avoid future hemorrhage.

33. The answer is E (Chapter 13, V D). Cases of diverticulitis complicated by perforation and abscess formation are best managed by percutaneous drainage in the absence of evidence of diffuse peritonitis. Young patients (typically considered as being less than 50 years of age) with a single severe case such as this should be considered for an interval resection of the diseased section of bowel because of the very high risk of subsequent severe episodes. Older patients are often referred after a second episode. Colonoscopy should not be routinely performed during the acute phase of an episode of diverticulitis but should be performed prior on an interval basis. Operative intervention during the acute phase is reserved for cases that either present with diffuse peritonitis, perforation or continued worsening of the clinical picture in spite of appropriate non-operative therapy. Primary anastomosis is typically avoided in the setting of severe infection and contamination.

34–36. The answers are 34-C (Chapter 14, II E 3 a), **35-D** (Chapter 14, II B 3), **36-A** (Chapter 14, II H 3 a–b, 4). Acute variceal bleeding commonly occurs because of portal hypertension from underlying cirrhosis. Other causes of upper gastrointestinal bleeding that must also be considered in these patients include gastritis and peptic ulcer disease. Upper gastrointestinal endoscopy is the most rapid way of making the diagnosis of the site and identifying the cause of upper gastrointestinal bleeding. Once the diagnosis has been made, sclerotherapy is the preferred method of managing acute variceal bleeding. It is successful in 90% of patients.

Portacaval shunt, mesocaval shunt, sclerotherapy, transjugular intrahepatic portosystemic shunt, and selective Warren shunt for recurrent bleeding would potentially be successful in preventing long-term hemorrhage. However, portacaval shunt would make a subsequent liver transplant extremely difficult and hazardous.

37. The answer is D (Chapter 14, III F). Cholangitis is a potentially life-threatening disease. This patient is present with Charcot's triad of pain, fever, and jaundice.

38–39. The answers are 38-D (Chapter 15, II C), **39-E** (Chapter 15, II C). Uncomplicated acute pancreatitis is best managed conservatively with nasogastric decompression, intravenous hydration, bowel rest, and pain medicine. Imaging with ultrasound, CT scan, magnetic resonance imaging, or magnetic resonance cholangiopancreatography can be useful in establishing a possible etiology (gallstones) or detecting complications. Endoscopic retrograde cholangiopancreatography (ERCP) should not be used routinely during the acute presentation due to the risk of ERCP-associated pancreatitis complicating the acute situation. ERCP should be reserved for specific cases where there is evidence of biliary obstruction. Evaluation of pancreatic duct anatomy can be helpful on an interval basis to help assess causes of chronic or recurrent pancreatitis.

40. The answer is A (Chapter 15, III A). When patients are unresectable due to distant metastases at the time of surgery, a surgeon must accomplish several things. A biliary bypass (hepaticojejunostomy) palliates the obstructive jaundice, and a cholecystectomy is performed in conjunction with this. A gastric bypass (gastrojejunostomy) prevents the gastric outlet obstruction observed in 19% of unresected periampullary cancer patients. A celiac axis nerve block has been shown to significantly reduce cancer-related pain. A surgeon must also make a tissue diagnosis, in this case by taking a biopsy of one of the liver metastases. An additional pancreatic biopsy is unnecessary and adds additional risks.

41. The answer is E (Chapter 15, III A). Findings that determine unresectability on preoperative CT scan include encasement of the superior mesenteric artery or proximal celiac axis and occlusion of the superiormesenteric vein or portal vein. Tumor abutting these vessels but not encasing or occluding them is not a contraindication to resection. The gastroduodenal artery is ligated during a pancreaticoduodenectomy, thus its occlusion does not preclude resection. A replaced right hepatic artery is not uncommon and must be preserved. This does not, however, preclude resection.

42–46. The answers are 42-C, 43-E, 44-A, 45-B, and 46-D (Chapter 11, I B 3; Chapter 11, II B 1). The blood supply of the viscera is important in gastrointestinal surgery. Three of the four main arteries can be sacrificed, and blood flow to the stomach will still be preserved through collateral circulation. The proximal lesser curvature is supplied by the left gastric artery (arising from the celiac axis). The right gastric artery (arising from the common hepatic artery) supplies the distal lesser curvature. The left and right gastroepiploic arteries supply the proximal and distal greater curvature, respectively. The duodenum and head of the pancreas are supplied by the superior and inferior pancreaticoduodenal arteries that arise from the gastroduodenal and superior mesenteric arteries, respectively. The body and tail of the pancreas are supplied by branches of the splenic artery.

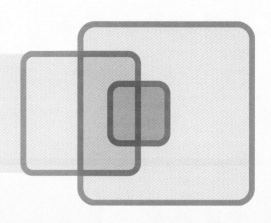

PART **V**

Endocrine Disorders

chapter 16

Thyroid, Adrenal, Parathyroid, and Thymus Glands

JOHN S. RADOMSKI · HERBERT E. COHN · JOHN C. KAIRYS

I THYROID GLAND

Indications for operations on the thyroid gland have varied since excision was first described by Kocher in the late 1800s. In early years, operations on the thyroid were performed primarily to relieve the pressure symptoms of large iodine-deficiency goiter, to control hyperthyroidism, or to remove thyroid neoplasms. With the advent of iodized salt, iodine-deficiency goiters have been almost eliminated, and hyperthyroidism is now controlled mainly by nonoperative means. However, surgery remains the mainstay of treatment for thyroid neoplasms and, in many instances, is important in their diagnosis.

A **Vasculature of the thyroid gland** (Fig. 16-1)
  1. **Arterial supply**
     a. The **superior thyroid artery,** which is the first branch of the external carotid artery, supplies the upper pole of the thyroid.
     b. The **inferior thyroid artery,** which arises from the thyrocervical trunk of the subclavian artery, supplies the lower pole of the gland.
     c. A **thyroidea ima artery** occasionally arises from the aortic arch and connects to the thyroid isthmus inferiorly.
  2. **Venous drainage** of the thyroid is an interconnecting system of veins without valves.
     a. The **superior thyroid veins** drain along the course of the superior thyroid arteries into the internal jugular vein.
     b. The **middle thyroid vein** drains directly into the internal jugular vein.
     c. The **inferior thyroid veins** drain from the lower pole and isthmus either directly into the internal jugular vein or into the innominate vein.
  3. **Lymphatic drainage**
     a. Lymphatics from the thyroid gland always drain to the ipsilateral cervical lymph nodes in either the anterior or posterior triangle of the neck, along the course of the internal jugular vein to the nodes in the tracheoesophageal groove, or to the paratracheal nodes in the mediastinum.
     b. The **nodes in the tracheoesophageal groove** are most important in the spread of thyroid malignancies because involvement of these nodes may cause tumor extension into the underlying recurrent nerve, trachea, or esophagus.

B **Nerves related to the thyroid gland**
  1. **Recurrent (inferior) laryngeal nerve**
     a. **Course.** The recurrent laryngeal nerve runs in the tracheoesophageal groove in intimate relationship to the posteromedial aspect of the thyroid gland.
        (1) **On the right,** the nerve recurs around the subclavian artery and runs an oblique course from lateral to medial, crossing the inferior thyroid artery before entering the tracheoesophageal groove.
        (2) **On the left,** the nerve recurs around the ligamentum arteriosum in the mediastinum and runs a course parallel to the tracheoesophageal groove throughout its course in the neck.

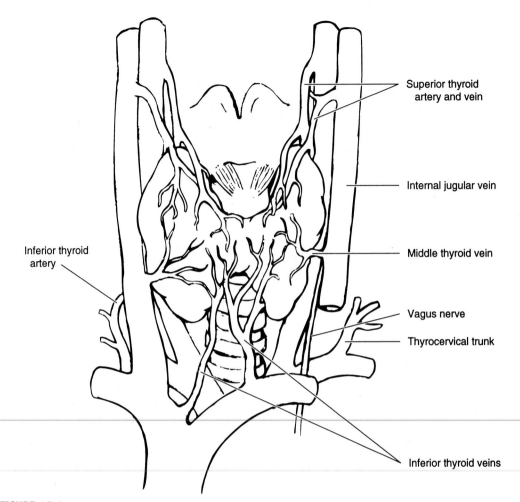

FIGURE 16-1 Blood supply of the thyroid. (Reprinted with permission from Edis AJ, Grant CS, Egdahl RH. *Comprehensive Manuals of Surgical Specialties—Manual of Endocrine Surgery*, 2nd ed. New York: Springer-Verlag; 1984:75.)

    b. Branches. The nerve divides into an external branch, which is sensory to the larynx, and an internal branch, which supplies the intrinsic muscles of the larynx.

    c. Injury to the recurrent laryngeal nerve most commonly occurs where the nerve crosses the inferior thyroid artery or where it penetrates the cricothyroid membrane, but injury can occur anywhere along its course (see I D 2 e [4] [d]). Injury can be avoided by visualizing the nerve throughout its course during operations requiring complete thyroid lobectomy.

  2. Superior laryngeal nerve

    a. Course. The nerve is intimately intertwined with the branches of the superior thyroid artery.

    b. Branches. The superior laryngeal nerve has an internal branch, which is sensory to the larynx, and an external branch, which is motor to the cricothyroid muscle.

    c. Injury. The superior laryngeal nerve can be injured during mobilization of the upper pole of the thyroid, especially when the lobe is enlarged.

      (1) Injury results in voice weakness, which is especially noticeable in singers or orators.

      (2) Injury can be avoided by ligation of the branches of the superior thyroid artery at their junction with the gland rather than along the course of the artery in the neck.

  3. Parathyroid glands

    a. Location

      (1) The superior parathyroids are typically located at the junction of the upper and middle third of the thyroid on the posteromedial aspect (Fig. 16-2).

      (2) The inferior parathyroids are located in relationship to the lower pole of the thyroid, either on the surface of the gland or within a 3-cm circle, the center of which is formed by the junction of the inferior thyroid artery and the recurrent laryngeal nerve.

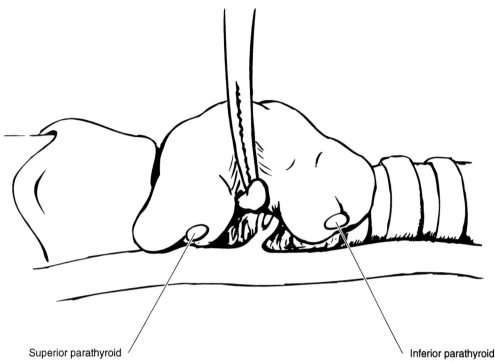

Superior parathyroid   Inferior parathyroid

FIGURE 16-2 Normal locations of the parathyroid glands, lateral view. The *superior parathyroid gland* on each side is almost always located on the dorsal surface of the thyroid gland at the proximate level of the cricoid cartilage. When not in its usual location, the superior gland may be found in a retroesophageal or retropharyngeal position; less often, it is alongside the superior thyroid vessels, above the upper pole of the thyroid gland. The *inferior parathyroid gland* is more variable in location. In approximately 50% of patients, it lies on the lateral surface at the lower pole of the thyroid, near the point of attachment of the thyrothymic ligament. In the other 50%, the inferior parathyroid glands are intimately associated with the thymus, either in the neck or in the superior mediastinum. (Reprinted with permission from Edis AJ, Grant CS, Egdahl RH. *Comprehensive Manuals of Surgical Specialties—Manual of Endocrine Surgery*, 2nd ed. New York: Springer-Verlag; 1984:2.)

      b. Injury to the parathyroids during thyroid surgery usually occurs during total lobectomy or total thyroidectomy and results from disruption of the blood supply to the parathyroids. If this occurs, the consequence is either temporary or permanent hypoparathyroidism, unless the parathyroids can be successfully reimplanted (see III A]).

C **Abnormalities of thyroid descent**   (see Chapter 18, III B)

  1. Route of descent
    a. Normal descent. The thyroid migrates downward from its point of origin at the foramen cecum at the base of the tongue. It descends to assume its normal position on either side of the trachea at the level of the thyroid and cricoid cartilages.
    b. Abnormal descent of the thyroid may result in ectopic placement of thyroid tissue in the tongue, in the midline of the neck, or in the mediastinum.

  2. Glottic (lingual) thyroid
    a. Location. Glottic (lingual) thyroid occurs when the thyroid does not descend into the neck and remains at the base of the tongue. It may be the only functioning thyroid tissue in the individual.
    b. Symptoms of obstruction or difficulty with speech are usually related to goiter formation in the lingual mass.
    c. Diagnosis is by inspection or indirect laryngoscopy. A radioiodine thyroid scan should be performed to identify the mass as thyroid tissue.
    d. Management
      (1) Suppression of thyroid-stimulating hormone (TSH) with thyroxine should be the first step in management because glottic thyroid tissue is usually hypofunctioning.
      (2) Surgical removal should be considered when a patient has obstructive symptoms, especially if hormonal therapy is ineffective.

3. Ectopic midline thyroid tissue
  a. Location. A diagnosis of ectopic midline thyroid tissue should be considered when a midline mass is encountered below the hyoid bone.
  b. Diagnosis. If there is no thyroid gland in the neck, the ectopic thyroid should be confirmed by radioiodine scan because removal of the ectopic tissue will leave the patient without functioning thyroid tissue.

4. Mediastinal thyroid (substernal goiter)
  a. Location. Most aberrant thyroids in the mediastinum are located in the anterosuperior mediastinum. They may represent **substernal extensions** from an enlarged thyroid or **normal thyroid tissue,** resulting from aberrant embryologic descent of the thyroid into the mediastinum.
    (1) Normal functioning thyroid tissue will take up radioiodine and, thus, can be confirmed by a radioiodine scan of the mediastinum.
    (2) Substernal extensions of the thyroid may be caused by adenomatous hyperplasia and, as a result, may not take up radioiodine.
      (a) Substernal goiters usually occur in older age-groups.
      (b) They usually result in tracheoesophageal compression.
      (c) They do not respond to nonoperative attempts to relieve pressure symptoms by suppressing TSH with thyroxine.
  b. Management. Operation is usually advised to relieve pressure symptoms or to diagnose an otherwise undiagnosed mediastinal mass. Substernal goiters can usually be removed through a cervical incision without the need for sternotomy because their blood supply is derived from the neck.

5. Thyroglossal duct cysts and sinuses
  a. Location. Thyroglossal duct cysts usually present as midline masses located between the hyoid bone and the thyroid isthmus. They are always connected to the base of the tongue, traversing the center of the hyoid bone.
  b. Signs or symptoms
    (1) They may be solid or cystic and may communicate with the skin, forming a sinus.
    (2) These lesions may present at any age, but most are found in children.
    (3) A history of redness and inflammation from infection in the cyst is present in one third of the cases.
  c. Management. Treatment involves excising the cyst or sinus along with a portion of the hyoid bone and the proximal duct extending to the base of the tongue (Sistrunk procedure).

D **Thyroid dysfunction requiring surgery**

1. Thyroid hormones
  a. Tri-iodothyronine and thyroxine. The **follicular cells** of the thyroid are derived primarily from the floor of the foregut. These cells produce the thyroid hormones triiodothyronine (T_3) and thyroxine (T_4; tetraiodothyronine).
    (1) Hormone synthesis and release
      (a) Iodine and tyrosine combine to form T_3 and T_4.
      (b) Both of these hormones bind with thyroglobulin and are stored in the gland until released into the bloodstream.
      (c) Release is under the control of TSH from the pituitary and thyrotropin-releasing hormone (TRH) from the hypothalamus.
      (d) A feedback mechanism regulating T_3 and T_4 release is related to the levels of the circulating hormones.
    (2) Hormonal action
      (a) The thyroid hormones activate energy-producing respiratory processes, resulting in an increase in the metabolic rate and an increase in oxygen consumption.
      (b) Increased glycogenolysis results in an increase in blood sugar levels.
      (c) The thyroid hormones also enhance metabolic, circulatory, and somatic neuromuscular actions of catecholamines.
        (i) The result is an increase in the pulse rate, cardiac output, and blood flow.

(ii) Nervousness, irritability, muscular tremors, and muscle wasting can also occur.

(iii) These effects can be blocked by the use of β-blockers, such as propranolol.

b. **Thyrocalcitonin.** The **parafollicular, or C, cells** are derived from the ultimobranchial body. These cells are part of the amine precursor uptake and decarboxylation (APUD) cell system (see Chapter 17, II A) and produce thyrocalcitonin.

2. **Graves' disease (diffuse toxic non-nodular goiter)**

a. **Pathogenesis.** Graves' disease is thought to be an autoimmune disease resulting from a defect in cell-mediated immunity.

(1) A substance known as **long-acting thyroid stimulator (LATS)** is produced, which increases the size of the thyroid and its production of thyroid hormone.

(2) A clinical syndrome of hypermetabolism with associated abnormal eye signs, and an unusual form of pretibial edema results.

b. **Clinical presentation**

(1) **Hypermetabolic state**

(a) Symptoms include palpitations, sweating, intolerance to heat, irritability, insomnia, nervousness, weight loss, and fatigue.

(b) Signs include an audible bruit over the gland, tremors of the hands and tongue, cardiac arrhythmias, and a widening of the palpebral fissure of the eye.

(2) **Abnormal deposition of mucopolysaccharide and round cell infiltration** in the tissues is characterized by exophthalmos, edema of the eyelids, chemosis, and pretibial edema.

c. **Diagnosis**

(1) Graves' disease is confirmed by the presence of an increased total serum T_4, an increase in the T_3 resin uptake (T_3RU), and an increase in T_3 by radioimmunoassay.

(2) An increase of the free thyroxine index (the T_3RU value times the total serum T_4) and an increase in radioiodine uptake distinguish this form of thyrotoxicosis from thyrotoxicosis without hyperthyroidism (caused by thyroiditis, factitious thyrotoxicosis, or struma ovarii).

(3) A thyroid scan shows an enlarged thyroid with uniform uptake throughout.

(4) The serum cholesterol level is decreased, and the blood sugar and alkaline phosphatase are increased.

d. **Medical treatment.** The preferred initial treatment is medical because the disease has a tendency to remit spontaneously after 1–2 years in adults or after 3–6 months in children.

(1) Radioiodine (^{131}I) administered orally is simple, safe, and inexpensive.

(a) It obviates the need for surgery and apparently does not increase the risk of carcinoma.

(b) It has, however, several disadvantages.

(i) It may produce hypothyroidism in the fetus if administered during pregnancy.

(ii) Because of its slow onset of effectiveness, concomitant use of antithyroid drugs may be necessary if the patient is severely symptomatic.

(2) **Antithyroid drugs** are effective in about 50% of patients, especially those with symptoms of short duration and with a small gland. They are rapidly effective and can reverse symptoms in a short time.

(a) These drugs act by altering various stages of iodine metabolism.

(i) Propylthiouracil and methimazole act through competitive inhibition of peroxidase, blocking the oxidation of iodide to elemental iodine. Propylthiouracil also interferes with the peripheral conversion of T_4 to T_3.

(ii) Iodine in high concentrations blocks the release of thyroid hormones by inhibiting proteolysis. However, glands treated with iodine suppression escape this therapeutic effect after 10–14 days of therapy.

(iii) Propranolol, a β-adrenergic blocker, reduces the secondary effects of hypermetabolism, such as tachycardia, without affecting the production of T_3 or T_4.

(b) Their main disadvantage is that the incidence of recurrence is high if the drugs are stopped, and prolonged therapy is required.

(c) They must be discontinued if drug toxicity occurs, manifested by fever, rash, arthralgia, a lupuslike syndrome, or agranulocytosis.

e. **Surgical treatment.** The preferred operation for Graves' disease is bilateral subtotal thyroidectomy.

(1) Indications. Thyroidectomy is indicated for Graves' disease under the following circumstances:

    (a) (1) When medical therapy has failed because remission has not occurred after treatment for 1 year in adults or for 3 months in children, (2) because the patient refuses to take the medication, or (3) because the patient develops an adverse reaction to the antithyroid drugs

    (b) When radioiodine therapy is not advisable because the patient is pregnant or the patient refuses radioiodine therapy

(2) Objectives of surgery are to remove enough thyroid tissue to correct the hyperthyroidism.

    (a) In the past, many endocrinologists and surgeons recommended bilateral subtotal thyroid lobectomy. Approximately 4–5 gm of tissue was left in situ in the hopes of rendering the patient euthyroid while minimizing the risk of hypoparathyroidism and nerve injury. However, as many as 40% of patients developed hypothyroidism postoperatively and required thyroid hormone supplementation. Another 40% of patients remained hyperthyroid to some extent and thus sometimes required further medical treatment of their disease.

    (b) Currently, most experts recommend performing either a near total thyroidectomy (total lobectomy on one side and a subtotal lobectomy on the other) or total thyroidectomy. Patients require supplementation thyroid hormone postoperatively, but the risk of persistent hyperthyroidism is greatly reduced.

(3) Preoperative preparation. To minimize the risk of thyroid storm (see I D 2 e [4] [a]), the patient should be euthyroid before operation.

    (a) Antithyroid drugs are usually given until the patient is euthyroid, and then Lugol's solution or saturated potassium iodide is given for 7–10 days before surgery.

        (i) This reduces the risk of thyroid storm both during and after surgery. It also reduces the size and vascularity of the thyroid gland, which increases the technical ease of surgery.

        (ii) However, it takes several weeks or longer to achieve the euthyroid state. Moreover, in a pregnant woman, thyroid drugs can cross the placenta and cause fetal goiter.

    (b) Propranolol can be given in conjunction with Lugol's solution if patients have had adverse reactions to antithyroid drugs.

        (i) This is effective in rapidly restoring the euthyroid state and in reducing thyroid size and vascularity. Moreover, it is not known to cause any fetal abnormalities if the patient is pregnant.

        (ii) Propranolol must be given for 4–5 days postoperatively to prevent thyroid storm because the half-life of circulating thyroid hormone is 5–10 days.

(4) Complications of thyroidectomy (*Note:* These complications are not unique to the management of Graves' disease. They may occur during thyroidectomy for other thyroid conditions as well.)

    (a) Thyroid storm is a severe hypermetabolic state that causes hyperpyrexia and tachyarrhythmias due to uncontrolled hyperthyroidism.

        (i) Thyroid storm is rarely found when the patient is adequately prepared preoperatively. It occurs most often when a patient has undiagnosed hyperthyroidism and has surgery for some unrelated emergency.

        (ii) Treatment is with large doses of antithyroid drugs, iodine, and propranolol.

    (b) Hemorrhage is possible due to increased vascularity in a hyperactive thyroid gland.

        (i) Postoperative hemorrhage can cause airway obstruction due to tracheal compression and laryngeal edema.

        (ii) Treatment is by opening the wounds, evacuating the clot, and controlling the bleeding.

    (c) Hypoparathyroidism usually develops within the first 24 hours after surgery and results in a subnormal serum calcium concentration.

        (i) Symptoms of hypocalcemia include numbness and tingling periorally or in the fingers and toes, nervousness, and anxiety. Increased neuromuscular transmission is evidenced by positive Chvostek's and Trousseau's signs.

        (ii) Treatment is with intravenous calcium gluconate, followed by oral calcium and vitamin D therapy after several days if hypocalcemia persists.

        (iii) Serum calcium levels should be checked daily for at least 3 days after thyroidectomy.

    (d) **Recurrent laryngeal nerve injury** produces vocal cord paralysis.

        (i) Unilateral injury is usually manifested by hoarseness. If the nerve is intact, the patient usually recovers a normal voice in 3 weeks to 3 months postoperatively.

        (ii) If the injury is bilateral, airway obstruction results due to paralysis of the vocal cords in the midline adducted position. This requires emergency intubation or tracheostomy. If the nerves are intact and the injury is temporary, recovery usually occurs in 3–6 months. If the injury is permanent, it will require either a permanent tracheostomy or lateral fixation of the arytenoid cartilages.

    (e) Injury to the external branch of the superior layrngeal nerve causes voice fatigue and a loss of timbre and projection.

        (i) This nerve is motor to the cricothyroid muscle and can be injured during ligation of the branches of the superior thyroid artery.

3. **Plummer's disease (toxic multinodular goiter)** is a hyperthyroid state caused by several hyperfunctioning nodules in a multinodular gland. This disorder is most commonly found in women older than 50 years of age and is usually associated with a history of pre-existing nontoxic multinodular goiter.

    a. **Clinical presentation**

      (1) Hypermetabolic symptoms tend to be more subtle than in Graves' disease. However, cardiovascular manifestations of hyperthyroidism, such as tachycardia, palpitations, and arrhythmias (atrial fibrillation) are more common.

      (2) Signs suggesting Plummer's disease are arrhythmias, occasional muscle wasting, and the presence of a multinodular goiter.

    b. **Laboratory studies**

      (1) T_3 and T_4 levels are increased.

      (2) Radioiodine uptake is increased in the hyperfunctioning nodules.

      (3) The nodules will not be suppressed by exogenously administered T_4 (thyroxine).

    c. **Treatment**

      (1) Options for treatment are as outlined for Graves' disease (I D 2 e). Radiolodine tends to be less effective for toxic multinodular goiter than for Graves' disease.

      (2) Preoperative preparation and perioperative management are the same as for Graves' disease except for the use of iodides, which may worsen the hyperthyroidism (see I D 2 e [1]–[3]).

4. **Toxic adenoma** causes hyperthyroidism due to an autonomously hyperfunctioning solitary nodule in an otherwise normal gland.

    a. **Clinical presentation**

      (1) **Symptoms.** Initially, the patient may be asymptomatic because hormone production by the rest of the gland will be suppressed. Eventually symptoms of hyperthyroidism can occur as the nodule continues to secrete thyroid hormone.

      (2) **Signs.** A solitary thyroid nodule may be palpable in an otherwise normal gland.

    b. **Laboratory studies.** T_3 and T_4 levels are increased; radioactive iodine uptake (RAIU) is increased in the nodule (hot nodule), and hormone secretion will not be suppressed by exogenously administered T_4.

    c. **Treatment.** Surgical excision of the nodule (lobectomy) is the safest and most expeditious treatment. Preparation for surgery is as outlined for Graves' disease.

E **Enlargements of the thyroid (goiters)**

1. **Overview.** Enlargements in the thyroid gland have been collectively referred to as **goiters**. Goiters may be **diffuse** or **focal** and may be either smooth or nodular. They may be associated with normal thyroid function or with thyroid hyperfunction or hypofunction.

    a. Diffuse non-nodular goiters with normal or decreased function are due to benign causes.

    b. Focal or nodular goiters with normal function may be due to thyroid neoplasms.

2. Diffuse thyroid enlargements
  a. Colloid and iodine-deficiency goiters
    (1) Incidence. They occur infrequently in the United States.
    (2) Clinical presentation. These are large, bulky, soft enlargements of the thyroid that may grow to sizable proportions. They occasionally produce compressive symptoms.
    (3) Treatment
      (a) Compressive symptoms may require surgery, but occasionally they are removed for cosmetic reasons.
      (b) Other treatment is medical and depends on the cause of the goiter.
  b. Thyroiditis. Inflammations of the thyroid can be acute, subacute, or chronic.
    (1) Acute suppurative thyroiditis is an uncommon disorder caused by the hematogenous spread of microorganisms into the thyroid gland.
      (a) Clinical presentation
        (i) The clinical picture is that of acute inflammation with pain and tenderness, swelling, and redness over one or both lobes.
        (ii) The condition may occur in an immunocompromised patient.
        (iii) Staphylococci and streptococci have been incriminated, but any organism can be causative.
      (b) Diagnosis is established by needle aspiration with appropriate bacteriologic studies.
      (c) Treatment is by open drainage or localized resection with administration of appropriate antibiotics.
    (2) Subacute thyroiditis (giant cell, granulomatous, or de Quervain's thyroiditis) is thought to be viral in origin and is often preceded by an upper respiratory infection.
      (a) Clinical presentation
        (i) It is characterized by sore throat, enlargement of the gland (which may be asymmetrical), and tenderness and induration over the gland.
        (ii) Patients may have symptoms of hyperthyroidism due to the release of thyroid hormone from the gland secondary to the inflammation, but the radioiodine uptake is always decreased, distinguishing it from Graves' disease.
        (iii) The disorder is self-limited, usually lasting from 2–6 months.
        (iv) Occasionally, subacute thyroiditis is painless, causing hyperthyroidism without symptoms of inflammation in the gland, so it may resemble Graves' disease clinically. This form is also distinguished from Graves' disease by the low radioiodine uptake. Painless thyroiditis frequently occurs during the postpartum period.
      (b) Treatment. Symptoms are controlled with either aspirin or corticosteroids.
        (i) β-adrenergic blockade may be used to relieve the symptoms of hyperthyroidism.
        (ii) Antithyroid drugs are ineffective because the hyperthyroidism is not caused by increased thyroid hormone synthesis.
    (3) Chronic thyroiditis occurs in two major forms, Hashimoto's and Riedel's.
      (a) Hashimoto's thyroiditis (struma lymphomatosa) is a relatively common autoimmune disorder that occurs predominantly in women. It is considered to be autoimmune because it coexists with other autoimmune conditions and is associated with the presence of antithyroid antibodies in the serum.
        (i) Clinical presentation. Because Hashimoto's thyroiditis is a rather common form of thyroid enlargement today, it should be considered in any woman who has a goiter and hypothyroidism. It is usually unassociated with any other symptoms. The enlargement in the thyroid is most commonly diffuse and is less commonly nodular or asymmetrical. There does not appear to be a predilection for thyroid cancer, but thyroid cancer should be suspected when the thyroiditis is associated with a dominant nodule. Needle biopsy is helpful in confirming the diagnosis.
        (ii) Diagnosis. Thyroid function studies are normal or indicate hypothyroidism. Radioiodine uptake and scans show decreased uptake with patchy distribution.
        (iii) Treatment. This form of thyroiditis is usually treated with long-term thyroxine therapy. The gland will usually regress in size unless there is considerable

fibrosis. Surgery is indicated when a dominant mass is not suppressed by thyroxine therapy, when the gland continues to enlarge despite thyroxine therapy, and when the history and physical findings or the needle biopsy are suggestive of thyroid malignancy.

  (b) Riedel's (fibrous) thyroiditis is a relatively rare form of thyroiditis in which the thyroid parenchyma is almost completely replaced with dense fibrous tissue.

    (i) Clinical presentation. Riedel's thyroiditis usually occurs during middle age and may cause pressure symptoms, such as cough, dyspnea, or dysphagia. Because the gland is usually stony hard, the condition is difficult to distinguish from thyroid malignancy.

    (ii) Treatment. Surgery (i.e., resection of the isthmus) is needed both to confirm the diagnosis and to relieve compression symptoms.

3. Nodular thyroid enlargements. Diffuse multinodular goiter is the most common form of thyroid enlargement. It is the cause of a palpable nodule in the thyroid in as many as 10% of the adult population.

  a. Clinical presentation. These goiters are caused by adenomatous hyperplasia of the thyroid gland.

    (1) The thyroid enlargement is thought to be due to long-standing stimulation of the thyroid by TSH during a period of suboptimal thyroid hormone production.

    (2) The progression to multinodularity occurs through a process of cyclic changes of hyperplasia and colloid formation.

    (3) Despite the relatively high incidence of adenomatous hyperplasia, the presence of biologically active thyroid cancer in multinodular goiters without clinical evidence of malignancy occurs in fewer than 1% of cases.

  b. Pathogenesis. The nodules in the glands show a wide variety of pathologic findings.

    (1) Some are filled with colloid, while others show evidence of cystic degeneration.

    (2) There may be focal calcification, hemorrhage, or scarring.

  c. Diagnosis

    (1) Most patients are asymptomatic, and the nodularity is detected on routine physical examination.

    (2) Occasionally, these glands may enlarge to the point where they may cause symptoms due to tracheal and/or esophageal compression. The patient may experience pain, dyspnea, or difficulty in swallowing if the nodules enlarge either spontaneously or due to hemorrhage.

    (3) Thyroid function studies are normal, as are thyroid antibodies. Radioiodine uptake is normal, but scanning shows variegated uptake of the radioiodine in the areas of multinodularity.

    (4) Patients with "cold" dominant nodules on radioiodine uptake should undergo fine-needle aspiration to rule out malignancy.

  d. Treatment

    (1) If there are no clinical signs of malignancy and the gland is not symptomatic, no treatment is necessary and simple observation is appropriate.

    (2) If the gland is cosmetically objectionable or if pressure symptoms develop, then exogenous thyroid hormone may be administered. The purpose of thyroxine therapy is to suppress endogenous TSH stimulation of the gland and to allow the gland to shrink. Lifelong therapy may be required.

    (3) Subtotal or total thyroidectomy is advisable if the glands are large enough to produce compressive symptoms, extend substernally, or do not regress with thyroxine therapy.

    (4) If patients develop clinical signs of malignancy, this should be confirmed by needle-aspiration biopsy, and appropriate surgery should be performed.

F **Thyroid neoplasms**

1. Overview. The most common reason for thyroid surgery today is to diagnose or treat a suspected thyroid neoplasm that cannot be diagnosed by other means. Frequently, a solitary or prominent thyroid nodule is detected on physical examination in an asymptomatic patient. The concern is that the nodule will be malignant, although most solitary thyroid nodules are

TABLE 16-1 Clinical Pathologic Classification of Primary Thyroid Malignant Lesions

Pathologic Variety	Local Invasion by Primary Lesion	Multicentric Thyroid	Regional Lymph Node Metastases	Distant Metastases
Carcinoma				
Well-differentiated				
Papillary*	Uncommon	Common	Common	Uncommon
Follicular*				
Low-grade, encapsulated	Rare	Rare	Uncommon	Occasional
High-grade, angioinvasive	Common	Occasional	Common	Common
Hürthle cell tumors	Uncommon	Common	Common	Occasional
Sclerosing ("occult" or minimal)	Uncommon	Rare	Occasional	Rare
Medullary (parafollicular C-cell origin)	Common	Constant in familial	Common	Common
Anaplastic	Always	Common	Common	Common

*Associated foci of anaplastic carcinoma convert this to virulence of anaplastic variety. (Reprinted with permission from Block MA, Cerny JC. Endocrine system. In: Beahrs OH, Beart RW Jr, eds. *General Surgery—Therapy Update Service.* Harwal Medical Publications: Media, PA; 1984:2–7.)

benign. **Clinical pathologic classification** of primary thyroid malignancies is shown in Table 16-1.

2. **Assessment of thyroid nodules**
   a. **Patient's age**
      (1) In children, 10%–15% of thyroid nodules are malignant.
      (2) During the childbearing years, most nodules are benign.
      (3) The incidence of cancer in nodules increases by about 10% per decade after age 40 years.
   b. **Patient's sex**
      (1) Thyroid cancer is more common in women than in men.
      (2) Benign thyroid nodules are also more common in women.
      (3) The likelihood that a nodule will prove to be malignant is greater in men than in women.
   c. **Family history of thyroid malignancy.** Medullary carcinoma of the thyroid may be transmitted as an autosomal dominant trait, but other thyroid cancers are not transmitted genetically.
   d. **History of radiation exposure**
      (1) Exposure of the head or neck region to therapeutic radiation has been found to increase the incidence of thyroid cancer 5- to 10-fold.
         (a) The radiation exposure required to induce neoplasia may be as low as 50 rad.
         (b) Radiation was previously given for a variety of disorders, such as an enlarged thymus in infancy, enlarged tonsils and adenoids during childhood, congenital hemangiomas of the head or neck region, acne vulgaris, and Hodgkin's disease.
      (2) Thyroid cancers from radiation exposure are no different from those that occur without a history of radiation, but the latent interval from the time of radiation exposure until the development of thyroid cancer varies with the age at which the radiation exposure occurred.
         (a) When the thyroid is irradiated during infancy, the mean interval until development of thyroid cancer is 10–12 years.
         (b) When the thyroid is irradiated during adolescence, the mean interval until development of thyroid cancer is 20–25 years.
         (c) When the thyroid is irradiated during adulthood, the mean interval until development of thyroid cancer is 30 years.

> > e. **Characteristics of the nodule**
> > > (1) **Consistency**
> > > > (a) Nodules that are firm in consistency suggest malignancy; however, malignant nodules may undergo cystic degeneration, so they may be somewhat soft to palpation.
> > > > (b) Soft nodules are likely to be benign; however, long-standing adenomatous hyperplasia may be associated with calcification in the nodule, making it firm.
> > > (2) **Infiltration** of the nodule into the surrounding thyroid or overlying structures, such as the strap muscles or trachea, suggests malignancy. However, malignant nodules may have no sign of infiltration and may mimic benign nodules.
> > > (3) **Nodulation. Solitary nodules** have a 20% chance of being malignant. **Multiple nodules** are present in as many as 40% of proven cases of thyroid malignancy.
> > > (4) **Growth patterns.** Nodules that suddenly appear or suddenly increase in size should be suspected of being thyroid neoplasms. Hemorrhage into a pre-existing nodule, such as adenomatous hyperplasia, can cause a sudden increase in the size of the nodule, but this is frequently associated with pain.

> > f. **Ipsilateral lymph node enlargement** suggests thyroid malignancy. In children, as many as 50% of thyroid cancers are first detected because of cervical lymph node enlargement.

> > g. **Mobility of the vocal cords** should be assessed preoperatively in all patients undergoing thyroid operations.
> > > (1) Ipsilateral vocal cord paralysis in a patient with a thyroid nodule is almost always diagnostic of a thyroid malignancy that has infiltrated the recurrent laryngeal nerve.
> > > (2) Because vocal cord paralysis may not be associated with voice changes, the cords should be examined by either indirect or direct laryngoscopy or by nasal pharyngoscopy.
> > > (3) Examination should be repeated postoperatively if voice abnormalities occur.

> 3. **Diagnostic studies.** Although clinical evaluation is the mainstay in distinguishing benign from malignant thyroid nodules, alone it may be insufficient, and other diagnostic studies may be needed.
> > a. **Thyroid function tests** are of little value in diagnosing thyroid cancer. Nearly all thyroid cancers are nonfunctioning, as are the nodules of adenomatous hyperplasia. Therefore, fewer than 1% of all thyroid malignancies will be associated with hyperfunction.

> > b. **Antithyroid antibody levels** may be increased in patients with Hashimoto's thyroiditis, but thyroid cancer may coexist with thyroiditis; thus, a positive antibody test does not preclude the diagnosis of thyroid cancer.

> > c. **Thyrocalcitonin assay** will show an increased level in patients who have medullary carcinoma of the thyroid. Patients who are diagnosed with medullary carcinoma should undergo genetic testing for abnormalities of the RET proto-oncogene as well. Their family members may require genetic testing and counseling as well.

> > d. **Radioisotope scanning** of the thyroid may be done with radioiodine or with technetium-99m (^{99m}Tc) pertechnetate.
> > > (1) Isotope tracers are taken up by normally functioning thyroid tissue, which appears as a "hot" area on a thyroid scan; nodules that do not take up the tracers appear as "cold" areas.
> > > > (a) Approximately 20% of cold nodules will be neoplastic, and approximately 40% of thyroid cancers will take up the radioisotope tracer to some degree.
> > > > (b) Radioisotope scanning may exclude nodules that are not malignant if they appear hot but does not discriminate benign cold nodules from malignant ones.
> > > (2) Iodine-123 (^{123}I) and -125 (^{125}I) give less radiation exposure than iodine-131 (^{131}I) because they have shorter half-lives than ^{131}I. They do not provide any better discrimination than ^{131}I between benign and malignant thyroid nodules.
> > > (3) ^{99m}Tc pertechnetate is trapped in but, in contrast to radioiodine, not organified by the thyroid gland.
> > > > (a) Nodules that are cold to radioiodine will also be cold to ^{99m}Tc.
> > > > (b) Tumors of the thyroid may take up ^{99m}Tc and appear hot on the scan due to the vascularity of the tumor. Thus, all nodules that are hot on a ^{99m}Tc scan should be scanned with radioiodine to determine their function.
> > > > (c) ^{99m}Tc delivers only a fraction of the radiation that is delivered by ^{131}I. It does not discriminate any better than does ^{131}I between benign and malignant thyroid nodules.

    e. Ultrasonography

       (1) Using an ultrasound probe, an image of the size and shape of the thyroid gland and the nodules that it contains can be mapped. Thus, thyroid nodules, can be identified as cystic, solid, or complex (i.e., a mixture of solid and cystic components).

       (2) Although ultrasonography can distinguish pure cysts of the thyroid, which are rarely malignant, from complex or solid masses, it cannot be used to absolutely distinguish benign from malignant complex or solid masses.

       (3) Features that may be suggestive of malignancy include the presence of micro- or macro-calcifications, solid echo-texture, appearance different from other nodules in the gland, indistinct borders, local invasion,or increased vascularity.

       (4) Ultrasonography is helpful in identifying thyroid nodules that are not clinically palpable and in directing a needle to a nonpalpable nodule for biopsy.

    f. Needle biopsy of the thyroid allows for the histopathologic or cytopathologic examination of cells as an aid in the diagnosis of thyroid nodules and in planning therapy. Needle biopsy is the most useful diagnostic tool, aside from surgery, for distinguishing benign from malignant thyroid nodules. However, none of these biopsy techniques can distinguish benign from malignant follicular neoplasms.

       (1) Fine-needle aspiration

         (a) Cells are aspirated from the nodule by applying suction to a syringe attached to a 21- to 25-gauge needle.

         (b) This technique obtains a specimen for cytopathologic examination of individual cells and clusters of cells.

         (c) The technique requires interpretation by a well-trained thyroid cytopathologist.

         (d) It has a good degree of accuracy and specificity in diagnosing thyroid malignant lesions and, due to the small size of the needle, is associated with virtually no complications.

         (e) Inadequate or nondiagnostic specimens must be repeated. Otherwise, operative excision of the nodule may be required to establish the diagnosis.

       (2) Large-needle biopsy

         (a) A plug of tissue is aspirated from the nodule by applying suction to a syringe attached to an 18- or 20-gauge needle that is inserted into the nodule. Fragments of tissue are obtained for cytopathologic and histopathologic examination.

         (b) This technique offers some of the advantages as core biopsy but has a lower rate of complications as compared with core biopsy due to the smaller size of the needle.

         (c) The combination of fine-needle and large-needle aspiration carries with it an adequacy in diagnosis of 90%–95% in experienced hands.

       (3) Core biopsy

         (a) Using a 14- or 18-gauge specially designed needle (Tru-Cut), this biopsy technique obtains a cylinder of tissue from the thyroid nodule. The specimen is then fixed and stained for histopathologic analysis.

         (b) It is the most accurate method of assessing the histologic nature of a thyroid nodule.

         (c) Because of the large size of the needle, it is unsuitable for biopsy of small nodules.

         (d) Due to a relatively high incidence of bleeding complications, the technique is rarely performed.

4. Operative approach to the thyroid nodule (Fig. 16-3)

    a. Overview. Operative removal is the mainstay of treatment for thyroid carcinoma.

       (1) The **extent of the operation** will depend on the:

         (a) Histologic type of thyroid cancer

         (b) Extent of the tumor as determined from the preoperative assessment and the operative findings. For a solitary nodule confined to one lobe, the minimal operation is total removal of that lobe and the isthmus.

         (c) Biologic aggressiveness of the tumor

       (2) A frozen section of the resected tissue must always be obtained to determine whether the nodule is benign or malignant.

         (a) If the lesion is grossly benign in appearance and the frozen section reports a benign lesion, but the permanent sections reveal it to be papillary or follicular carcinoma,

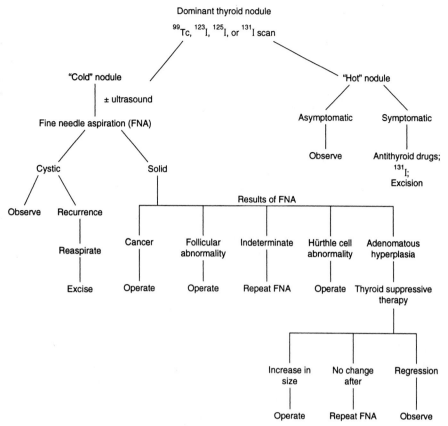

FIGURE 16-3 Algorithm for evaluation and management of an asymptomatic thyroid nodule discovered on routine physical examination.

the extent of further surgery is determined by the biologic aggressiveness of the lesion.

   (b) If the lesion appears to be grossly malignant and is confined to one lobe without invasion of surrounding tissues, then total removal of that lobe and the isthmus, and near-total removal of the opposite lobe are appropriate therapy.

   (c) If the lesion appears grossly malignant and extends beyond the thyroid or involves both lobes, then total thyroidectomy is indicated.

(3) Lymph node resection is indicated when nodes appear to be grossly involved.

   (a) The resection should generally concentrate on nodes in the interjugular location, especially in the tracheoesophageal groove.

   (b) Prophylactic removal of uninvolved lymph nodes is of no proven benefit.

(4) The parathyroid glands and the recurrent laryngeal nerve should be identified in all operations. The parathyroid glands should be reimplanted in an appropriate skeletal muscle site if their blood supply is compromised during thyroidectomy.

(5) The complication rate after total thyroidectomy, and especially the incidence of permanent hypoparathyroidism, is significantly greater than the rate after near-total thyroidectomy. Therefore, total thyroidectomy should not be performed unless it is of proven clinical benefit.

 b. Biologic aggressiveness of thyroid cancers. Two risk groups have been defined for patients with well-differentiated thyroid cancer, based on an analysis by the Lahey Clinic and the Mayo Clinic.

(1) Low-risk group. This group consists of women who are younger than 50 years of age and men who are younger than 40 years of age with intrathyroidal papillary carcinoma or follicular carcinoma with minimal vascular or lymphatic invasion, both of which are less than 5 cm in size and are not associated with distant spread.

   (a) Unless both lobes are grossly involved with tumor, patients in this group do as well with near-total thyroidectomy as with total thyroidectomy. The remaining thyroid remnant may be ablated postoperatively with ^{131}I.

    (b) After surgery, patients should receive exogenous thyroid hormone for life to suppress endogenous TSH production.

    (c) With comparable treatment, the recurrence rate and death rate in this group have been found to be significantly lower than in the high-risk group.

   (2) High-risk group. This group consists of patients of any age with evidence of distant spread or with extrathyroidal papillary carcinoma, follicular carcinoma with significant vascular invasion (tumors greater than 5 cm in size), or women who are older than 50 years of age and men who are older than 40 years of age with either papillary or follicular carcinoma.

    (a) In this group, the tumors are much more aggressive and require a more aggressive initial approach because local recurrences are more difficult to treat and the mortality rate is significantly greater. Thus, total thyroidectomy is indicated in these patients.

    (b) Lymph node dissection of palpable nodes should be more extensive than in the low-risk groups.

    (c) Radioiodine ablation of any tissue showing radioiodine uptake postoperatively should be performed, and exogenous thyroid hormone should be administered to suppress TSH production.

 5. Types of thyroid malignancy

  a. Papillary carcinoma

   (1) Incidence

    (a) Papillary carcinoma accounts for 80% of all thyroid cancers in children and 60% in adults.

    (b) It affects women twice as often as men and is the most common histologic type found in patients who have a history of radiation exposure.

   (2) Characteristics

    (a) The tumor is characterized by a slow rate of growth and spread to regional lymphatics in 50% of the cases. It spreads by way of the bloodstream in fewer than 5% of cases.

    (b) Tumors range in size from occult (less than 1.5 cm in diameter) to tumors that involve an entire lobe or both lobes.

    (c) In 40% of cases, the tumor is multicentric in origin.

     (i) Microscopic multicentric lesions rarely develop into clinical carcinoma.

     (ii) Macroscopic multicentric lesions will usually be biologically similar to papillary cancer.

    (d) Some tumors are well encapsulated with minimal invasion of adjacent normal thyroid. Others are poorly encapsulated with invasion to perithyroidal structures.

   (3) Prognosis

    (a) Prognosis is excellent with occult or well-encapsulated intrathyroidal carcinoma. Patients with these tumors have a 20-year survival rate of better than 90%.

    (b) Prognosis is poor when the tumor is poorly encapsulated and extends by extrathyroidal invasion. The 20-year survival rate is less than 50%.

    (c) Prognosis is also poorer as the patient's age increases beyond 40 years.

    (d) Survival does not appear to be adversely affected by lymphatic spread.

  b. Follicular carcinoma

   (1) Incidence

    (a) Follicular carcinoma accounts for approximately 20% of all thyroid malignancies. It is more common in areas of the world where iodine-deficiency goiter is in evidence.

    (b) It also affects women twice as often as men.

    (c) Its relative frequency increases after 40 years of age.

   (2) Characteristics

    (a) Follicular carcinoma spreads primarily through the bloodstream by way of angioinvasion. It rarely spreads to regional lymph nodes except for locally invasive nodules that extend into the perithyroidal tissue.

    (b) The tumor is slow growing and usually unifocal.

    (c) When found cytologically to be combined with papillary elements, it is biologically similar to papillary carcinoma.

(3) Prognosis

(a) Prognosis is good when there is minimal vascular invasion, with a better than 80% 20-year survival rate.

(b) Prognosis is poor when there is gross invasion, with a less than 20% 20-year survival rate.

c. Medullary carcinoma

(1) Incidence

(a) Medullary carcinoma of the thyroid accounts for fewer than 10% of all thyroid cancers.

(b) It occurs at all ages without predilection for either sex.

(c) It most commonly occurs sporadically but also can be genetically transmitted.

(i) When it occurs sporadically, it usually appears as a solitary lesion.

(ii) When transmitted genetically, it may occur as a solitary lesion or may be a part of multiple endocrine neoplasia (MEN) syndrome type II; (see Chapter 17, I B 2, C 2, D 2).

(2) Characteristics

(a) Early spread to the lymphatics is characteristic, and spread by way of the bloodstream is also common.

(b) There are two types of medullary carcinoma that are indistinguishable histologically:

(i) Those characterized by aggressive, rapid growth, rapid spread, and early metastasis

(ii) Those characterized by slow growth and a prolonged course despite metastasis

(c) Because these tumors arise from the C cells of the thyroid, they produce thyrocalcitonin.

(i) This hormone can be detected by radioimmunoassay in early stages of tumor development.

(ii) In patients with hereditary MEN type II, the disease can be detected in this way before the development of clinically evident malignancy.

(3) Prognosis is poorer than for papillary or follicular carcinoma and is related to the stage of the tumor at the time of its initial diagnosis.

(a) Stage I medullary carcinoma has a 50% 20-year survival rate.

(b) Stage II has a less than 10% 20-year survival rate.

(c) Death results from generalized metastasis.

(d) Medullary thyroid carcinoma occurring in MEN syndrome is curable by total thyroidectomy if detected and treated before the development of clinically evident malignancy.

d. Anaplastic carcinoma

(1) Incidence

(a) This tumor accounts for fewer than 10% of all thyroid cancers.

(b) It is most common between the ages of 50 and 70 years and shows no predilection for either sex.

(2) Characteristics

(a) Anaplastic carcinomas are characterized by small cells, giant cells, or spindle cells.

(b) They usually arise from a pre-existing, well-differentiated thyroid neoplasm, such as a follicular lesion.

(c) They grow rapidly into local structures, such as the trachea and esophagus, and metastasize early by way of the lymphatics and the bloodstream, so they are usually incurable at the time of initial presentation.

(3) Prognosis

(a) Prognosis is poor with a fatal outcome in almost all instances, regardless of the type of treatment.

(b) When treatment appears successful, the lesion may well have been a lymphoma instead of a small cell anaplastic carcinoma, and the histologic nature of the neoplasm should be confirmed by electron microscopy or immunohistochemistry.

e. Lymphoma and lymphosarcoma

(1) Incidence. This tumor accounts for fewer than 1% of all thyroid malignancies and affects mostly women 50–70 years of age.

(2) Characteristics

(a) Fine-needle aspiration alone may not be able to establish this diagnosis. Core biopsy or open biopsy may be required.

(b) Pathologically, these are usually small cell tumors and may be difficult to distinguish from small cell anaplastic carcinoma except by electron microscopy.

(c) The lesion may occur primarily in the thyroid gland as an extranodal growth, or it may be part of a generalized lymphomatous process.

(d) The local type is best treated by radiation therapy, whereas the diffuse type will probably require systemic multidrug chemotherapy. Unless the tumor is small and confined to the thyroid lobe, surgical excision is generally not indicated.

(3) Prognosis is variable and depends on the cell type and whether the tumor is local or diffuse.

II   ADRENAL GLAND

A **Introduction**   The adrenal glands are the source of several tumors, benign and malignant, and of hyperplasias, primary and secondary. Some of these lesions produce syndromes due to the overproduction of normal adrenal hormones, including Cushing's syndrome, Conn's syndrome, and pheochromocytomas. The diagnosis and treatment of these disease states require a thorough knowledge of the production, action, and metabolism of the adrenal hormones.

1. Embryology. The adrenal gland consists of two distinct parts, the **cortex** and the **medulla,** each of which has a different embryologic origin.

  a. The **adrenal medulla** originates from ectodermal cells of neural crest origin.

  (1) These cells migrate from the sympathetic ganglion and combine to form the medulla, which is surrounded by mesodermal cortex.

  (2) Additional **collections of adrenal medullary tissue** can form. These are most frequently found in the paraganglia, in the organ of Zuckerkandl just below the origin of the inferior mesenteric artery, and in the mediastinum.

  b. The **adrenal cortex** is derived from mesodermal cells near the genital ridge.

  (1) These cells coalesce to form a complete layer around the ectodermal cells that will form the adrenal medulla.

  (2) Occasionally, these cells become separated from the main cortex and form **adrenocortical rests.** These are most commonly found in the ovary or testis and near the adrenal glands and kidneys.

2. Anatomy. There are two adrenal glands, each one lying on the medial aspect of the superior pole of a kidney. The normal combined weight of the two glands is about 10 g.

  a. Histology. Three distinct areas can be recognized in the cortex.

  (1) The **zona glomerulosa** is the outer zone, where the production of mineralocorticoids such as aldosterone takes place.

  (2) The **zona fasciculata** is the intermediate zone, where cortisol and the other **glucocorticoids** are produced.

  (3) The **zona reticularis** is the inner zone, where **androgens** and **estrogens** are made.

  b. Vasculature of the adrenal glands

  (1) Arterial supply to the adrenals varies but arises from three primary sources (i.e., the phrenic artery, aorta, and renal artery).

  (2) Venous drainage is more constant. There is usually a large single vein on each side of the body. The right adrenal vein drains into the vena cava, and the left adrenal vein empties into the left renal vein. Small accessory veins can occur.

  (3) Adrenal portal system. Venous blood from the cortex, containing high levels of glucocorticoids, drains into the medulla, helping to induce the enzyme phenylethanolamine-*N*-methyltransferase. This enzyme methylates norepinephrine to form epinephrine.

B **Adrenal hormones and catecholamines**

1. Steroid hormones. The adrenal cortex produces three main classes of steroid hormones: the glucocorticoids, the mineralocorticoids, and the sex steroids (androgens and estrogens).

a. Glucocorticoids. The most important glucocorticoid physiologically is **cortisol.** Production of cortisol takes place primarily in the **zona fasciculata.** There is a diurnal variation, with the highest levels occurring around 6:00 A.M. and the lowest levels at 8–12 P.M.

(1) Regulation

(a) Adrenocorticotropic hormone (ACTH; corticotropin) is produced by the anterior pituitary gland. ACTH stimulates the production of cortisol by the adrenal. **Cortisol,** in turn, exerts a negative feedback on ACTH production at the hypothalamic-pituitary level.

(b) Corticotropin-releasing factor (CRF) is produced by the hypothalamus and stimulates the release of ACTH from the pituitary.

(c) Free cortisol is the active hormone. Normally, most circulating cortisol is bound to **corticosteroid-binding globulin (CBG).** When large amounts of cortisol are produced, the binding sites become saturated, and the levels of free hormone will increase.

(2) Metabolism. Cortisol is metabolized in the liver by conjugation with glucuronide. This renders it water soluble for urinary excretion. The level of urinary 17-hydroxycorticosteroids reflects glucocorticoid production and metabolism. However, in states of hypercortisolism, the urinary free cortisol is more accurate.

b. Mineralocorticoids. The major mineralocorticoid produced by the adrenal gland is **aldosterone,** which is produced in the **zona glomerulosa** of the adrenal cortex.

(1) Regulation

(a) Aldosterone production is regulated chiefly by the **renin-angiotensin system** and changes in plasma concentrations of sodium and potassium.

(i) Renin is released by the juxtaglomerular cells of the kidney in response to a decrease in blood pressure.

(ii) Renin converts **angiotensinogen** (made in the liver) to **angiotensin I.**

(iii) Angiotensin I is converted to **angiotensin II** by **angiotensin-converting enzyme,** which is produced by endothelial cells.

(iv) Angiotensin II stimulates the adrenal cortex to release **aldosterone.**

(b) Aldosterone production is minimally controlled by ACTH.

(c) The sympathetic nervous system can also stimulate the release of aldosterone.

(2) Metabolism. Aldosterone is metabolized in a similar manner to cortisol. It is excreted in the urine in small quantities and can be measured by radioimmunoassay.

c. Sex steroids. Androgens and **estrogens** are produced in the **zona reticularis** of the adrenal cortex. The urinary level of 17-ketosteroids reflects the androgen production. Estrogens can also be measured in the urine.

2. Catecholamines. The **adrenal medulla** is the site of catecholamine production, including dopamine, norepinephrine, and epinephrine.

a. Regulation. Catecholamine production is under the control of the sympathetic nervous system.

b. Metabolism

(1) The pathways of catecholamine production and metabolism in the adrenal medulla are summarized in Figure 16-4. Dopamine can also be metabolized by an alternate pathway to homovanillic acid (HVA).

(2) The levels of metanephrine, normetanephrine, vanillylmandelic acid (VMA), and the individual catecholamines can be measured in the urine to evaluate the function of adrenal tumors.

C Congenital virilizing adrenal hyperplasia

1. Pathogenesis

a. If an enzyme is missing from the pathway of cortisol production, the consequent shortage of cortisol will cause an increase in ACTH activity, and adrenal hyperplasia will result. The cortisol precursors will then be shunted into the production of androgens.

b. Although several different enzymes can be congenitally absent, the most common defect is a block in hydroxylation at C-21 of the cortisol molecule.

2. Clinical presentation

a. Virilization results from the hormonal defect. In the female, this produces **pseudohermaphroditism,** and in the male, **macrogenitosomia precox.**

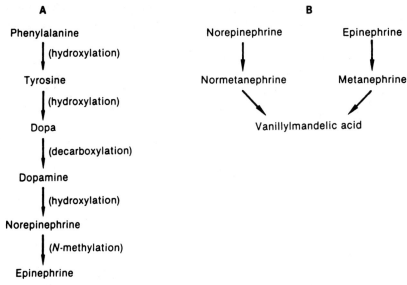

FIGURE 16-4 Pathways of **(A)** catecholamine production and **(B)** metabolism.

    b. In a minority of cases, the block is more complete, and a severe salt-losing state with vascular collapse results from the aldosterone deficiency.

  3. Diagnosis. The diagnosis can be suspected from the characteristic virilization and the excess levels of 17-ketosteroids in the urine.

  4. Treatment

    a. The metabolic deficiency is treated with steroid replacement.

    b. In females, plastic surgical procedures are often necessary to correct the genital deformities.

    c. An accurate sex assignment must be made in female pseudohermaphrodites by means of karyotyping and Barr body analysis.

D **Adrenocortical insufficiency (Addison's disease)**　This condition is important to the practicing surgeon because patients who have Addison's disease are not capable of undergoing the stress of surgery without receiving corticosteroid support.

  1. Types. Addison's disease may be primary or secondary.

    a. Primary adrenocortical insufficiency results in diminished or absent function of the adrenal cortex because of adrenal pathology. **Causes** include:

      (1) An autoimmune attack on the adrenal gland

      (2) Bilateral adrenal tuberculosis

      (3) Adrenal fungal infections

      (4) Bilateral adrenal hemorrhage, which can occur:

        (a) Secondary to meningococcal septicemia

        (b) Postpartum

        (c) In patients on anticoagulant therapy

    b. Secondary adrenocortical insufficiency is due to atrophy of the adrenal cortex secondary to a decreased pituitary production of ACTH. **Causes** include:

      (1) ACTH suppression by corticosteroid drugs, which is **the most common cause of adrenal insufficiency** encountered in the surgical patient

      (2) Primary pituitary pathology, which is a **less common cause**

  2. Clinical presentation

    a. Cortisol deficiency, which occurs in both the primary and secondary forms, is manifested by:

      (1) Anorexia, malaise, and weight loss

      (2) Poor tolerance of stress

      (3) Hypoglycemia

      (4) Hypotension

      (5) Occasionally, hyperpigmentation of the skin

    b. Aldosterone deficiency occurs only in the primary form because aldosterone production is not primarily under feedback control via ACTH. It causes a tendency for:

        (1) Volume depletion

        (2) Hyponatremia and hyperkalemia

        (3) Azotemia and acidosis

3. Preparation for surgery

    a. A patient who has taken steroids regularly for any period during the past year is assumed to have inadequate adrenal reserve.

    b. Perioperative steroid replacement is handled on an individual basis and depends on how long the patient was taking steroids, the dosage that was taken, and the magnitude of the planned procedure. The following is a general **guideline** for a patient undergoing a major operation who is a **chronic steroid user:**

        (1) The target is 100–150 mg of hydrocortisone intravenously daily for 2–3 days.

        (2) The steroid dosage is then returned to the preoperative oral dosage.

E Hyperadrenocorticalism (Cushing's syndrome)

1. Types. Cushing's syndrome results from the effects of chronically increased cortisol levels. Different mechanisms cause two types of Cushing's syndrome.

    a. ACTH dependent

        (1) Pituitary Cushing's syndrome, or **Cushing's disease,** accounts for approximately 70% of the cases of Cushing's syndrome and is more common in middle-aged women.

            (a) It results from an overproduction of ACTH by the pituitary, which results in bilateral adrenal hyperplasia.

            (b) The source of the excess ACTH has been debated.

                (i) Pituitary tumors, either chromophobic or basophilic adenomas, probably account for the majority of cases. Some autopsy series have shown pituitary tumors in at least 90% of patients who have Cushing's disease.

                (ii) However, in the remaining patients no tumor was found. This raises the possibility of an abnormality in the hypothalamic-pituitary axis, resulting in increased ACTH secretion.

        (2) Ectopic Cushing's syndrome also represents approximately 15% of the cases and is more common in older men.

            (a) In this form, ACTH is produced by an extra-adrenal, extrapituitary neoplasm. The result is a hyperplasia of the adrenocortical tissue with consequent hypercortisolism.

            (b) The cause is most commonly a small cell carcinoma of the lung, but the syndrome can also occur with bronchial carcinoids, thymomas, and tumors of the pancreas and liver.

    b. ACTH independent. Adrenal Cushing's syndrome accounts for approximately 15% of the cases.

        (1) It is caused by an excess of cortisol that is produced autonomously by the adrenal cortex. This can be due to an adenoma, a carcinoma, or bilateral nodular dysplasia and ectopic cortisol-producing tumors.

        (2) The remaining adrenocortical tissue atrophies, and ACTH levels are low because of suppression by the excess cortisol.

2. Clinical presentation. The presentation of Cushing's syndrome is extremely variable and consists of any combination of various features. The most common manifestations are listed in Table 16-2.

3. Diagnosis. No one test is conclusive for Cushing's syndrome. However, the normal **diurnal rhythm** of cortisol secretion is usually lost in Cushing's syndrome. The laboratory test results and the clinical presentation must be considered together to make an accurate diagnosis (Table 16-3).

    a. Plasma total cortisol is the most direct measurement, since Cushing's syndrome is a state of hypercortisolism.

        (1) The accuracy of this determination is increased by measuring morning and afternoon samples as well as a morning sample after a suppressing dose of dexamethasone the night before.

TABLE 16-2	Common Manifestations of Cushing's Syndrome
Hypertension	Peripheral muscle wasting
Diabetes	Striae
Hypokalemic alkalosis	Easy bruising
Osteoporosis	Hirsutism
Buffalo hump	Acne
Truncal obesity	Menstrual irregularities
Muscle weakness	Emotional lability

    (2) Plasma cortisol levels are suggestive of Cushing's syndrome if they exceed 30 μg/dL at 8:00 A.M. and 15 μg/dL at 5:00 P.M., or 10 μg/dL at 8:00 A.M., following a midnight dose of 1 mg dexamethasone, especially if these results are reproducible on several different days.

    (3) The overnight dexamethasone suppression test is not fully reliable, as both false-positive and false-negative results occur. Adjusting the dose of dexamethasone on the basis of the patient's weight may reduce the number of false-positive and false-negative results.

  b. **24-Hour urinary free cortisol** is the most reliable urinary index of hypercortisolism due to the increased renal clearance of unmetabolized cortisol, if further confirmation is needed.

4. Pathogenesis. Once the diagnosis of Cushing's syndrome has been made, the underlying pathophysiologic mechanism (see II E 1) must be identified.

  a. The **plasma ACTH level** gives a good indication of the type of Cushing's syndrome.

    (1) Extremely low values are found with adrenal Cushing's syndrome due to the suppressive effects of cortisol.

    (2) Very high levels occur with ectopic Cushing's syndrome due to the autonomous ACTH production.

    (3) In pituitary Cushing's syndrome, the values are normal in 50% of the cases but are increased in the other 50%.

  b. **Differentiating ectopic from pituitary Cushing's syndrome** when the ACTH level is in the intermediate range can be difficult. Four methods are helpful in making this distinction:

    (1) **High-dose dexamethasone suppression test.** After the diagnosis of Cushing's syndrome has been made, the patient is given dexamethasoiie, 8 mg/day for 2 days, and the urine is collected for measurement of 17-hydroxycorticosteroids. In pituitary Cushing's syndrome, the 17-hydroxycorticosteroid levels will usually decrease to less than 50% of normal, whereas they will show no suppression in the ectopic syndrome. However, there have been enough recorded exceptions in both cases to make this test of questionable value.

    (2) Corticotropin-releasing hormone (CRH) test. Response to CRH stimulation can be used instead of high-dose dexamethasone suppression (Table 16-4).

    (3) Jugular versus peripheral ACTH levels. Samples of venous blood are drawn from a peripheral site and, by catheterization, from the inferior petrosal sinus. Ratios of petrosal to peripheral ACTH greater than 2.0 have correlated with a pituitary source for the Cushing's syndrome and ratios less than 1.5 with an ectopic source.

TABLE 16-3	ACTH Determinations for Sources of Cushing's Syndrome		
Type of Cushing's Syndrome	Plasma ACTH Level	ACTH after High-dose Dexamethasone Suppression Test	CRH Stimulation Test
Pituitary Cushing's syndrome (Cushing's disease)	Normal to increased	Decreased	Increased
Adrenal Cushing's syndrome	Low or undetectable	Baseline	Baseline
Ectopic Cushing's syndrome	Increased	Baseline	Baseline

ACTH, adrenocorticotropic hormone; CRH, corticotropin-releasing hormone.

TABLE 16-4   Corticotropin-releasing Hormone Stimulation Test Response

Disease State	Plasma ACTH	Plasma Cortisol
Normal	Increased	Increased
Cushing's disease	Increased	Highly increased
Adrenal or ectopic Cushing's disease	Baseline	Baseline

CRH, corticotropin-releasing hormone; ACTH, adrenocorticotropic hormone.

    (4) Plasma lipotropic hormone (LPH, lipotropin) concentration. This tends to be higher than the ACTH concentration with ectopic Cushing's syndrome, while the opposite holds true for pituitary Cushing's syndrome.

5. Localization of the tumor
    a. Pituitary Cushing's syndrome. Polytomography of the sella turcica has localized some pituitary tumors, but computed tomography (CT) and magnetic resonance imaging (MRI) are more sensitive and are specific for detecting small adenomas.
    b. Ectopic Cushing's syndrome. A chest film usually shows the offending neoplasm; however, a technique such as CT or MRI may be needed to detect pancreatic or hepatic tumors.
    c. Adrenal Cushing's syndrome. Several techniques are available.
        (1) CT or MRI can correctly identify more than 90% of adrenal lesions, including adenomas larger than 1 cm in diameter, carcinomas, and bilateral hyperplasia.
        (2) Radioisotope scanning. A radiocholesterol analogue, **NP-59** (iodomethylnorcholesterol), can successfully localize functioning adrenocortical tumors in 70%–75% of these patients.
        (3) Arteriography can localize adrenal tumors and is helpful in assessing the arterial supply of a neoplasm before its surgical removal.
        (4) Retrograde adrenal venography can also localize adrenal tumors and allows for bilateral cortisol measurements. However, there is a 5% risk of adrenal hemorrhage and possible infarction.
        (5) Venacavography is helpful if a malignancy is suspected to assess the intravenous extension of the tumor.

6. Treatment
    a. Curative therapy
        (1) Pituitary Cushing's syndrome. Treatment depends on the cause.
            (a) Trans-sphenoidal resection of the tumor is the procedure of choice if a pituitary adenoma is localized.
            (b) Pituitary irradiation from an external source has been effective in up to 80% of children. However, the cure rate is only about 15%–20% for adults.
                (i) Implantation of yttrium-90 may improve results, but this requires a separate operation for implantation and may cause progressive hypopituitarism.
                (ii) There is a lag period with radiation therapy of up to 18 months before effects are seen.
            (c) Bilateral total adrenalectomy
                (i) With the advent of effective trans-sphenoidal removal of pituitary adenomas, bilateral adrenalectomy is now reserved for cases in which no pituitary adenoma is found, radiation has failed, or when the patient is too sick to tolerate the prolonged radiation process or to await its ultimate effect.
                (ii) The advantage of bilateral adrenalectomy is its immediate and complete control of the cushingoid state.
                (iii) The disadvantages are the increased morbidity and mortality secondary to the operative procedure. It produces a permanent addisonian state, and in at least 15% of the cases, an ACTH-secreting pituitary tumor develops (**Nelson's syndrome**). Therefore, all patients treated for Cushing's disease with bilateral total adrenalectomy must be monitored yearly with visual field examination and sellar tomography or head CT scans.

(2) **Ectopic Cushing's syndrome.** Treatment is directed toward the underlying neoplasm secreting ACTH. Removal of the tumor is curative. However, because of the diffuse nature of small cell lung cancers, often only palliative therapy can be offered.

(3) **Adrenal Cushing's syndrome.** Treatment involves total adrenalectomy via laparopscopic or open techniques.

(a) Laparoscopic adrenalectomy has become the preferred approach for most benign adenomas less than 6 cm in size. The gland may be approached transabdominally or retroperitoneally via the flank or back.

(b) Open adrenalectomy via an anterior or flank approach is advisable for lesions greater than 6 cm or for those with aggressive characteristics on imaging studies (significant heterogeneity, nodal involvment, local soft tissue or vascular invasion). Even if all of the malignant tissue cannot be removed, palliative therapy is easier if as much tumor as possible is resected.

b. **Palliative chemotherapy** can be offered to those patients who have unresectable or incompletely resected malignancies and, during the lag phase, to those undergoing radiation treatment. Remissions can be obtained in about 60% of the cases, but relapse is rapid after drug cessation. Two groups of drugs exist with differing sites of action.

(1) Drugs acting on the adrenal cortex, inhibiting steroid synthesis, include mitotane (formerly called o,p'-DDD), metyrapone, trilostane, and aminoglutethimide.

(2) Centrally acting drugs appear to be fast acting and less toxic. They apparently act by affecting the hypothalamic release of CRF and, therefore, pituitary ACTH production. These drugs include cyproheptadine (a serotonin antagonist) and bromocriptine (a dopamine agonist).

F **Primary hyperaldosteronism (Conn's syndrome)**

1. **Overview.** Conn's syndrome is due to the excess secretion of aldosterone by the adrenal cortex as a result of a unilateral adenoma of the adrenal gland in 85% of the cases and to bilateral adenomas in fewer than 5%. Bilateral hyperplasia causes about 5%–10% of the cases. Rarely, the syndrome is due to an adrenocortical carcinoma.

2. **Types.** It is important to **distinguish primary from secondary hyperaldosteronism.** It is also important to distinguish hyperaldosteronism due to an adenoma from that due to hyperplasia because surgical excision is curative for most cases of adenoma, but the response is not as good in hyperplasia.

a. **In the primary form,** plasma renin levels are normal or low.

b. **In the secondary form,** there is an increase in plasma renin and, subsequently, in aldosterone. This results from a decrease in pressure on the juxtaglomerular cells of the kidney. Common causes include renal artery stenosis, malignant hypertension, and edematous states, such as congestive heart failure, cirrhosis, and the nephrotic syndrome.

3. **Signs and symptoms.** The increased secretion of aldosterone leads to hypertension, muscle weakness, fatigue, polyuria and polydipsia, and headaches.

4. **Diagnosis.** Most of the laboratory abnormalities follow from the hypersecretion of aldosterone but can be influenced by antihypertensive drugs. Therefore, antihypertensive drugs should be discontinued before laboratory testing.

a. **Plasma electrolytes.** Frequently, the potassium level is low, and the sodium level is slightly elevated. The carbon dioxide content may be increased due to alkalosis.

b. **Sodium loading.** Hypokalemia and a significant increase in urinary potassium may be induced (or will persist if already present) by giving the patient a high-sodium diet (200 mEq/day).

c. **Plasma and urinary aldosterone levels**

(1) One of the most common causes of a missed diagnosis is the measurement of aldosterone before potassium repletion. Hypokalemia inhibits aldosterone secretion and may lead to a false-negative result.

(2) After potassium repletion, the serum and 24-hour urinary aldosterone levels are markedly increased in most patients who have Conn's syndrome.

d. **Plasma renin activity.** This helps to distinguish primary from secondary hyperaldosteronism. The activity is very high in the secondary form but low, even undetectable, in the primary disease.

e. **Postural response of aldosterone.** The response of aldosterone production to 4 hours of upright posture after overnight recumbency is helpful in distinguishing hyperaldosteronism due to an adenoma from that due to hyperplasia. In patients with an adenoma, there is no change or a decrease in aldosterone production. With hyperplasia, there is an increase in aldosterone levels.

5. **Localization of adenomas**
   a. **Selective sampling of the adrenal venous blood** to determine aldosterone concentration is the most accurate means of identifying an adenoma. However, this test is very difficult to perform and frequently provides incomplete results. Nonetheless, it is currently recommended for most patients to help rule out the possibility of bilateral nodular hyperplasia (seen in as many as 40% of patients) or to detect small functional adenomas that may not be identified with other techniques.
   b. **CT** and **MRI** have been shown to be at least 80% accurate in detecting adrenal adenomas and are much less invasive than adrenal venous sampling. However, these tests may either miss small adenomas or may identify adrenal lesions that are actually nonfunctional. This could lead to improper surgical planning.
   c. **Iodocholesterol scintigraphy** (see II E 5 c [2]) can also be used to localize aldosterone-producing adenomas.

6. **Treatment**
   a. **Surgical treatment**
      (1) For patients who have primary hyperaldosteronism due to an adrenocortical adenoma, the treatment of choice is laparopscopic adrenalectomy. Either total adrenalectomy of the involved gland or partial adrenalectomy to include the nodule may be considered.
      (2) It is important to restore potassium levels to normal before surgery.
   b. **Medical management**
      (1) **Spironolactone,** a direct antagonist to aldosterone at the kidney tubule, gradually leads to a reduction in blood pressure and a return to normal potassium levels.
         (a) Spironolactone is used in patients with primary hyperaldosteronism caused by adrenal hyperplasia because the results of surgery have been disappointing in these patients.
         (b) Spironolactone is also used in the preoperative restoration of normal serum potassium levels in patients who have adenomas.

G **Pheochromocytoma**   (Table 16-5)

1. **Overview.** Pheochromocytomas are functionally active tumors that develop from the neural crest-derived chromaffin tissue.
   a. Pheochromocytomas produce excess amounts of catecholamines, particularly norepinephrine and epinephrine.
   b. Most of these tumors (approximately 90%) are benign, but some (10%) are found to be malignant. There is a higher incidence of malignancy with extra-adrenal tumors.
      (1) Histologic examination is not an accurate means of determining the malignancy of a pheochromocytoma.
      (2) Malignancy is determined by the presence of metastases or direct invasion by the tumor.
   c. Pheochromocytomas can occur as part of the syndrome of multiple endocrine neoplasia type II (Sipple's syndrome—see Chapter 17, I B 2). The adrenal medullary abnormality is bilateral in up to 80% of these cases.

2. **Location**
   a. Approximately 90% of all pheochromocytomas are found in the adrenal medulla. Approximately 10% of these are bilateral.

TABLE 16-5 **Pheochromocytoma: The Ten-percent Tumor**	
10% malignant	10% multiple
10% bilateral	10% familial
10% extra-adrenal	10% children

    b. Of the extra-adrenal tumors, most are found in the organs of Zuckerkandl, the extraadrenal paraganglia, the urinary bladder, and the mediastinum.

3. Signs and symptoms

    a. Hypertension results from the excess production of catecholamines.

        (1) The hypertension is sustained in about half the patients and intermittent in the others.

        (2) However, patients with the sustained variety can have paroxysms of more severe hypertension superimposed on the baseline hypertension.

    b. Other findings include attacks of headaches, sweating, palpitations, tremor, nervousness, weight loss, fatigue, abdominal or chest pains, polydipsia and polyuria, and convulsions.

4. Diagnosis

    a. Urinary levels of metanephrine and VMA are the most reliable diagnostic screening tests. These levels are increased in 90%–95% of the cases.

    b. Fractionated plasma and urinary catecholamine levels can increase the accuracy of the diagnosis to virtually 100%.

    c. The need for potentially hazardous provocative tests using histamine, tyramine, and glucagon has been greatly reduced. These tests are used only in the rare patient who has equivocal biochemical findings.

5. Localization of the tumor

    a. CT and **MRI** have emerged as the most accurate, minimally invasive means of localizing pheochromocytomas. They are accurate in more than 95% of cases.

    b. Arteriography should be used only after adequate α-adrenergic blockade because it can precipitate a hypertensive crisis.

    c. Scintigraphy with radioiodine-labeled *m*-iodobenzylguanidine (MIBG), which structurally resembles norepinephrine, has been helpful for cases in which CT has not localized the tumor, especially with small extra-adrenal tumors.

    d. Vena cava sampling. If the pheochromocytoma still has not been localized, samples of blood can be taken by catheter from different parts of the vena cava and other veins for catecholamine analysis.

6. Surgical treatment

    a. Preparation for surgery should include adrenergic blockade with both α- and β-blockers.

        (1) Adrenergic blockade is helpful for three reasons.

            (a) It provides preoperative control of hypertension.

            (b) It reduces the risk of dramatic swings in blood pressure during surgery.

            (c) It provides vasodilation, allowing restoration of a normal blood volume (blood volume can be about 15% less than normal in patients who have pheochromocytomas).

        (2) Alpha-blockade is achieved first. Phenoxybenzamine therapy is begun 2 weeks before surgery, starting with 40 mg/day and adjusting the dose until hypertension and associated symptoms are controlled.

        (3) β-**blockade** is then obtained with propranolol, starting about 3 days before surgery, to control tachycardia. A starting dose of 40 mg/day may need adjustment if tachycardia persists.

    b. Operation

        (1) The patient should be monitored with an arterial and a central venous pressure line because of the potential for wide blood pressure changes and the large fluid requirements. A Swan-Ganz catheter should be used in elderly patients and in those with cardiac disease.

        (2) The approach may be transabdominal because of the high incidence of multiple and extra-adrenal tumors. However, with more accurate imaging techniques, the laparoscopic approach can be used for smaller tumors.

        (3) Total adrenalectomy is the procedure of choice for pheochromocytomas.

    c. Special situations

        (1) Malignant pheochromocytomas are treated by surgical excision of the tumor. If this cannot be accomplished, then as much tumor as possible is resected, and pharmacologic control of the catecholamine excess is started. Chemotherapy can be used for extensive metastatic disease.

(2) When pheochromocytoma is a component of **multiple endocrine neoplasia,** a bilateral total adrenalectomy should be performed. If only one gland is removed, there is a high incidence of recurrence on the other side.

H **Adrenal cysts and other adrenal tumors**

1. **Adrenal cysts** occur infrequently, showing up in fewer than 0.1% of autopsies.
   a. **Types.** Most adrenal cysts are either endothelial cysts (lymphangiomatous or angiomatous) or pseudocysts, resulting from hemorrhage into normal adrenal tissue or into an adrenal neoplasm. Rarely are they retention cysts or cystic adenomas.
   b. **Symptoms.** A large cyst can present as a palpable mass and can cause dull aching or gastrointestinal symptoms due to pressure. With cystic neoplasms, symptoms are those of the underlying process.
   c. **Diagnosis.** CT and MRI are the best methods available for diagnosing adrenal cysts.
   d. **Treatment.** Because a neoplasm cannot be excluded, these cysts should be surgically excised.

2. **Virilizing tumors of the adrenal cortex** are either adenomas or carcinomas.
   a. **Symptoms**
      (1) **In females,** hirsutism, amenorrhea, and an enlarged clitoris are characteristic. In female patients, it is important to exclude other causes of virilization, particularly congenital virilizing hyperplasia in the young and an arrhenoblastoma of the ovary in older patients.
      (2) **In males,** pseudoprecocious puberty occurs.
      (3) **In all patients,** some of the features of Cushing's syndrome may be evident. The urinary excretion of 17-ketosteroids is increased.
   b. **Diagnosis.** CT or MRI provides the best localization of the tumor.
   c. **Treatment** consists of complete surgical excision. Mitotane is used for metastatic disease.

3. **Feminizing tumors of the adrenal cortex** are either adenomas or carcinomas.
   a. **Symptoms.** In females, the tumor causes rapid premature sexual development. In males, there will be gynecomastia, decreased libido, and testicular atrophy.
   b. **Diagnosis.** Localization is by CT or MRI.
   c. **Treatment.** Complete surgical excision offers the only hope for cure. Mitotane is used for metastatic disease.

4. **Nonfunctioning adrenal masses** have been discovered at autopsy in up to 9% of patients. With the growing use of CT and MRI scanning, an increased number of these "incidentalomas" are being discovered during life.
   a. Although adenomas cannot be distinguished from carcinomas except by excision and inspection, carcinomas are rare when lesions are nonfunctional and smaller than 6 cm in diameter.
   b. These patients should probably be followed up with a repeat CT or MRI in 6 months. However, if a nonfunctioning mass is larger than 6 cm or is enlarging, surgical excision is the safest course to take.
   c. A CT-directed needle biopsy of nonfunctional tumors less than 6 cm in diameter may be considered to establish a diagnosis. However, risks include bleeding (which could make any subsequent laparoscopic approach more difficult) or dissemination of tumor cells (which could make subsequent extirpation of the disease more difficult).

III PARATHYROID GLANDS

A **Introduction** The parathyroid glands are important to surgeons for two reasons. First, because surgeons treat patients with symptomatic hyperparathyroidism, they must know the cause and management of various hyperparathyroid conditions, and second, during operations for the neck, it is imperative that the integrity of the parathyroids be preserved to avoid injury, the consequence of which can be permanent hypoparathyroidism. There is no satisfactory replacement for endogenously produced parathyroid hormone, and the patient with hypoparathyroidism is doomed to a lifelong process of episodic, symptomatic hypocalcemia despite calcium and vitamin D therapy.

1. **Embryology.** In most individuals, there are two superior and two inferior parathyroid glands that differ in their embryologic origin.

a. Superior parathyroid glands

(1) The superior parathyroid glands arise from the fourth branchial pouch in close proximity to the origin of the thyroid (the floor of the foregut) and descend into the neck.

(2) Because of the embryologic origin, abnormal parathyroid locations may be either intrathyroidal or within the posterior mediastinum near the tracheoesophageal groove or the esophagus.

b. Inferior parathyroid glands

(1) The inferior parathyroids arise from the third branchial pouch in relationship to the thymic anlage. They cross the superior glands in their descent into the neck.

(2) Frequently, they are associated with the thymus gland in the anterosuperior mediastinum.

2. Anatomy (Fig. 16-5)

a. Clinical presentation. Some 85%–95% of individuals have four parathyroid glands, but as few as three glands and as many as five have been identified in 10%–15% of the population. The average parathyroid gland weighs from 40–70 mg.

b. Location

(1) **The superior parathyroid glands** usually lie at the junction of the upper and middle third of the thyroid gland on its posteromedial surface or in the tracheoesophageal groove.

(a) They usually lie posteriorly to the recurrent laryngeal nerve and are in close proximity to the thyroid gland.

(b) Occasionally, they may even be intrathyroidal.

(2) **The inferior parathaoid glands** lie within a circle with a 3-cm diameter, the center of which is the point where the recurrent laryngeal nerve crosses the inferior thyroid artery.

(a) The inferior parathyroids usually lie in a plane anterior to the recurrent laryngeal nerve.

(b) They may be in close proximity to or within the cervical limb of the thymus gland.

c. Vasculature

(1) **Arterial supply**

(a) The arterial supply is derived mainly from the inferior thyroid artery, arising from the thyrocervical trunk of the subclavian artery.

(b) Since the superior parathyroid glands have been reported to receive their blood supply from the superior thyroid artery in 10% of autopsies, this artery should always be left intact when the superior parathyroid glands are exposed so that their blood supply is not disrupted.

(2) **Venous drainage** from the parathyroid glands is into the superior, middle, and inferior thyroid veins. These veins can be cannulated to provide blood specimens for parathyroid hormone analysis as a means of localizing sources of increased parathyroid hormone production.

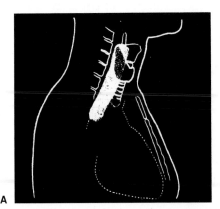 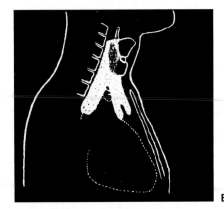

FIGURE 16-5 Variations in position of normal parathyroids. **A** (left) is location of superior parathyroids; **B** (right) is location of inferior parathyroids.

   d. Histopathology
   (1) The normal parathyroid gland has a significant amount of fat interspersed with chief and oxyphil cells.
   (2) Hypercellular glands, found in hyperparathyroid states, have a paucity of fat. The hypercellularity is mostly oxyphil-cell hyperplasia, but occasionally chief-cell hyperplasia may also be noted.
   (3) Histologically, one cannot distinguish the hypercellularity of a hyperplastic gland from that of a gland harboring an adenoma.

B **Parathyroid hormone (parathormone, PTH)**
1. **Calcium metabolism regulation.** PTH is a major regulator of calcium metabolism.
   a. It acts in conjunction with calcitonin and activated vitamin D_3 to regulate the plasma concentration of the ionized form of calcium. There is normally a reciprocal relationship between the serum calcium concentration and PTH secretion.
      (1) As serum calcium levels decrease, the secretion of PTH increases.
      (2) As serum calcium levels increase, the secretion of PTH decreases.
   b. PTH exerts its biologic effect on bone, intestine, and kidney.
      (1) It increases the mobilization of calcium and phosphorous from bone by stimulating osteoclastic and osteolytic activity.
      (2) It acts synergistically with 1, 25-dihydroxyvitamin D_3 to increase the absorption of calcium and phosphorus from the gut.
      (3) **Renal effects**
         (a) PTH raises the renal threshold for calcium by promoting the active reabsorption of calcium in the distal nephron.
         (b) It also lowers the renal threshold for phosphate by inhibiting phosphate reabsorption in the proximal tubule.
         (c) PTH secretion and phosphate depletion stimulate the activation of 1,25-dihydroxyvitamin D_3 via the activation of 1 α-hydroxylase.

2. **Increased, unopposed PTH secretion** has the following clinical effects on bone, intestine, and kidney:
   a. Hypercalcemia
   b. Altered calcium excretion
      (1) Initially, hypocalciuria occurs due to increased calcium reabsorption.
      (2) This reverts to hypercalciuria in chronic hyperparathyroid states when the hypercalcemia exceeds the renal threshold for calcium.
   c. Hypophosphatemia
   d. Hyperphosphaturia

3. **Laboratory tests.** Serum PTH levels can be measured by radioimmunoassay. Normal values vary from laboratory to laboratory, depending in part on whether the intact molecule or the C or N terminal of the PTH molecule is used in the assay. The intact molecule assay is more reliable.

C **Hyperparathyroidism**
1. **Primary hyperparathyroidism**
   a. **Incidence.** Primary hyperparathyroidism is a relatively common disorder and is the most common cause of hypercalcemia in patients outside the hospital. It most commonly occurs sporadically but may occur as:
      (1) Part of a MEN syndrome (see Chapter 17)
      (2) Familial hyperparathyroidism
      (3) Ectopic or pseudohyperparathyroidism due to the production of a PTH-like substance from an extraparathyroidal tumor
   b. **Etiology and pathology**
      (1) Between 85% and 90% of primary hyperparathyroidism cases are due to a solitary adenoma of one of the four glands.
      (2) Approximately 10%–15% are due to four-gland hyperplasia. The hyperplasia may be asymmetrical with one or two glands grossly enlarged. Microscopically, however, all glands show hypercellularity.

(3) Parathyroid carcinoma accounts for less than 1% of primary hyperparathyroidism cases.

(4) About 0.4% of cases are due to multiple adenomas involving more than one gland.

(5) Microscopically, the glands have a paucity of fat and appear hypercellular (see III A 2 d).

c. Clinical presentation

(1) Most patients with primary hyperparathyroidism are asymptomatic, and the altered state is discovered only because an increased serum calcium level is noted on routine multichannel biochemical screening.

(2) When patients are symptomatic, the symptoms follow the mnemonic **"stones, bones, moans, and abdominal groans."**

(a) **Stones.** Renal lithiasis occurs in 50% of patients with symptomatic primary hyperparathyroidism (although primary hyperparathyroidism occurs in fewer than 10% of all patients who have renal lithiasis).

(b) **Bones.** Osteitis fibrosa cystica (von Recklinghausen's disease of bone) is found mostly in patients who have secondary and tertiary hyperparathyroidism, which are due to chronic renal disease (see III C 2, 3).

(c) **Moans.** Psychiatric manifestations—personality disorders or frank psychosis—may accompany primary hyperparathyroidism but are relatively uncommon.

(d) **Abdominal groans**

(i) The incidence of peptic ulcer disease is increased in primary hyperparathyroidism, usually associated with hypergastrinemia that results from the hypercalcemia.

(ii) Cholelithiasis or pancreatitis may also occur, accounting for abdominal symptoms.

(3) Most patients have nonspecific symptoms, such as weakness, easy fatigability, lethargy, constipation, and arthralgia.

d. Diagnosis

(1) **Laboratory studies**

(a) An increased serum calcium level is the cornerstone of diagnosis.

(i) This should be shown on at least three blood specimens, drawn on different occasions.

(ii) While primary hyperparathyroidism is a relatively common cause of hypercalcemia, other causes must be excluded, such as metastatic bone disease, myeloma, sarcoidosis, the use of thiazide diuretics, milk-alkali syndrome, hypervitaminosis, thyrotoxicosis, and Addison's disease.

(b) A serum PTH level that is disproportionately high for the serum calcium level (measured concomitantly) is diagnostic for primary hyperparathyroidism (Fig. 16-6).

(i) In patients who have metastatic bone disease, hypercalcemia occurs without a disproportionate increase of PTH level.

(ii) In patients who have secondary hyperparathyroidism, the serum PTH level is increased and the serum calcium is low.

(iii) In patients who have hypoparathyroidism, the serum calcium and serum PTH levels are both low.

(iv) The serum PTH level can also be increased in patients who have **pseudohyperparathyroidism,** a disorder characterized by an extraparathyroidal source of PTH. For example, tumors arising from the APUD cell system (see Chapter 17, II A 2) may produce a PTH-like substance that is indistinguishable from PTH by normal laboratory means.

(c) The serum phosphorus level is decreased, and the serum chloride:phosphorus ratio usually exceeds 33:1.

(d) The tubular reabsorption of phosphorus is less than 80%, resulting in hyperphosphaturia.

(e) Measurement of urinary cyclic adenosine monophosphate shows increased levels.

(f) Urinary calcium excretion is increased when the patient is on a calcium-restricted diet.

(2) **Radiographic studies**

(a) Radiographs of the skull may show a "ground-glass" appearance in the outer two thirds of the skull. Skull radiographs are also obtained to search for enlargement of the sella turcica due to a pituitary tumor, which may connote multiple endocrine neoplasia.

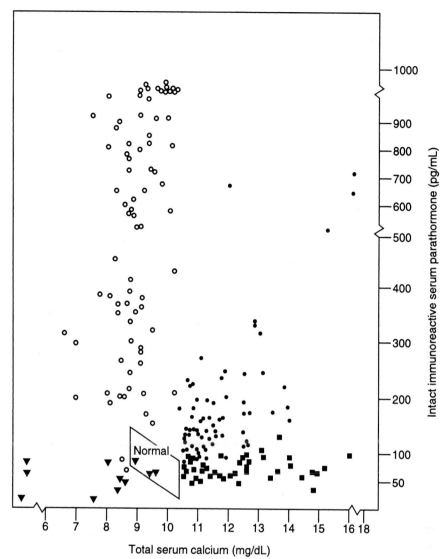

FIGURE 16-6 The relationship between serum calcium and serum parathormone levels in primary hyperparathyroidism surgically proven (●), secondary hyperparathyroidism (○), hypoparathyroidism (▼), and hypercalcemia due to metastatic bone disease (■).

(b) Radiographs of the proximal ends of the long bones may show bony reabsorption or brown tumors of the bone.

(c) Radiographs of the fingers may show subperiosteal absorption on the radial side of the middle phalanges and in the tufts of the terminal phalanges. Abnormal calcification in the digital vessels may also be found.

e. Indications for surgery. Once the diagnosis of primary hyperparathyroidism is confirmed biochemically, patients should be selected for operation.

(1) All symptomatic patients with biochemically proven hyperparathyroidism should be considered for surgery.

(2) Operation is also advised for an asymptomatic patient younger than 50 years of age or any patient whose serum calcium levels exceed 11 mg/dL, especially if the patient has a decrease in bone density, hypercalciuria, or a decrease in renal function due to other diseases such as hypertension or diabetes mellitus.

f. Preoperative localization of the parathyroid glands

(1) Localizing the abnormal parathyroids preoperatively is helpful for several reasons.

(a) It permits a minimal access approach and reduces the operating time for many patients.

(b) It helps to define the anatomy of the neck in patients who have had prior surgery, in whom the normal anatomy may be distorted.

(c) It aids in defining the pathology in patients who have had prior unsuccessful surgery for primary hyperparathyroidism and who still have either persistent or recurrent hypercalcemia.

(2) Methods of preoperative localization

(a) Scintigraphy using Tc sestamibi is helpful in localizing 75%–90% of parathyroid adenomas.

(i) Tc sestamibi is taken up by the thyroid and parathyroid glands on initial images. Delayed images show persistent uptake by enlarged parathyroid glands but rapid washout from the thyroid. It is less accurate in imaging patients with multiglandular disease.

(ii) Sestamibi scanning is useful in imaging enlarged parathyroid glands in ectopic locations such as the mediastinum.

(iii) SPECT (single positron emission computerized tomography) may reveal anatomic relationships that traditional planar imaging does not.

(iv) Combination SPECT-CT may provide additional localizing information in subtle or difficult cases.

(b) Ultrasonography will define an enlarged parathyroid in 70%–80% of the cases. The ultrasound criteria for an enlarged parathyroid gland include:

(i) A hypoechoic area in close proximity to either pole of the thyroid gland

(ii) The presence of internal echoes that exclude a pure cyst or vascular structure

(c) CT and MRI

(i) CT is particularly successful in localizing enlarged parathyroids in the mediastinum. In addition, it allows visualization of parathyroids that may not be visible by ultrasound or dual-tracer imaging.

(ii) MRI seems to be as successful as CT in localizing parathyroids. It reveals enlarged parathyroids on the T_2-weighted image.

(iii) Used alone or in combination, CT and MRI are the most accurate of the noninvasive localization studies but are also the most expensive.

(d) Selective venous sampling and PTH assay. The Seldinger technique can be used in the venous system to obtain blood samples from different venous sites for PTH assay. Because the study is costly and time consuming, it is reserved only for patients in whom initial surgery was unsuccessful or who had a recurrence of hyperparathyroidism after initial successful treatment.

(i) Retrograde injection of the thyroid veins is performed, and each of the draining thyroid veins is selectively cannulated.

(ii) A disproportionately high PTH level in one or more of the venous samples helps to localize the lesion to one side of the neck or the other.

(iii) Significant increase in samples obtained from veins on both sides of the neck suggests four-gland hyperplasia.

(e) Thyrocervical angiography

(i) If the thyrocervical trunk is selectively cannulated, and angiograms of the thyroid and parathyroid are obtained, enlarged glands in the neck can be seen.

(ii) If the internal mammary artery is selectively cannulated, enlarged parathyroids in the mediastinum can be found.

(iii) Stroke has been reported as a complication of thyrocervical angiography; therefore, this technique should not be used indiscriminately.

(iv) It is reserved primarily for patients who have previously had unsuccessful surgery, who develop recurrent hyperparathyroidism after operation, and who have had no success with other localization techniques.

g. Surgical treatment

(1) Successful surgery requires a thorough knowledge of the anatomy of the normal parathyroids and their abnormal locations. When possible, all four parathyroid glands should be identified at surgery.

(2) When a solitary adenoma is present, it should be completely excised.

(a) In the past, routine full neck exploration was performed. Visualization of the other three glands and biopsy of at least one of those glands was needed to to rule out the presence of multiple adenomas or four-gland hyperplasia.

(b) Currently, improved localization techniques and the use of a rapid intraoperative assay of PTH levels allows for a minimal access approach to parathyroid adenomas in most patients.

  (i) A PTH level is drawn at the beginning of the operation, and then a limited dissection is performed through a small incision to identify and excise the previously localized adenoma.

  (ii) Injection of sestamibi may be performed preoperatively and a hand-held gamma probe used intraoperatively to aid in the localization of the adenoma. However, this technique is limited by a low signal to background noise ratio and is generally not needed in most cases.

  (iii) Following excision of the adenoma, additional PTH levels are drawn at specific intervals (various protocols can be followed, but levels drawn at 0, 5, and 10 minutes after excision are generally sufficient).

  (iv) Due to the very short half-life of PTH in the circulation (about 2 minutes), a significant drop in the PTH level should be seen if all abnormal parathyroid tissue has been removed. A drop of the PTH level to less than 50% of the highest level (either preoperatively or at the time of excision) or a clear drop into the normal range is associated with a 95%–98% cure rate. If the levels do not drop sufficiently, then additional levels should be obtained and/or further exploration performed to ensure that all abnormal parathyroid tissue has been removed.

(3) **Management of four-gland hyperplasia.** Two options are currently available.

  (a) **Subtotal parathyroidectomy,** leaving a well-vascularized remnant (100 mg of parathyroid tissue in the adult and 150 mg in the child) to provide for normal parathyroid function. Once again, intraoperative PTH levels are obtained to ensure that an adequate excision of parathyroid tissue has been performed. If the levels do not drop despite three and a half gland excision, supernumery parathyroid glands should be sought out and removed. There is a 5% recurrence rate after subtotal parathyroidectomy.

  (b) **Total parathyroidectomy** with autotransplantation of minced parathyroid tissue into a well-vascularized, accessible forearm muscle so that recurrence can be treated without reoperation on the neck. There is a real danger of permanent hypoparathyroidism after total parathyroidectomy and reimplantation if the autotransplant does not survive.

h. **Postoperative management. Postoperative hypocalcemia** usually develops after successful therapy.

(1) Asymptomatic postoperative hypocalcemia requires no treatment.

(2) Symptomatic hypocalcemia always requires treatment.

  (a) In severely symptomatic patients, treatment should begin with intravenous calcium gluconate.

  (b) Mildly symptomatic patients may be given oral calcium in the form of calcium lactate, calcium carbonate, or calcium gluconate. Doses ranging from 4–20 g/day may be required.

(3) If hypocalcemia remains symptomatic despite calcium supplementation, additional therapy with vitamin D may be needed. Supplemental calcium and vitamin D therapy should be continued until serum calcium levels return to normal.

(4) Patients with significant bone disease will require prolonged calcium therapy to permit remineralization of the calcium-depleted skeleton.

2. **Secondary hyperparathyroidism**

  a. **Etiology and pathology**

   (1) Secondary hyperparathyroidism is found in patients who have chronic renal failure. These patients are unable to synthesize the active form of vitamin D; and, therefore, they develop chronic hypocalcemia, hyperphosphatemia, and impaired calcium absorption from the gut.

    (2) If untreated, secondary hyperparathyroidism may result in symptomatic bone demineralization, metastatic calcification in soft tissues, and accelerated vascular calcification. It occasionally can cause severe pruritus and painful skin ulcerations.

  b. Treatment

    (1) Medical treatment. Initial treatment is with:

      (a) Dialysis with a high-calcium bath

      (b) Phosphate-binding antacids

      (c) Calcium supplements plus the active form of vitamin D

    (2) Surgical treatment. In patients who are refractory to medical therapy, subtotal parathyroidectomy or total parathyroidectomy with autotransplantation of parathyroid tissue is indicated because secondary hyperparathyroidism is always associated with four-gland hyperplasia.

3. Tertiary hyperparathyroidism

  a. Etiology. This term refers to the hyperparathyroidism that persists in patients who have chronic renal disease despite a successful renal transplant.

    (1) Apparently, the parathyroid hyperplasia of long-standing renal disease becomes autonomous despite the return of normal kidney function.

    (2) Patients are often hypercalcemic, hypophosphatemic, and hypercalciuric.

    (3) Tertiary hyperparathyroidism may produce the same symptoms as those found in secondary hyperparathyroidism.

  b. Surgical treatment. When persistent, tertiary hyperparathyroidism is treated by subtotal parathyroidectomy or total parathyroidectomy with autotransplantation.

IV   THYMUS GLAND

A **Introduction** The thymus is important to the surgeon because it is the origin of a variety of tumors and is significantly involved in the development of cellular immunity. As such, it has been implicated in a variety of disease states.

1. Embryology

  a. The thymus arises from the third branchial pouch and descends into the anterosuperior mediastinum.

  b. It is a multilobulated structure with many fibrous septa. Each lobule has a **cortex** and a **medulla.**

    (1) The **cortex** consists primarily of lymphocytes, which appear to migrate to the medulla and then emigrate from the thymus.

    (2) The **medulla** also contains Hassall's corpuscles, which are composed of concentric layers of epithelial cells. Their function is unknown.

2. Anatomy

  a. Development

    (1) Because of the bilateral origin of the thymus gland, it develops two lobes and a roughly **H-shaped** configuration.

    (2) Two limbs of the thymus extend into the neck and are often associated with the inferior parathyroid glands.

    (3) The inferior limbs extend along the surface of the pericardium and abut the pleura.

    (4) The thymus reaches maximal size shortly after birth and then begins to involute during adolescence and early adult life.

  b. Functions

    (1) Cellular immunity. The thymus is essential for the development of cellular immunity, which controls such processes as delayed hypersensitivity reactions and transplant rejection.

      (a) The thymic-dependent portion of the immune system consists principally of the thymus and a circulating pool of small lymphocytes that produce cell-mediated immune reactions.

        (i) While removal of the neonatal thymus in certain strains of mice leads to significant impairment in immunologic capacity, it has no such effect in the human newborn.

        (ii) However, impaired thymic development may be associated with immunologic deficiency disorders.

     (b) The thymus is the first organ to manufacture lymphocytes during fetal life, but most of the cells produced in the thymus die there.

    (2) Immune system function and thymic lesions. Histologic abnormalities in the thymus, such as lymphoid hyperplasia or thymic tumors, are frequently found in association with certain autoimmune diseases, suggesting a relationship between thymic function and immune system disorders. The autoimmune diseases are:

     (a) Myasthenia gravis (see IV C)

     (b) Systemic (disseminated) lupus erythematosus

     (c) Erythroid agenesis

     (d) Hypogammaglobulinemia

     (e) Rheumatoid arthritis

     (f) Dermatomyositis

  c. Vasculature

    (1) Arterial supply to the thymus is derived from small branches of the internal mammary or pericardiophrenic arteries.

    (2) Venous drainage is primarily to a single thymic vein that drains into the left innominate vein.

B **Thymic tumors**

1. Incidence. Thymic tumors (**thymomas**) are among the most common tumors of the anterosuperior mediastinum in the adult.

  a. While thymic tumors can occur at any age, they are most common in the fifth and sixth decades of life.

  b. Males and females are equally affected.

  c. Some 40%–50% of patients with thymomas have associated myasthenia gravis.

2. Pathology

  a. While thymic tumors have been described according to their cell of origin as lymphoid, epithelial, spindle cell, or mixed, it is almost impossible to distinguish benign from malignant thymic tumors microscopically.

    (1) Two thirds of thymic tumors are considered benign, and of these, 10% are simple cysts (see Chapter 18, III A 1).

    (2) Spindle cell thymomas appear to have a better prognosis than epithelial thymomas, which have a poor prognosis.

  b. The best index of the benign or malignant nature of the tumor is its tendency to invade contiguous structures.

    (1) Benign tumors are well encapsulated.

    (2) Malignant tumors are invasive, spreading by direct invasion of contiguous structures and onto adjacent pleural surfaces. Distant spread is extremely rare.

3. Diagnosis

  a. Most patients who have thymomas are asymptomatic, and the tumor is discovered incidentally on a routine chest radiograph. Symptoms, when present, are related to invasion by malignant thymomas and consist of chest pain, dyspnea, or superior vena cava syndrome.

  b. The existence of a thymoma is suggested by either:

    (1) An abnormality on chest radiograph, CT scan, or MRI (Fig. 16-7)

    (2) The presence of myasthenia gravis

     (a) This condition should prompt a search of the mediastinum for a thymic tumor.

     (b) A lateral chest radiograph is most helpful because small tumors may be obscured by the great vessels in standard posteroanterior chest radiographs.

  c. Recently, CT and MRI have been helpful in identifying the degree of invasion of thymic tumors.

4. Surgical treatment. Most thymic tumors are removed through a sternal-splitting median sternotomy.

A

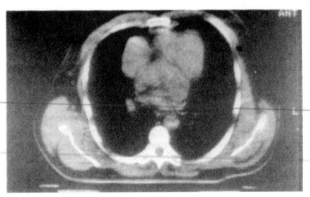

B

FIGURE 16-7 **A:** Posteroanterior and lateral chest radiograph, showing an anterior mediastinal mass in the right hemithorax in a patient with a thymoma. **B:** A CT scan from the same patient showing an anterior mediastinal mass without fixation to the underlying pericardium.

   a. Thymic tumors that are not associated with myasthenia gravis or another clinical syndrome require mediastinal exploration and total removal of the tumor.
      (1) Benign tumors can be removed by local excision or thoracoscopically (video-assisted thoracic surgery) with sternotomy.
      (2) Malignant tumors
         (a) If possible, all areas of invasion should be removed.
         (b) When invasive thymic tumors are nonresectable or cannot be removed completely, postoperative radiation may be valuable. Chemotherapy using iphosphamide, etopiside, cisplatinum, and paclitaxel (Taxol) has been useful as has somatostatin analogue.
   b. Thymic tumors that are associated with myasthenia gravis or other clinical syndromes should be removed, including the entire remaining thymus gland.

C Myasthenia gravis

   1. Overview. Myasthenia gravis is an autoimmune disease of neuromuscular transmission that causes skeletal muscle weakness. It is characterized by spontaneous remissions and by exacerbations that are often precipitated by an upper respiratory infection. The most common symptoms are ptosis, double vision, dysarthria, dysphagia, nasal speech, and weakness of the arms and legs.

2. **Pathophysiology**
    a. **Normal neuromuscular transmission**
        (1) The neurotransmitter acetylcholine is produced at the nerve terminal of the myoneural junction.
        (2) The acetylcholine binds to receptor sites on the muscle end plates.
        (3) This action triggers muscle contraction.
    b. **Neuromuscular transmission in myasthenia gravis.** It appears that antibodies to acetylcholine receptors develop, which decrease the available number of receptor sites on the muscle end plates, resulting in reduced muscle contraction.

3. **Treatment**
    a. **Medical treatment.** Patients who have myasthenia gravis respond to drugs that stimulate the neuromuscular junction, such as neostigmine and pyridostigmine.
    b. **Surgical treatment**
        (1) In patients who have thymic tumors, surgical removal of the tumor is advised, although the effect on the myasthenia is unpredictable. However, even in patients without thymic tumors, thymectomy appears to be the treatment of choice for all forms of myasthenia except purely ocular myasthenia. Thymectomy seems to:
            (a) Increase the percentage of permanent remissions
            (b) Decrease the morbidity and mortality of the disease
            (c) Improve the response to medication in patients who do not undergo complete remission
        (2) **Preoperative and postoperative management** have significantly reduced the morbidity and mortality rates of surgery.
            (a) Surgery in patients with myasthenia gravis creates several problems.
                (i) The sternal-splitting incision reduces the ability of patients with impaired muscle strength to ventilate properly and to mobilize secretions.
                (ii) The use of parasympathomimetic drugs improves muscle strength but also increases pharyngeal and tracheobronchial secretions.
            (b) Preoperative plasmapheresis has been used with good results.
                (i) It eliminates the need for parasympathomimetic drugs and eliminates circulating acetylcholine receptor antibodies.
                (ii) This produces significant improvement in perioperative muscle strength and virtually eliminates the need for prolonged ventilatory support.
        (3) Thymectomy can be performed by a transcervical route, thoracoscopically, or through a sternal-splitting incision—the former for normal thymus glands, the latter for large benign glands and most thymic tumors.
    c. **Results of medical and surgical treatment**
        (1) Without surgery, spontaneous remissions occur in 18% of patients with myasthenia gravis, whereas thymectomy induces complete remission in approximately 38% of patients.
        (2) Sustained improvement is achieved with medication in only 33% of patients without surgery and in 85% of patients after thymectomy.
        (3) The best results from thymectomy are usually found in younger patients who have myasthenia of relatively short duration who have become increasingly refractory to medication.

chapter 17

Multiple Endocrine Neoplasia and Tumors of the Endocrine Pancreas

JOHN S. RADOMSKI · HERBERT E. COHN · RONALD J. WEIGEL

I   MULTIPLE ENDOCRINE NEOPLASIA

A **Overview** Multiple endocrine neoplasia (**MEN**) syndromes, formerly known as multiple endocrine adenomatosis, are characteristic patterns of endocrine hyperfunction inherited as autosomal dominant traits.

1. Many of the endocrine cell types involved originate from the neuroectoderm and have the ability to secrete peptide hormones, amines, or both, but no unifying molecular defect is currently known.

2. Certain features are present in all MEN syndromes.
   a. All are autosomal dominant traits with significant phenotypic variability.
   b. The involved endocrine glands develop hyperplasia, adenoma, or carcinoma.
   c. The neoplasias in the involved glands can develop simultaneously or at different times.
   d. Ectopic hormone production is common.

B **Types** Three types of MEN have been identified (Table 17-1).

1. **Type 1 (Wermer's syndrome)** involves the parathyroid glands, pancreatic islets, and pituitary gland and is caused by inheritance of a mutation of the menin gene on chromosome 11q13.
   a. **Hyperparathyroidism** (see Chapter 16, III C) is present in 90% or more of the patients, with most having hyperplasia of multiple parathyroid glands.
   b. **Pancreatic tumors** are present in 80% of patients.
      (1) These are usually nonbeta islet cell tumors, which can cause the Zollinger-Ellison syndrome (see II C).
      (2) However, other syndromes can occur (see II and Chapter 15, III).
   c. **Pituitary tumors** are present in 65% of cases. These are usually chromophobe adenomas, which produce acromegaly, galactorrhea, amenorrhea, or Cushing's syndrome.
   d. Approximately 90% of patients present with hypercalcemia, hypoglycemia, peptic ulcer, or complaints secondary to a pituitary mass.

2. **Type 2A (Sipple's syndrome)** comprises medullary carcinoma of the thyroid, pheochromocytoma, and, in MEN 2A, parathyroid hyperplasia. MEN2 is caused by mutation of the Ret gene, which maps to 10q11.2.
   a. **Medullary thyroid carcinoma** (see Chapter 16, I F 5 c) occurs in all patients.
      (1) It is usually multifocal and is preceded by nonmalignant hyperplasia of the parafollicular, or C, cells.
      (2) Serum calcitonin levels are increased, although in the premalignant state, stimulation with calcium or pentagastrin may be necessary to identify this.
   b. **Pheochromocytomas** (see Chapter 16, II G) occur in approximately 40% of patients.
      (1) They are usually bilateral and occasionally are malignant.
      (2) They often present later than the medullary thyroid cancer.

TABLE 17-1 Multiple Endocrine Neoplasia Syndromes

Pathologic Entities	1	2A	2B
Hyperparathyroidism (usually 4-gland hyperplasia)	+	+	−
Pancreatic islet cell tumor (insulinoma or gastrinoma)	+	−	−
Pituitary tumor	±	−	−
Adrenocortical involvement	±	−	−
Adrenomedullary pheochromocytoma	−	+	+
Medullary carcinoma of the thyroid	−	+	+
Mucosal neuromas	−	−	+

+, present; −, absent.

    c. Parathyroid hyperplasia, with consequent hyperparathyroidism, develops in 60% of patients with MEN 2A and is often milder than the parathyroid hyperplasia of MEN 1.

  3. Type 2B (mucosal neuroma syndrome)

    a. As in type 2A, patients develop medullary thyroid carcinoma and pheochromocytoma.

    b. However, the features most characteristic of type 2B are a marfanoid body habitus and the development of multiple neuromatous mucosal nodules.

    c. In addition, type 2B presents at a much earlier age, usually in the first or second decade of life, and assumes a much more aggressive course.

C **Diagnosis**

  1. MEN 1 (Wermer's syndrome)

    a. Most patients with MEN type 1 present with symptoms of peptic ulceration related to the pancreatic gastrinoma (see II C 1 a) or with symptoms related to the pituitary tumor (see I B 1 c).

    b. The hyperparathyroidism is typically asymptomatic and is usually detected by an increased serum calcium level.

  2. MEN 2A (Sipple's syndrome)

    a. The diagnosis should be suspected in all kindred of any patient with **medullary carcinoma of the thyroid.**

      (1) The inherited trait can be diagnosed in the premalignant stage, when **C-cell hyperplasia** is present before the medullary carcinoma develops by testing for mutation of the ret proto-oncogene.

      (2) Finding an increased serum calcitonin level leads to the diagnosis. Infusion of calcium and pentagastrin helps to stimulate an abnormal thyrocalcitonemia in those with C-cell hyperplasia or occult medullary carcinoma before either is clinically detectable.

    b. Hyperparathyroidism is usually detected by increases in the serum calcium and parathyroid hormone levels.

    c. Pheochromocytomas or **adrenal medullary hyperplasia** may be asymptomatic but should be detectable by biochemical screening for increased serum and urine catecholamines.

  3. MEN 2B (mucosal neuroma syndrome)

    a. Since MEN 2B assumes such an aggressive course, early diagnosis is important so that effective treatment can begin promptly.

    b. The diagnosis is similar to that for MEN 2A. The early appearance of mucosal neuromas and the marfanoid body habitus should help in making the diagnosis.

D **Treatment**

  1. MEN 1

    a. If only the pancreatic and parathyroid components of this syndrome are present, the **hyperparathyroidism** is treated first. This may reduce the production of gastrin and relieve the peptic ulceration.

(1) Subtotal or total parathyroidectomy with arm reimplantation is required because the parathyroid disorder is usually four-gland hyperplasia.

(2) If the hypergastrinemia and peptic ulceration persist, treatment is directed toward the **Zollinger-Ellison syndrome** (see II C 5). This involves removal of the gastrin-producing tumor, if possible, or, rarely, removal of the end organ (i.e., total gastrectomy) if the tumor cannot be removed and if the use of histamine$_2$ (H$_2$)-receptor antagonists or proton pump inhibitors (e.g., omeprazole) do not control the ulceration.

b. **Pituitary tumors** are usually treated medically with bromocriptine. Trans-sphenoidal hypophysectomy, using an operating microscope to minimize the risk of injury to the posterior pituitary, may be needed in some cases.

2. **MEN 2A**
   a. **Medullary carcinoma** should be treated in the premalignant stage, when only C-cell hyperplasia is present, at which time total thyroidectomy is curative.
   b. **Pheochromocytoma or adrenal medullary hyperplasia,** if present, should be treated before thyroidectomy because these hormone-producing disorders can lead to hypertensive crises during thyroidectomy. Simultaneous approaches have also been used.
   c. **Hyperparathyroidism** can be treated at the time of total thyroidectomy by the protocol described in Chapter 16, III C 1, 2.

3. **MEN 2B** is treated similarly to MEN 2A. Since MEN 2B assumes such an aggressive course, prompt and effective treatment is important.

II ■ TUMORS OF THE ENDOCRINE PANCREAS

A Pathophysiology

1. The pancreatic islet cells and the endocrine cells of the gut (known as the **a**mine **p**recursor **u**ptake and **d**ecarboxylation cell system or **APUD cells**) originate from embryonic cells that have certain cytochemical properties in common.
   a. They have a high amine content.
   b. They have the ability for amine precursor uptake.
   c. They produce the enzyme amino acid decarboxylase.

2. Tumors that arise from these APUD cells are termed **apudomas.** The various kinds of apudomas arising in the pancreas include:
   a. **Insulinomas**
   b. **Gastrinomas (Zollinger-Ellison syndrome)**
   c. **Glucagonomas**
   d. **Vipomas** (for **v**asoactive **i**ntestinal **p**eptide, or **VIP**)
   e. **Somatostatinomas**

B Insulinomas

1. **Overview.** An insulinoma is a tumor originating from the beta cells of the pancreatic islets that releases abnormally high amounts of insulin.
   a. Approximately 80%–90% of insulinomas are solitary, benign adenomas.
   b. About 10% are malignant with the potential to metastasize.
   c. The remainder are islet cell hyperplasia (termed **nesidioblastosis** in children).

2. **Clinical presentation.** The abnormally increased insulin levels and the resultant hypoglycemia produce the following clinical picture.
   a. Bizarre behavior; unconscious episodes
   b. Palpitations, nervousness, and other symptoms of sympathetic discharge
   c. **Whipple's triad:**
      (1) Episodes of illness precipitated by fasting
      (2) Hypoglycemia during the episodes, usually with blood glucose levels less than 60 mg/dL
      (3) Relief of hypoglycemic symptoms by oral or intravenous administration of glucose

3. Diagnosis. Once suspected, the diagnosis must be confirmed by documenting the abnormal circulating insulin levels.

    a. Measurement of fasting insulin and glucose levels. An effective screening test is to have the patient fast for 72 hours or until symptoms of hypoglycemia appear and then to test the insulin and glucose levels. An increased insulin level in the presence of a low glucose level (insulin:glucose ratio greater than 0.25) effectively confirms an insulinoma. The presence of an elevated insulin C peptide is used to rule out iatrogenic insulin overdose.

        (1) Essentially, all patients with insulinomas will become hypoglycemic within 72 hours.

        (2) As many as 40% will develop symptoms within 2 hours of beginning the fast.

    b. Comparing insulin and proinsulin levels can be helpful.

        (1) Proinsulin is the single-chain intracellular precursor that is cleaved, before secretion, into insulin and C peptide.

        (2) Normally, less than 20% of the total circulating immunoreactive insulin is proinsulin.

        (3) In patients who have insulinoma, proinsulin levels frequently represent more than 20% of the total circulating insulin.

    c. Provocative tests rarely may be necessary to prove the diagnosis.

        (1) Tolbutamide or glucagon may be infused intravenously: An increased insulin level is diagnostic of insulinoma.

        (2) Fish insulin may be infused: Endogenous insulin levels will be suppressed in the normal individual but not in the insulinoma patient. (Fish insulin is not immunoreactive with human insulin.)

        (3) Calcium may be infused. This will cause the release of insulin and proinsulin in insulinoma patients, resulting in symptoms of hypoglycemia.

4. Treatment

    a. Surgical treatment

        (1) Surgical management is based on preoperative localization of the tumor.

            (a) More than 75% of all insulinomas are smaller than 1.5 cm, so arteriography, computed tomography (CT), and magnetic resonance imaging (MRI) are less sensitive for detecting insulinomas than for larger tumors. Selective arteriography may detect 50% of these tumors.

            (b) Percutaneous catheterization of the portal vein with serial insulin measurements can also help to localize the area of the tumor.

            (c) Endoscopic ultrasound is probably the best imaging test for insulinomas.

        (2) Exploration of the entire pancreas for a palpable mass is undertaken first.

            (a) If the tumor is palpable or is visible as a reddish-brown discoloration, it should be either enucleated or removed as part of a distal pancreatectomy.

            (b) Intraoperative ultrasound is helpful to localize small insulinomas (Fig. 17-1).

            (c) If lymph nodes adjacent to the tumor are firm and enlarged, suggesting carcinoma, or if the tumor feels malignant (i.e., firm and infiltrative), then a standard form of resectional therapy should be performed, such as pancreaticoduodenectomy or total pancreatectomy with lymphadenectomy.

        (3) The combination of careful palpation plus the use of intraoperative ultrasound should demonstrate the tumor in approximately 90% of patients. If the tumor is not localized, then the management is debatable.

            (a) The classic procedure is to resect the tail of the pancreas and examine the specimen pathologically. If a tumor is still not found, all of the pancreas but the head and the uncinate process is removed, and the operation is terminated.

            (b) The surgeon may proceed to total pancreatectomy if the tumor is not found in the tail of the pancreas.

            (c) The surgeon may resect only 80%–90% of the pancreas and then observe the patient for hyperinsulinism postoperatively. If medical measures then do not control the patient's symptoms, a total pancreatectomy may be necessary.

        (4) When islet cell hyperplasia is present, an 80%–90% subtotal pancreatectomy will usually control the symptoms.

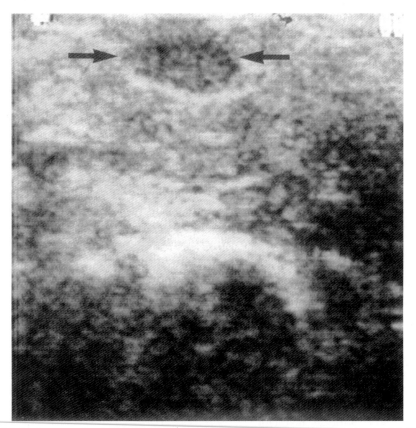

FIGURE 17-1 Intraoperative ultrasound of an islet cell tumor producing hyperinsulinism in a 34-year-old woman.

      (5) Blood glucose levels should be monitored in the operating room to prevent hypoglycemia.

  b. **Medical treatment** is limited to patients who are incurable operatively or who have malignant disease.

5. Prognosis

  a. Approximately 65% of patients are cured by surgery.

  b. The operative mortality rate is 10%.

  c. Patients who have malignant insulinomas have a 60% 2-year survival rate.

C **Gastrinomas (Zollinger-Ellison syndrome)**

1. Pathogenesis

  a. Symptoms in this disorder result from oversecretion of gastrin, the consequence of which is peptic ulceration because of high gastric acid secretion.

  b. The cause is usually a nonbeta islet cell tumor of the pancreas (i.e., a D-cell or δ-cell tumor).

  c. Zollinger-Ellison syndrome may be a component of MEN type I.

2. Clinical presentation

  a. Abdominal pain secondary to the peptic ulceration is present in more than 90% of the patients.

  b. Diarrhea is common, resulting from:

    (1) Gastric hypersecretion, which creates a low duodenal pH and inactivates pancreatic enzymes, resulting in steatorrhea

    (2) Gastrin-stimulated intestinal motility, which impairs fluid and electrolyte absorption

  c. Gastrointestinal (GI) hemorrhage from the peptic ulceration occurs in up to 40% of patients.

  d. Ulcer perforation and gastric outlet obstruction also occur.

  e. Profound dehydration and malnutrition may be present.

3. **Diagnosis**
   a. The following conditions should alert the physician to the possibility of Zollinger-Ellison syndrome:
      (1) Recurrent ulcer symptoms
      (2) Recurrent ulcer after a standard surgical procedure for peptic ulcer disease
      (3) An ulcer that is refractory to intensive treatment with antacids, H_2-receptor blockers, or omeprazole
   b. **Laboratory findings** provide the diagnosis.
      (1) **Gastric acid hypersecretion** is present in 70%–80% of patients. It is manifested by:
         (a) A 12-hour overnight basal acid output (BAO) of more than 100 mmol of hydrochloric acid
         (b) A 1-hour BAO of more than 15 mmol
         (c) Little or no increase in gastric acid secretion after stimulation of pentagastrin or betazole
            (i) This test shows that the parietal cells are under maximal stimulation.
            (ii) Results are expressed as the ratio of basal:maximal acid output (BAO:MAO), which usually exceeds 0.6 in patients who have Zollinger-Ellison syndrome.
      (2) **Increased levels of serum gastrin** are the key to the diagnosis.
         (a) Gastrin levels are determined by radioimmunoassay, which measures both the heptadecapeptide itself and its precursor form, G-34 or "big gastrin."
         (b) Most patients who have Zollinger-Ellison syndrome have a fasting serum gastrin level of 500 pg/mL or more (the normal level is 20–150 pg/mL).
         (c) Some patients have an intermediate serum gastrin level of 200–500 pg/mL. A gastrin stimulation test may then aid in the diagnosis.
            (i) In Zollinger-Ellison syndrome, an infusion of calcium will increase the gastrin level by more than 300 pg/mL, and an infusion of secretin will increase it by 100 pg/mL or more.
            (ii) Peptic ulcer patients and normal persons will not show this response.
         (d) Extremely high gastrin levels (more than 5000 pg/mL) or the presence of α-chain human chorionic gonadotropin in the serum strongly suggests a malignant gastrinoma.
         (e) Serum gastrin levels also may be increased by pathologic processes other than nonbeta islet cell carcinoma of the pancreas, including:
            (i) Nonbeta islet cell adenomas
            (ii) Antral G-cell hyperplasia
            (iii) Gastric outlet obstruction
            (iv) A retained gastric antrum after incomplete antrectomy for peptic ulcer disease
            (v) Conditions that cause gastric hypoacidity (which is a stimulus for gastrin production), including pernicious anemia, atrophic gastritis, and gastric carcinoma
         (f) Another innovative technique combines selective injection of secretin into mesenteric arteries with simultaneous measurement of gastrin.
   c. **Radiographs** will usually show upper GI ulceration.
      (1) Frequently, multiple ulcers are found.
      (2) Ulcers are sometimes found in the distal duodenum and jejunum.

4. **Localization of the tumor.** Localization studies are the same as described for insulinomas. Arteriography is less accurate for gastrinomas because these tumors are less vascular than insulinomas.

5. **Treatment** of Zollinger-Ellison syndrome is centered around removal of the causative tumor plus control of the end-organ (gastric mucosal) response.
   a. The tumor should be removed if possible because approximately 60% are malignant.
      (1) Unfortunately, the tumor is frequently multifocal or difficult to identify at laparotomy.
      (2) Only about 20% are resectable.
      (3) Lesions in the wall of the duodenum (present in greater than 25% of cases) and in the tail of the pancreas are the most common types of resectable tumors.

(4) Most gastrinomas are located in the **"Gastrinoma triangle,"** which is an anatomic triangle defined by the junction of the cystic and common bile ducts superiorly, the junction of the second and third portions of the duodenum inferiorly, and the junction of the neck and body of the pancreas medially.

b. The end-organ response (i.e., gastric hypersecretion) and the complications it causes may be treated either by surgical means or by the use of H_2-receptor blockers or omeprazole.

(1) Total gastrectomy is the classic treatment of choice.

(a) It should be performed even in the presence of metastasis because of the slow-growing nature of the tumor.

(b) It results in control of the severe GI hypersecretion and ulceration, and it is well tolerated by most patients.

(2) Prolonged H_2-receptor blockade with cimetidine or the use of proton pump inhibitors (PPI) such as omeprazole may control the GI manifestations of Zollinger-Ellison syndrome, but the failure rate is as high as 15%.

6. Prognosis for Zollinger-Ellison syndrome is good if the GI hyperacidity can be controlled by surgical or medical measures. Although two thirds of the causative tumors are malignant, they are very slow growing, and patients may live a long time.

D **Pancreatic cholera** is a syndrome of severe diarrhea associated with hypersecretion of a pancreatic nonbeta islet cell tumor.

1. Symptoms. The syndrome has been called **WDHA syndrome** because of the following symptoms.

a. **W**atery **d**iarrhea

b. **H**ypokalemia and a resultant profound muscular weakness due to the high potassium content in the stool

c. **A**chlorhydria

2. Pathogenesis. The probable cause is an increase in the secretion of VIP due to a pancreatic tumor.

a. The tumor is solitary in 80% of cases and is usually localized to the body or tail of the pancreas.

b. One half of the tumors are malignant and frequently have metastasized by the time of surgery.

3. Treatment is surgical excision when possible. If not, "debulking" the tumor may improve the diarrhea.

4. Prognosis is poor. The average length of survival after surgery is 1 year.

E **Glucagonomas** are tumors of the pancreatic alpha$_2$ islet cells that cause hypersecretion of glucagon.

1. The patient is usually diabetic and has weight loss, dermatitis, anemia, and stomatitis.

2. Sixty-five to 70% of these tumors are malignant.

CRITICAL POINTS

MEN1: Parathyroid hyperplasia, pancreatic endocrine tumors, pituitary adenomas

MEN2: Medullary thyroid cancer, pheochromocytoma

MEN2A: Parathyroid hyperplasia

MEN2B: Mucosal neuromas and marfanoid habitus

Treatment of MEN1

1. The primary concern is treating the hyperparathyroidism, which is more severe than in MEN2A. Surgical treatment with subtotal or total parathyroidectomy with arm reimplantation and cryopreservation.

2. Resection of pancreatic islet cell neoplasm, if symptomatic

3. Treat pituitary tumors with bromocriptine, which is adequate in most cases.

Treatment of MEN2

1. Total thyroidectomy for medullary thyroid cancer. Early operation for affected family members is done in early childhood before development of carcinoma.

2. Pheochromocytoma is treated with adrenalectomy after appropriate alpha blockade.

3. Hyperparathyroidism occurs in MEN2A, is milder than MEN1, and can be treated with subtotal parathyroidectomy.

Tumors of Endocrine Pancreas

1. Half are nonfunctional and half are functional (gastrinoma or insulinoma most common).

2. May be sporadic (occuring as solitary tumor) or with MEN1 (multifocal with tumors in pancreas and duodenal wall)

3. Insulinoma: 10% malignant; patients present with bizarre neurologic symptoms due to hypoglycemia; diagnose with high insulin in setting of hypoglycemia; imaging with CT and endoscopic ultrasound; treat by surgical enucleation; intraoperative ultrasound helpful to localize

4. Gastrinoma: 60% malignant; causes Zollinger-Ellison Syndrome; peptic ulcer disease and diarrhea common symptoms; confirm diagnosis with elevated gastrin; localize tumors with CT and endoscopic ultrasound; resect pancreatic tumors and excise duodenal tumors; most gastrinomas are located in the gastrinoma triangle, defined by the junction of the cystic and common bile ducts superiorly, the junction of the second and third portions of the duodenum inferiorly, and the junction of the neck and body of the pancreas medially; if unresectable, debulking will help symptoms (treat medically with H_2 blockers or PPI); gastrectomy option to treat uncontrolled acid.

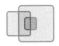

Study Questions for Part V

Directions: *Each of the numbered items in this section is followed by several possible answers. Select the ONE lettered answer that is BEST in each case.*

1. A 40-year-old man has a subtotal thyroidectomy performed for Graves' disease. Several hours later, he complains of difficulty breathing. On examination, he has stridor and a markedly swollen, tense neck wound. What should be one of the first steps in the management of this patient?

- A Intubate with an endotracheal tube
- B Perform a tracheostomy
- C Control the bleeding site in the operating room
- D Open the wound to evacuate the hematoma
- E Aspirate the hematoma

2. A 50-year-old hypertensive man has definitive biochemical evidence of a pheochromocytoma. Computed tomography (CT) scan and magnetic resonance imaging (MRI) do not reveal any abnormalities, and *m*-iodobenzylguanidine scanning is not readily available. What should be the next step in the management of this patient?

- A Abdominal exploration
- B Continued clinical observation
- C Mediastinoscopy
- D Selective venous sampling
- E Mediastinal exploration

3. A 55-year-old woman with progressive but episodic muscle weakness is diagnosed as having myasthenia gravis. Her chest radiograph is normal and reveals no evidence of mediastinal mass or tumor. What is the most definitive treatment that can be offered this patient?

- A Prednisone
- B Neostigmine
- C Thymectomy
- D Plasmapheresis
- E Atropine

4. A first-degree relative of a patient found to have advanced medullary carcinoma of the thyroid gland is referred for further evaluation. Which screening measure is the choice for detection of medullary thyroid pathology?

- A Careful physical examination
- B Serum calcitonin level
- C Stimulated serum calcitonin level (calcium and pentagastrin)
- D Gastrin level
- E Carcinoembryonic antigen (CEA) level

5. If a first-degree relative of a patient with MEN-2 A syndrome is found to have medullary pathology requiring surgical exploration of the thyroid gland, what should the preoperative screening include?

- A Serum cortisol level
- B Fasting glucose and insulin
- C CT scan of the head
- D Urinary aldosterone and renin
- E Urinary vanillylmandelic acid and metanephrines

6. A 60-year-old female patient has a workup for episodic symptoms of palpitations, nervousness, and bizarre behavior, all of which tend to occur during fasting states. Biochemically, she is diagnosed as having an insulinoma. What is the best choice for localizing this tumor?

- [A] CT scan
- [B] MRI
- [C] Selective arteriography
- [D] Percutaneous catheterization of the portal vein with selective venous sampling
- [E] Surgical exploration and intraoperative ultrasound

7. A 55-year-old female patient is evaluated for new onset of diabetes mellitus. Her medical history is largely unremarkable. Her physical examination is unrevealing except for the presence of an erythematous skin rash. Her further evaluation should include an investigation of the possibility of which of the following?

- [A] Insulinoma
- [B] Glucagonoma
- [C] Gastrinoma
- [D] Carcinoid tumor
- [E] Pancreatic cholera

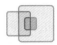

Answers and Explanations

1. The answer is D (Chapter 16, I D 2 e [4] [b] [ii]). Postoperative bleeding after thyroidectomy can cause airway compromise due to tracheal compression. The first step should be to open the wound to evacuate the hematoma, followed by a return to the operating room to control the bleeding site. Attempts to perform either endotracheal intubation or tracheostomy may be difficult until the external compression of the hematoma is relieved.

2. The answer is D (Chapter 16, II G 5 d). Although 90% of pheochromocytomas are located in the adrenal glands, they can occur in any tissue that is derived from neuroectoderm. When computed tomography (CT) scan and magnetic resonance imaging (MRI) do not identify a tumor, *m*-iodobenzylguanidine scanning can be helpful; however, this is not always available. Selective measurements of catecholamines drawn at various levels from the vena cava and its major branches should be obtained before surgical exploration.

3. The answer is C (Chapter 16, IV C 3 b). Myasthenia gravis is an autoimmune disease of neuromuscular transmission that causes skeletal muscle weakness. Parasympathomimetic drugs have been found to improve muscle strength in these patients. Prednisone has also been used with some success because of the autoimmune nature of this disease. Plasmapheresis may be effective in preparing the patient preoperatively. The treatment of choice for all forms of myasthenia, except purely ocular, appears to be thymectomy. An increased percentage of patients have permanent remission. The response to medication is improved in patients who do not achieve a complete remission.

4. The answer is C (Chapter 16, I F 5 c [2] [c]). All first-degree relatives of patients with medullary carcinoma of the thyroid gland should be screened for this disorder because it can occur in a familial pattern. Physical examination of the thyroid gland should be performed for the detection of any nodules. An increased serum calcitonin or an increased stimulated serum calcitonin test will also indicate underlying medullary pathology, either hyperplasia or carcinoma. The stimulated tests will detect disease at an earlier, more curable stage. Increased gastrin levels are associated with Zollinger-Ellison syndrome and are not part of this multiple endocrine adenomatosis (MEN) type 2 syndrome. Carcinoembryonic antigen (CEA) is elevated in some gastrointestinal malignancies.

5. The answer is E (Chapter 16, II G 4 a; Chapter 17, I B 2). Medullary carcinoma of the thyroid gland may present as a sporadic or familial form associated with MEN type 2A or 2B. Both are associated with pheochromocytomas. If a pheochromocytoma is present, it should be diagnosed and treated first to avoid the morbidity of cervical exploration in a patient with untreated pheochromocytoma. Urinary vanillylmandelic acid and metanephrines should be evaluated preoperatively.

6. The answer is E (Chapter 17, II B 4 a [2]). The patient has had a definitive biochemical diagnosis of insulinoma. These tumors can be present anywhere in the pancreas. Because they are usually small in size, arteriography, CT, and MRI are less sensitive than they would be for larger tumors. With careful surgical exploration and intraoperative ultrasound, approximately 90% of these tumors can be localized at the time of surgery.

7. The answer is B (Chapter 17, II E 1). Glucagon-producing tumors of the pancreas secrete glucagon in large amounts. Patients tend to present with new onset of diabetes mellitus (hyperglycemia). Affected individuals also characteristically have a migratory erythematous skin rash.

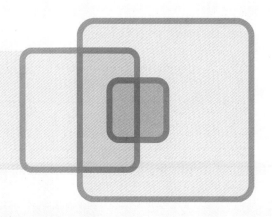

PART **VI**

Head and Neck Disorders

chapter 18

Benign Lesions

JOSEPH R. SPIEGEL · ROBERT T. SATALOFF · DAVID A. ZWILLENBERG

I · INTRODUCTION

Familiarity with the benign conditions reviewed in this chapter is essential to the physician who must distinguish life-threatening illnesses from those of little consequence, choose appropriate therapy, and avoid injudicious surgery.

A Overview

1. The most common neck mass is a reactive node, and these masses are most often secondary to bacterial or viral infections of the ear, nose, paranasal sinuses, teeth, tonsils, or skin and soft tissues of the head and neck.

2. Most neck masses in children are benign.

3. In adults, neck masses are more likely to be malignant.

4. The **"rule of sevens"** is a useful guide:
   a. A mass that has been present for 7 days is inflammatory.
   b. One present for 7 months is malignant.
   c. One present for 7 years is congenital.

B Workup for acquired lesions (see IV)

1. The **history** should be detailed, especially regarding:
   a. **Family history** of malignancy
   b. **Past malignancy** in the patient
   c. **Risk factors** associated with malignancy, such as:
      (1) Smoking
      (2) Alcohol consumption
      (3) Exposure to radiation, certain fumes, sawdust, or other potential carcinogens
   d. **Recent relevant illnesses,** such as:
      (1) Upper respiratory infection, sinusitis, or tonsillitis
      (2) Otitis or conjunctivitis
      (3) Dental problems

2. **Physical examination** should include careful inspection and palpation of the scalp, eyes, ears, nose, mouth (including the teeth and tonsils), hypopharynx, and nasopharynx for signs of infection, ulceration, or unsuspected abnormalities.

3. **Laboratory tests** may include:
   a. Complete blood count and differential
   b. Chest radiograph
   c. Tuberculin test for tuberculosis
   d. A heterophil titer (monospot test) for mononucleosis
   e. Thyroid function tests or thyroid scan
   f. Serologic tests for syphilis
   g. Viral titers, especially for Epstein-Barr virus, which is associated with nasopharyngeal carcinoma and Burkitt's lymphoma

4. **Radiologic studies** may include soft tissue radiographs of the neck, xeroradiograms, a barium swallow, and a complete gastrointestinal series or scanning procedures such as computed

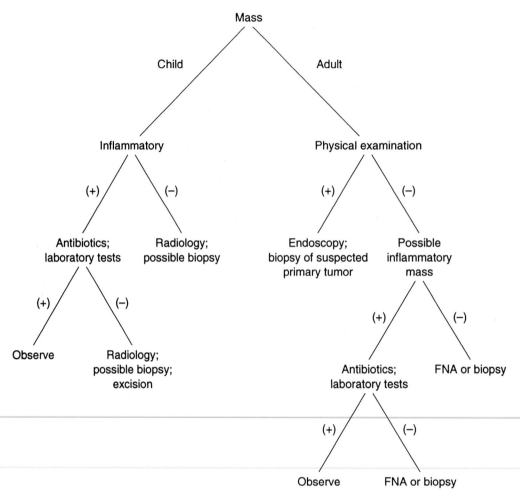

FIGURE 18-1 Algorithm for evaluation and treatment of a neck mass. FNA, fine-needle aspiration; PE, physical examination.

tomography (CT), magnetic resonance imaging (MRI), bone scan, or other radioisotope scans.

5. **Endoscopy** is indicated to search for the tumor if a primary neoplasm is suspected. Endoscopic biopsy and radiologic studies should precede any incision in the neck (see Chapter 19, II B)

6. Treatment depends on the findings during the workup (Fig. 18-1).
   a. Antibiotics should be administered if a bacterial infection is suspected.
   b. Antituberculous drugs may be needed.
   c. Consultation with a specialist in another field may be helpful.
      (1) A dental consultation may be useful if the teeth seem to be the source of a problem.
      (2) If dandruff, scabies, or another dermatologic condition is noted, a dermatology consultation is indicated.
   d. If a mass does not shrink significantly or disappear within a reasonable time (usually 6 weeks), then surgical treatment or biopsy may be indicated.
      (1) If cervical adenopathy persists, then:
         (a) The presence of enlarged or cryptic tonsils is believed by many to be an indication for tonsillectomy.
         (b) Equivocal or abnormal dental findings are an indication for dental treatment.
      (2) If a source of infection is not found, then persistent cervical adenopathy is an indication for excisional biopsy after a complete evaluation for malignancy.
      (3) A neck mass biopsy is the last step in a proper workup. Fine-needle aspiration can be used to diagnose carcinoma, but it is usually inadequate to define lymphoma.

TABLE 18-1 Neck Abscesses
Signs and Symptoms Pain Swelling Dysphagia Dyspnea Leukocytosis Fever Air in soft-tissue radiograph
Treatment Airway protection Incision and drainage Antibiotics

II NECK ABSCESSES

A **Overview** A patient presenting with fever and a painful, fluctuant neck mass most probably has an abscess (Table 18-1).

1. The source of infection should be identified, and **drainage** should be carried out.

2. Owing to the **danger to the carotid artery, airway, and cranial nerves,** deep neck abscesses should be treated only by those knowledgeable in the standard techniques and anatomy of the area. They should be treated on an emergency basis.

B **Types of abscesses**

1. **Bezold's abscesses** are neck abscesses that arise from infection in the middle ear or mastoid.

2. **Ludwig's angina** is an abscess that occupies the sublingual space.
   a. It generally arises from a dental source.
   b. It can cause death from airway obstruction and, therefore, frequently requires tracheostomy.

3. **Parapharyngeal space abscesses** arise from the posterior teeth or tonsils and can affect the carotid sheath structures and multiple cranial nerves. They can cause mediastinitis and carotid "blowout" (i.e., erosion of the artery wall leading to massive hemorrhage).

4. **Retropharyngeal abscesses** arise from infected retropharyngeal nodes or extension from other spaces. They can lead to airway obstruction or mediastinitis.

5. **Peritonsillar abscesses (quinsy)** arise as a complication of acute tonsillitis.
   a. They present with ipsilateral palatal edema, contralateral deviation of the uvula, "hot potato" voice, trismus, and dysphagia. The patient may have only a low-grade fever or be afebrile.
   b. They are the most common abscesses in the parapharyngeal space.

III CONGENITAL MASSES (Table 18-2)

A **Parenchymal cysts**

1. **Thymic cysts**
   a. **Embryology.** The thymus arises from the third pharyngeal pouch and migrates caudally and medially to descend into the superior mediastinum.
      (1) During this descent, an attachment may remain in the neck.
      (2) Thymic tissues may present in the neck as separate nodules of mature thymus or may occur in association with ciliated or columnar epithelial remnants of the pharyngeal outpouching.
      (3) Thymic cysts may occur anywhere on a line from the mandibular angle to the suprasternal notch.
   b. **Characteristics**
      (1) Approximately 95% of thymic cysts are unilateral, and 90% of thymic ectopias are cystic.
      (2) They are generally found in children, and there is a male predominance.

TABLE 18-2 Congenital Neck Masses

Type	Location	Examination	Treatment
Thymic cysts	Anterior triangle	Firm, nontender	Surgical excision
Parathyroid cysts	Paratracheal	Firm, nontender	Surgical excision
Thyroglossal cysts	Midline	Firm, nontender	Surgical excision
Teratoma	Anywhere	Firm	Surgical excision
Hemangioma	Anywhere	Diffuse	Observation; laser treatment
Cystic hygroma	Posterior triangle	Diffuse	Partial excision
Branchial cleft cyst	Preauricular anterior triangle	Firm, nontender	Surgical excision

       (3) They may be unilocular or multilocular.

       (4) Loculated cysts generally contain amber to brown fluid, which may be clear or turbid.

    c. Complications

       (1) Cysts are often asymptomatic but may be painful if they are infected or if they grow suddenly.

       (2) Midline cysts may cause dysphagia.

       (3) Both benign and malignant hyperplasia have been reported in these cysts.

       (4) Myasthenia gravis is not found in association with cervical thymic cysts.

    d. Differential diagnosis

       (1) Branchial cleft cysts seldom extend inferiorly to the clavicle and often present with signs of acute inflammation.

       (2) Cystic hygromas are lateral, spongy, and more diffuse. They are seen generally in infants.

    e. Treatment. Surgery is the treatment of choice.

  2. Parathyroid cysts

    a. Characteristics

       (1) These unusual cysts generally present in adults from 30–50 years of age as a solitary mass at either inferior pole of the thyroid gland.

       (2) Tracheal deviation is usual and causes a variable degree of respiratory obstruction.

       (3) Hoarseness may occur because of pressure on the recurrent laryngeal nerve.

    b. Treatment consists of surgical excision.

B Lesions of thyroid origin

  1. Overview. The thyroid gland originates at the foramen cecum and descends centrally to the thyroid and cricoid cartilages.

    a. The thyroglossal duct may pass in front of, through, or behind the hyoid bone. It is generally obliterated but may persist.

    b. Elements of thyroidal primordium may remain at any site in its passage.

       (1) These elements may give rise not only to cysts and fistulas but also to accessory thyroid tissue and neoplasms.

       (2) Most cystic remnants occur in the midline around the hyoid bone.

       (3) Solid tumors of thyroglossal duct origin occur almost exclusively within the tongue and above the hyoid bone.

  2. Thyroid rests

    a. Characteristics

       (1) Thyroid rests may be lingual or may occur in the neck.

       (2) Endotracheal ectopias may occur.

       (3) Palpation of the normal position of the thyroid often reveals easily palpable tracheal rings in patients with these rests.

    b. Treatment is dictated by the degree of obstruction present and by the presence of other thyroid tissue.

       (1) A thyroid scan should be performed before the removal of lesions suspected of being thyroid rests to ensure that there is functional thyroid tissue in the usual location.

       (2) Between 70% and 80% of patients have no other functional thyroid.

3. Thyroglossal cysts, sinuses, and fistulas

   a. Anatomy

      (1) These occur in the midline, unless previous surgery has produced distortion.

      (2) Approximately 20% are suprahyoid, 15% occur at the hyoid, and 65% are infrahyoid.

   b. Characteristics

      (1) Fistulas are almost always the result of infection with spontaneous or surgical drainage. Fistulas can drain internally, externally, or both (complete fistulas).

      (2) Thyroglossal duct cysts present by age 10 in 50% of cases.

         (a) There is no sexual predominance, but there is a racial predominance; the cysts occur most often in whites.

         (b) Cysts usually measure 2–4 cm in diameter and gradually increase in size, although the size may fluctuate.

         (c) They rise and fall with the larynx during swallowing.

   c. Treatment is total surgical excision (Sistrunk procedure), including the:

      (1) Cyst and sinus to the base of the tongue

      (2) Whole fistula if one is present

      (3) Middle third of the hyoid bone

C **Cutaneous branchiogenic cysts** are rare, asymptomatic nodules that are noted soon after birth and gradually increase in size.

   1. Anatomy. They are located in the suprasternal notch.

   2. Treatment is by local surgical excision.

D **Teratomas** are growths that consist of multiple tissues that are foreign to the part of the body in which they arise.

   1. Types

      a. Epidermoid cysts, the most common type, are lined by squamous epithelium and have no adnexa.

      b. Dermoid cysts are epithelium-lined cavities containing skin appendages (e.g., hair, glandular tissue, and follicles).

      c. Teratoid cysts are lined with simple stratified squamous epithelium or respiratory epithelium and contain cheesy keratinous material. They are rare in the head and neck.

   2. Cervical teratomas are most commonly present at birth. Appearance after the age of 1 year is rare.

      a. Characteristics

         (1) The lesions are usually 5–12 cm in their long axis and are semicystic, although they may be solid. They are usually unilateral.

         (2) Infants with cervical dermoids usually have stridor, apnea, or cyanosis because of tracheal compression or deviation. Dysphagia may also be present.

         (3) Some infants are asymptomatic at birth but become symptomatic within weeks or months.

      b. Associated anomalies. There is an increased incidence of maternal hydramnios, but affected infants show no increase in associated anomalies.

      c. Treatment. Early excision in infants is mandatory.

   3. Malignant teratomas of the neck are rare and occur exclusively in adults. The prognosis is very poor.

   4. Nasal dermoids are often apparent shortly after birth.

      a. Anatomy. The nasal dorsum is the most common site, but they may occur in the tip of the nose or the columella.

      b. Characteristics

         (1) They show a male predominance of 2:1.

         (2) They must be differentiated from encephaloceles and gliomas.

      c. Treatment. Early removal is important. Recurrences secondary to incomplete removal are common.

E **Vascular tumors**   (see Chapter 26, II B 3 a)

1. **Hemangiomas** are the most common tumors of the head and neck in children. Girls are more often affected than boys, and the lesions are usually solitary.

   a. **Types**

      (1) **Capillary hemangiomas,** such as nevus flammeus (port-wine stain) and strawberry nevus are characteristically found in the dermis.

         (a) They rarely appear in adults.

         (b) They have an early period of evolution, after which they often regress. They may develop suddenly and grow quite large.

      (2) **Cavernous hemangiomas** are more permanent. Spontaneous regression is more likely for hemangiomas present at birth than in those appearing later.

      (3) **Arteriovenous hemangiomas** occur almost exclusively in adults and have a predilection for the lips and perioral skin.

      (4) **Invasive hemangiomas** occur in the deep subcutaneous tissues, deep fascial layers, and muscles.

         (a) These hemangiomas present as neck masses, predominantly in children.

         (b) They tend to recur long after excision but do not metastasize.

         (c) The masseter and trapezius are the muscles most commonly involved in the head and neck.

         (d) Intramuscular hemangiomas most commonly present in young adults as palpable, mobile, noncompressible masses.

            (i) They are generally without thrills, pulsations, or bruits.

            (ii) Pain secondary to compression of other structures is usually present.

      (5) **Subglottic hemangiomas** are usually capillary in type. Owing to their location, they often present at birth (or soon thereafter) with stridor and usually with cutaneous involvement as well.

   b. **Treatment**

      (1) **Congenital cutaneous hemangiomas** are generally not treated initially.

         (a) When patients reach school age, cosmetically deforming lesions may be excised.

         (b) Steroids may be used to slow a rapid growth phase if necessary.

         (c) Tunable dye and copper vapor lasers have shown promise in the treatment of cutaneous lesions.

      (2) **Subglottic lesions** may require tracheotomy, steroids, and, in some cases, laser excision.

      (3) Surgery may be needed for extensive lesions.

      (4) Radiation therapy has been used to suppress tumor growth. However, radiation alone will not effect a cure, and its use in these lesions is controversial.

2. **Cystic hygromas** are found predominantly in the neck and are usually noted at birth or soon thereafter.

   a. **Anatomy.** They are more common in the posterior triangle.

      (1) They may reach up into the cheek or parotid region and down into the mediastinum or axilla.

      (2) Large masses extend past the sternocleidomastoid muscle into the anterior compartment and may cross the midline.

      (3) They may involve the floor of the mouth and the base of the tongue.

   b. **Symptoms and signs** may include:

      (1) Difficulty in nursing

      (2) Facial or neck distortion

      (3) Respiratory distress

      (4) Brachial plexus compression with pain or hyperesthesia

      (5) A sudden increase in size secondary to spontaneous hemorrhage, which can be fatal

   c. **Characteristics**

      (1) There is no predilection for either sex or for either side of the body.

      (2) The hygromas can be progressive, static, or regressive.

      (3) Small lesions are unilocular and firm.

      (4) Large tumors are loculated, shiftable, and compressible.

     (5) The hygromas generally transilluminate.

     (6) The cyst walls are usually tense, and because the loculi tend to communicate, rupture of one locule can cause all of them to partially collapse.

   d. Treatment. Surgery is the mainstay of treatment.

     (1) Recurrences are common because the cysts insinuate themselves into adjacent structures, so resection is often incomplete.

     (2) The greater the lymphangiomatous component of a hygroma, the more likely it is to recur.

3. Oral and perioral lymphangiomas are relatively common lesions that are usually found at birth or soon thereafter. They behave very much like cystic hygromas.

F **Branchial cleft anomalies**

1. Embryology

   a. In the fourth week of gestation, five ridges appear on the ventrolateral surface of the embryonic head, with a groove between each. These ridges and grooves form the branchial arches and clefts, respectively.

   b. The pharyngeal pouches develop internally at the same level as the external grooves.

2. Types

   a. A **sinus,** or **incomplete fistula,** has either an internal or an external opening.

   b. A **complete fistula** has both an internal and an external opening.

   c. A **cyst** has neither an internal nor an external opening.

   d. Combinations of any of the preceding types can occur.

3. Anatomy. Branchial cleft anomalies are generally located along the anterior border of the sternocleidomastoid muscle or deep to it. They can occur anywhere between the external auditory canal and the clavicle.

   a. First branchial cleft anomalies are always superior to the hyoid bone.

     (1) If a fistula is present, it courses superiorly to end near the external auditory canal.

     (2) The cyst and tract may lie in the parotid gland, with a variable relationship to the facial nerve.

   b. Second cleft anomalies are the **most common** type.

     (1) An external opening, when present, is about two thirds of the way down the sternocleidomastoid anteriorly.

     (2) The fistula, if present, ascends with the carotid sheath and crosses over the hypoglossal and glossopharyngeal nerves and between the external and internal carotid arteries to end at the tonsillar fossa.

   c. Third cleft anomalies are rare.

     (1) The external opening occurs in the same position as in a second cleft fistula.

     (2) The tract ascends along the carotid sheath posteriorly to the internal carotid artery, over the hypoglossal nerve, under the glossopharyngeal nerve, and over the vagus nerve to open in the piriform sinus.

   d. Fourth branchial cleft anomalies have never been seen in their entirety.

     (1) Theoretically, they would have an external opening anterior to the sternocleidomastoid muscle in the lower neck.

     (2) They would descend along the carotid sheath into the chest, passing under the subclavian artery on the right and the aortic arch on the left, ascend into the neck to cross the hypoglossal nerve, then descend to open into the esophagus.

4. Characteristics

   a. Branchial cleft cysts are generally smooth, round, nontender masses.

   b. An increase in size during upper respiratory infections is common.

   c. An infected branchial cleft cyst may abscess or rupture spontaneously to form a sinus.

   d. The size and the location of a branchial cleft anomaly determine the symptoms.

     (1) Large cysts may cause dysphagia, stridor, and dyspnea.

     (2) Small cysts are often not discovered until adulthood because of their slow rate of growth and minor symptoms.

5. **Treatment**
    a. Complete excision without damage to the surrounding vital structures is the definitive treatment. Antibiotics are given if the lesion is infected.
    b. Incision and drainage are avoided, if possible, because they make subsequent excision more difficult.

G **Encephaloceles** are congenital brain herniations, which may be confused with nasal dermoids or polyps. Meningitis or cerebrospinal fluid leaks are not uncommon, particularly with manipulation.

1. **Anatomy**
    a. They are usually discovered early in life. Approximately 75% are occipital, 15% are sincipital, and 10% enter the nose or nasopharynx.
    b. These lesions may or may not communicate centrally. Communicating lesions increase in size and tension when the infant cries; noncommunicating ones generally do not.

2. **Treatment** should include total removal. The lesions do not need to be treated as emergencies if there is no imminent threat of meningitis.

IV ACQUIRED LESIONS

A **Leukoplakia and keratosis** are white lesions that occur on the mucosa of the mouth, pharynx, or larynx. **Erythroplakia** is a similar red patch.

1. **Etiology.** These lesions are associated with repeated trauma (e.g., from poorly fitting dentures, decayed teeth), smoking, or use of alcohol. There is little correlation between the clinical appearance of the lesions and their histology. Erythroplakia is somewhat more likely to be carcinoma.

2. **Diagnosis.** Biopsy, to rule out squamous cell carcinoma, should be performed:
    a. In high-risk patients (smokers and drinkers)
    b. If the lesion persists after the removal of an irritative focus

3. **Treatment.** Benign leukoplakic lesions require no treatment but do require continued observation.

B **Papillomas**

1. **Squamous papillomas of the oral cavity** usually occur singly but may be multiple. They are common on the palate and faucial arches.
    a. They are usually pedunculated and cauliflowerlike in appearance.
    b. Recurrence is rare after excision.

2. **Nasal papillomas**
    a. **Squamous papillomas of the nasal cavity** are warts that are similar in appearance and behavior to cutaneous warts elsewhere on the body.
    b. **Cylindrical and fungiform papillomas** are other forms of benign nasal papillomas.
    c. **Inverted papillomas**
        (1) **Anatomy**
            (a) The lesions typically arise from the lateral nasal wall and can invade the sinuses and orbits.
            (b) Grossly, the lesions appear bulky and deep red to gray in color. They vary in consistency.
            (c) Unlike nasal polyps of allergic origin (see IV C), they are unilateral.
        (2) **Characteristics**
            (a) Patients generally present with nasal obstruction, a postnasal drip, and headaches. A few have epistaxis. These lesions occur mainly in men between 50 and 70 years of age.
            (b) The reported incidence of malignant degeneration is about 2%. The incidence of associated malignancy in adjacent tissue is as high as 15%.
        (3) **Treatment** is complete excision. Recurrence is common because excision is often incomplete.

3. **Laryngeal papillomas** are the most common laryngeal tumors of childhood and may be found at any age.
   a. **Juvenile type.** This type occurs predominantly in childhood and tends to involute at puberty.
      (1) **Etiology.** The etiology is viral.
      (2) **Characteristics**
         (a) **Multiple papillomas** are the most common characteristic. They may involve the airway from the epiglottis to the bronchi. The vocal folds are usually involved.
         (b) **Hoarseness** is an early sign, and **obstruction** is a later one.
      (3) **Treatment**
         (a) A tracheotomy may be necessary but should be avoided if possible because it predisposes to tracheal seeding of the papillomas.
         (b) Laryngoscopic removal, often by the use of a carbon dioxide laser, is the mainstay of therapy.
         (c) Interferon therapy has not proved to be as useful as early reports predicted. Other medical therapies are under investigation.
         (d) Recurrence and spread are currently common.
   b. **Adult type.** In this form, the papilloma is generally single.
      (1) As in the juvenile form, the papilloma tends to recur following excision.
      (2) Recurrent lesions can undergo malignant transformation, particularly in patients exposed to radiation.

C **Nasal polyps** are rare before 5 years of age and occur more commonly in men.
   1. **Etiology.** Nasal polyps are believed to be an allergic response, but this etiology has not been clearly established.
      a. They may be associated with asthma and an idiosyncratic reaction to aspirin.
      b. In children, the presence of nasal polyps should prompt a sweat test to rule out cystic fibrosis.
   2. **Characteristics**
      a. Inflammatory polyps are almost always bilateral and may recur frequently.
      b. Involvement of the paranasal sinuses is common.
   3. **Treatment.** Polyps are excised if they obstruct the nasal airways or the sinus drainage pathways.

D **Fibrous lesions**
   1. **Nodular (proliferative) fasciitis** presents as a rapidly growing, discrete soft tissue mass.
      a. **Etiology**
         (1) Probably a reactive, non-neoplastic response to injury, it may occur at any time from childhood to age 70.
         (2) The lesions may be mistaken for sarcoma.
      b. **Characteristics.** Fascia is the primary tissue involved.
      c. **Treatment.** The lesions generally do not recur after excision.
   2. **Proliferative myositis** occurs in adults and appears to be post-traumatic in origin.
      a. **Characteristics**
         (1) Like nodular fasciitis, it can be confused with sarcoma.
         (2) The lesion involves muscle diffusely.
         (3) Occasionally, spontaneous regression occurs.
      b. **Treatment.** Lesions do not recur after excision.
   3. **Traumatic myositis ossificans,** bony deposits in muscle due to trauma, generally presents as a painful mass in the muscle 1–4 weeks after a single severe trauma.
      a. **Characteristics**
         (1) In the head and neck, the masseter or sternocleidomastoid is generally involved.
         (2) Radiography reveals feathery opacities or irregular radiodensities.
         (3) The condition must be differentiated from **myositis ossificans progressiva,** which is a progressive, systemic illness that begins early in life and results in the conversion of muscle tissue to bony tissue.
      b. **Treatment.** Persistent painful masses are excised. Local recurrence is common.

4. **Desmoid tumors** are benign, locally invasive, encapsulated tumors.
   a. **Etiology**
      (1) They arise from the muscle fascia and are often associated with prior trauma.
      (2) These tumors are uncommon in the head and neck but, when found, usually arise from the sternocleidomastoid muscle.
   b. **Treatment.** Complete surgical excision is the treatment of choice.

E **Tumors of skeletal muscle**

1. **Characteristics**
   a. **Extracardiac rhabdomyomas** have a predilection for the head and neck.
   b. They show a slight male predominance.

2. **Signs and symptoms** depend on the site and size of the tumor.

3. **Treatment.** Rhabdomyomas are treated with complete surgical excision, if possible, followed by chemotherapy and radiation.

F **Tumors of peripheral nerves** (see Chapter 26, II B 6)

1. **Schwannomas** are solitary, encapsulated tumors attached to or surrounded by a nerve. They are primarily located centrifugally and are often painful and tender. They are not associated with von Recklinghausen's disease or with malignant change, in contrast to neurofibromas.

2. **Acoustic neuromas** constitute a type of schwannoma.
   a. **Etiology.** They arise from the eighth cranial nerve, usually start within the internal auditory canal, and can involve the cerebellopontine angle.
   b. **Characteristics.** Signs and symptoms may include hearing loss, tinnitus, imbalance, and vertigo. Asymmetric sensorineural hearing loss is common and requires that acoustic neuroma be ruled out.
   c. **Evaluation.** Testing includes an audiogram, an auditory brain stem response test, and an MRI with gadolinium enhancement.
   d. **Treatment.** Early discovery is important because it results in earlier resection, with a consequent decrease in morbidity and mortality.

3. **Von Recklinghausen's neurofibromatosis (NF I)**
   a. **Etiology.** It is caused by a nerve growth factor gene on chromosome 17q11.2. Inheritance is autosomal dominant.
   b. **Characteristics**
      (1) Neurites (axons) pass through the tumor.
      (2) Lesions are usually multiple and unencapsulated.
      (3) In 8% of patients, neurofibromas undergo malignant changes.
      (4) Usually, these lesions are located centripetally and are characteristically asymptomatic.
      (5) Café au lait spots, vitiligo, gliomas (especially optic), osseous changes, Lisch nodules (iris hamartomas) meningitis, spina bifida, syndactyly, hemangiomas, axillary or inguinal freckling, NF I in a first-degree relative, or retinal and visceral manifestations may be present.

4. **Central neurofibromatosis (NF II)**
   a. **Etiology.** It is caused by an abnormality on chromosome 22q11.21-13.1 and involves encoding of a suppressor protein called *schwannomin*. Inheritance is autosomal dominant, but almost 50% of cases are new mutations.
   b. **Characteristics**
      (1) Classically, slow-growing, bilateral acoustic neuromas or neurofibromas cause hearing loss or dizziness and lead to a diagnosis by age 20.
      (2) The diagnosis may also be established by a unilateral eighth nerve mass and:
         (a) A relative with NF II or,
         (b) Any two of the following: glioma, juvenile posterior subscapular lenticular opacity, meningioma, neurofibroma schwannoma
      (3) Café au lait spots, posterior lens cataracts, and cutaneous neurofibromas are uncommon. Lisch nodules are not found.

(4) Wishart type: Early onset rapid growth, other fibromatous tumors in addition to eighth nerve masses

(5) Gardner type: Later onset, slow growth rate, usually bilateral acoustic neuromas only

5. **Traumatic neuromas** are reactive hyperplasias due to a nerve's attempts at regeneration after injury. They are generally oval or oblong, gray, firm, and unencapsulated. Persistent hyperesthesia and tenderness are the usual signs.

6. Most neurogenous tumors of the head and neck can be excised safely without sacrificing nerves. If an important nerve must be cut, it should be generally reanastomosed or a nerve graft should be interposed.

G **Granular cell tumors**

1. **Congenital epulis** occurs on the gum pads of newborns in the region of the future incisors. The lesion can be quite large, does not recur after excision, and may spontaneously regress. The female:male ratio is 8:1.

2. **Nonepulis form of granular cell tumors** occurs mainly in young adults, especially in blacks.

H **Paragangliomas (chemodectomas)** can occur in the head or neck (see Chapter 19, XII).

I **Nondental lesions of the jaw**

1. **Giant cell granuloma**
   a. **Types.** This jaw lesion can occur in two forms:
      (1) **Central granulomas** occur within the jaw.
      (2) **Peripheral granulomas,** occurring on the gingival or alveolar mucosa, are four times more common.
   b. **Characteristics.** The mucosa is generally intact, but radiographs of the central lesions show radiolucent areas.
   c. **Treatment.** Excision or curettage is the treatment of choice.

2. **Fibrous dysplasia of the jaw** is noted early in life.
   a. **Characteristics**
      (1) It shows active growth in childhood and stabilization in adulthood.
      (2) Enlargement of the bone is the most common sign and may be either minor or significant enough to cause obvious facial asymmetry.
      (3) The maxilla is more commonly involved than the mandible.
      (4) Radiographs reveal sclerosis, lytic lesions, or unilocular lesions.
   b. **Treatment**
      (1) Obvious deformity, pain, or interference with function suggests the need for surgery.
      (2) Malignant transformation is possible but uncommon, and conservative resection appears to be the best treatment.

3. **Torus** is a benign bony growth, occurring at the midline of the palate (**maxillary torus**) or bilaterally lingual to the bicuspid (**mandibular torus**). Tori grow slowly and generally have no significance except that they may interfere with the fitting of dentures.

4. **Osteomas** are slow-growing, benign tumors in the sinuses, jaws, or external ear canals. They may require excision if they produce a headache or an occlusion of drainage.

J **Laryngeal lesions**

1. **Laryngocele** is a dilatation of the laryngeal saccule, producing an air sac that communicates with the laryngeal ventricle. Anything that increases intralaryngeal pressure increases the size of a laryngocele (e.g., coughing, straining, playing a wind instrument). A **laryngopyocele** is an infected laryngocele. It can be fatal if it results in asphyxia or if the purulent contents are aspirated into the tracheobronchial tree.
   a. **Anatomy.** Laryngoceles may be unilateral or bilateral. They may also be internal (within the larynx), external (presenting in the neck), or both (combined).
      (1) An **internal laryngocele** causes bulging of the false cord and aryepiglottic fold.
      (2) An **external laryngocele** appears as a neck swelling at about the level of the hyoid bone and anterior to the sternocleidomastoid.

  b. Characteristics

    (1) Internal laryngoceles cause hoarseness, breathlessness, and stridor on enlargement.

    (2) External laryngoceles increase in size with coughing or the Valsalva maneuver.

      (a) They are tympanic to percussion.

      (b) A hissing may be heard as the laryngocele empties air into the larynx when the air pressure is reduced.

  c. Diagnosis

    (1) Plain films may show cystic spaces that contain air.

    (2) Tomograms may help to demonstrate the continuity between the internal and external components.

    (3) CT and MRI scans show these lesions well.

  d. Treatment

    (1) Symptomatic laryngoceles are treated by surgical excision.

    (2) Laryngopyoceles should be treated by incision, drainage, and subsequent excision. Antibiotics are also appropriate.

2. Laryngeal webs

  a. Characteristics

    (1) They may be congenital or may follow bilateral vocal fold trauma.

    (2) When extensive, they present with stridor, weak phonation, and feeding problems in infants.

  b. Treatment. Excision or division is now generally the preferred treatment, and placement of a stent or keel is often required.

3. Vocal nodules

  a. Anatomy. Vocal nodules are bilateral benign masses that usually occur at the junction of the anterior and middle thirds of the true vocal folds.

  b. Etiology. They are associated with vocal abuse.

  c. Treatment

    (1) Vocal nodules are best treated by modifying the patient's speaking or singing technique through voice therapy.

    (2) Surgery is rarely necessary and is generally performed only after failure of voice therapy.

4. Vocal polyps

  a. Characteristics. Vocal polyps are usually unilateral and often do not regress with speech therapy—two important points in distinguishing the polyps from vocal nodules.

  b. Treatment

    (1) The recommended therapy is careful excision with microscopic visualization and avoidance of injury to the underlying lamina propria.

    (2) In selected cases, the laser may be helpful.

5. Laryngeal granulomas

  a. Anatomy. Laryngeal granulomas occur over the vocal processes of the arytenoid cartilages.

  b. Etiology. They are generally the result of trauma, usually from an endotracheal tube, and are usually associated with reflux laryngitis. Voice abuse may be a factor.

  c. Treatment

    (1) Antireflux therapy is often helpful.

    (2) They can regress as a result of treatment with antireflux medication and speech therapy.

  d. They are best treated by excision of persistent granulomas after a period of voice and medical therapy.

  e. Botulinum toxin is used for selected, recurrent cases.

6. Arytenoid dislocation

  a. Etiology. Arytenoid dislocation generally is the result of endotracheal tube or external trauma.

  b. Characteristics. A soft, breathy voice after extubation should arouse suspicion.

  c. Treatment. Prompt reduction is advisable; otherwise, the arytenoid usually becomes fixed in the dislocated position. However, late reduction (after months or years) can be successful and should be attempted when diagnosis or treatment has been delayed.

7. **Contact ulcers**
   a. **Anatomy.** Contact ulcers are mucosal disruptions usually located posteriorly on the vocal folds.
   b. **Etiology.** They sometimes result from trauma (e.g., from intubation), occasionally from vocal abuse, and often from gastric reflux laryngitis or heavy coughing.
   c. **Treatment** with antireflux medication and behavioral changes such as elevation of the head of the bed; avoidance of caffeine, chocolate, late-night snacks, and fried or fatty foods; and antacid therapy will usually result in prompt resolution of the ulcers. Antibiotics may be helpful.

V INFECTIONS OF THE HEAD AND NECK

A **Common head and neck infections** (e.g., otitis media, mastoiditis, and sinusitis) are now controlled with antibiotics, which must be given at high doses and over long periods for these sequestered spaces.

B **Tonsillar and adenoidal hypertrophy and infection** Tonsillectomy with adenoidectomy was once the most common operation performed in the United States. It remains quite prevalent but is now performed for these specific indications:

1. **Obstructive hypertrophy**
   a. Patients benefiting from tonsillectomy with adenoidectomy are those with airway obstruction, sleep apnea, cor pulmonale, dysphagia, or failure to thrive.
   b. **Adenoidectomy** is performed in children with chronic nasal obstruction, especially when they also demonstrate chronic serous otitis media or orthodontic problems.

2. **Recurrent infection.** Patients with documented recurrent adenotonsillitis are improved after tonsillectomy with adenoidectomy. A history of three to six episodes annually is a relative indication.

3. Tonsillectomy is often suggested after treatment for **peritonsillar abscess** in patients with a history of previous tonsillitis.

C **Atypical mycobacteria infection** presents as an inflamed mass or draining sinus in the head and neck. It is most common in children and adolescents.

1. Pulmonary involvement is rare.

2. It is commonly associated with the parotid or submandibular glands, but it is not isolated to these sites.

3. Fixation of overlying skin and sinus formation are common. Biopsy can lead to a chronically draining sinus tract.

4. Treatment is by surgical excision or curettage and drainage. Antimycobacterial drug therapy is not indicated.

chapter 19

Malignant Lesions of the Head and Neck

JOSEPH R. SPIEGEL · ROBERT T. SATALOFF · DAVID A. ZWILLENBERG

I OVERVIEW

Table 19-1 shows the basic characteristics of head and neck cancer.

A Epidemiology

1. Primary malignant neoplasms of the head and neck, excluding skin cancer, account for 5% of new cancers each year in the United States.

2. The male:female ratio is 3:1 to 4:1, and most lesions occur in patients older than 40 years of age.

3. Approximately 80% of primary head and neck malignancies are squamous cell carcinomas. The remainder are thyroid cancers, salivary neoplasms, lymphoma, and other less common tumors.

4. The number of patients with a second primary malignancy at the time of initial presentation has been reported to be as high as 17%.

B Risk factors

1. Tobacco use (chewing or smoking), alcohol consumption, and exposure to radiation are etiologic factors in most squamous cell carcinomas of the head and neck.

2. Approximately 85% of patients with head or neck cancer smoke or formerly smoked cigarettes at the time of diagnosis.

C Evaluation of the patient starts with a careful history and physical examination.

1. **History.** The patient should be questioned about:
   a. **Exposure to etiologic agents** (e.g., tobacco, alcohol, sawdust, other toxins, and irradiation)
   b. **Associated symptoms,** including hoarseness or sore throat of more than 3 weeks' duration, dysphagia, dyspnea, nonhealing ulcers, hemoptysis, and neck mass
   c. Any **history of head or neck malignancy**
   d. **Nutritional status, family history, and psychosocial status**
      (1) The patient's nutritional status is of prime concern when choosing therapy. **Many patients are malnourished,** either because of alcoholism or an obstructive tumor.
      (2) Treatment is sometimes delayed or limited because of the **need for hyperalimentation.** In most patients, this requirement can be met with nutritional supplements or tube feedings into the stomach, but parenteral nutrition is sometimes required.
      (3) The **family history** is critical in some head and neck tumors with inherited factors (i.e., medullary thyroid cancer)

2. **Physical examination** must include an inspection of all the skin and mucosal surfaces of the head and neck.
   a. An **intranasal examination** and **indirect mirror examination** of the nasopharynx and hypopharynx are included.
   b. Careful **palpation** of the oral cavity, base of the tongue, and oropharynx is mandatory.
   c. **Fiberoptic examination** of the nose, pharynx, and larynx is indicated in all patients who are being evaluated for head and neck cancer.

TABLE 19-1 **Basic Characteristics of Head and Neck Cancer**

Location	Most Prominent Symptom	Risk Factor	Risk of Cervical Metastases
Nose and sinus	Mass	Nickel, wood	Moderate
Nasopharynx	Neck mass; serous otitis media	Epstein-Barr virus	High
Oral cavity	Pain	Tobacco, alcohol	Moderate
Oropharynx	Dysphagia	Tobacco, alcohol	High
Larynx	Hoarseness	Tobacco	Glottic, low; supraglottic, high
Hypopharynx	Dysphagia	Tobacco, alcohol	High
Salivary glands	Mass	Radiation	High-grade, high; other, low

D **Treatment** is based on the site and pathology of the primary cancer and the extent of the local, regional, and distant disease (Fig. 19-1).

1. **Surgery** is the indicated treatment for many patients with head and neck cancer. The time for treatment is short, and careful pathologic examination of the tissue removed is possible. In addition, the effects of radiation are avoided, and radiation can be saved for recurrent disease or other primary cancers. The **choice of surgery can be influenced by many factors.**
   a. **Malnourishment** can increase the perioperative risk of morbidity and mortality.
   b. The patient may have a **coexistent systemic disease** (e.g., diabetes, chronic obstructive pulmonary disease, or coronary artery disease), which increases the surgical risk.
   c. The necessary procedures can be **disfiguring** and can leave the patient with **severe functional deficits.**
      (1) Resection of the larynx, for example, alters communication.
      (2) Surgery on the tongue, oropharynx, hypopharynx, or mandible can alter or prevent swallowing.
      (3) This type of surgery is best performed in institutions that can provide the full range of rehabilitative services.
   d. **Contraindication.** Surgery for a cure is generally contraindicated in patients with distant metastases.

2. **Radiation therapy**
   a. Radiation alone is adequate treatment for many early lesions.
      (1) It can provide a cure without the functional or cosmetic deficits associated with surgery.
      (2) It can treat multiple primary lesions simultaneously.
      (3) It can prophylactically treat regional nodes that are clinically negative.

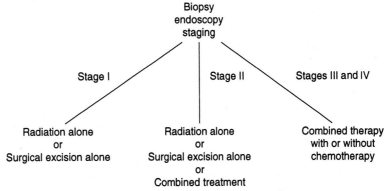

FIGURE 19-1 Basic algorithm for treatment of head and neck cancer.

b. Planned postoperative radiation can significantly increase the survival rate for patients with advanced lesions.

c. Recent studies show that the response to radiation therapy can be enhanced (even in advanced tumors) by using hyperfractionation (more than one daily treatment) and concomitant chemotherapy. These techniques increase the risk and severity of local side effects.

d. Complications of radiotherapy include mucositis, xerostomia, loss of taste, dermal and soft tissue fibrosis, dental caries, and bone and soft tissue necrosis. A dental examination is required before radiotherapy. Dental treatment during and up to 2 years after radiotherapy can be hazardous because of decreased vascularity and consequent delayed healing.

3. Chemotherapy is not curative as a single treatment modality in head and neck squamous cell carcinoma. Cisplatin is the most effective agent. It is often combined with 5-fluorouracil (5-FU), paclitaxel (Taxol), and other drugs. Methotrexate is also an effective single agent and is used primarily for palliation.

a. Chemotherapy is used in neoadjuvant treatment to reduce the tumor burden before radiation or surgery.

b. Chemotherapy is used with concomitant radiation therapy to increase response rates in advanced tumors.

c. Chemotherapy is being evaluated as adjuvant therapy to reduce recurrence rates.

d. Chemotherapy is used for palliation in patients with unresectable tumors or distant metastases.

E **Rehabilitation** should be planned at the same time as treatment.

1. Cosmetic and functional defects are reconstructed at the time of the cancer resection whenever possible. The use of **surgical flaps** (see Chapter 26, I C) has greatly facilitated reconstruction. The flaps may be:

a. Local flaps (nasolabial, forehead)

b. Distant pedicled skin flaps (deltopectoral, omocervical)

c. Pedicled myocutaneous flaps (pectoralis major, latissimus dorsi, trapezius)

d. Free microvascular flaps

2. Prosthetic rehabilitation is necessary when portions of the maxilla, orbit mandible, or palate are resected.

3. When the larynx is removed, intensive rehabilitation is required to re-establish the voice.

a. Initially, patients are taught to speak with an electrolarynx that is applied to the neck surface and positioned intraorally or incorporated within dentures.

b. Later, patients learn to speak with regurgitated air (esophageal speech) or with a prosthesis (a one-way valve) placed in a surgically created tracheoesophageal fistula.

4. Many patients who undergo partial laryngectomy, pharyngectomy, or glossectomy require training to facilitate swallowing and to avoid aspiration.

II   CANCER OF THE NECK

A **Anatomy**

1. Divisions. The neck is divided into anterior and posterior triangles.

a. The **anterior triangle** is bounded by the midline of the neck, the inferior border of the mandible, and the anterior border of the sternocleidomastoid muscle. It can be subdivided further into submandibular, submental, superior carotid, and inferior carotid triangles.

b. The **posterior triangle** is bounded by the posterior border of the sternocleidomastoid muscle, the anterior border of the trapezius, and the clavicle. It is divided further into supraclavicular and occipital triangles.

2. Lymphatic drainage

a. Fascial planes of the neck enclose the lymphatic system.

(1) The **superficial fascia** is subcutaneous and envelops the platysma.

(2) The **deep fascia** has three parts:

(a) Superficial layer, which invests the sternocleidomastoid and trapezius muscles

        (b) Pretracheal fascia (middle)

        (c) Prevertebral fascia (deep)

    b. There are approximately 75 **lymph nodes** on each side of the neck.

      (1) Most lie within the deep jugular and spinal accessory chains.

      (2) The jugular chain is divided into superior, middle, and inferior groups.

      (3) Cervical lymph node levels:

        (a) **Level 1** contains the submental and submandibular nodes.

        (b) **Level 2** is the upper third of the jugular nodes medial to the sternocleidomastoid muscle, and its inferior boundary is the plane of the hyoid bone (clinical) or the bifurcation of the carotid artery (surgical).

        (c) **Level 3** describes the middle jugular nodes and is bounded inferiorly by the plane of the cricoid cartilage (clinical) or the omohyoid (surgical).

        (d) **Level 4** is defined superiorly by the omohyoid muscle and inferiorly by the clavicle.

        (e) **Level 5** contains the posterior cervical triangle nodes.

        (f) **Level 6** contains the paratracheal and pretracheal nodes.

B **Evaluation of a neck mass** A workup for malignancy should be undertaken in all adults with a persistent neck mass.

    1. **History and physical examination.** A careful history is taken, and the head and neck are examined for evidence of a possible primary cancer (see I C).

    2. **Diagnosis.** If the primary cancer is not identified on the initial examination, the **workup** that follows should include:

      a. A chest x-ray, barium swallow, and computed tomography (CT) scan of the neck are indicated in most patients. Magnetic resonance imaging (MRI) of the neck and other x-ray or nuclear medicine studies are guided by findings on the history and physical examination.

      b. MRI is particularly useful in defining deeply invasive tumors of the tongue, pharynx, and larynx.

      c. CT of the sinuses can be used to search for primary tumors. CT or MRI of the chest and abdomen are often used for staging.

      d. Panendoscopy (direct laryngoscopy, esophagoscopy, bronchoscopy, and nasopharyngoscopy)

      e. If the result of the endoscopic survey is negative, random **biopsies** of the nasopharynx (right, middle, and left) are performed. A random biopsy of the tongue base or a tonsillectomy may also be worthwhile.

      f. If all biopsies have negative results, the next step is to proceed with open neck biopsy and frozen section.

C **Staging of metastatic neck disease**

    1. **Stage N0:** No clinically positive node

    2. **Stage N1:** A single clinically positive node homolateral to the primary tumor and 3 cm or less in its greatest diameter

    3. **Stage N2a:** A single clinically positive homolateral node larger than 3 cm but less than 6 cm in its greatest diameter

    4. **Stage N2b:** Multiple clinically positive homolateral nodes, with none larger than 6 cm in its greatest diameter

    5. **Stage N2c:** Bilateral or contralateral clinically positive nodes, with none larger than 6 cm in its greatest diameter

    6. **Stage N3:** Any node greater than 6 cm in greatest diameter

D **Treatment** If a primary cancer is identified and confirmed with biopsy, the metastatic neck disease is treated in conjunction with this primary cancer.

    1. **Types of neck dissection** (Fig. 19-2)

      a. **Radical neck dissection** is an en bloc dissection of the cervical lymphatics.

        (1) It includes removal of the sternocleidomastoid muscle, internal jugular vein, or spinal accessory nerve.

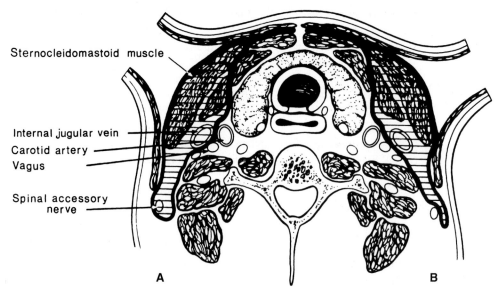

Sternocleidomastoid muscle

Internal jugular vein
Carotid artery
Vagus

Spinal accessory
nerve

A   B

FIGURE 19-2 Types of neck dissection, including traditional neck dissection and various levels of modification. In a radical neck dissection **(A)**, the sternocleidomastoid muscle, internal jugular vein, and spinal accessory nerve are removed. In the most conservative modification **(B)**, only the fascial compartment with the lymphatic tissue is removed, and all of the structures are spared.

      (2) It is performed when squamous cell carcinoma is found in a neck mass with an unknown primary cancer or in conjunction with excision of the primary tumor.

    b. Modified (functional, conservative) neck dissection removes the cervical lymphatics within their fascial compartments.

      (1) It spares the sternocleidomastoid muscle, internal jugular vein, and spinal accessory nerve.

      (2) Indications include:

        (a) Elective neck dissections

        (b) A single node less than 3 cm in diameter that is to be treated postoperatively with radiation

        (c) Differentiated thyroid cancers with neck metastases

        (d) Simultaneous bilateral neck dissections

    c. Segmental neck dissection refers to removal of less than all five nodal groups on one side of the neck (e.g., submandibular triangle dissection, supraomohyoid dissection)

  2. Elective neck dissection refers to surgical treatment of **N0** disease.

    a. There is controversy about when and whether to use elective neck dissection, because radiation therapy can provide prophylaxis for metastatic neck disease in many cases.

    b. The choice between surgery and radiation usually depends on the treatment of the primary tumor.

    c. In general, when elective neck dissection is performed, it is done for a primary cancer that has a 30% or greater chance of occult metastasis.

III CANCER OF THE NASAL CAVITY AND PARANASAL SINUSES

A Anatomy

  1. Basic structure

    a. All sinuses are paired, and all are contiguous with the nasal cavity through their natural ostia.

    b. The nose and sinuses are lined with a respiratory mucosa, which is pseudostratified columnar with goblet cells and cilia.

  2. Lymphatic drainage is to the parapharyngeal or retropharyngeal nodes. Secondary lymphatics are the subdigastric nodes of the internal jugular chain.

B Classification

  1. Location. Most tumors (59%) are in the maxillary sinus, 24% are in the nasal cavity, 16% in the ethmoid sinuses, and 1% in the frontal and sphenoid sinuses.

2. Approximately 80% of the malignancies are **squamous cell carcinoma.**

3. Tumors that arise anteriorly tend to be well differentiated.

4. Tumors arising from the posterior nasal cavity and ethmoids are generally poorly differentiated.

5. Nasal and sinus cancers are locally invasive. Nodal metastases are unusual and tend to occur late, even with extensive local disease.

6. Approximately 10%–14% of the malignancies are **adenocarcinomas,** including adenoid cystic carcinoma.

7. **Inverted papilloma** is a benign tumor (see Chapter 18, IV B 2 c [2] [b]). The reported incidence of malignant degeneration is approximately 2%. The incidence of associated malignancy in adjacent tissue is as high as 15%.

C **Clinical evaluation**

1. **Presenting symptoms** can include nasal obstruction; epistaxis; localized pain; tooth pain; cranial nerve deficits; a mass in the face, palate, or maxillary alveolus; proptosis; and trismus.

2. **Diagnosis.** The **extent of the disease** is determined by physical examination and radiographic studies.
   a. A CT scan is useful for identifying bony erosions and orbital or intracranial extension.
   b. MRI can be used to determine intraorbital and intracranial invasion.
   c. Arteriography is useful in patients with skull base invasion or rare vascular tumors.
   d. Most biopsies can be performed under local anesthesia.

D **Staging** is available for maxillary sinus cancer.

1. **Stage TX:** Cannot be assessed

2. **Stage T0:** No evidence of a primary cancer

3. **Stage T1:** Tumor confined to the inferior antrum without bone erosion

4. **Stage T2:** Tumor confined to the superior antrum without bone erosion of the inferior or medial walls

5. **Stage T3:** Extensive tumor involving the skin of the cheek, the orbit, the anterior ethmoids, or the pterygoid muscles

6. **Stage T4:** Massive tumor involving the cribriform plate, posterior ethmoids, sphenoid, nasopharynx, pterygoid plates, or base of the skull

E **Treatment**

1. **Maxillary sinus cancer**
   a. **Stage T1 and T2 tumors** are treated with subtotal or radical maxillectomy. Radiation is used when cancer may have been left at the surgical margins and when tumors recur.
   b. **Stage T3 and T4 tumors** receive radiotherapy followed by re-evaluation for surgical resection. Orbital exenteration and skin resection are performed when necessary.

2. **Ethmoid sinus or nasal cavity tumors** are usually treated with radiation therapy followed by surgery for residual disease.

3. **Extensive cancers** are treated with combined craniofacial resection for selected patients. Chemotherapy is often utilized either in conjunction with surgery and radiation or for palliation.

4. **Inverted papillomas** are treated by en bloc resection that includes the lateral nasal wall and ethmoid sinus.

5. **Cervical lymph node metastases** are treated with radiotherapy followed by radical neck dissection for residual disease.

F **Prognosis**

1. The overall cure rate is approximately 30%–35%.

2. The 5-year survival rate for patients with stage T1 and T2 lesions is 70%.

3. The 5-year survival rate for patients with stage T3 and T4 lesions is 15%–20%.

IV   CANCER OF THE NASOPHARYNX

A **Anatomy**

1. **Basic structure.** The nasopharynx is the most cephalad portion of the pharynx.
   a. Its **roof** is formed by the basioccipital and sphenoid bones, and its **posterior wall** is formed by the atlas.
      (1) These walls are covered by mucosa, and the adenoid tissue is embedded within.
      (2) The lateral wall contains the orifice of the eustachian tube, and, just posterior to that, the fossa of Rosenmüller.
   b. The choanae define the **anterior limit,** and the free edge of the soft palate provides the **inferior limit.**
2. **Lymphatic drainage** is to the lateral retropharyngeal, jugulodigastric (tonsillar), and high spinal accessory nodes.

B **Epidemiology and classification**

1. Nasopharyngeal cancer has a high incidence among people from the Kwan Tung province of China.
2. Elevated Epstein-Barr virus titer has a high incidence among persons with cancer of the nasopharynx.
3. Nasopharyngeal cancer occurs at younger ages than do most solid head and neck tumors.
4. Approximately 85% of nasopharyngeal tumors are epithelial: 7.5% are lymphomas. Epithelial tumors commonly arise in the fossa of Rosenmüller.

C **Clinical evaluation**

1. **Presenting symptoms** are anterior or posterior epistaxis, cervical adenopathy, serous otitis media, and nasal obstruction. Headache, diplopia, facial numbness, trismus, ptosis, and hoarseness may also be present. At presentation, 60%–70% of patients will have nodal disease, and 38% will have cranial nerve involvement.
2. **Diagnosis**
   a. Diagnosis is confirmed by endoscopic biopsy or by biopsy of a metastatic lymph node.
   b. Nasopharyngeal cancer can best be staged and monitored with CT and MRI.
   c. When a patient presents with an elevated Epstein-Barr virus titer, monitoring of the titer should show a decrease with successful treatment and an increase with recurrences.

D **Staging**

1. **Stage TIS:** Carcinoma in situ
2. **Stage T1:** Tumor confined to the nasopharynx
3. **Stage T2:** Tumor extends to the oropharynx or nasal cavity
4. **Stage T2a:** Tumor with no parapharyngeal extension
5. **Stage T2b:** Tumor with a parapharyngeal extension
6. **Stage T3:** Tumor invades bone or paranasal sinuses
7. **Stage T4:** Tumor with intracranial extension or involvement of cranial nerves, infratemporal fossa, hypopharynx, or orbit

E **Treatment**

1. Radiation is the primary treatment for all epithelial nasopharyngeal tumors. The dose (usually 65–75 gy) is delivered to the nasopharynx and to both sides of the neck. Improved responses are possible with combined chemotherapy and radiation in patients who can tolerate the increased toxicity.
2. Radical neck dissection is performed for residual nodes if the primary tumor is controlled.

F **Prognosis**   The 5-year survival rate is 40% in patients without positive nodes and 20% in patients with positive nodes.

V   **CANCER OF THE ORAL CAVITY**

A   Anatomy

1. **Basic structure.** The oral cavity extends from the lip anteriorly to the faucial arches posteriorly. It includes the lips, buccal mucosa, gingivae, retromolar trigones, hard palate, anterior two thirds of the tongue (the oral tongue), and floor of the mouth.

2. **Lymphatic drainage** is to the submental, submandibular, and deep jugular nodes.

B   Etiology

1. Approximately 90% of patients are heavy users of tobacco (either smoking or chewing).

2. Approximately 80% of patients are heavy drinkers.

3. Syphilis accounts for a few cases.

4. Herpes simplex virus type 1 is currently under investigation as a cause.

C   Clinical evaluation

1. **Presenting symptoms** can include loose teeth, painful or nonhealing ulcers, odynophagia, otalgia (with posterior lesions), and cervical adenopathy. The lip is the most common site of oral cavity carcinoma, followed by the oral tongue and floor of the mouth.

2. **Diagnosis**
   a. **Mandibular radiographs** should be taken to assess the bony involvement by adjacent tumors.
   b. **Pain,** which is often a late symptom, occurs after ulceration develops.
   c. **Nodal metastases** (up to 30% of which are occult, microscopic metastatic disease) are found in 50% of patients with squamous cell carcinoma of the anterior tongue and in 58% of patients with cancer of the floor of the mouth (occult metastases in up to 12% of the patients).
   d. **Metastases** are uncommon and usually occur late in cancer of the lip or the buccal mucosa.

D   Staging

1. **Stage T1:** Tumor less than 2 cm in its greatest diameter

2. **Stage T2:** Tumor 2–4 cm in its greatest diameter

3. **Stage T3:** Tumor more than 4 cm in its greatest diameter

4. **Stage T4:** Massive tumor that involves the mandible, pterygoid muscles, antrum, root of the tongue, or skin

E   Treatment

1. **Stage T1, N0 tumors** can be treated with either local excision or radiotherapy.

2. **Stage T2 or larger lesions** should be treated with combined surgery and radiation.
   a. **Surgery** involves an **en bloc resection** of the tumor and radical neck dissection.
   b. Either a **partial mandibulectomy** is included or the tumor is "pulled through" medially to the mandible into the neck (i.e., the tumor is removed en bloc with the radical neck specimen, leaving the mandible intact).

3. **Tumors attached to the mandible** may be removed with a partial thickness of mandible (i.e., the lingual plate or alveolar process). The mandibular arch is kept intact when possible.

4. **Tumors demonstrating bony erosion in the mandible** are removed with a full-thickness portion of bone.

F   Prognosis

1. The **overall 5-year survival rate** for cancer of all oral cavity sites is approximately **65%.**

2. For **lip cancer,** 5-year survival rates as high as **90%** have been reported.

3. The prognosis for **tongue lesions** is worse if the lesion is posterior. Because anterior (mobile) tongue lesions are often diagnosed when they are small, the overall 5-year survival rate is higher

than 65%. Posterior (tongue base) lesions are often stage III or stage IV at diagnosis, and the overall 5-year survival rate is less than 40%. Posterior lesions involving the tongue base can invade the pre-epiglottic space, necessitating laryngectomy.

VI CANCER OF THE OROPHARYNX

A Anatomy

1. Basic structure
   a. **Boundaries.** The oropharynx is bounded by the free edge of the soft palate superiorly, the tip of the epiglottis inferiorly, and the anterior tonsillar pillar anteriorly.
   b. **Contents.** The oropharynx contains the soft palate, tonsillar fossae and faucial tonsils, lateral and posterior pharyngeal walls, and base of the tongue.
   c. The **parapharyngeal space** is directly lateral to the oropharynx.
      (1) It contains the glossopharyngeal, lingual, and inferior alveolar nerves; pterygoid muscles; internal maxillary artery; and carotid sheath.
      (2) It is a site of early extension of an oropharyngeal tumor.
      (3) It also provides a pathway for the tumor to spread to the base of the skull.

2. **Lymphatic drainage** is primarily to the jugulodigastric (tonsillar) nodes.
   a. Tumors of the soft palate, lateral wall, and tongue base also spread to the retropharyngeal and parapharyngeal nodes.
   b. Retromolar trigone lesions can drain to submaxillary nodes.

B Etiology

1. **Alcohol and tobacco use** are commonly found together in patients with oropharyngeal cancer. There appears to be a synergistic effect between the two substances, but it has not been defined.

2. **Local mucosal irritation, malnutrition, and immune defects** have also been implicated.

C Clinical evaluation

1. **Presenting symptoms**
   a. The most common presenting symptom is a **persistent sore throat.**
   b. This symptom is frequently accompanied by ipsilateral otalgia (referred pain via the tympanic branch of the glossopharyngeal nerve).
   c. A vague sensation of throat irritation, restriction of tongue motion ("hot potato voice"), odynophagia, and bleeding may also be noted.
   d. Most patients (especially those with large lesions) are significantly malnourished.
   e. Many patients present with **cervical adenopathy.** Nodal metastases are found in 76% of patients with cancer of the base of the tongue and in 60% of patients with tonsillar cancer. Most of these nodes are palpable.

2. **Initial examination** must include careful palpation of the tonsils and base of the tongue. Many small tumors are difficult to see but may be palpated easily.

3. **Diagnosis** is often made late in the course.
   a. Many patients are asymptomatic until tumors are quite large and ulcerated.
   b. Other patients are treated conservatively for incorrectly diagnosed lesions.
   c. All lesions should be evaluated by endoscopy under general anesthesia before treatment is chosen.
   d. CT and MRI are useful in determining tumor extension

D Staging (Table 19-2)

1. **Stage TIS:** Carcinoma in situ

2. **Stage T1:** Lesion 2 cm or less in its greatest diameter

3. **Stage T2:** Lesion larger than 2 cm but less than 4 cm in its greatest diameter

4. **Stage T3:** Lesion larger than 4 cm in its greatest diameter

5. **Stage T4:** Lesion larger than 4 cm, with invasion of bone or soft tissues of the neck or the root of the tongue

TABLE 19-2   International College of Surgeons Staging of Oropharyngeal Cancer

Stage	T	N	M
I	T1	N0	M0
II	T2	N0	M0
III	T3	N0	M0
	T4	N0	M0
	Any T	N1	M0
	Any T	N2	M0
IV	Any T	N3	M0
	Any T	Any N	M1

T, tumor; N, nodes; M, metastases.

E Treatment

1. **T1 and T2 lesions** are treated with radiotherapy.

2. **Combined therapy** offers improved survival rates for most large lesions and is indicated when nodal metastasis is present.

3. **Composite resection** (the jaw-neck or commando procedure) is most commonly used to resect T3 and T4 lesions of the oropharynx Fig. 19-3).
   a. It involves a radical neck dissection and a partial mandibulectomy in conjunction with excision of the tumor.
   b. A tracheotomy is routine treatment.
   c. Occasionally, the larynx is spared after total glossectomy in young and otherwise healthy patients. A laryngectomy is performed when either:
      (1) The tumor invades the pre-epiglottic space
      (2) The entire tongue base and both hypoglossal nerves are removed

F Prognosis   The poor prognosis of oropharyngeal cancers is directly related to their late diagnosis.

1. In **tonsillar cancers,** 5-year survival rates range from 63% for patients with T1 tumors to 21% for those with T4 disease.

2. Patients with **tumors of the base of the tongue** have 5-year survival rates of 40%–60% for T1 disease and 10%–20% for T4 disease. A high incidence of late presentation is reflected in the large number of patients with T4 disease.

3. For patients with **tumors of the palatal arch,** the 5-year survival rates range from 77% for T1 disease to 20% for T4 disease.

4. The presence of nodal metastases reduces the 5-year survival rate significantly: For N0, the survival rate is 75%; for N1, 25%.

VII   CANCER OF THE HYPOPHARYNX AND CERVICAL ESOPHAGUS

A Anatomy

1. **Basic structure**
   a. **Boundaries.** The hypopharynx extends from the pharyngoepiglottic fold to the inferior border of the cricoid area, excluding the larynx.
   b. **Contents.** It includes the piriform sinuses, the postcricoid area, and the posterior pharyngeal wall.

2. **Lymphatic drainage.** The hypopharynx has a rich lymphatic network.
   a. The **piriform sinuses** drain to jugulocarotid and midjugular nodes.
   b. The **posterior pharyngeal wall** drains primarily to retropharyngeal nodes.
   c. **Lower hypopharyngeal areas** drain to paratracheal and low jugular nodes.
   d. The **cervical esophagus** is drained by mediastinal nodes.

A

B

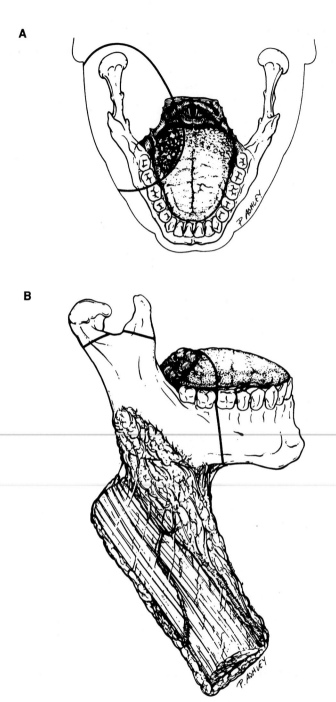

FIGURE 19-3 **A:** Level of resection in an en bloc composite resection of the oral cavity, oropharynx, or both (the classic commando procedure). **B:** The specimen includes the primary cancer, a segmental mandibulectomy, and the radical neck dissection.

B **Classification and etiology**

1. Ninety-five percent of the tumors in this region are **epithelial cancers.**

2. Approximately 60%–75% arise in the piriform sinuses and 20%–25% on the posterior pharyngeal wall; tumors rarely arise in the postcricoid area.

3. As with other head and neck tumors, the tumors are related to **heavy use of alcohol and tobacco.**

C **Clinical evaluation**

1. **Presenting symptoms.** The triad of throat pain, referred otalgia, and dysphagia is present in more than 50% of patients.

2. **Hoarseness and airway obstruction** indicate laryngeal involvement.

3. Small postcricoid tumors often present with mild symptoms of sore throat, a "lump in the throat," and throat clearing.

4. **Cervical lymph node metastases** (41% occult) are found in 75% of patients with piriform sinus cancers and in 83% of patients with pharyngeal wall tumors (66% occult).

5. **Diagnosis.** A barium swallow and endoscopy with biopsy complete the workup.

D **Staging**

1. **Stage TIS:** Carcinoma in situ

2. **Stage T1:** Carcinoma confined to one subsite of the hypopharynx and 2 cm or less in greatest diameter

3. **Stage T2:** Tumor extends to an additional subsite of the hypopharynx or to an adjacent site without fixation of the hemilarynx (vocal fold) or measures more than 2 cm but less than 4 cm in greatest diameter

4. **Stage T3:** Tumor measures more than 4 cm in greatest diameter or with fixation of the hemilarynx

5. **Stage T4:** Massive tumor, with invasion of bone, cartilage, or the soft tissues of the neck

E **Treatment**

1. **Laryngopharyngectomy and radical neck dissection followed by radiotherapy** are necessary for most T3 and T4 lesions.

2. If the tumor is **T1 or T2** and spares the apex of the piriform sinus, a supraglottic laryngectomy can be considered.

3. Some **small T1 tumors** can be treated by radiation therapy alone or by surgical resection via a lateral pharyngotomy.

4. **Cancers of the cervical esophagus** can require removal of the pharynx, esophagus, and larynx.

5. **Reconstruction of circumferential defects of the hypopharynx and cervical esophagus can be accomplished by multiple methods.** The ideal procedure to reconstruct swallowing function and to reduce operative morbidity is chosen on an **individual basis.** The following types of reconstruction are available for consideration:
   a. **Regional skin flaps,** such as deltopectoral or cervical (requires multiple stages)
   b. **Pedicled myocutaneous flaps** (pectoralis major, latissimus dorsi)
   c. **Esophagectomy,** followed by gastric "pull-up" (raising the stomach into the chest or neck to replace the esophagus)
   d. **Colon interposition**
   e. A **free intestinal graft or soft tissue flap** with microvascular anastomosis (Fig. 19-4)

F **Prognosis** is poor because of extensive submucosal spread and the high incidence of cervical metastasis.

1. The **overall 5-year survival rate** is approximately 30% for patients with hypopharyngeal tumors.

2. The 5-year survival rate rises to 50% for those who qualify for supraglottic laryngectomy.

3. Chemotherapy is used with radiation therapy in organ-sparing protocols.

VIII **CANCER OF THE LARYNX**

A **Anatomy**

1. **Divisions.** The larynx is divided into three regions.
   a. The **supraglottis** extends from the tip of the epiglottis to include the false vocal folds and roof of the ventricle.

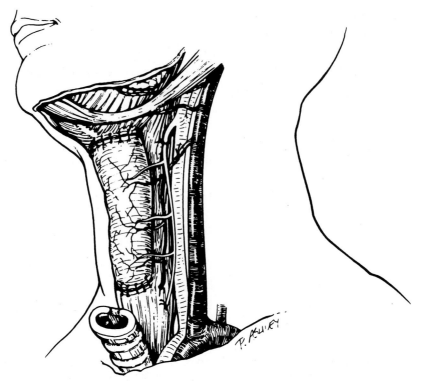

FIGURE 19-4   Reconstruction of a circumferential pharyngeal defect with a jejunal free graft. The vascular pedicle has been anastomosed to branches of the external carotid artery and internal jugular vein.

  b. The **glottis** extends from the depth of the ventricle to 1 cm below the free edge of the true vocal fold.
  c. The **subglottis** extends from 1 cm below the free edge of the true vocal fold to the inferior border of the cricoid cartilage.
 2. Lymphatic drainage
  a. The **supraglottis** has a rich network that crosses the midline and drains to the deep jugular nodes.
  b. The **glottis** has poorly developed, sparse lymphatics.
  c. The **subglottis** drains through the cricothyroid membrane to the prelaryngeal (delphian) and pretracheal nodes.

B **Etiology**
 1. More than 90% of patients have a significant history of **smoking.**
 2. Heavy **alcohol** consumption is a common but not definite etiologic factor.

C **Classification**
 1. Squamous cell carcinomas account for 95%–98% of the tumors.
 2. Verrucous carcinoma is a variant of squamous cell carcinoma that is locally invasive but almost never metastasizes. It can undergo malignant transformation to a more aggressive malignancy, especially after radiotherapy.

D **Clinical evaluation**
 1. Presenting symptoms
  a. The most common symptom is hoarseness.
  b. Stridor, cough, hemoptysis, dysphagia, and aspiration also occur.
  c. Neck masses are uncommon at the time of presentation in glottic tumors.
 2. Diagnosis
  a. All patients require direct laryngoscopy and biopsy.
  b. Laryngograms, a barium swallow, stroboscopic laryngoscopy, and CT scan may be helpful.

E **Staging**

1. **Stage TIS:** Carcinoma in situ
2. **Stage T1:** Tumor confined to the site of origin
3. **Stage T2:** Tumor has spread to an adjacent laryngeal site or has impaired vocal fold mobility
4. **Stage T3:** Tumor confined to the larynx, with fixation of the hemilarynx
5. **Stage T4:** Tumor has destroyed cartilage or extends beyond the larynx

F **Treatment**

1. **Carcinoma in situ** is treated by **excision of the involved vocal fold mucosa** and is then monitored closely.
2. Most **T1 lesions** are treated with **radiation** because the resultant voice is usually of better quality than the one after surgical excision (at least initially). However, surgery is still indicated for many patients, and long-term results on the voice after radiation and surgery have not been studied adequately.
   a. **Removal of the involved vocal fold** by traditional techniques or by carbon dioxide laser yields equivalent local control.
   b. Some glottic lesions that involve the **anterior commissure** may be treated by **hemilaryngectomy** (vertical laryngectomy) because of the increased risk of cartilage involvement.
   c. Some **small lesions** of the tip of the epiglottis can also be treated with **limited surgical resection.**
3. **Large supraglottic tumors** are treated with a **supraglottic (horizontal) laryngectomy.** This procedure **spares the true vocal folds** but removes the epiglottis, aryepiglottic folds, and false vocal folds.
4. For **transglottic tumors** (supraglottic tumors that spread to a true vocal fold), a **suprahemilaryngectomy** may be considered. Radical neck dissection, radiation, or both are often necessary because nodal metastases (30% of which are occult) are found in 55% of supraglottic cancers.
5. **T3 and T4 lesions** usually require a **total laryngectomy,** often combined with radical neck dissection. Postoperative radiotherapy is usually indicated (Fig. 19-5).
6. **Verrucous carcinoma** is treated surgically by using a conservation laryngectomy, when possible. There is no need for elective radical neck dissection, and radiotherapy has been implicated as one cause of anaplastic transformation.
7. Current **adjuvant chemotherapy protocols** achieve cure rates comparable to those for traditional combined therapy and allow some patients to avoid total laryngectomy. Figure 19-6 shows a protocol example.

G **Prognosis** is better for patients with laryngeal cancer than with cancer of other head and neck sites. Five-year survival rates by stage are as follows:

1. **Stage T1:** 85%–90% with surgery or radiation
2. **Stage T2:** 80%–85%
3. **Stage T3:** 75%
4. **Stage T4:** 30%

IX **CANCER OF THE EAR**

A **Anatomy**

1. **Basic structure.** The **tympanic membrane** separates the external canal from the middle ear. The portions of the ear most susceptible to tumors include the external ear (pinna), external auditory canal, and middle ear. The mastoid and other parts of the temporal bone may also be involved.
2. **Lymphatic drainage** of the external ear and canal is anterior through the parotid, posterior to the mastoid nodes, and deep to the jugulodigastric nodes.

A

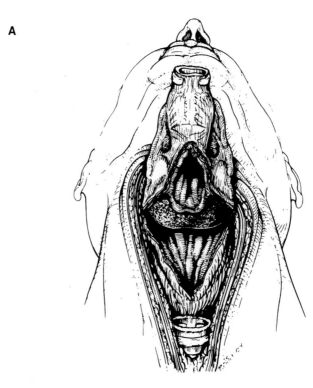

B

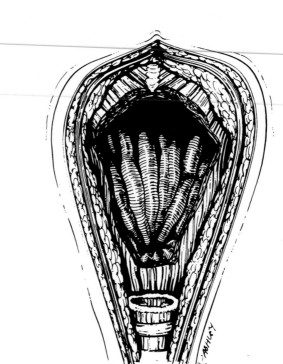

FIGURE 19-5 **A:** Total laryngectomy specimen ready for removal, attached only to the tongue base. **B:** Pharyngeal defect following total laryngectomy. Closure is usually accomplished in layers in a T fashion.

B **Classification and etiology**   Cancer of the ear is rare.

1. The **etiology** has been related to thermal burns, chronic suppurative infection, and exposure to radium. Cancer of the pinna may come from actinic radiation.

2. Approximately 86% are **epithelial cancers.** Basal cell carcinomas comprise 8%; melanoma and adenocarcinoma comprise 2% each; and rhabdomyosarcoma and spindle cell sarcoma comprise 1% each. Other malignancies, such as osteogenic sarcoma, are rare.

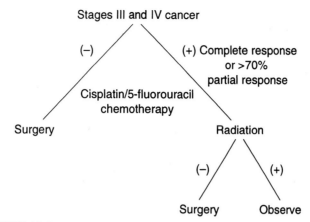

FIGURE 19-6 Example of organ-sparing neoadjuvant chemotherapy protocol.

3. Approximately 80% of ear cancers arise on the **auricle,** 15% in the external canal, and 5% in the middle ear.

4. **Lytic lesions** deep in the temporal bone should be worked up as possible metastases and may be from an adenocarcinoma, hypernephroma, melanoma, or other primary tumor.

C **Clinical evaluation**

1. **Presenting symptoms**
   a. Most ear tumors present as an infected, painful, chronically draining ear.
   b. If a mass is present in the external canal, it is usually friable.
   c. Vertigo and facial paralysis are ominous signs.

2. **Diagnosis**
   a. **Biopsy.** When cancer is suspected, the mass is biopsied under controlled conditions. Significant hemorrhage may occur.
   b. **CT and MRI scanning** are necessary in most cases to evaluate the extent of tumor invasion.

D **Treatment**

1. Cancers of the auricle can usually be treated with **wedge excision.**

2. In deeper, more advanced cancers, **radical surgery** provides the best chance for a cure.
   a. Tumors of the canal that are at least 5 mm lateral to the eardrum can be treated by **excision of the external canal.**
   b. Cancers that impinge on the tympanic membrane without middle ear invasion are treated with **partial (lateral) temporal bone resection.** This procedure removes the external canal, eardrum, incus, and malleus, while sparing the facial nerve.
   c. Cancers that involve the middle ear or pneumatized spaces are probably treated best by **total en bloc temporal bone resection.**

3. **Radiation therapy** has not produced satisfactory cure rates and is used best to treat recurrent or residual disease.

4. **Combined therapy** may be indicated in some cases.

E **Prognosis** Results are difficult to evaluate because of the small number of cases reported.

1. For patients requiring temporal bone resection, 5-year survival rates range from 25%–35%. However, many of these operations have transgressed the tumor, leaving gross tumor behind. The newly described en bloc procedure should improve these statistics.

2. For lesions confined to the pinna, an 80% cure rate can be expected after treatment.

X **CANCER OF THE SKIN** (see Chapter 26, II C–F)

Cancers of the skin account for 25% of all cancers, and squamous cell carcinomas account for 30%.

A **Basal and squamous cell carcinomas** Basal cell carcinoma accounts for 60% of skin cancers, and squamous cell carcinoma accounts for 30%.

1. **Etiology**
   a. Sunlight
   b. Radiation
   c. Arsenic
   d. Burns, scars
   e. Genetic disorders (xeroderma pigmentosum, basal cell nevus syndrome, albinism)

2. **Clinical evaluation**
   a. Skin cancers usually present as slowly enlarging cutaneous or subcutaneous lesions. Some lesions form nonhealing ulcers.
   b. Nodal metastasis is uncommon.

3. **Treatment.** Therapy includes electrodesiccation, curettage, cryosurgery, excision, Mohs' surgery, radiation, and topical fluorouracil.
   a. Surgical excision is preferred for **squamous cell carcinoma** because it allows removal of a margin.
   b. **Basal cell carcinomas** of the nasolabial folds, medial and lateral canthi, or postauricular regions are especially aggressive. They can invade multiple tissue planes and, therefore, require an extensive surgical resection.
   c. **Mohs' surgery** involves the precise mapping and frozen-section control of the entire resection bed. It is especially useful for cancers in areas known for aggressive patterns of spread and recurrence. It allows for early reconstruction because of reliable surgical margins.
   d. **Radiation therapy** is usually reserved for advanced lesions in areas where surgical excision leaves a cosmetically unacceptable defect (e.g., the nose, eyelid, lip).
      (1) Radiation should probably not be used when tumors invade bone or cartilage.
   e. All **positive nodes** should be treated with **radical neck dissection or radiotherapy.**

B **Malignant melanoma**

1. **Epidemiology**
   a. Malignant melanoma accounts for 1% of all cancers.
   b. Approximately 20%–30% of all melanomas arise in the head and neck.
   c. Melanoma occurs predominantly in whites. It commonly occurs in people between 30 and 60 years of age and is rare in children.

2. **Etiology**
   a. **Sun exposure and heredity** play important roles in the causes of melanoma.
   b. Melanomas may arise from **junctional nevi** (see Chapter 26, II D 2 a).
      (1) These nevi are usually present at birth.
      (2) Nevi that undergo malignant transformation are usually in an irritated or exposed area.
      (3) Melanomas can also arise on the mucosal surfaces of the head and neck.

3. **Pathologic variants** include:
   a. Lentigo maligna melanoma
   b. Superficial spreading melanoma
   c. Nodular melanoma

4. **Staging** is by depth of invasion.
   a. **Stage T1:** Up to 0.75 mm deep
   b. **Stage T2:** 0.76–1.5 mm
   c. **Stage T3:** 1.51–3 mm
   d. **Stage T4:** More than 3 mm

5. **Treatment** is by wide excision of the melanoma.
   a. A **radical neck dissection** is performed for positive nodes.
      (1) A **parotidectomy** is added to the radical dissection for lesions of the anterior scalp, eyelids, auricles, and cheeks because the first-level lymphatic drainage is to the periparotid nodes.
      (2) Elective radical neck dissection is usually performed on patients with T3 and T4 tumors.
   b. **Radiation therapy** is usually reserved for palliative treatment of recurrent disease.
   c. **Chemotherapy,** primarily with dacarbazine, is used for disseminated melanoma.

6. Prognosis

  a. The survival rate is related to the depth of invasion.

   (1) T1 lesions have a 5-year survival rate of 90%; T4 lesions, 10%.

   (2) N0 lesions have a 5-year survival rate of 90%; N1 and N3 lesions, 10%.

  b. The prognosis in patients with mucosal melanoma is extremely poor.

XI LYMPHOMA OF THE HEAD AND NECK

A Epidemiology

  1. Approximately 80% of all malignant lymphomas arise from nodes, many of which are in the head and neck.

  2. About 65%–70% of patients with Hodgkin's lymphoma have cervical lymph node involvement.

  3. Extranodal presentation is rare in Hodgkin's disease but occurs in 20% of patients with non-Hodgkin's lymphoma.

B Classification

  1. **Non-Hodgkin's lymphoma** is really a group of diseases, which are classified into favorable and unfavorable types on the basis of therapeutic response.

   a. **Favorable types** include:

    (1) Nodular lymphomas

    (2) Well-differentiated lymphocytic lymphoma

   b. **Unfavorable types** include:

    (1) Diffuse, poorly differentiated lymphocytic lymphoma

    (2) Diffuse histiocytic lymphoma

    (3) Diffuse undifferentiated lymphoma

    (4) Nodular histiocytic lymphoma

  2. **Hodgkin's lymphoma.** The histology of Hodgkin's disease influences the prognosis.

   a. **Favorable types:**

    (1) Lymphocyte predominant

    (2) Nodular sclerosing

   b. **Guarded type:** Mixed cellular

   c. **Unfavorable type:** Lymphocyte depleting

C Clinical evaluation

  1. **Presenting symptoms**

   a. The **usual presentation** is a single, enlarged cervical node.

    (1) The initial workup is aimed at discovering an extranodal primary lesion.

    (2) The enlarged node must be differentiated from squamous cell carcinoma.

   b. Most **lymphomatous nodes** are firm and rubbery.

    (1) Non-Hodgkin's lymphoma typically presents in upper cervical nodes.

    (2) Hodgkin's disease is discovered in nodes throughout the cervical chain.

   c. The most common **sites of extranodal involvement** in non-Hodgkin's lymphoma are in the head and neck, particularly in Waldeyer's tonsillar ring. Other sites include the nasal cavity, paranasal sinuses, orbit, and salivary glands.

   d. Approximately 40% of patients with Hodgkin's lymphoma have **systemic symptoms** of fever, sweats, weight loss, and malaise.

  2. **Diagnosis** is usually made by **excisional biopsy of a lymph node.**

   a. If a possible extranodal source has been discovered, it should be biopsied first.

   b. **Endoscopy should always precede lymph node biopsy** to rule out a primary epithelial tumor.

   c. For a node biopsy, one of the largest nodes should be removed in its entirety.

   d. **Frozen-section diagnosis is of little value** except to exclude squamous cell carcinoma.

D **Staging** is aimed at determining the extent of spread of the lymphoma.

  1. **Further tests.** After the diagnosis is made, all patients undergo a chest radiograph, CT scan of the abdomen, and bone marrow biopsy.

    a. A CT scan of the chest, intravenous pyelography, and lymphangiography are sometimes added, depending on the initial findings.

    b. All patients with non-Hodgkin's lymphoma require staging radiologic studies of the abdomen, usually by CT or MRI.

    c. **Staging laparotomy** is often necessary for patients with an early stage of lymphoma when treatment with radiotherapy alone is contemplated. Laparoscopy can be substituted when patients also receive chemotherapy.

  2. **Stages** are as follows:

    a. **Stage I:** Involvement of a single lymph node region or a single extralymphatic site

    b. **Stage II:** Either of the following:

      (1) Involvement of two or more lymph node regions on the same side of the diaphragm

      (2) Localized involvement of an extranodal site and one or more lymph node regions on the same side of the diaphragm

    c. **Stage III:** Involvement of lymph node regions or extranodal sites on both sides of the diaphragm

    d. **Stage IV:** Diffuse or disseminated involvement of one or more distant extranodal organs

E **Treatment**

  1. Patients with **stage I or II Hodgkin's disease** can be treated with radiotherapy alone.

  2. Patients with **more advanced stages** are treated with **MOPP** (mechlorethamine, vincristine [Oncovin], procarbazine, and prednisone) **chemotherapy,** usually combined with nodal irradiation.

  3. Treatment of **non-Hodgkin's lymphoma** is much less clear-cut.

    a. In general, early stages (I and II) are treated with radiotherapy, and later stages (III and IV) are treated with chemotherapy.

    b. Combined treatment with radiation and chemotherapy is usually used for advanced unfavorable lesions.

F **Prognosis**

  1. **Hodgkin's disease**

    a. **Favorable prognostic factors** include:

      (1) Localized disease

      (2) A limited number of anatomic sites

      (3) Absence of massive disease

      (4) A favorable histology (lymphocyte predominant and nodular sclerosing)

    b. **Survival rates**

      (1) **Stages I and II** have 5-year, relapse-free rates of 80%–90%. The rate falls to 60%–80% in patients with advanced disease (stage III) treated with combined therapy.

      (2) Rates as low as 30% have been reported in **stage IV** lesions.

  2. **Non-Hodgkin's lymphoma**

    a. Radiation therapy for patients with stage I and II lesions yields 50%–70% cure rates.

    b. With more advanced lesions, patients with a favorable histology can have a 60%–70% 5-year survival rate and a 30% cure rate.

    c. Patients with an unfavorable histology face a 24%–40% 5-year survival rate with little chance for a cure.

XII   **UNUSUAL TUMORS**

A **Chemodectomas (paragangliomas)** arise from chemoreceptor tissue.

  1. They are **rarely malignant** (2%–6% are malignant), but they have a propensity for extensive local invasion.

  2. Paragangliomas are **often multicentric and associated with other malignancies.**

  3. **Location.** They are found in the carotid body, ganglion nodosum of the vagus nerve, aortic arch, and jugular bulb, and they are also found within the middle ear, orbit, nose, nasopharynx, or larynx. Morbidity and mortality depend on the type and extent of the tumor.

    a. Carotid body tumors usually present as slow-growing, painless neck masses.

      (1) Characteristics

        (a) Approximately 3% are bilateral. This tumor increases to 26% in patients with a familial tendency for paragangliomas.

        (b) Large tumors can cause dysphagia, airway obstruction, and cranial nerve palsies.

        (c) The mass may be pulsatile and may have a bruit.

      (2) Diagnosis is by **angiography,** which shows a tumor blush at the carotid bifurcation that splays the internal and external carotids.

      (3) Treatment is by surgical excision. Large tumors may require carotid bypass.

    b. Glomus jugulare and glomus tympanicum tumors

      (1) Characteristics

        (a) Glomus jugulare tumors arise in the jugular bulb. They can invade the middle ear, labyrinth, and cranium. They commonly affect multiple cranial nerves (CNs), especially CN VII, CN IX, CN X, CN XI, and CN XII.

        (b) Glomus tympanicum tumors arise in the middle ear, along the tympanic nerve. Most patients have pulsatile tinnitus and present with an aural "polyp" or a middle ear mass that can be seen with pneumatic pressure on the tympanic membrane. Hearing loss and vertigo are common.

        (c) Other rare sites of glomus tumor formation are along the vagus nerve in the neck (**glomus vagale**) and in the larynx.

        (d) Glomus tumors present predominantly in the fifth decade of life or later and occur rarely in children.

      (2) Evaluation includes angiography, retrograde jugular venography, and CT scan. Biopsy should be avoided.

        (a) Up to 10% of patients with a glomus tumor will have associated bilateral glomus tumor, carotid body tumor, thyroid carcinoma, or other neural crest tumors.

        (b) Four-vessel carotid arteriography should be done.

        (c) Some tumors have endocrine activity that can lead to serious problems such as hypertensive crises during anesthesia. Serum and urine tests should be obtained to screen for endocrine activity and should also include screening for catecholamine, vanillylmandelic acid, and metanephrine.

      (3) The **treatment** of choice is surgical excision.

        (a) This procedure is easily carried out for **small tympanicum tumors** but can carry significant morbidity in patients with large tumors because of intracranial extension, hemorrhage, facial paralysis, and recurrence.

        (b) Glomus tumors are radiosensitive but not radiocurable.

        (c) New **skull base surgical techniques** have rendered essentially all lesions in this area resectable, and radiation should probably be reserved for recurrences, minimal residual disease, and patients who are physically unfit for surgery.

B **Other rare malignant vascular lesions** are found in the head and neck.

  1. Angiosarcomas arise from the vascular endothelial cells.

    a. Characteristics. They grow quickly, extend through the dermis, and frequently metastasize. The most common site on the head or neck is the **scalp.**

    b. Treatment. The only chance for a cure is **complete excision.**

  2. Hemangiopericytoma arises from the pericytes of Zimmermann, which are wrapped around precapillary arterioles.

    a. Characteristics. Approximately 25% are found in the head and neck. They are locally invasive and display an inconsistent malignant potential. Distant metastasis is not uncommon, but nodal spread is rare.

    b. Treatment is by surgical excision. Local recurrence is common.

  3. Kaposi's sarcoma (see Chapter 26, II G 2 d) is a rare tumor that arises in the skin or mucous membranes and presents as a bluish-red macule.

    a. Kaposi's sarcoma is a manifestation of acquired immunodeficiency syndrome (**AIDS**).

    b. Treatment. Head and neck neoplasms in these patients tend to be multiple and have usually been treated with radiotherapy.

C **Esthesioneuroblastoma (olfactory neuroblastoma)** is a rare neurogenic lesion that arises from the olfactory mucosa at the roof of the nose.

1. **Presenting symptoms**
   a. It presents as a nasal mass, with the usual symptoms of epistaxis and obstruction.
   b. Involvement of the cribriform plate is routine, and intracranial extension is common.

2. **Diagnosis.** Pathologic diagnosis can be difficult. The workup includes a CT scan and, occasionally, angiography.

3. **Treatment and prognosis**
   a. Treatment is done with combined intracranial and intranasal resection and radiotherapy in selected cases.
   b. Local recurrence rates are high (50%), but metastasis is uncommon (20%).
   c. The 5-year survival rate is approximately 50%.
   d. However, because most of the literature predates the current mode of therapy, recurrence and survival statistics should improve.

D **Tumors of the bone and soft tissue**

1. **Osteogenic sarcoma**
   a. **Characteristics.** Osteogenic sarcoma is the most common malignant tumor of bone. It rarely occurs in the head and neck. The most common site in the head and neck is the jaw. Reports include only about 12 cases that were primary to the temporal bone.
   b. **Etiology.** Previous bone disease and prior irradiation have been implicated as etiologic factors.
   c. **Treatment** is by radical excision.
      (1) The efficacy of adjuvant radiation therapy is controversial.
      (2) The most recent literature suggests that chemotherapy should be reserved for metastatic disease, but this suggestion is also controversial.
   d. **Prognosis.** The 5-year survival rate is very poor.

2. **Ewing's sarcoma**
   a. **Characteristics.** Ewing's sarcoma occurs in the skull and facial bones in approximately 9% of patients. It is usually a painful, swollen lesion.
   b. **Treatment** is with radiation and adjuvant chemotherapy.
   c. **Prognosis.** The 5-year survival rate is about 50%.

3. **Ameloblastoma** is a locally invasive tumor that arises from the odontogenic apparatus.
   a. **Presenting symptoms.** Ameloblastoma usually presents as a painless swelling and is much more common in the mandible than in the maxilla.
   b. **Treatment** is by conservative local excision. Radiation can be used for the rare malignant case.

4. **Rhabdomyosarcoma** (see Chapter 26, II G 2 c) is primarily a disease that occurs in children.
   a. **Characteristics.** Rhabdomyosarcoma can occur in the orbit, oral cavity, pharynx, face, neck, ear, paranasal sinuses, or salivary glands.
   b. **Treatment.** It is treated with radiation and chemotherapy.
   c. **Prognosis.** Except for tumors in the orbit, which have an 80% 2-year survival rate, the prognosis is poor.

5. **Soft tissue sarcomas (fibro-, lipo-, and chondrosarcomas** [see Chapter 26, II G]) are quite rare in the head and neck.
   a. **Etiology.** They are associated with prior irradiation.
   b. **Treatment** is with surgery and radiation. Local recurrence rates are high.

6. **Chordoma** is a rare tumor that arises from the embryonic notochord.
   a. **Characteristics.** One half of these tumors occur in the craniocervical region.
   b. **Presenting symptoms**
      (1) They are slow-growing, locally invasive tumors that cause bone and soft tissue destruction.
      (2) They can present as a nasopharyngeal mass.
   c. **Treatment** is with surgical excision, radiation therapy, or both. Local recurrence rates are high.

chapter 20

Parotid Gland

R. ANTHONY CARABASI III · JOHN C. KAIRYS

I INTRODUCTION

A Anatomy

1. **Embryology.** The parotid gland is the largest of the salivary glands. The average gland weighs 25 g. It appears in the fourth week of gestation and originates from the epithelium of the oropharynx.

2. **Description**
   a. The gland covers the masseter muscle, extends posteriorly beyond the vertical ramus of the mandible, and abuts the external auditory meatus.
   b. The gland is enclosed by a dense **fascial sheath.** The tightness of this fascia is responsible for the severe pain that accompanies acute swelling of the gland (**acute parotitis**).
   c. Classically, the parotid gland was thought to have two lobes, superficial and deep. Anatomically, this is probably not the case, but it is useful to think of the gland in this way when discussing the surgical treatment of parotid disease.

3. **Drainage** of saliva is via Stensen's duct. This duct exits anteriorly, pierces the buccinator muscle, and enters the oral cavity opposite the second upper molar. The opening is marked by the parotid papilla, which may be felt by the tongue or a finger.

B Innervation of the parotid gland (Fig. 20-1)

1. The **facial nerve** enters the posterior part of the gland immediately after emerging from the stylomastoid foramen. This nerve divides within the substance of the gland into two parts, the zygomaticofacial and the cervicofacial, which eventually split into five major **branches:**
   a. Temporal
   b. Zygomatic
   c. Buccal
   d. Mandibular
   e. Cervical

2. The facial nerve and its branches separate the superficial and deep portions of the gland (Fig. 20-2).

3. The muscles of expression are supplied by the facial nerve on the ipsilateral side of the face.

II BENIGN NEOPLASMS

Approximately 80% of parotid tumors are benign. The most common presenting feature of these tumors is a painless mass. Many are multicentric and have a high incidence of local recurrence. Facial paralysis is rare. Very careful identification and surgical treatment, which consist of excision that includes a margin of normal gland, are required. Extension into the deep lobe requires a total parotidectomy. The facial nerve should be spared, if possible, during surgery for benign parotid neoplasms. A discussion of the different types of benign tumors follows.

A Mixed tumors are so named because they contain both stromal and epithelial components.

1. Mixed tumors are the most common benign salivary tumors and account for 60% of all parotid tumors.

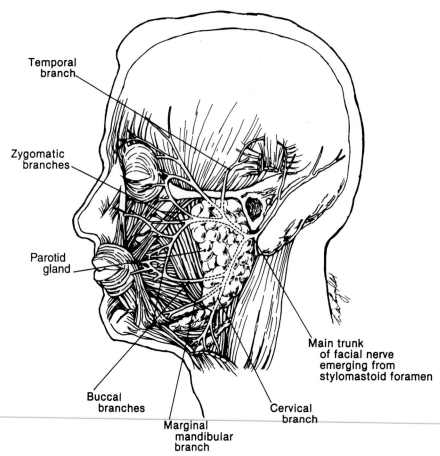

FIGURE 20-1   Innervation of the parotid gland.

2. They are slow-growing tumors but may be quite large at the time of presentation.

3. At surgery, mixed tumors often appear to "shell out" easily; that is, they seem easy to remove from the surrounding normal tissue. However, this excision invariably leaves nests of residual tumor, resulting in a recurrent tumor that requires re-excision.

4. Radiation therapy has no substantial effect.

B **Papillary adenocystoma (cystadenoma) lymphomatosum (Warthin's tumor)**

1. These tumors consist of both epithelial and lymphoid elements.

2. They are soft (cystic) when palpated.

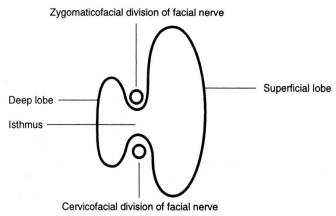

FIGURE 20-2   Frontal cross section of the parotid gland.

3. When cut, these tumors are found to contain mucoid material, which appears purulent. However, despite their appearance, the tumors are neoplastic and noninflammatory.

4. Malignant degeneration is rare but may occur in patients who have had prior neck irradiation.

5. This tumor is found in men five times as frequently as in women. It usually occurs in people between 40 and 60 years of age.

C **Benign lymphoepithelial tumor (Godwin's tumor)**

1. This uncommon tumor occurs most frequently in middle-aged or older women.

2. It is characterized by slowly progressive lymphoid infiltration of the gland.

3. Care must be taken not to confuse this lesion with a malignant lymphoma.

4. Occasionally, Godwin's tumor is unencapsulated. When this occurs, the tumor mimics an inflammatory process.

5. Recurrences may be treated with small doses of radiation.

D **Oxyphil adenomas** consist of acidophilic cells called **oncocytes.**

1. These tumors occur most frequently in elderly patients.

2. They grow slowly and do not usually grow larger than 5 cm.

E **Miscellaneous lesions,** such as **hemangiomas** and **lymphangiomas,** also occur. Hemangiomas that do not regress are treated by resection.

III **MALIGNANT NEOPLASMS**

Malignant tumors constitute 20% of all parotid neoplasms. They are often characterized by pain and facial nerve paralysis, which are features that are rarely, if ever, found in benign tumors.

A **Mucoepidermoid carcinoma**

1. This interesting tumor arises from the ducts of the gland. It is the most common parotid malignancy and constitutes 9% of all parotid tumors.

2. **Types**
   a. **Low-grade tumors** are the more common form and are the tumors seen most frequently during childhood.
      (1) They generally feel soft when palpated and appear encapsulated at surgery.
      (2) They are treated by excision, with preservation of those facial nerve branches that are not directly involved by the lesion.
      (3) When low-grade tumors are treated properly, the 5-year survival rate is approximately 95%.
   b. **High-grade tumors** are extremely aggressive, unencapsulated tumors that invade the gland widely.
      (1) Treatment must be radical and includes total parotidectomy, including the facial nerve, plus radical neck dissection (see Chapter 19, II D 1). Neck dissection is done even without palpable nodes, because there is a high incidence of microscopic nodal metastasis.
      (2) Surgery is usually supplemented by postoperative radiation.
      (3) The 5-year survival rate is 42% with optimal treatment.

B **Malignant mixed tumors**

1. These tumors are the second most common type of malignancy and are responsible for 8% of all parotid tumors.

2. The treatment is total parotidectomy; a radical neck dissection is also done for either palpable adenopathy or a high-grade tumor.

C **Squamous cell carcinoma** is a rare tumor in the parotid gland.

1. It is very hard on palpation and is usually accompanied by pain and nerve paralysis.

2. It is important to differentiate this lesion from a metastasis arising from a primary tumor elsewhere in the head and neck.

3. The 5-year survival rate is approximately 20%.

D Other lesions include **adenocystic carcinoma (cylindroma), acinic cell adenocarcinoma,** and **adenocarcinoma.**

1. Treatment is by total parotidectomy.

2. Neck dissection is added when obvious nodal disease for high-grade lesions is present.

3. High-grade, recurrent, and inoperable tumors should be treated with radiation.

E **Malignant lymphoma** may arise as a primary tumor in the gland. The treatment is the same as for other lymphomas (see Chapter 19, XI).

IV PAROTID TRAUMA

A **Lacerations** in the area of the parotid may damage the parenchyma of the gland, Stensen's duct, or the facial nerve.

1. **Parenchymal damage** without injury to Stensen's duct usually heals spontaneously.

2. **Stensen's duct.** If this duct is lacerated or transected, it should be repaired over a small catheter. This catheter is sutured to the oral mucosa and left in place for 10 days.

3. **Facial nerve injuries**
   a. These nerves may recover spontaneously if only a distal branch is injured.
   b. If a main trunk is injured, it requires meticulous repair by primary anastomosis or nerve grafting.
   c. If the injured area is hard to expose, a superficial parotidectomy should be done to facilitate repair.

B **Foreign bodies** (e.g., bullets) should be removed.

V INFLAMMATORY DISORDERS

A **Acute suppurative parotitis** is usually found in patients who are debilitated and dehydrated and who have poor oral hygiene.

1. **The offending organism** is usually *Staphylococcus aureus.*
   a. It most likely enters the gland from the mouth via Stensen's duct.
   b. The dehydrated patient whose salivary glands are not secreting actively is susceptible to rapid growth of the organism in this favorable environment.
   c. The bacterial proliferation leads to an intense inflammatory reaction in the gland, with edema and severe pain.

2. **Initial treatment** includes hydration, antibiotics, and measures to promote salivation, such as occasionally sucking on a lemon.
   a. Cultures are taken from Stensen's duct.
   b. Antibiotics are initially directed against *S. aureus* and are later adjusted as indicated by the results of the cultures.

3. **Surgical drainage** is required if the process is not arrested by the preceding measures.
   a. An incision is made around the angle of the mandible, and multiple horizontal incisions are made in the parotid fascia.
   b. There are usually multiple abscesses, and each must be drained.
   c. The wound is left open to ensure adequate drainage.

B **Calculous sialadenitis** is a condition caused by stones in the salivary ducts. If obstruction of the duct occurs, inflammation and intermittent painful swelling of the gland follow.

1. **Diagnosis**
   a. **Radiographs** may show the stones.
   b. A **sialogram,** in which contrast dye is injected into the draining duct, also shows areas of obstruction and is useful in patients when the stone is not radiopaque.

2. **Surgery**
   a. When the stone is near the end of the duct, it can be removed transorally.

b. If it is deep in the gland, it can be removed by an external incision.

c. If multiple stones are present and pain recurs, the entire gland should be removed.

3. **Variants.** Sialadenitis can occur without stones.

a. If there is a stricture of the duct on the sialogram, it should be dilated.

b. If symptoms persist, surgery may be necessary to remove the gland.

VI EVALUATION AND MANAGEMENT OF PAROTID MASSES

A **History and physical examination** can often differentiate among benign, malignant, and inflammatory processes.

1. A slowly enlarging, distinct mass can be either a benign neoplasm or a malignant neoplasm.

2. A rapidly enlarging, firm distinct mass associated with firm, ipsilateral adenopathy suggests a malignancy.

3. A mass associated with pain or facial nerve paralysis usually indicates a malignancy.

4. Acute, painful swelling in one or both glands, associated with fever or systemic symptoms, indicates an inflammatory process.

5. Intermittent pain and swelling in the gland suggest calculus sialadenitis. A stone may occasionally be palpable on intraoral examination.

6. A careful head and neck examination must be performed. Metastatic disease in a parotid lymph node (drainage from the upper two thirds of the face and the anterior scalp) may present as a mass in or near the parotid gland.

B **Diagnostic studies** may provide information that dictates the extent of surgery required, thus permitting better counseling of the patient preoperatively. However, some surgeons argue that no diagnostic studies are required because operation is indicated in most cases, and the extent of resection is dictated by the pathology encountered.

1. **Radiologic studies**

a. **Magnetic resonance imaging (MRI)** can establish whether the superficial or deep lobes are involved, whether suspicious lymphadenopathy is present, or whether there is invasion of the facial nerve. It may also help to differentiate individual histologic lesions.

b. **Computed tomography (CT) scans** discern many of the same structural details but are not nearly as successful in differentiating histologic lesions.

c. **Ultrasound** can localize the lesion to the superficial or deep lobe but otherwise adds little information.

d. **Plain radiographs** or **sialograms** may be useful for imaging stones.

2. **Invasive tests**

a. **Fine-needle aspiration** has a good accuracy rate (87%) and a low risk of spreading malignant cells. It may be helpful when planning the extent of surgery needed.

b. **Core-needle biopsy** or **open biopsy** carries the risk of spreading tumor cells and generally is not indicated.

C Surgical management

1. **Benign lesions**

a. Because most masses are found in the larger, superficial lobe, **superficial parotidectomy** is usually sufficient.

b. **Complete excision** is required. "Shelling out" a mass is unacceptable and often leads to a recurrence.

2. **Malignant lesions**

a. If the lesion is small, low grade, and completely confined to the superficial lobe, then resection of only that lobe may be sufficient. Otherwise, total parotidectomy should be performed.

b. The facial nerve should be sacrificed if it is involved. Nerve grafting allows restoration of some function in 6–12 months.

c. **Radical neck dissection** or **modified radical neck dissection** is indicated for high-grade lesions.

d. Postoperative radiation therapy may be used for unfavorable high-grade lesions or in patients in whom a limited dissection was performed.

CRITICAL POINTS

1. The parotid is the largest of the salivary glands. It covers the masseter muscle and extends posteriorly behind the ramus of the mandible. Thus, masses palpated in the region just in front of the ear may actually be located in the parotid, and appropriate workup must be undertaken.

2. The gland is enclosed by a dense fascial sheath and consists of a larger superficial and a smaller deep "lobe" with branches of the facial nerve passing between the two. Drainage of the gland is via Stenson's duct.

3. The majority of neoplasms (80%) arising in the parotid are benign. The most common presentation is that of a painless mass without evidence of nerve involvement.
   a. Pleomorphic adenomas or "mixed tumors" are the most common benign neoplasm, making up about 60% of parotid tumors overall.
   b. Papillary adenocystoma (cystadenoma) lymphomatosum or Warthin's tumor are typically soft, contain mucoid material, and are more common in women between 40 and 60 years of age.
   c. Benign lymphoepithelial tumor, or Godwin's tumor, may mimic a lymphoma or inflammatory process.

4. Only 20% of neoplasms are malignant tumors and are more frequently associated with pain or facial paralysis.
   a. Mucoepidermoid tumors, which may be either low grade or high grade, are the most common malignant neoplasms.
   b. Malignant mixed tumors are the second most common malignancy.
   c. Squamous cell carcinomas are rare. An effort must be made to rule out the parotid lesion as a mestastasis from some other site in the head and neck.

5. Trauma to Stensen's duct should be primarily repaired over a stent.

6. Acute suppurative parotitis is usually seen in debilitated patients and is typically caused by *S. aureus.* Initial treatment is hydration, antibiotics, and stimulation of salivation. Surgical therapy is wide drainage.

7. Calculus sialadenitis is caused by stones in the salivary ducts. Treatment involves either extraction through Stensen's duct or surgical removal via an external excision.

8. Evaluation of a parotid mass involves a detailed head and neck examination. The constellation of symptoms and physical examination findings typically differentiate among the pathologic possibilities (see VI A). Axial imaging (either MRI or CT) may give additional useful information. Fine-needle aspirations may be helpful in clarifying the clinical situation but are not always necessary. Core biopsy or open biopsy should not be performed.

9. Surgery for benign lesions is usually limited to superficial lobectomy. "Shelling out" a lesion is never acceptable.

10. Surgery for malignant lesions may include only a superfical lobectomy if the lesion is small, low grade, and confined to the superficial lobe. Otherwise, total parotidectomy should be performed. The facial nerve is sacrificed, if involved. Neck dissection is included for high-grade lesions. Radiotherapy may be given for high-grade lesions or where an incomplete dissection is performed.

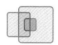

Study Questions for Part VI

Directions: *Each of the numbered items in this section is followed by several possible answers. Select the ONE lettered answer that is BEST in each case.*

1. A 35-year-old man presents with left unilateral tinnitus and mild left sensorineural hearing loss. Which of the following statements is true?

- [A] Such signs and symptoms are common and should not be worked up unless they worsen.
- [B] An MRI scan should be obtained, but gadolinium enhancement and its attendant risks are not necessary.
- [C] Brain stem evoked response audiometry is likely to be normal.
- [D] The patient should be assumed to have an acoustic neuroma until proven otherwise.
- [E] Conditions that cause such problems do not affect the other ear.

QUESTIONS 2–3

A 35-year-old man has right-sided serous otitis media and a right upper neck mass.

2. It is most important to evaluate this patient for which of the following?

- [A] Cancer of the right ear
- [B] Cancer of the right tonsil
- [C] Cancer of the right maxillary sinus
- [D] Cancer of the nasopharynx
- [E] Hodgkin's lymphoma

3. Which of the following will be the primary treatment for this tumor?

- [A] Local excision to negative margins
- [B] Wide local excision and radical neck dissection
- [C] Neoadjuvant chemotherapy followed by resection of residual tumor
- [D] Unilateral radiotherapy with combined chemotherapy
- [E] Bilateral radiotherapy

QUESTIONS 4–5

A 65-year-old man is found to have a small invasive squamous cell carcinoma of the right vocal cord. The right vocal cord is paralyzed, and a lymph node in the right anterior neck is 4 cm in diameter.

4. The stage of the tumor is which of the following?

- [A] T2N1
- [B] T2N2a
- [C] T3N1
- [D] T3N2a
- [E] T4N3

5. Optimal treatment of the primary tumor should include which of the following?

- [A] Total laryngectomy
- [B] Vertical hemilaryngectomy
- [C] Supraglottic (horizontal) laryngectomy
- [D] Right cordectomy
- [E] Chemotherapy

QUESTIONS 6–7

A 55-year-old woman presents with complaint of a mass overlying the angle of the right mandible. She says the mass has been slowly enlarging over the past 2–3 years and that the mass is painless. On physical examination, it is firm and overlies the angle of the right mandible and the area between the angle and the tragus of the ear. Neurologic examination of the head and neck is completely normal.

6. Which of the following does this mass most likely represent?
   - [A] Mucoepidermoid cancer of the parotid gland
   - [B] Acute parotitis
   - [C] Benign mixed tumor of the parotid gland (pleomorphic adenoma)
   - [D] Malignant mixed tumor of the parotid gland
   - [E] Hemangioma of the parotid gland

7. What will be the optimal treatment for this lesion?
   - [A] Radiation therapy
   - [B] Total parotidectomy with preservation of the facial nerve
   - [C] Total parotidectomy including resection of the facial nerve
   - [D] Superficial parotidectomy
   - [E] Enucleation

Answers and Explanations

1. The answer is D (Chapter 18, IV F 2). These are common presenting systems of an acoustic neuroma. Evaluation for acoustic neuroma is indicated in all cases of unilateral hearing complaints, especially when hearing loss is documented. Magnetic resonance imaging (MRI) of the brain with internal auditory canal views and gadolinium contrast is sensitive in 98% of patients with acoustic neuroma. Complications associated with gadolinium are exceedingly rare, and this contrast should always be used in an MRI to look for a tumor. Brain stem auditory response testing may or may not be normal in cases such as this. The differential diagnosis with this presenting complaint is quite extensive, and it includes processes that result in bilateral hearing loss.

2–3. The answers are 2-D and 3-E (Chapter 19, IV C; Chapter 19, IV B 2, C 2 b). The two most common presenting symptoms of cancer of the nasopharynx are enlarged posterior cervical lymph nodes and unilateral serous otitis media. Cancer of the right ear, right tonsil, or right maxillary sinus or Hodgkin's lymphoma generally do not cause otitis media and usually occur in an older age group. Hodgkin's lymphoma will lead to serous otitis media only if Waldeyer's ring involvement has led to eustachian tube dysfunction, which is a rare occurrence.

Bilateral radiotherapy is the primary treatment for all epithelial nasopharyngeal tumors.

4–5. The answers are 4-D and 5-A (Chapter 19, II C 3, VIII D 3; Chapter 19, VIII E 4). Any carcinoma of the vocal cord that leads to fixation of the cord or of the hemilarynx is at least T3. Massive involvement of surrounding soft tissues will make the tumor stage T4. The presence of a single homolateral lymph node greater than 3 cm but less than 6 cm in diameter makes the stage of the neck node N2a. Multiple small lymph nodes on the same side of the neck as the primary tumor are classified N2b, and lymph nodes involving the opposite side of the neck change the staging to N3.

T3 tumors cannot be adequately treated with partial laryngectomy in most cases; total laryngectomy is required. Radiation therapy is used postoperatively as a planned combined treatment in most cases. Chemotherapy is used for inoperable cases or in experimental protocols.

6–7. The answers are 6-C and 7-D (Chapter 20, II A 1–4). The history given is most consistent with a benign neoplasm of the parotid gland. Benign mixed tumors are the most common benign tumors of the salivary glands. Benign salivary tumors account for 60% of all parotid tumors. Malignant tumors, such as a mucoepidermoid cancer, usually grow more rapidly and are more often associated with facial nerve paralysis. The absence of pain makes acute parotitis unlikely. Hemangiomas of the parotid gland are much rarer than benign mixed tumors.

The optimal treatment for a benign mixed tumor is removal of the tumor with a margin of normal parotid gland. This usually can be accomplished with a superficial parotidectomy. Although these tumors often appear to shell out, removal by simple enucleation results in a very high recurrence rate. Excision of the entire gland with or without the facial nerve is indicated for malignant tumors. Radiation therapy does not have a role in the management of this lesion.

PART **VII**

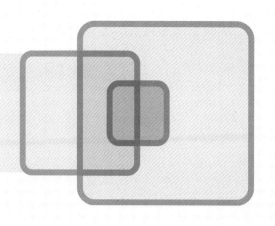

Special Subjects

chapter 21

Trauma and Burns

MURRAY J. COHEN • MICHAEL WEINSTEIN • KRIS R. KAULBACK •
JEROME J. VERNICK • NASIM AHMED

I TRAUMA

A Overview

1. **Incidence**
   a. Trauma is the leading cause of death for people 1–44 years of age.
   b. More than 150,000 people die from trauma every year.
   c. Half of these deaths result from motor vehicle accidents.
   d. For every death, three people are permanently disabled.
   e. Trauma-related costs exceed 400 billion dollars annually.

2. **Trauma management**
   a. Mortality can be greatly reduced by efficient handling of the injured, which involves three major components:
      (1) A **trauma center** with professional personnel who are trained in delivering rapid care and with facilities capable of handling a large number of patients at once
      (2) A **transportation system** capable of rapid transport to a trauma center
      (3) **Emergency medical technicians** who are capable of maintaining vital functions until the trauma surgeon can take over
   b. **Priorities.** The management of trauma requires adherence to an established order of priority, ensuring that the most life-threatening injuries will be treated first but that less serious injuries will not be neglected after resuscitation. The **order of priorities** in evaluating trauma patients is based on the advanced trauma life support (ATLS) course administered by the American College of Surgeons (ACS).
      (1) **Primary survey.**
         A—**Airway**
         B—**Breathing** (ventilation)
         C—**Circulation**
         D—**Disablility** (neurologic deficit)
         E—**Exposure/Enviroment**
      (2) The physician or emergency medical technician is urged to:
         A—**Establish a patent airway**
         B—**Ensure that both lungs are ventilated**
         C—**Restore circulating volume and compress external bleeding sites**
         D—**Check for neurologic deficit**
         E—**Fully expose (undress) the patient and cover with warmed blankets**
      (3) Diagnosis of immediately life-threatening injuries, followed by rapid treatment
      (4) Reassessment of the patients' status
      (5) **Secondary survey, "AMPLE"** history (Table 21-1), head-to-toe physical exam, **Glasgow Coma Scale (GCS)** (Table 21-2)
      (6) Definitive treatment, including surgery, prophylactic antibiotics, and tetanus prophylaxis (see Chapter 2, VI)

B Mechanisms of injury
Knowing the mechanism of injury allows the physician to anticipate lesions that may otherwise remain undiagnosed and to decide on the appropriate management for lesions that may be more extensive than they might initially appear.

TABLE 21-1   Points Covered in the "AMPLE" History
Allergies
Medications
Previous illnesses
Last meal
Events surrounding injury

1. **Acceleration–deceleration injuries** are typically caused by falls from heights, blunt trauma, or vehicular accidents.
   a. Obvious injuries result from direct contact with the landing site (i.e., the ground or the vehicle).
   b. Subtle injuries result from shearing forces produced by the momentum when heavy organs are suddenly halted or accelerated by a crash.
      (1) Heavy organs include fluid-filled loops of bowel, the blood-filled thoracic aorta, and mobile parenchymal organs such as the liver and spleen. The momentum of these organs is maintained after the motion of the victim has been stopped.
      (2) Damage occurs because force is exerted on the tethered portion of the viscus by the mobile portion of the viscus, which continues to move. For example:
         (a) The aortic arch shears at the fixed ligamentum arteriosus.
         (b) The small bowel tends to pull away from its mesenteric attachments, creating a "bucket-handle" tear with massive bleeding from mesenteric vessels.
         (c) Avulsion of the spleen at its hilus or peritoneal reflection is common.
         (d) Renal pedicle avulsion

2. **Missile injuries**
   a. **Low-velocity missile injuries** include most civilian gunshot wounds.
      (1) Missiles fired from handguns have a velocity in the range of 600–1,100 ft/second.
      (2) Wounds from this type of missile are generally restricted to the path and the residual cavity created by the missile as it penetrates tissues, such as blood vessels and organs. However, secondary injuries can occur.
         (a) External articles (buttons or keys) may be driven into the wound by the missile.
         (b) Bone fragments, produced when the missile strikes a large bone, can also cause secondary injury.
   b. **High-velocity missile injuries** can be recognized by a small entrance wound and a large exit wound with severe underlying tissue damage. These wounds may cause damage remote from the apparent tract of the missile as a large temporary cavity is created when the tissue recoils from the path of the bullet.
   c. **Shotgun injuries**
      (1) **Close-range** shotgun injuries can be devastating. Large soft tissue defects are created with widespread damage. In addition, these wounds often introduce nonopaque foreign material, which originates from the wadding used in the manufacture of the shotgun shell.
      (2) **Long-range** shotgun injuries consist of multiple low-velocity pellet injuries. These cause widespread penetration but are generally not severe unless the missile happens to strike a major blood vessel or organ.

TABLE 21-2 Revised Trauma Score			
Glasgow Coma Scale	Systolic Blood Pressure	Respiratory Rate	Coded Value
8–15	>89	10–29	4
8–12	76–89	>29	3
6–8	50–75	6–9	2
4–5	1–49	1–5	1
3	0	0	0

RTS = 0.9368 GCS_c + 0.7326 SBP_c + 0.2908 RR_c, where the subscript c refers to coded value.

    d. The **shocking, "knock-down" effect** of a missile depends on factors that influence the energy transferred to the victim by the impact.

        (1) Striking energy is directly proportional to the weight of a missile and the square of its velocity.

        (2) Missiles that completely penetrate the victim expend much of their energy on the objects beyond the victim. Maximum energy transfer results from the missile that remains in the victim.

        (3) Penetration is diminished when a bullet is used that expands or tumbles after impact.

    e. Treatment. All missile tracts should be debrided, but missiles need not be removed unless they cause symptoms or are in proximity to a vital structure where body movements or tissue erosion could cause further injury.

C Management of trauma victims

1. The **initial assessment** of the patient's state, performed when the patient arrives in the emergency room, determines the extent of injury and the need for immediate care. Obviously, inebriated patients often have serious injuries, but the presence of alcohol does not diminish the trauma team's responsibility to diagnose all injuries properly. The initial assessment can be performed by an experienced physician within seconds.

2. Airway

    a. Assessment

        (1) The mouth and upper airway should be inspected for obstruction from foreign bodies (teeth, blood) or maxillofacial instability.

        (2) Stridor or hoarseness implies laryngeal obstruction or injury.

        (3) Examine the neck for asymmetry, cyanosis, subcutaneous emphysema, and fractures.

        (4) The chest should be auscultated for bilateral equal breath sounds.

    b. Treatment. Rapid measures are necessary to correct unsatisfactory ventilation.

        (1) Supplemental oxygen should be administered to all trauma victims until stable.

        (2) Basic manuevers for relieving obstruction and maintaining ventilation include:

            (a) Finger sweep

            (b) Chin lift/jaw thrust

            (c) Oropharyngeal airway

            (d) Nasopharyngeal airway

        (3) Provide definitive airway.

            (a) Early intubation is important in unstable patients due to the propensity for apnea and sudden circulatory collapse. Some indications for rapid intubation include:

                (i) Depressed mental status (**GCS** <8)

                (ii) Major head, face, or neck injury

                (iii) Impaired ventilation from paralysis

            (b) Oral tracheal intubation is the most common modality used to provide a definitive airway. Patients are preoxygenated with a bag-valve mask and then intubated with in-line **cervical stabilization. Rapid-sequence induction** with **cricoid pressure** should be utilized.

            (c) Nasotracheal intubation is acceptable only in a spontaneously breathing patient without a suspected basilar skull fracture.

            (d) Surgical airway should be performed if standard intubating techniques are unable to be performed or are contraindicated.

                (i) Jet ventilation via a 12- or 14-gauge catheter in the cricothyroid membrane

                (ii) Cricothyroidotomy is contraindicated in children less than 12 years of age or in patients with laryngeal fractures.

                (iii) Tracheostomy

3. Breathing

    a. Assessment

        (1) Ventilation should be assessed by auscultation of the chest, followed by entidal CO_2 monitoring to check for endotracheal tube misplacement. Continuous pulse oximetry and arterial blood gas analysis is also useful.

(2) Inspect the thorax for sucking chest wounds, subcutaneous emphysema, tracheal deviation, and diminished breath sounds.

b. Treatment

(1) Pneumothorax is diagnosed by absent breath sounds, tracheal deviation away from the affected side, and hypotension.

(a) Needle decompression in the second intercostal space, midclavicular line

(b) Chest tube placement

(2) Hemothorax (volume replacement and chest tube)

(3) Open chest wound (placement of a semiocclusive dressing and chest tube)

4. Circulatory support. Once adequate ventilation has been established, the physician should rapidly proceed to the next critical stage of resuscitation, namely, establishment of tissue perfusion or circulatory support.

a. Assessment of the circulatory status should include appraisal of:

(1) Character of the pulse

(a) A rapid, faint pulse suggests profound hypovolemia in most cases.

(b) A slow, full pulse may be indicative of severe neurologic injury with increasing intracranial pressure or hypercarbia.

(2) Peripheral perfusion, as indicated by level of consciousness, rate of capillary refilling, urine output, and body temperature

(3) Tachycardia may be an early compensatory sign of hypovolemia.

(4) Blood pressure. The presence of a mild hypotension may be associated with inadequate tissue perfusion. A narrowed pulse pressure with diastolic hypertension is one of the earliest signs of hypovolemia.

(5) Stable vital signs with major injury. The condition of patients with major injury and seemingly stable vital signs is dangerous and deceptive.

(a) Previously healthy trauma patients, especially if young, are able to maintain a normal pulse and blood pressure, despite a continuing occult hemorrhage, until vasomotor response fails. When this occurs, the patient "crashes," which is manifested by a rapid loss of blood pressure and unconsciousness.

(b) These patients maintain stable hemodynamic parameters and may remain quietly pale or become excitable with progressive mental deterioration until overt shock develops, at which point they may not respond to further volume replacement.

(c) Beta-blockers and pacemakers may block tachycardia due to hypovolemia.

(6) Search for obvious **external hemorrhage.**

b. Treatment

(1) Venous access

(a) Lines should be inserted by a reliable method with which the physician is comfortable.

(i) Large-bore peripheral catheters (typically 14- or 16-gauge in the antecubital position) should be the primary route of access.

(ii) Subclavian catheterization should be learned in controlled settings, not on unstable trauma patients.

(iii) Subclavian lines and a saphenous cut-down are the quickest for venous access.

(iv) The saphenous vein often looks empty and may look pale and tendonlike in a hypovolemic patient. It should be recognized rather than divided.

(b) Two lines are usually inserted simultaneously.

(i) It is best to keep one on each side of the diaphragm so that volume replacement is effective in case of vena caval or subclavian venous trauma.

(ii) Shock patients often require between two to four separate lines for volume replacement to increase the blood pressure to more than 100 mm Hg in less than 10 minutes.

(iii) The first intravenous insertion should include the withdrawal of 20 mL of blood for crossmatching and for laboratory studies, including a **type and cross.**

(iv) Femoral artery punctures should be performed early for blood gas analyses.

(c) All resuscitation lines should be replaced in 12–24 hours. The urgent insertion of these lines leaves sterility in question, and catheter sepsis can become a serious problem after 24 hours.

(2) Volume resuscitation

(a) The initial fluid replacement should be **isotonic saline** or **lactated Ringer's** solutions. The amount infused is based on the initial judgment of shock and blood loss and is usually given in 500-cc boluses in adults.

(b) Once 2 L of crystalloid has been infused, blood transfusion should be strongly considered.

(c) Unmatched O-positive blood should be used in emergent situations when time is not available for formal blood typing and crossmatching. O negative blood should be used in female patients of childbearing age.

(d) If time is available, the use of type-specific crossmatched packed red blood cells is optimal.

(e) Fresh frozen plasma, cryoprecipitate and platelets are reserved for known or suspected coagulopathies.

(3) Control of hemorrhage must accompany fluid resuscitation.

(a) External bleeding

(i) Applying direct pressure on bleeding wounds with manually held gauze pads is safe and usually effective.

(ii) Proximal and distal digital compression of bleeding superficial vessels may allow visualization of the bleeding point and accurate clamping. Blind clamping is never indicated.

(iii) Pressure dressings may be used to control diffuse bleeding from abrasions and avulsions that involve large areas.

(iv) Temporary packing of missile tracts and stab wounds can slow the blood flow until surgical exposure is obtained.

(v) Pneumatic splints and medical antishock trousers (MAST) help in tamponading bleeding and increasing peripheral resistance to increase the blood pressure. The antishock trousers provide increased peripheral resistance without the pharmacologic effects of pressor agents. MAST should be reserved for certain cases where long transport times are anticipated or in pelvic fractures when tamponade and relative immobilization may be important.

(vi) Tourniquets should be avoided if personnel are available for direct compression.

(b) Internal bleeding requires early diagnosis and prompt treatment by appropriate surgical intervention (see C 7).

(4) Cardiac resuscitation

(a) Closed chest cardiac massage should be performed while fluid resuscitation is begun if the patient is asystolic or demonstrates evidence of poor cardiac function.

(b) Emergency room thorocotomies for **open cardiac massage** have few indications and should only be performed by trained surgeons.

(c) Indications for emergency room thoracotomy are:

(i) Hypovolemic cardiac arrest despite vigorous blood volume replacement plus closed chest massage and defibrillation

(ii) Cardiac arrest with penetrating injury to the chest

(d) Relative contraindications include:

(i) Major obvious injuries to the central nervous system (i.e., decapitation, extruding brain tissue)

(ii) Failed external cardiac massage lasting more than 10 minutes

(iii) Major blunt trauma

(5) Monitoring circulating blood volume and resuscitative therapy is based on the signs and symptoms of shock. Examination of pulses, skin color, capillary refill, heart rate, blood pressure, and mental status should occur continuously. Adjuncts to hemodynamic monitoring useful in trauma include urine output and central venous pressure (CVP).

(a) Urine output measured hourly is an important guideline to the accuracy of fluid resuscitation. Output exceeding 30 cc/hour implies adequate perfusion to all vital organs.

(b) CVP can be useful when its trend is observed over time and in patients with significant preexisting cardiac and pulmonary disfunction. Pulmonary artery (Swan-Ganz) catheter monitoring may be more appropriate in these patients.

5. Assessment of neurologic injury. After adequate ventilation and tissue perfusion have been restored, immediate attention must be given to the patient's neurologic condition.

  a. Head trauma

    (1) Assessment

      (a) Loss of consciousness signifies a head injury until such an injury has been ruled out.

      (b) Intracranial trauma cannot be adequately assessed while the patient is in shock.

      (c) If hypotension is present in a patient with a head injury, it is rarely secondary to the head trauma, and the physician must look for another cause of the hypotension.

      (d) The neurologic evaluation should assess the following factors rapidly:

        (i) Level of consciousness. Is the patient alert, lethargic and disoriented, comatose but responsive to pain, or unresponsive?

        (ii) Motor activity and tactile sensation

        (iii) Obvious head trauma, such as a depressed skull fracture, gunshot wound, or leaking cerebrospinal fluid

        (iv) Pupil size and response to light

        (v) Oculocephalic ("doll's eye") reflex. Because testing involves rotating the patient's head, it should only be done after spinal cord injury has been ruled out.

      (e) Evolving hypertension and bradycardia (Cushing's phenomenon) indicate increasing intracranial pressure and a worsening neurologic problem.

    (2) Treatment

      (a) Consultation with a neurosurgeon is imperative for proper management of patients with head injuries. However, if one is not available, then a telephone consultation should be obtained and initial treatment begun, followed by transfer of the patient to a center with a neurosurgeon.

      (b) Initial management includes the following considerations:

        (i) Sterile saline-soaked gauze should be placed over open injuries.

        (ii) Mannitol and other drugs to lower intracranial pressure should be given after consultation with the neurosurgeon.

        (iii) Hypotension and hypoventilation seriously injure brain cells. It is, therefore, important to assess adequately fluid requirements and ventilation.

        (iv) Overhydration increases intracranial pressure and should be avoided once fluid requirements have been met and the patient is stable.

  b. Spinal cord trauma

    (1) Assessment

      (a) Until proven otherwise, the spine should be considered unstable and the cord, therefore, liable to injury in all patients with major blunt trauma.

      (b) The **cervical spine** should be considered unstable in:

        (i) Every unconscious patient

        (ii) Every patient with face and head contusions or vertebral tenderness

        (iii) Every patient with decreased mentation, which precludes adequate neurologic examination

      (c) Radiographic films showing all seven cervical vertebrae intact should be obtained before allowing the patient's neck to be extended for any reason. At least three views need to be obtained, including cross-table lateral, anterior-posterior, and odontoid views.

      (d) Evidence of injury to the spinal cord should be sought.

        (i) It should be recognized that the cord may not yet be injured although the spine is unstable. A negative neurologic examination does not prove the absence of injury to the cervical spine.

        (ii) Appropriate spinal stabilization must be performed until proper studies have been done.

        (iii) Findings, such as absence of motor or sensory function below the injury, loss of muscle tone, and loss of anal sphincter tone, should be sought.

        (iv) Hypotension may be present if there is a loss of vascular tone (arterial and venous) within the affected region.

(2) Treatment. The required stabilization and reduction of the injury must be performed under the supervision of a neurosurgeon or an orthopedic surgeon experienced in treating these injuries.

6. **Exposure**
   a. **Assessment.** All patients should be removed of clothing from head to toe. This allows for complete visualization of the entire body surface, which helps to limit missed injuries. Chemical and enviromental contamination and chemical burning is also lessened by removing contaminated clothing.
   b. **Treatment.** Hypothermia must be addressed rapidly to avoid complicating the patient's hemodynamic status. Heated blankets, warmed IV fluids, and raising the ambient room temperature are excellent ways to limit hypothermia.

7. **Secondary survey.** After the primary survey is complete and immediate life-threatening manuevers are under way, the physcian should perform a detailed head-to-toe assessment to evaluate minor injuries and to diagnose occult life- or limb-threatening injuries. In brief, the physcian should place a finger or instrument in every orifice. Constant reevalutation of the patient's **ABCDE's** is vital (see C I 5).
   a. **Head and neck.** Pupil size and character, tympanic membranes, and facial stability should all be assessed. Fractures should be evaluated for airway compromise. Rhinorrhea and otorrhea should be suspected with clear drainage. **Raccoon eyes** and **Battle's sign** indicate a base of skull fracture. Computed tomography (CT) is the imaging of choice for these injuries.
   b. **Thorax.** Tension pnuemothorax and massive hemothorax are often diagnosed and treated on the primary survey. Pulmonary contusion, rib fractures, small effusions, and small pneumothoraxes are found on chest radiographs, which should be performed early on during the resuscitation.
      (1) Tamponade is decreased cardiac output secondary to poor right ventricular filling that is impaired by fluid (blood) around the heart.
         (a) Echocardiography is a noninvasive means to look for pericardial fluid and right ventricular collapse.
         (b) Pericardial window is a surgical procedure where the pericardium is directly visualized from a subxyphoid approach.
         (c) Pericardial centesis should only be used to decompress a tamponade that is awaiting surgery.
      (2) Blunt aortic tears and penetrating great vessel injury
         (a) Chest x-ray. Widened mediastinum, deviation of nasogastric (NG) tube, depressed left mainstem bronchus, pleural cap, blurring of aortic knob, and first and second rib fractures all could indicate great vessel injury. Knowing the mechanism of injury is important because the chest x-ray can also be normal.
         (b) Transesophageal echocardiography, which is operator dependent, is useful as a screening tool while the patient undergoes emergent surgery.
         (c) Angiography is the gold standard. May be replaced eventually with CT or magnetic resonance (MR) angiography.
      (3) Esophageal perforation must be evaluated with esophagoscopy and contrast swallow.
   c. **Abdomen.** Assessment of the abdomen for intracavitary injury can be difficult on the polytrauma patient. Subtle exam findings are often masked due to pain from extremity or spine fractures. Patients may be under the influence of various drugs and alcohol, making the exam unreliable. Tests for abdominal injury are chosen based on the injury pattern, stability of the patient, and index of suspicion.
      (1) Diagnostic peritoneal lavage is an invasive test in which a surgeon places a catheter in the peritoneal cavity and irrigates with 1 L of saline. The test is considered positive if the fluid cell count is greater than 100,000 red blood cells or greater than 500 white blood cells or if vegetative matter or bacteria is present. The lavage is sensitive but not specific to the organ injured.
      (2) Ultrasound is a noninvasive exam performed by the trauma surgeon in the emergency department. The study is quick and sensitive but not specific.

(3) CT scan is a noninvasive test with excellent sensitivity and specificity. The exam is also the only modality that evaluates the retroperitonium. The test often requires transfer of the patient out of the resuscitation area.

(4) Surgery. Once ongoing bleeding or perforation is diagnosed, prompt laparotomy should be performed. Solid organ injury (liver/spleen) can be managed nonoperatively, depending on the clinical situation in relatively stable patients.

 d. Genitourinary injuries (see Chapter 25, VII)

  (1) Urethral injury

   (a) Blood at the meatus is an indication for retrograde urethrography. Even gentle insertion of a Foley catheter can disrupt a partially divided urethra.

   (b) Major injuries should be repaired surgically.

  (2) Bladder injuries usually heal spontaneously if adequate urinary drainage is established. (Generally, intraperitoneal bladder ruptures require operative repair.)

  (3) Kidneys are commonly injured organs.

   (a) Most renal injuries can be managed nonoperatively; however, renal pedicle disruption or major parenchymal damage with hemorrhage are the primary indications for surgery.

   (b) Intravenous pyelography provides a good test of renal function, but it is not adequate for determining anatomic continuity of the organ. Extravasated contrast medium is an indication for drainage of the area where the leakage occurred.

 e. Soft tissue injuries

  (1) Debridement is the key to avoiding infection and promoting rapid healing.

   (a) All devitalized tissue must be removed during debridement.

   (b) It is helpful to understand how different tissues respond to injury. The degree of injury often depends on the density of the tissue and its water content.

    (i) The lung tends to receive relatively minor degrees of damage remote from the missile tract.

    (ii) By contrast, muscle or liver, because of their greater density and water content, develop large temporary cavities and require extensive debridement beyond the apparent missile tract.

  (2) Muscle

   (a) Wide areas of devitalized tissue occur in high-velocity wounds and require debridement.

   (b) Viable muscle tissue visibly contracts when touched with an electrosurgical instrument set on a low power. It also contracts when gently pinched with forceps.

   (c) Muscle that does not react must be removed, although weakness and deformity will result.

  (3) Arteries

   (a) Palpable pulses do not rule out arterial injury.

   (b) Grossly injured vascular areas that exhibit intramural bleeding or disruption require removal. It is not necessary to remove apparently normal areas of arteries.

   (c) Repair should be done with autogenous material, if at all possible. There is an increased incidence of infection and failure when prosthetic material is used (see Chapter 7, VIII).

   (d) Fasciotomies are almost always required in conjunction with vascular repair if there has been prolonged ischemia or concomitant venous injury. It is far better to do a fasciotomy early in anticipation of swelling and tension in muscle compartments than to wait until tissue loss has occurred.

   (e) Stab wounds and missile tracts in proximity to major vascular structures require either surgical exploration or, at a minimum, emergency arteriography.

  (4) Major **veins** should be repaired when injured.

  (5) Nerves. It is not necessary to debride nerves that are injured. Exposed nerves should be covered with normal muscle or fat, leaving definitive repair for a future time.

  (6) Bone. Contaminated small pieces of bone that are not attached to soft tissue may be removed. Attached bones should generally be left in situ to speed healing.

  (7) Lung tissue is usually resistant to remote damage. Because of its spongy nature, the lung absorbs shock without injury, so a missile tract generally contains all of the injury.

(8) Parenchymal organs, such as the **liver and kidney**
    (a) Bleeding is the major problem. Devitalized tissue should be removed with as much functional tissue left as possible.
    (b) An effort should be made to salvage an injured **spleen,** particularly in a child. There is evidence that a small spleen slice, reimplanted in the omentum, will grow and provide some splenic function.

(9) Genitalia. Very conservative debridement is indicated. Exposed testicular tissue should be covered with scrotal skin or reimplanted under attached skin, if possible.

  f. Fractures (see Chapter 28, II A 3)
    (1) A fracture is seldom a major priority in the presence of other life-threatening injuries.
      (a) Hemorrhage or vascular compromise associated with a fracture gives it a higher priority, as does a threat to the viability of an extremity.
      (b) Bleeding associated with a fracture can account for a large portion of a patient's circulating blood volume, and hypovolemic shock is commonly associated with bilateral femoral fractures.
    (2) Early fractures that are open can be treated in accordance with the associated soft tissue injury.
      (a) Debridement, vascular repair, and other soft tissue surgery should be performed before stabilization of the fracture.
      (b) However, adequate splinting and stabilization should be accomplished because it decreases the risk of fat embolism syndrome.
      (c) Internal fixation devices are generally hazardous in the presence of extensive soft tissue injury and should be avoided, if possible.

  g. Tendon injuries require conservative debridement only. Tendons should be covered with normal tissue; otherwise, they become devitalized and useless.

  h. Special situations
    (1) Pediatrics. Young children have different injury patterns due to their pliable skeletons and head-to-body ratio. Intravenous access is sometimes difficult and requires intramedullary access. Pediatrics should be involved early in the management.
    (2) Pregnancy. Assessment and treatment is directed toward the mother, as her health is primarily important to the fetus. Early obstetrical input as well as fetal ultrasounds and monitoring are vital. Emergent cesarean section for fetal deterioration is performed in conjuction with the trauma surgeons. Elevation of the right hip displaces the gravid uterus from the inferior vena cava for increased cardiac return.

8. Transfer to definitive care. After the initial resuscitation, all patients who have injuries or suspicion of injury that exceeds the institution's capability should be transferred. Physician-to-physician transfer to state-accredited trauma centers is optimal. Most hospitals have preexisting transfer agreements.

D | **Trauma severity scoring and quality assurance** Trauma centers are required to maintain trauma registries, which are used for quality assurance and center accreditation. It is necessary to provide an objective means of identifying patients whose injuries were apparently not of sufficient magnitude to justify death or a poor outcome (i.e., unexpected deaths). It is also helpful to identify patients who have survived injuries that predictably should have caused death (i.e., survivors). The scoring systems are based on anatomic or physiologic data.

1. The **revised trauma score** (RTS) is the most commonly used physiologic estimate of injury.
  a. The RTS is based on the **GCS,** systolic blood pressure, and respiratory rate (Table 21-3).
  b. The RTS ranges from 1 to 8. A score of 4+ is associated with a probability of survival of 60%.

2. The **GCS** (Table 21-2) is uniquely important and is a key component of RTS. It is important to the **secondary survey.**

3. The **anatomic score** is based on the abbreviated injury scale (AIS), which is a list of hundreds of injuries assigned values of 1 (minor) to 6 (usually fatal).
  a. The AIS is summarized in the injury severity score (ISS). The ISS is calculated by summing the squares of the three highest AIS scores in different regions: head/neck, face, throat, abdomen and pelvis, intestines, and external.

TABLE 21-3 Glasgow Coma Scale

1. **Eye opening**
   Spontaneous _____ 4
   To voice _____ 3
   To pain _____ 2
   None _____ 1
2. **Verbal response**
   Oriented _____ 5
   Confused _____ 4
   Inappropriate words _____ 3
   Incomprehensible sounds _____ 2
   None _____ 1
3. **Motor response**
   Obeys commands _____ 6
   Localizes pain _____ 5
   Withdraw (pain) _____ 4
   Flexion (pain) _____ 3
   Extension (pain) _____ 2
   None _____ 1
   Total Glasgow Coma Scale points (1 + 2 + 3) _____

   b. The ISS ranges from 1 to 75. An AIS 6 injury receives an ISS score of 75. An ISS in the 40+ range is associated with approximately a 50% survival.

4. The above methodology (i.e., trauma score and ISS) is combined in outcome evaluation using the trauma and injury severity score (**TRISS**) **methodology** (Fig. 21-1).
   a. **Revised trauma score (RTS) is plotted against ISS** (Fig. 21-1), and a 50% probability of survival (PS) isobar is drawn.
   b. Deaths should be above the PS 50 isobar, and survivors below it. Outliers are cases worthy of audit; they are not necessarily truly unexpected survivors or deaths unless the audit confirms the TRISS-predicted outcome.
   c. Many statistical methods have been developed to compare the probable outcome of a given injury to the actual outcome seen in the trauma center. The ultimate statistical tool has yet to be developed.

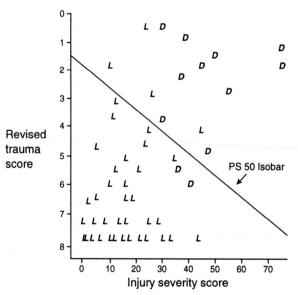

FIGURE 21-1 "TRISS" methodology combines the revised trauma score and the injury severity score. Deaths are plotted above the 50% probability of survival (PS 50) isobar, whereas survivors fall below the isobar. However, there are some unexpected deaths, which are plotted below the PS 50 isobar, and some unexpected survivors, which are plotted above the PS 50 isobar.

II **BURNS**

A **Overview**   The initial treatment of burns is based on the same principles and priorities as for other forms of trauma (see I A 2 b [1]). However, one **special priority** is to stop any continuing burn injury caused by smoldering clothes or corrosive chemicals by using neutral solutions to flush away all garments from the injured area. It is also mandatory to assess any concomitant injuries. The management of the burned patient depends on the depth, extent, and location of the burned area. Transfer of the burn patient to a burn center or consultation with the center should be considered for all but minimal burn injuries.

1. **Depth of burns**
   a. **First-degree burns (involvement of epidermis only).** Clinical findings are limited to erythema.
   b. **Second-degree (partial-thickness or intradermal) burns**
      (1) Clinical findings include vesicles, swelling, and a moist surface.
      (2) Partial-thickness burns are painful and are hypersensitive to a light touch or even the movement of air.
      (3) Epithelial remnants (skin appendages) are spared.
      (4) Second-degree burns are categorized into superficial and deep dermal burns.
   c. **Third-degree (full-thickness, entire depth of dermis) burns**
      (1) These burns have a charred, waxen, or leathery appearance and may be white or grayish in color. They usually appear dry. Thrombosed vessels may be evident.
      (2) The burn surface is pain free and is anesthetic to a pinprick or to touch.
2. **Extent of burns.** This is determined by the **"rule of nines"** (Fig. 21-2).
   a. **Inpatient treatment** is required for a patient with either:
      (1) Full-thickness burns extending over 2% or more of the body surface area (BSA)
      (2) Partial-thickness burns extending over 10% or more of the BSA

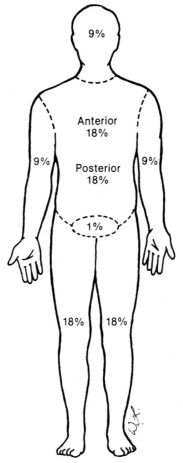

Figure 21-2   Rule of nines. The body surface area is divided into anatomic areas, each of which is 9% (or a multiple thereof) of the total BSA. This is a simple method of estimating the total burn surface.

    b. Intravenous fluid resuscitation is required for all partial- or full-thickness burns extending over 20% or more of the BSA.

  3. Location of burns

    a. Inpatient treatment is required for second- or third-degree burns of the face, hands, feet, or genitalia.

    b. Second- or third-degree burns involving major flexion creases usually require hospital treatment to minimize contractures and other late problems.

    c. Second and third-degree burns exceeding 20% BSA.

B **Airway control and ventilation**

  1. Airway obstruction may develop rapidly after inhalation injury or may be delayed. **Delayed airway obstruction** is due to progressive swelling and is apt to develop 24–48 hours after the injury. The possibility should be suspected if any of the following conditions are present:

    a. A history of being burned in a confined space

    b. A facial burn or singed facial hair

    c. Charring or carbon particles in the oropharynx

    d. Carbonaceous sputum

    e. Circumferential burns of the trunk, especially those with a thick eschar (which may require emergency excision—see II D 5)

  2. Measurement of arterial blood gases (see Chapter 1, VII C 5 f) is indicated as well as measurement of carbon monoxide level (carboxyhemoglobin value over 10% is significant) (Rx: F_iO_2 100%).

  3. Endotracheal intubation should be performed before the patient develops respiratory problems. Intubation is preferable to a tracheostomy in the patient with burns of the face, neck, or respiratory tract because tracheostomy through a burn carries a high mortality.

C **Circulatory support and fluid resuscitation**   Major burns—those involving 20% or more of the BSA—call for fluid resuscitation.

  1. Intravenous fluids should be administered through a 14- or 16-gauge intravenous catheter.

    a. The catheter may be placed through the burn wound, if required.

    b. Intravenous fluids should not be given via a lower extremity because the site is prone to sepsis and its increased mortality risk.

  2. Fluid resuscitation should begin with lactated Ringer's solution.

    a. The **volume to be given** is calculated as follows:

      (1) For adults: % BSA burned $\times$ kg body weight $\times$ 2–4 mL electrolyte solution

      (2) For children: % BSA burned $\times$ kg body weight $\times$ 3 mL electrolyte solution

      (3) The percentage of the BSA that is burned is estimated by the "rule of nines" (Fig. 21-2).

    b. Half of the calculated amount of fluid is given in the first 8 hours, and the remaining half is distributed over the succeeding 16 hours.

    c. The volume and rate of fluid administration should be varied, if necessary, depending on the central venous pressure, urine output, and other vital signs.

      (1) **Optimal urine output** is 30–50 mL/hour in adults and 1 mL/kg of body weight/hour in children.

      (2) To aid urine flow and to allow monitoring of output, an indwelling urethral catheter should be inserted early, even in children.

    d. Evaporative hypotonic fluid loss is evident after the first 24 hours.

      (1) Intravenous fluids at a rate to maintain serum sodium concentration at 140 mEq/L (approximately 4–5 L in a 70-kg patient with 50% burn)

      (2) Colloid (controversial) at a rate of 0.3–0.5 mL plasma/kg body weight/% burn

D **Burn wound care**

  1. Cold compresses may be applied to relieve the pain of partial-thickness burns if the burns cover less than 10% of the BSA. If burns cover a large area, cold compresses or immersion in water will cause an unacceptable lowering of the body temperature with associated problems.

  2. Maintenance of body temperature is important, especially in children, who have a high evaporative heat loss and may rapidly become hypothermic.

3. **Shielding the burn from air movement** by covering it with a clean, warm linen dressing will help to relieve the pain of partial-thickness burns.

4. **Topical antimicrobial treatment** with agents such as silver nitrate solution is usually recommended for deep second-degree and third-degree burns. However, only specific antibacterial burn wound medications should be applied to the burn.

5. **Debridement and escharectomy** are best performed in specialized centers; however, escharotomy may be urgently required in circumferential extremity wounds, causing distal circulatory impairment, and in circumferential trunk or neck wounds, causing respiratory impairment.

E **Other considerations** in the care of burn patients

1. **NG intubation** is indicated for any patient with nausea or vomiting and for most patients with burns covering 25% or more of the BSA.

2. **Analgesia** should be confined to conservative use of intravenous narcotics in small, frequent doses.

3. **Systemic antibiotics** are usually not indicated. However, in some situations, particularly in the early treatment of patients with partial-thickness burns, prophylaxis against β-hemolytic streptococci is warranted.

4. **Tetanus toxoid** with or without hyperimmune human globulin should be given if the patient's immunization status is not current (according to ACS guidelines).

5. **Chemical burns**
   a. Alkali burns are generally deeper and more serious than acid burns.
   b. All chemical burns should be treated by flushing with neutral solutions.
      (1) Immediate drenching in a shower or with a hose is helpful.
      (2) Burns of the eye require extensive flushing over an 8-hour period.

6. **Electrical burns** are usually deeper and more severe than indicated by the surface appearance.
   a. **Muscle and soft tissue injury.** Electrical energy is converted to heat as it traverses the body along the path of least resistance (i.e., blood vessels and nerves). Thus, muscles closest to bone—which has a high resistance and, therefore, generates the most heat—incur the most damage.
      (1) **Muscle involvement** may be markedly underestimated by attention to the surface wounds alone (e.g., fluid requirements are about 50% higher than estimated by surface wounds).
         (a) Brawny edema is characteristic.
         (b) Early escharotomy, fasciotomy, and debridement are often necessary, and repeated explorations at 24–48 hours may be needed.
      (2) Serious **soft tissue injury** results from **high-voltage electrical burns** (generally considered more than 1,000 volts); **low-voltage electrical burns** (household outlets) cause less soft tissue injury but may cause asystole and apnea.
   b. **Surface burns** occur at both the entrance and exit points of the current. Unsuspected exit sites, including the scalp, feet, or perineum, should be sought.
   c. **Oliguria** is common, as is **acidosis.**
      (1) Urine output should be maintained at high levels—at least 100 mL/hour in adults. Mannitol administration is usually needed to maintain this level and is mandatory in the presence of myoglobinuria.
      (2) Arterial blood pH should be monitored and maintained with intravenous bicarbonate, given as 50 mEq every half hour until the pH reaches normal levels.
   d. **Myocardial infarction** (immediate or delayed) is well-described postinjury, thus making continuous cardiac monitoring essential in all patients with electrical burns.
   e. **Transverse myelitis** and **cataracts** are long-term sequelae.

chapter 22

Spleen

R. ANTHONY CARABASI III • JOHN C. KAIRYS • JOHN S. RADOMSKI

I INTRODUCTION

A **Anatomy**

1. **Developmental considerations**
   a. The spleen develops from mesenchymal tissue in the dorsal mesogastrium. This tissue rotates to the left as development progresses. By the end of the third gestational month, the organ is formed. The point at which the spleen remains attached to the dorsal mesogastrium becomes the **gastrosplenic ligament.**
   b. The organ itself consists of an outer capsule and trabeculae, which enclose the pulp. The pulp consists of three zones:
      (1) The **white pulp** is essentially a lymph node. It contains lymphocytes, macrophages, and plasma cells in a reticular network.
      (2) The **red pulp** consists of cords of reticular cells with sinuses in between.
      (3) The **marginal zone** is a poorly defined vascular space between the pulps.
   c. The adult spleen weighs between 100 g and 150 g and measures $12 \times 7 \times 4$ cm.

2. **Location.** The spleen is located in the left upper quadrant of the abdomen and is protected by the eighth to the eleventh ribs. It is bordered by the left kidney posteriorly, the diaphragm superiorly, and the fundus of the stomach and the splenic flexure of the colon anteriorly.

3. **Vasculature**
   a. The main blood supply is the **splenic artery,** which is a branch of the celiac axis. It travels along the superior border of the pancreas. At the hilus, it branches into trabecular arteries, which terminate in small vessels to the splenic pulp.
   b. The **splenic vein** crosses behind or at the lower border of the pancreas. It joins the superior mesenteric vein to form the portal vein (Fig. 22-1).

B **Physiology**   The spleen has multiple functions, some of which remain poorly understood. Its most important functions are its ability to act as a **blood filter** and its role in the **immunologic process** of the body.

1. **Filtering functions. Splenic blood flow** is approximately 350 L/day of blood. Most blood elements pass through rapidly and uneventfully.
   a. **Removal of old or abnormal red blood cells**
      (1) The spleen removes about 20 mL/day of aged or abnormal red blood cells.
      (2) Cells that have immunoglobulin G (IgG) on their surfaces are removed by monocytes in the spleen. This removal of cells may be the mechanism of increased cell destruction in some diseases, such as idiopathic thrombocytopenic purpura and autoimmune hemolytic anemia.
   b. **Removal of abnormal white blood cells, normal and abnormal platelets, and cellular debris**

2. **Immunologic functions**
   a. **Opsonin production.** The entire reticuloendothelial system is capable of removing well-opsonized bacteria from the circulation, but the spleen, with its highly efficient filtering mechanism, is particularly suited to removing poorly opsonized or encapsulated pathogens.

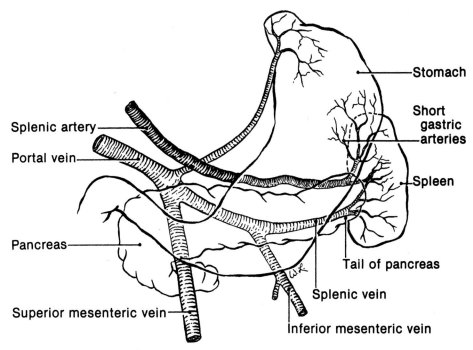

FIGURE 22-1 Anatomic relationships of the spleen.

    b. Antibody synthesis. This synthesis occurs mainly in the white pulp, where soluble antigens stimulate the production of immunoglobulin M (IgM).

    c. Protection from infection. It is well established that splenectomy leaves some patients more susceptible to infection.

3. Storage functions. Approximately one third of the body's **platelets** are stored in the spleen. In some pathologic states, the percentage is increased.

II   **HYPERSPLENISM**

Hypersplenism refers to the exaggerated destruction or sequestration of circulating red blood cells, white blood cells, or platelets by the spleen. The term should not be confused with **splenomegaly**, which refers only to physical enlargement of the spleen.

A **Primary hypersplenism** is uncommon.

B **Secondary hypersplenism** is caused by an identifiable underlying disease, such as:

1. Disorders of splenic blood flow

2. Hematopoietic disorders leading to increased red blood cell turnover

3. Immune disorders

4. Infiltrative disorders

5. Infectious diseases

6. Neoplastic diseases

C **Presentation**

1. **Anemia, leukopenia, or thrombocytopenia** may be noted on a routine laboratory workup.
    a. Anemia may lead to pallor, fatigue, and dyspnea.
    b. Leukopenia may lead to increased susceptibility to infection.
    c. Thrombocytopenia is characterized by easy bruising and epistaxis.

2. **Splenomegaly** may be found incidentally during the physical examination or in a radiologic imaging study.

3. The patient may present with **pain** secondary to splenic enlargement or rupture.

D **Evaluation**

1. **Peripheral blood smears** may demonstrate a decreased number of red blood cells, white blood cells, or platelets.
   a. **Reticulocytosis** is frequently observed if the hypersplenism is causing an increased turnover of red blood cells.
   b. **Abnormal red blood cell morphology** is sometimes diagnostic for the underlying hematologic disorder (e.g., spherocytosis).

2. **Bone marrow aspirate**
   a. A compensatory increase in megakaryocytes should be observed if there is sequestration of platelets in the spleen.
   b. Abnormalities of hematopoiesis may be identified as well.

3. **Radiologic imaging**
   a. An **ultrasound** or a **computed tomography (CT) scan** can accurately document the size of the spleen as well as determine any structural abnormalities. Other findings on the scans may suggest an underlying disease process.
   b. **Radioisotope scans** may demonstrate a shortened half-life for circulating blood elements and their sequestration in the spleen.

4. **Immunologic tests** using specific antibodies may be diagnostic for certain diseases, particularly those with an autoimmune basis.

E **Treatment** depends on the underlying condition. Table 22-1 summarizes the role of surgery in various pathologic conditions.

TABLE 22-1   Absolute and Relative Indications for Splenectomy

Type of Pathology	Absolute Indications	Relative Indications
Primary splenic disorders	Splenic cyst	Primary hypersplenism
Disorders of splenic blood flow	Bleeding esophagogastric varices associated with splenic vein thrombosis	Portal hypertension with severe hypersplenism
Hematopoietic disorders	Heriditary spherocytosis	Hereditary elliptocytosis
		Thalassemia major
		Sickle cell anemia
		Congenital erythropoietic porphyria
Immune disorders	None	Idiopathic autoimmune hemolytic anemia
		Idiopathic thrombocytopenic purpura
		Thrombotic thrombocytopenic purpura
		Felty's syndrome
		Systemic lupus erythematosus
Infiltrative disorders	None	Myeloid metaplasia
		Sarcoidosis
		Gaucher's disease
Infectious diseases	Splenic abscess Echinococcal cyst	
Neoplastic diseases	Primary splenic tumors	Staging laparotomy for Hodgkin's disease or non-Hodgkin's lymphoma
		Chronic lymphocytic leukemia
		Chronic myelogenous leukemia
		Hairy cell leukemia
Miscellaneous	Massive splenic trauma Spontaneous rupture	

III **PATHOLOGIC CONDITIONS AFFECTING THE SPLEEN**

A **Primary splenic disorders**

1. **Primary hypersplenism** is essentially a **diagnosis of exclusion;** it is made only after possible causes of secondary hypersplenism have been ruled out.
   a. It is rare, and it affects mainly women.
   b. There is an exaggerated destruction or sequestration of circulating blood elements.
      (1) Any one or all of the formed blood elements may be involved.
      (2) The hematologic findings may be accompanied by recurrent fevers and infections.
   c. Splenomegaly is almost always present.
   d. It may, in some cases, actually be an early manifestation of lymphoma or leukemia.
   e. The **treatment** is **splenectomy.** Steroids do not improve the condition.

2. **Splenic cysts** may be idiopathic or, more commonly, may result from previous trauma. Surgery is indicated if the cysts become large enough to cause pain or torsion or if they exert a significant mass effect on surrounding structures. With simple cysts, unroofing is sufficient, thus preserving splenic function.

B **Disorders of splenic blood flow**

1. **Portal hypertension** may cause passive splenic congestion.
   a. It is the **most common mechanism** of secondary hypersplenism.
   b. Causes of portal hypertension include alcoholic cirrhosis, viral hepatitis, Budd-Chiari syndrome, and congestive heart failure.
   c. Hypersplenism associated with portal hypertension is usually mild and clinically insignificant. Only 15% of patients develop significant hypersplenism; therefore, isolated splenectomy is generally not indicated.

2. **Splenic vein thrombosis** can cause secondary hypersplenism with massive splenomegaly.
   a. **Cause.** Pancreatitis is the usual cause of the thrombosis.
   b. **Presentation.** The patient may present with bleeding from esophageal or, more characteristically, proximal gastric varices.
   c. **Treatment.** The hypersplenism and bleeding varices are cured by splenectomy.

3. **Splenic artery aneurysm** (see Chapter 7)

C **Hematopoietic disorders**

1. **Hereditary spherocytosis** is one of a group of hereditary hemolytic anemias that cause the most severe symptoms.
   a. **Characteristics**
      (1) Hereditary spherocytosis is characterized by a defect of the red blood cell membrane that results in loss of red blood cell surface area, which causes the cell to be spherical (hence the name), small, and more susceptible to lysis than normal red blood cells.
      (2) The cell membrane is thick and rigid, which causes the cells to be held in the splenic pulp. This holding of cells leads to cell lysis, due to deprivation of glucose and adenosine triphosphate (ATP), and occurs only in the spleen.
      (3) It is transmitted as an autosomal dominant trait.
   b. **Symptoms**
      (1) Symptoms of hereditary spherocytosis include malaise, abdominal discomfort, jaundice, anemia, and splenomegaly.
      (2) The disease may be complicated by gallstones (which are rare in patients younger than 10 years of age) and by chronic leg ulcers that heal only after splenectomy.
   c. **Diagnosis** is based on the preceding clinical findings and the results of laboratory studies, which include a demonstration of the following:
      (1) Spherocytes and an elevated reticulocyte count on a Wright-stained blood smear
      (2) Increased osmotic fragility of the red blood cells
      (3) Chromium 51 (^{51}Cr)-tagged red blood cells, which have a greatly shortened half-life and are sequestered in the spleen

    d. Treatment is splenectomy.

       (1) This procedure cures the anemia and jaundice in all patients. Failure of splenectomy to cure the patient is normally caused by an accessory spleen that has been overlooked during the operation.

       (2) The operation should be delayed until 4 years of age, if possible, to decrease the chance of postsplenectomy sepsis (see V F 1).

       (3) The gallbladder should be removed at the time of splenectomy if gallstones are present.

2. Other congenital hemolytic anemias. Although splenectomy is not curative, it is indicated occasionally because it reduces the need for multiple transfusions in the following conditions:

  a. Enzyme deficiencies, such as glucose-6-phosphate dehydrogenase (G6PD) deficiency and pyruvate kinase deficiency

  b. Hereditary elliptocytosis, in which most of the patient's erythrocytes are misshapen (i.e., they are elliptical) and there are varying degrees of anemia and red blood cell destruction

  c. Thalassemia major, which is transmitted as a dominant trait and is characterized by defective hemoglobin synthesis that causes homozygotes to have severe anemia and hepatosplenomegaly

3. Sickle cell anemia

  a. Most patients with sickle cell anemia "autosplenectomize" because of multiple infarcts caused by stagnation and stasis of the abnormal red blood cells.

  b. These patients may require splenectomy in rare cases in which excessive splenic sequestration of red blood cells is documented or when areas of infarction develop an abscess.

4. Congenital erythropoietic porphyria is a rare autosomal recessive defect of pyrrole metabolism that leads to deposition of porphyrins in the skin and other tissues.

  a. Patients have photosensitivity, bullous dermatitis, and hemolytic anemia.

  b. Splenectomy improves the hemolytic anemia and decreases tissue levels of porphyrins.

D **Immune disorders**

1. Idiopathic autoimmune hemolytic anemia occurs most commonly in persons older than 50 years of age and occurs twice as often in women than in men.

  a. Clinical presentation

    (1) In this disorder, both warm and cold hemolytic antibodies have been described. These antibodies presumably shorten the life of the red blood cells.

    (2) The anemia is accompanied by reticulocytosis. There is splenomegaly in 50% of the patients, and there may be mild jaundice.

  b. Diagnosis. The direct Coombs' test result is positive. ^{51}Cr-tagged red blood cells may demonstrate sequestration in the spleen.

  c. Treatment. The disease may run a self-limited course that requires no treatment.

    (1) Steroids and **azathioprine** are administered in more persistent cases.

    (2) Splenectomy is helpful in some patients, especially if they have demonstrated excessive splenic sequestration of ^{51}Cr-tagged red blood cells, and if steroids are ineffective or contraindicated.

2. Idiopathic thrombocytopenic purpura (ITP)

  a. The **etiology is unknown** but is presumed to be immunologic because most patients with chronic disease have platelet-agglutinating antibodies that rapidly destroy transfused platelets.

    (1) The **acute form** is more common in children younger than 16 years. Eighty percent of affected individuals recover spontaneously.

    (2) The **chronic form** is most common in adults, and women predominate in a ratio of 3:1.

  b. Clinical presentation

    (1) This disease is characterized by a decreased platelet count accompanied by increased megakaryocytes in the bone marrow. **The spleen is usually not enlarged.**

    (2) The disease presents as unexplained ecchymoses or petechiae, often accompanied by bleeding from the gums or hematuria.

  c. Treatment

    (1) Steroids induce remission in 75% of patients; approximately 20% of these patients have a sustained response.

(2) Splenectomy is commonly indicated in individuals who do not respond to steroids or in those who have a relapse after steroids are tapered off. It is also indicated if central nervous system bleeding occurs. It produces a sustained remission in 70% of patients.

3. **Thrombotic thrombocytopenic purpura (TTP)** is a rapidly progressive and usually fatal disease. It is also thought to have an immunologic basis.

   a. **Clinical presentation includes** fever, thrombocytopenic purpura, hemolytic anemia, neurologic disturbances, and renal failure.

   b. **Diagnosis** is confirmed only by biopsy of a purpuric lesion. This characteristic vascular lesion consists of occlusion of arterioles and capillaries by a hyaline membrane.

   c. **Treatment.** The most effective treatments are **splenectomy** and **steroid therapy.** Plasmapheresis, antiplatelet agents (e.g., dextran), or exchange transfusions with fresh blood have resulted in survival in a few patients.

   d. **Prognosis.** The long-term survival rate is less than 10%, even with optimal therapy.

4. **Felty's syndrome**

   a. **Clinical presentation**

      (1) Felty's syndrome is a **triad** consisting of chronic rheumatoid arthritis, splenomegaly, and granulocytopenia.

      (2) Spontaneous serious infections can occur due to neutropenia, and splenectomy is helpful in this group of patients.

   b. **Treatment. Splenectomy** may also be indicated for management of intractable leg ulcers, severe thrombocytopenia, and anemia.

5. Although **systemic lupus erythematosus** affects neither blood cells nor the spleen directly, patients with significant anemia or thrombocytopenia may benefit from splenectomy.

E **Infiltrative diseases**

1. **Myeloid metaplasia** is thought to be related to polycythemia vera and myelogenous leukemia.

   a. **Clinical presentation**

      (1) It is characterized by connective tissue proliferation in the bone marrow, liver, spleen, and lymph nodes and is accompanied by proliferation of the hematopoietic tissue of the liver, spleen, and long bones.

      (2) The usual symptoms are anemia and splenomegaly, which usually appear in middle-aged or older adults. Secondary hypersplenism may develop.

   b. **Treatment**

      (1) Primary treatment consists of **alkylating agents** to reduce the size of the spleen and **male hormones** to stimulate failing bone marrow and to treat anemia.

      (2) **Splenectomy** does not change the course of the disease, but it may help to control the hypersplenism.

2. **Sarcoidosis**

   a. Patients typically have diffuse lymphadenopathy, skin lesions, and pulmonary abnormalities. Approximately 25% of patients develop hypersplenism.

   b. There is no specific treatment, but patients with significant hypersplenism may experience resolution of their hematologic abnormalities after splenectomy.

3. **Gaucher's disease** is an inborn error of metabolism characterized by deposition of glucosylceramide lipids throughout the reticuloendothelial system, which causes hepatosplenomegaly and bone pain.

   a. Significant hypersplenism is an indication for splenectomy.

   b. Because the diagnosis is often made in childhood, partial splenectomy may be indicated to preserve some immunologic function.

F **Infectious diseases** may cause splenomegaly and hypersplenism. Treatment is generally medical, although surgery may be indicated for abscess or disease localized to the spleen.

1. **Bacterial infections** may cause abscess formation or transient splenic enlargement. **Splenic abscess** is uncommon but has a high mortality rate when it occurs.

    a. Causes include the following:

      (1) Infection of a pre-existing lesion, such as a hematoma or an infarct

      (2) Direct spread from adjacent structures, such as the pancreas or colon

      (3) Hematogenous seeding from a remote size (especially in users of intravenous drugs) or during overwhelming bacteremia (e.g., in endocarditis)

      (4) Most common organisms causing infection are *Staphylococcus aureus* or streptococcus. Less common pathogens include Salmonella or anarobes.

    b. Diagnosis should be suspected if signs of abscess, such as fever and an elevated white blood cell count, occur in association with left upper quadrant fullness or tenderness. It can be confirmed by CT scan and scanning with technetium-99m (^{99m}Tc).

    c. Treatment is broad spectrum antibiotics and splenectomy. Percutaneous drainage may be considered in select cases, but hemorrhage is a potential complication.

2. Viral infections including mononucleosis, human immunodeficiency virus, and hepatitis may cause transient splenomegaly and hypersplenism.

3. Parasitic infections including malaria, leishmaniasis, or trypanosomiasis affect blood cells and may cause splenomegaly. An echinococcal cyst may develop in the spleen. Partial or total splenectomy is curative.

4. Fungal infection with histoplasmosis produces characteristic areas of calcification within the spleen.

G Neoplastic diseases

1. Primary splenic tumors are rare.

    a. They include lymphoma, sarcoma, hemangioma, and hamartoma.

    b. Symptoms are caused by the enlarged spleen, and there may be associated hypersplenism.

    c. Treatment is splenectomy.

2. Metastatic disease from solid tumors is uncommon, probably owing to its efficient immune mechanism.

3. Hodgkin's disease. Advances in therapy have greatly improved chances for the cure or long-term survival of patients with this disease. Treatment may include radiation therapy alone, chemotherapy alone, or a combination of both.

    a. Types of staging (see Chapter 19)

    b. Staging laparotomy consists of liver biopsy, splenectomy, complete abdominal exploration, and sampling of lymph nodes from multiple areas but is now performed only rarely.

      (1) Indications for staging laparotomy in patients with Hodgkin's disease are changing.

        (a) Traditionally, patients with clinical stage I or II disease and sometimes stage IIIA disease were considered for staging laparotomy.

        (b) Studies suggest that laparotomy may not be needed for many patients.

          (i) Current imaging techniques have improved diagnostic accuracy.

          (ii) Oncologists are now treating more stages of Hodgkin's disease with chemotherapy alone or in combination with radiation therapy, thus obviating laparotomy.

          (iii) There is no evidence that splenectomy improves the survival rate.

          (iv) There appears to be an increased risk of secondary leukemias in patients who have undergone staging laparotomy and splenectomy.

          (v) There is a risk of morbidity and mortality with laparotomy.

        (c) Laparotomy is clearly not indicated in patients with stage IIIB or IV disease. Chemotherapy is the treatment of choice.

4. Non-Hodgkin's lymphoma

    a. Staging for non-Hodgkin's lymphoma uses the same classification as for Hodgkin's disease. Careful evaluation reveals stage III or IV disease in most patients.

    b. Laparotomy is not frequently used in non-Hodgkin's lymphoma. Percutaneous liver biopsy, laparoscopy, or bone marrow biopsy frequently reveals diffuse disease.

    c. Splenectomy may be useful in some of these patients to treat hypersplenism or to relieve symptoms of massive splenomegaly.

5. **Leukemias**
   a. Patients with **chronic lymphocytic leukemia (CLL)** or **chronic myelogenous leukemia (CML)** may develop thrombocytopenia and massive splenomegaly. Splenectomy is indicated for symptomatic relief.
   b. Patients with **hairy cell leukemia** and hypersplenism may benefit from splenectomy.

H **Miscellaneous lesions**

1. **Rupture of the spleen** may follow either penetrating or nonpenetrating trauma as well as iatrogenic injury, or rupture may occur spontaneously.
   a. **Traumatic rupture** (see Chapter 21 I C 7e–8b)
   b. **Iatrogenic (intraoperative) trauma** accounts for 20% of all splenectomies. The trauma results from excessive traction on the splenic attachments or from misplacement of retractors.
   c. **Spontaneous rupture** usually occurs because of massive splenomegaly due to an associated disease.

2. **Splenosis is autotransplantation** of splenic fragments throughout the abdominal cavity.
   a. Autotransplantation has been attempted to preserve splenic immunologic function following splenectomy for trauma. No benefit has ever been proved.
   b. Splenosis may occur spontaneously after rupture of the spleen. When splenectomy is being performed for disease, splenosis may lead to resumption of the hypersplenic state.

3. **Aneurysms of the splenic artery** (see Chapter 7)

4. **Ectopic and accessory spleens**
   a. An **ectopic spleen** is caused by a long splenic pedicle, which allows the spleen to "wander" about the abdomen.
   b. **Accessory spleens** are found in approximately 10% of autopsies. These spleens are usually located near the hilus or the tail of the pancreas and less frequently in the mesentery. They are significant only if they are overlooked during splenectomy for hematologic disease.

IV. TECHNICAL ASPECTS OF SPLENECTOMY

A Traditionally, the spleen has been removed through a **laparotomy** incision, either through a midline or a left subcostal incision.

1. There are two basic approaches for removing the spleen.
   a. The spleen is lifted up along with the tail of the pancreas by dividing the splenophrenic and splenocolic ligament. The blood supply in the hilum is then controlled and divided.
      (1) This approach is particularly effective in a patient with splenic rupture and hemorrhage.
   b. Alternatively, the splenic vessels are first approached through the lesser sac and ligated. The hilar dissection is then completed, and the remaining ligamentous attachments are divided.
      (1) This approach is often preferred in a patient with massive splenomegaly.
      (2) Another benefit is that by ligating the artery first, the patient receives an "autotransfusion" of the red blood cells and platelets sequestered in the spleen.

B More recently, surgeons skilled in advanced laparoscopic techniques have advocated the use of **laparoscopic splenectomy.**

1. The technique is especially suited to conditions where the spleen is not massively enlarged, especially idiopathic thrombocytopenic purpura.

2. The spleen is mobilized by dividing its attachments and elevating it so that the hilum is exposed. The vessels are then secured and divided by using a stapling device.

3. The spleen is placed in a sturdy plastic bag and is broken up into small fragments. The organ is then extracted through a port incision.
   a. Care must be taken to avoid rupture of the bag; otherwise, splenosis may result.
   b. Some surgeons have also demonstrated that even massively enlarged spleens can be removed in this fashion.

V COMPLICATIONS AFTER SPLENECTOMY

A **Atelectasis** of the left lower lung is the most common complication.

B **Injury to surrounding structures**

1. The **gastric wall** may be injured in the course of controlling the short gastric vessels. In extreme cases, this injury may lead to necrosis of the gastric wall with delayed perforation.

2. The **tail of the pancreas** may be injured during attempts to secure hemostasis of the splenic pedicle. This injury may result in postoperative pancreatitis, abscess, or phlegmon formation.

C **Postoperative hemorrhage** may result from inadequate hemostasis of the splenic pedicle or the short gastric vessels.

D **Subphrenic abscess** may develop and is usually accompanied by a left pleural effusion.

E **Thrombocytosis** postoperatively is common. If the platelet count exceeds 1 million, anticoagulation may be required to prevent spontaneous thrombosis.

F **Postsplenectomy sepsis**

1. **Overview.** Some patients are susceptible to **overwhelming sepsis** following splenectomy. The syndrome begins with nonspecific, mild, influenzalike symptoms and progresses to high fever, shock, and death.
   a. In general, the younger the patient and the more serious the disease requiring the splenectomy, the greater is the risk for the development of overwhelming sepsis. The risk is greatest if splenectomy occurs during the first 2–4 years of life, particularly if it is done for a disease of the reticuloenclothelial system.
   b. In healthy adults who have the spleen removed for trauma, the incidence of overwhelming sepsis is low (<0.5%), but it is still higher than that in the normal population (0.01%).
   c. Approximately 80% of septic episodes occur within 2 years after splenectomy.
   d. Typically, the causitive organisms are encapsulated bacteria, including *Streptococcus pneumoniae*, *Neisseria meningitidis*, and *Haemophilus influenzae*.

2. **Prevention and treatment**
   a. **Polyvalent pneumococcal vaccine** should be given to all splenectomized patients, which will protect them from 80% of pathogenic pneumococci (the organisms that most commonly cause the sepsis).
   b. Vaccines for ***N. meningitidis*** and ***H. influenza****e* should be administered as well.
   c. **Prophylactic penicillin** may be given to high-risk pediatric patients.
   d. Patients should be instructed to seek medical attention immediately if symptoms begin, and penicillin therapy should be started in an attempt to prevent the full-blown syndrome from developing.

VI CRITICAL POINTS

1. The spleen is an important but not essential organ that has a role in filtering and sequestering circulating blood elements.

2. The spleen has an important immunologic role, filtering opsonized bacteria from the circulation and providing a site for antibody synthesis.

3. **Hypersplenism** should **not** be confused with **splenomegaly.**
   a. Hypersplenism refers to the exaggerated destruction of sequestration of circulating red blood cells, white blood cells, or platelets.
   b. Splenomegaly refers to physical enlargement of the spleen only.

4. **Primary** hypersplenism is uncommon and is a diagnosis of exclusion, occurring mostly in women.

5. Most cases of hypersplenism are **secondary** to other pathologic conditions.
   a. **Disorders of splenic blood flow,** including portal hypertension or splenic vein thrombosis
   b. **Hematopoietic disorders,** including hereditary spherocytosis, hemolytic anemias, sickle cell disease, or congenital erythropoietic porphyria

 c. Immunologic disorders, including idiopathic autoimmune hemolytic anemia, ITP, TTP, or Felty's syndrome.

  (1) ITP is one of the most common reasons for elective splenectomy. In this condition, the spleen is generally normal in size.

 d. Infiltrative diseases, including myeloid metaplasia, sarcoidosis, or Gaucher's disease

 e. Infection diseases, including bacterial, viral, parasitic, or fungal infections

  (1) *S. aureus* and streptococci are the most common etiologic agents.

 f. Neoplastic diseases of the spleen are uncommon but may include primary tumors, metastatic tumors, or hematologic disorders such as lymphoma. Staging laparotomies are now uncommonly performed.

6. **Traumatic rupture** of the spleen can often be managed nonoperatively. Splenectomy is reserved for those patients who are unstable or who have additional, massive injuries.

7. **The management of most cases of hypersplenism is medical. Splenectomy** usually has only a secondary role, when symptoms are significant or medical therapy fails to control the disease.

 a. The conditions where surgery is clearly indicated are bleeding esophagogastric varices associated with splenic vein thrombosis, hereditary spherocytosis, splenic abscess, echinococcal cyst, primary splenic tumors, massive splenic trauma, or spontaneous rupture (Table 22-1).

8. **Surgery** is frequently performed through a **laparotomy** incision but may also be performed **laparoscopically**, when the skill of the surgeon and the size of the spleen permit.

9. Patients undergoing splenectomy are at risk for developing **overwhelming postsplenectomy sepsis.** This risk is greatest in young children. The risk can be decreased by prophylactically immunizing patients preoperatively or postoperatively, if necessary.

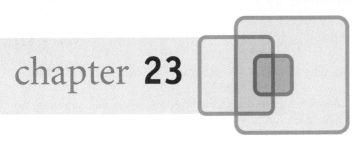

chapter 23

Breast

KAREN A. CHOJNACKI • DIANE R. GILLUM • KANDACE PETERSON •
FRANCIS E. ROSATO

I INTRODUCTION

A **Anatomy** (Tear-drop shape)

1. **Four quadrants**
   a. Upper inner quadrant
   b. Upper outer quadrant (includes the axillary tail of Spence), most common site for breast cancer
   c. Lower inner quadrant
   d. Lower outer quadrant

2. **Parenchyma**
   a. **Alveoli** (10–100) form each lobule.
   b. **Lobules** (20–40) form each lobe.
   c. **Lobes** (15–20) are radially arranged segments that are each drained by a duct; all lobes converge at the nipple.

B **Vasculature**

1. **Arterial supply**
   a. Internal mammary artery (60%)
   b. Lateral thoracic artery (30%)

2. **Venous return**
   a. Axillary vein (primary)
   b. Intercostal vein
   c. Internal mammary veins

3. **Lymphatic drainage** follows venous drainage.
   a. The **axillary chain** is important drainage for neoplastic disease and is divided into three levels (Fig. 23-1).
      (1) **Level 1** nodes are lateral to the pectoralis minor muscle.
      (2) **Level 2** nodes are behind the pectoralis minor muscle.
      (3) **Level 3** nodes are medial to the pectoralis minor muscle.
   b. **Rotter's nodes** consist of interpectoral nodal tissue. These nodes lie between the pectoralis major and minor muscle, and they have no major role in staging or prognosis.
   c. The **internal mammary chain** has relatively minimal drainage from the breast. Rarely, this chain may be the primary drainage from the breast, and the sentinel node will be found here.

II BREAST EVALUATION

A **Self breast examination (SBE)**   A **monthly SBE** is recommended, ideally just after the menses.

B **Physical examination** is done by a physician.

1. **Visual inspection.** The patient sits and raises her arms upward, then presses on her hips to contract the pectoralis major muscle.
   a. Check for **symmetry.**
   b. Observe for **skin changes:** color, texture, dimpling, edema (peu d'orange), and ulceration (visible tumor).
   c. Look for **nipple retraction and drainage.**

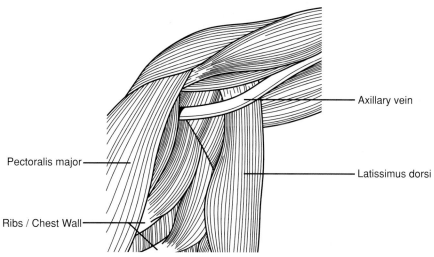

FIGURE 23-1 The borders of axillary dissection. Apex, axillary vein; lateral, latissimus dorsi muscle; medial, the lateral border of the pectoralis major muscle; inferior, the fifth to sixth rib.

2. **Palpation.** With the patient in a supine position and with the ipsilateral arm above the head and a pillow under the ipsilateral shoulder, the physician palpates the breast for masses or asymmetric densities.

3. The **axilla and supraclavicular region** should be examined for adenopathy.

C **Radiologic exam**

1. **Mammogram**
   a. A baseline mammogram is advised when the woman is 40 years of age and then yearly as long as the patient is in good health.
   b. The mammogram is done sooner if the patient has a family history of early breast cancer. For these patients, the first mammogram should be done 5 years earlier than the age of the family member when diagnosed with breast cancer. For example, a patient whose sister developed breast cancer at age 39 should have her first mammogram at age 34.
   c. Mammography can reveal the following: breast architecture, asymmetry, skin thickening, irregular masses, and microcalcifications.

2. **Ultrasound**
   a. Ultrasound is not recommended for routine screening.
   b. It is useful as a targeted exam for a symptomatic patient.
   c. It can further characterize abnormalities seen on mammogram or found on physical exam (i.e., cyst vs. solid mass).

3. **Magnetic resonance imaging (MRI)**
   a. Also not used for routine screening
   b. Very sensitive but not specific evaluation of the breast
   c. Especially useful in the evaluation of patients with mammographically dense breasts, patients with axillary disease, and negative mammogram
   d. MRI can detect the extent of tumor within the breast and residual tumor within the breast after lumpectomy and can differentiate between tumor and postsurgical scar.

D **Biopsy** is necessary to make a diagnosis.

1. **Fine-needle aspiration (FNA)** is useful in the evaluation of palpable lesions.
   a. **Cyst** aspiration is both diagnostic and therapeutic.
      (1) Cyst must be drained completely.
      (2) Cyst fluid must be nonbloody. If fluid is bloody, excision is recommended to rule out malignancy.
   b. If the lesion is **solid,** a fine-needle aspirate can extract cells, which can be examined cytologically. If cytology reveals atypia, excisional biopsy is recommended. If cytology reveals malignancy, further surgery is necessary.

2. **Core-needle biopsy** is used to evaluate palpable solid lesions.

3. **Incisional** biopsy may be useful for diagnosis of inflammatory breast cancer.

4. **Excisional** biopsy
   a. Completely removes the lesion
   b. It may be the only surgical treatment of breast tissue if the margins are adequate.
   c. It can be done using a local anesthetic with mild sedation.

5. **Nonpalpable radiographic abnormalities**
   a. A **needle-guided biopsy** is performed by excising the lesion after the radiologist places a localizing wire in the breast to identify the site. The lesion must be visible on two mammographic views to allow accurate needle placement.
   b. A **stereotactic or mammotome biopsy** uses computed mammographic equipment to deploy a core needle into mammographic abnormalities. This biopsy accurately samples nonpalpable lesions. This less invasive biopsy technique is indicated for patients with small nonpalpable radiodensities, single or multiple foci of calcifications, lesions seen on only one mammographic view, and lesions adjacent to breast implants.

III BENIGN BREAST DISEASE

A Infectious and inflammatory breast diseases

1. **Cellulitis, mastitis**
   a. Infection of the breast is usually associated with lactation.
   b. Bacteria enter through the nipple (*Staphylococcus* or *Streptococcus*). Treatment is a 10- to 14-day course of antibiotics to cover *Staphylococcus* and *Streptococcus*.
   c. Patient can continue to breast feed during treatment. If breast feeding is too painful, a breast pump should be used.

2. **Abscess** is a collection of purulent fluid within breast parenchyma. It is treated by surgical drainage.

3. A **chronic subareolar abscess** occurs at the base of the lactiferous duct. Squamous metaplasia of the duct may occur.
   a. A sinus tract to the areola develops.
   b. **Treatment** requires complete excision of the sinus tract.
   c. **Recurrences** are common, especially if the entire tract is not excised.

4. **Mondor's disease** is phlebitis of the thoracoepigastric vein.
   a. A palpable, visible, tender cord runs along the upper quadrants of the breast along the course of the vein.
   b. Disease is self-limited, but anti-inflammatory agents and warm compresses improve patient comfort and shorten disease course.

B Benign lesions of the breast

1. **Fibrocystic change** (chronic cystic mastitis). This term is used for a broad spectrum of benign breast changes. It is characterized by nodularity with or without pain. Any dominant masses must be biopsied.

2. **Fibroadenoma**
   a. Fibroadenoma is a well-defined tumor of the breast.
   b. It consists of fibrous stromal tissue with an epithelial component.
   c. Fibroadenoma is most common in younger women.
   d. It is mobile and well circumscribed.
   e. Usually, it is well visualized by ultrasound.
   f. FNA, core biopsy, or excision is used to establish diagnosis.

3. **Phyllodes tumors** were previously referred to as cystosarcoma phyllodes.
   a. These tumors are giant fibroadenomas that are rarely malignant.
   b. They consist more of a cellular stroma than a fibroadenoma.
   c. **Malignancy** is determined in part by an increased number of mitoses per high-power field compared with **benign** phyllodes tumors.

         (1) Treatment is with a wide local excision. Inadequate local excision is associated with higher rates of local recurrence.

4. **Sclerosing adenosis** is a proliferation of acini in the lobules, which may appear to have invaded the surrounding breast stroma.

5. **Atypical hyperplasia** has three to six times higher the risk of breast cancer.

6. **Fat necrosis** is associated with trauma or radiation therapy to the breast but may simulate cancer with a mass or skin retraction. (The biopsy is diagnostic.)

7. **Mammary duct ectasia**
   a. It can be found in older women.
   b. Dilatation of the subareolar ducts can occur.
   c. A palpable retroareolar mass, nipple discharge, or retraction can be present.
   d. Treatment involves excision of the area.

8. **Cysts.** The diagnosis is made by needle aspiration.
   a. **Color**
      (1) A **simple cyst** has clear or green fluid and is benign.
      (2) A **milk-filled cyst,** called a galactocele, is benign.
      (3) A **bloody cyst** may represent atypia or malignancy, and excision should be considered.
   b. **Cyst resolution**
      (1) **Complete resolution.** Perform follow-up exam to determine if cyst recurs.
      (2) **Incomplete resolution.** Treat as a breast mass and excise.

9. **Intraductal papilloma**
   a. A true polyp of the breast duct that often presents as bloody nipple discharge; treated by central duct excision

C **Nipple discharge**

1. Usually a benign condition secondary to fibrocystic change or papilloma
   a. Features of **benign** discharge:
      (1) Bilateral
      (2) Clear, green, white fluid
      (3) Occurs with stimulation/palpation of breast
   b. Features of **malignant** discharge:
      (1) Unilateral
      (2) Bloody fluid
      (3) Occurs spontaneously

2. **Evaluation and treatment**
   a. **Cytologic examination** can be performed on the discharge.
   b. A **mammogram** should be obtained to rule out an associated mass.
   c. The **drainage** is usually from an isolated nipple duct, which should be excised.

D **Mastalgia** refers to breast pain.

1. **Cyclic pain**
   a. This pain correlates with the menstrual cycle and is usually worse just before the menses.
   b. Treatment includes support with a bra and analgesics, if severe.

2. **Noncyclic pain** has no such pattern.
   a. **Treatment**
      (1) Restrict caffeine intake.
      (2) Wear a supportive bra.
      (3) Nonsteroidal anti-inflammatory drugs (NSAIDS)
      (4) Vitamin E (400 IU/day) and evening primrose oil (3 g/day) may provide symptomatic relief in some patients.
      (5) Severe cases may require treatment with tamoxifen or danazol.

3. **Cancer** must be excluded as a cause of pain. Though cancer rarely presents as pain, all patients should have a thorough exam and mammogram. Ultrasound is indicated if the pain is focal.

IV MALIGNANT DISEASES OF THE BREAST

A Epidemiology

1. A woman has a one in eight chance of developing breast cancer at some point in her life.

2. In 2004, it was estimated that 217,440 new cases of breast cancer (215,900 women and 1,450 men) would be diagnosed in the United States.
   a. 215,990 women
   b. 1,450 men

3. There will be 40,580 deaths from breast cancer.
   a. 40,110 women
   b. 470 men

4. An increased incidence of 1% each year is partly related to early detection.

5. The mortality rate decreased significantly in the last decade.

B Risk factors (Table 23-1)

1. **Family history** for breast carcinoma produces a two to three times higher risk.
   a. **First-degree relatives** (i.e., mother, daughter, sister) are affected. Risk is higher if the relative is premenopausal.
   b. **Hereditary breast cancer (HBC).** The **breast cancer gene (BRCA)** has two forms:
      (1) **BRCA-1**: 60%–80% lifetime risk of developing breast cancer
      (2) **BRCA-2**: 30%–80% lifetime risk

2. **Prior contralateral breast cancer** doubles the patient's risk.

TABLE 23-1 Risk Factors for Breast Cancer

Factor	High Risk	Low Risk
More Than Four Times Relative Risk		
Age	Old	Young
History of cancer in one breast	Yes	No
Family history of premenopausal bilateral breast cancer	Yes	No
Two to Four Times Relative Risk		
Any first-degree relative with breast cancer	Yes	No
History of primary cancer of ovary or endometrium	Yes	No
Age at first full-term pregnancy	Older than 30 years	Younger than 20 years
Oophorectomy	No	Yes
Body habitus, postmenopausal	Obese	Thin
Country of birth	North America, northern Europe	Asia, Africa
Socioeconomic class	Upper	Lower
History of fibrocystic disease	Yes	No
One to Two Times Relative Risk		
Marital status	Single	Married
Place of residence	Urban, northern United States	Rural, southern United States
Race	White	Black
Age at menarche	Early	Late
Age at menopause	Late	Early

Adapted with permission from Kelsey JL, Gannon MD. The epidemiology of breast cancer. *CA Cancer J Clin* 1991;41(3):157.

3. **High socioeconomic status**

4. A **nulliparous** woman's risk is increased two to three times.
   a. The risk is lowest in women who become pregnant before 23 years of age.

5. **Exogenous estrogen** has been shown to increase the risk of breast cancer in postmenopausal women.

C Symptoms

1. **Masses** are the presenting symptom in 85% of patients with carcinoma. Approximately 60% of breast masses are discovered by patients on SBE.

2. **Pain** is rarely a symptom but should be completely evaluated to eliminate the possibility of a malignancy.

3. **Metastatic disease** may also be the initial symptom.
   a. **Axillary nodes.** Two percent of patients with breast cancer present with axillary node enlargement but no palpable primary breast tumor.
      (1) Hodgkin's disease; lung, ovarian, or pancreatic cancer; and squamous cell carcinoma of the skin must be ruled out.
      (2) If the results of all studies (including MRI) are negative, a blind mastectomy (i.e., removal of the breast without evidence of malignancy) is indicated.
   b. **Distant organ**

4. **Asymptomatic patients.** High-risk patients (i.e., family or personal history of breast cancer) should be followed closely with mammography and physical examination. They should also be advised to practice SBE.

D Noninvasive breast cancers constitute 10% of all types of breast cancer. The diagnosis has increased with early detection through mammography. The prognosis is good. Treatment is aimed at preventing the development of an invasive breast cancer.

1. **Ductal carcinoma in situ (DCIS)**
   a. DCIS is confined to ductal cells.
   b. No invasion of the underlying basement membrane occurs. Risk of axillary metastasis is <1%.
   c. **Treatment options**
      (1) Excision with clear margins
         (a) Twenty-five percent risk of recurrence within 5 years
         (b) Recurrence may be invasive (50%) or DCIS (50%)
      (2) Excision with clear margins and radiation
         (a) Reduces risk of recurrence to 8%
      (3) Total (simple) mastectomy
         (a) Removal of breast tissue and areolar/nipple complex
         (b) No need to sample axillary nodes
         (c) Less than 1% chance of recurrence
         (d) Reconstruction can be done at the time of mastectomy.

2. **Lobular carcinoma in situ (LCIS)**
   a. This type is most commonly found incidentally.
   b. The risk of invasive cancer within 20 years is 15%–20% **bilaterally.**
   c. Treatment involves careful follow-up, because the lesion is considered to be a marker for increased future risk of invasive cancer in both breasts. Bilateral total mastectomy may be considered if other risk factors are present (i.e., family history, other hormone-sensitive tumor, prior breast cancer).

3. **Paget's disease**
   a. This uncommon lesion involves the nipple.
   b. Histologically vacuolated cells (Paget's cells) are seen in the epidermis of the nipple and result in an eczematous dermatitis of the nipple.
   c. This lesion may be associated with an invasive component in the underlying ducts.
   d. Mammography should be performed to look for a mass.
   e. **Mastectomy is the standard treatment.**
   f. Eighty percent 10-year survival for patients with no axillary involvement.

TABLE 23-2	Staging of Breast Cancer		
Stage I	T1	N0	M0
Stage IIA	T1	N1	M0
	T2	N0	M0
Stage IIB	T2	N1	M0
	T3	N0	M0
Stage IIIA	T0	N2	M0
	T1	N2	M0
	T2	N2	M0
	T3	N1	M0
	T3	N2	M0
Stage IIIB	T4	Any N	M0
	Any T	N3	M0
Stage IV	Any T	Any N	M1

T, tumor; N, node; M, metastases.

E **Invasive breast cancer**

1. **Favorable histologic types.** (There is an 85% 5-year survival rate.)
   a. Tubular carcinoma (grade 1 intraductal)
   b. Colloid or mucinous carcinoma
   c. Papillary carcinoma

2. **Less favorable lesions**
   a. **Medullary cancer.** This type involves lymphocytic infiltration and a well-circumscribed lesion.
   b. **Invasive lobular cancer.** Small cells infiltrate around benign ducts.
      (1) The prognosis is slightly better than for invasive ductal cancer.
      (2) There is a higher incidence of bilaterality.

3. **Least favorable histologic type**
   a. **Inflammatory breast cancer.** The histology involves tumor-plugged subdermal lymphatics. The prognosis is a 5-year survival rate in approximately 30% of patients. Inflammatory signs are seen (e.g., warmth, swelling and pain).

F **Staging and prognosis of breast cancer**   After the diagnosis of breast cancer is made, the next step is to determine the extent of disease. This process of staging guides treatment and also predicts survival.

1. **Clinical staging.** Based on physical exam and mammogram. Distant disease is evaluated with chest x-ray, bone scan, liver function tests (LFT).
   a. A **mammogram** is useful to determine both additional foci in the involved breast and the presence of metastatic or synchronous disease.
   b. A **chest radiograph** detects pulmonary parenchymal or bone metastasis.
   c. A **computed tomography (CT) scan** of the chest should be obtained for stage III patients to evaluate the supraclavicular area and mediastinum or if the chest radiograph is abnormal.
   d. LFTs
      (1) Alkaline phosphatase is the most sensitive in detecting hepatic metastasis.

TABLE 23-3	Breast Cancer Prognosis Based on Stage
Stage I	93% 5-year survival rate
Stage II	72% 5-year survival rate
Stage III	41% 5-year survival rate
Stage IV	18% 5-year survival rate

(2) An ultrasound or a CT scan of the liver should be performed if the alkaline phosphatase level is abnormal or if other evidence of distant metastasis is present.

e. A **bone scan** should be performed if nodes are clinically positive or if nodes are clinically negative but the patient has symptoms of bone pain (patients in stages II, III, and IV).

f. A CT scan of the head should be done if neurologic signs or symptoms are present.

2. Clinical/pathologic staging

  a. Tumor (T)

    Tis = carcinoma in situ

    T1 = Tumor 2 cm or less in greatest dimension

    T2 = Tumor greater than 2 cm but no more than 5 cm

    T3 = Tumor greater than 5 cm in greatest dimension

    T4 = Tumor of any size with direct extension to chest wall (not pectoralis major) or skin

    (1) Poor prognostic features include:

      (a) Edema or ulceration of the surrounding skin.

      (b) Tumor fixed to the chest wall or overlying skin.

      (c) Satellite skin nodules

      (d) Dermal lymphatic invasion. **Peau d'orange** is an orange-peel consistency of breast skin.

      (e) Skin retraction and dimpling (shortening of tumor-involved Cooper's ligaments) occur.

  b. Axillary node status (N) remains the best source of predicting survival or outcome.

    N0 = No axillary metastasis

    N1 = Metastases to movable axillary nodes

    N2 = Metastases to fixed, matted axillary nodes

    N3 = Metastases to ipsilateral internal mammary nodes

    (1) Poor prognostic features include:

      (a) Capsular invasion

      (b) Extranodal spread

      (c) Edema of the arm

  c. Distant disease/metastasis (M)

    M0 = No distant metastases

    M1 = Distant metastases, including ipsilateral supraclavicular nodes

    (1) Sites of metastasis

      (a) Lung

      (b) Liver

      (c) Bone

      (d) Brain

      (e) Adrenal

G **Treatment of breast cancer** Multimodality therapy that can include surgery, chemotherapy, radiation and/or hormonal therapy

1. Surgery

  a. Most women are candidates for breast conservation or mastectomy. Much of the decision making, when medically appropriate, involves patient preference.

  b. Breast Conservation. There is no survival difference between breast conservation (with or without radiation) and mastectomy. There is an increase in recurrence with breast conservation.

    (1) Lumpectomy with negative margins

      (a) Lumpectomy alone: 25% rate of recurrence

      (b) Lumpectomy with radiation: 8% rate of recurrence

    (2) Must include axillary sampling to accurately stage patient

      (a) Axillary lymphadenectomy (Fig. 23-1)

        (i) Level I and II nodes are removed in relation to the axillary vein (Fig. 23-2).

        (ii) Skip metastasis (i.e., involved level III nodes with negative level I and II nodes) occurs in fewer than 5% of cases.

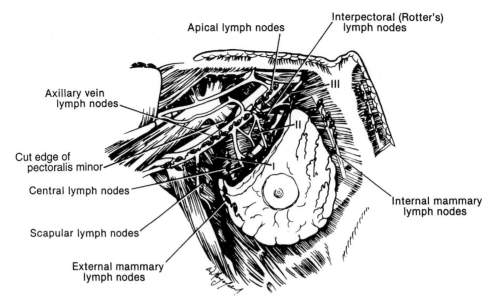

Apical lymph nodes

Interpectoral (Rotter's) lymph nodes

Axillary vein lymph nodes

Cut edge of pectoralis minor

Central lymph nodes

Scapular lymph nodes

External mammary lymph nodes

Internal mammary lymph nodes

FIGURE 23-2 The lymphatic drainage of the breast, showing lymph node groups and levels. Level I lymph nodes, lateral to lateral border of the pectoralis minor muscle; level II lymph nodes, behind the pectoralis minor muscle; level III lymph nodes, the medial to medial border of the pectoralis minor muscle.

- (b) **Sentinel node biopsy**
    - (i) This biopsy allows minimal dissection with a substantial decrease in morbidity (lymphedema).
    - (ii) Nuclear scanning or vital blue dye is used to identify the first node drained by the breast.
    - (iii) This node is then examined for the presence of axillary disease. If the sentinel node is negative for metastatic disease, no further lymphadenectomy is performed. If the sentinel node is positive for metastatic disease, a standard lymphadenectomy is performed to stage the axilla.
    - (iv) The **long thoracic nerve** should be carefully preserved to prevent denervation of the serratus anterior muscle, which results in a winged scapula. The thoracodorsal nerve and blood supply to the latissimus muscle are also preserved.
- (3) Patients who choose breast conservation therapy should also undergo radiation therapy to decrease the risk of recurrence. Breast conservation **cannot** be performed for patients who have undergone chest radiation, have diffuse multicentric disease, collagen vascular disease, or persistent positive margins after lumpectomy. These patients are more effectively treated by mastectomy. Patients with a large tumor in relation to breast size may have superior cosmetic result with mastectomy.
- c. **Mastectomy** is removal of the breast tissue and nipple/areolar complex.
    - (1) **Modified radical mastectomy** includes axillary dissection/sentinel lymph node biopsy (Fig. 23-3).
    - (2) **Skin-sparing mastectomy** (nonareolar breast skin is preserved) with immediate reconstruction provides more cosmetic result and does not increase the risk of recurrence.
    - (3) **Radical mastectomy** includes the pectoralis major muscle. It is used in the therapy of tumors invading that muscle.
- d. Patients who are **not** candidates for surgery include those with:
    - (1) Extensive edema of the breast
    - (2) Satellite nodules of carcinoma
    - (3) Inflammatory carcinoma
    - (4) A parasternal tumor, indicating spread to the internal mammary nodes
    - (5) Supraclavicular metastasis
    - (6) Edema of the arm
    - (7) Distant metastasis

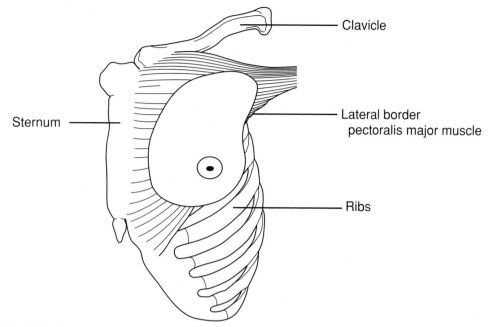

Clavicle

Sternum

Lateral border
pectoralis major muscle

Ribs

FIGURE 23-3 The borders of a mastectomy. Superior, clavicle; lateral, lateral border of the pectoralis major muscle; inferior, the inframammary fold (fifth to sixth rib); medial, the sternum.

2. **Radiation**
   a. Whole breast radiation involves 4,500 rads. A boost of 2,000 rads is given to the tumor site.
   b. Radiation therapy can be useful as adjuvant therapy after mastectomy in high-risk patients or in those with chest wall involvement.

3. **Chemotherapy**
   a. Candidates for chemotherapy include node-positive patients, patients with tumor >1 cm, and estrogen receptor/progresterone receptor (ER/PR)-negative patients
   b. Common chemotherapy drugs include cyclophosphamide (C), methotrexate (M), fluorouracil (F), and adriamycin (A)
   c. Different combination drug regimens, given together for 3 to 6 months, include CMF, CAF, AC, and AC followed by paclitaxel (Taxol).
   d. The results show improvement in both the diseasefree interval and the overall survival of premenopausal women.
   e. **Side effects**
      (1) **Myelosuppression** requires monitoring of bone marrow function.
      (2) **Alopecia**
      (3) **Cardiomyopathy** (with adriamycin only)
   f. **Chemotherapy** and **hormone therapy** are also used to treat recurrent and metastatic disease.

4. **Neoadjuvant therapy** is chemotherapy given before surgical therapy of local disease.
   a. **Inflammatory breast cancer.** Diffuse intraductal invasive breast cancer requires chemotherapy treatment immediately.
   b. Large fixed tumors or fixed nodal disease
      (1) Can downstage disease and enable resectability
      (2) Can also decrease tumor size and allow breast conservation
      (3) Can increase overall survival

5. **Hormonal therapy**–for ER/PR-positive patients. ER/PR-positive patients in general have better prognosis.
   a. Tamoxifen or raloxifene (antiestrogens) or anastrozole (Arimidex) (aromatase inhibitor) are taken for 5 years.
   b. Hormonal therapy is as effective as chemotherapy in postmenopausal patients.

c. This therapy is an excellent choice of treatment in elderly persons who cannot tolerate chemotherapy.

d. Adding tamoxifen decreases recurrence rates by 47% and death rates by 20%.

e. Side effects can include vaginal bleeding, hot flashes, thromboembolic events, and increased risk of endometrial cancer.

H Follow-up (ipsilateral and contralateral breast)

1. **Observation** is made for tumor recurrence and complications.
   a. **Monthly SBE**
   b. **Annual breast examination** by a physician
   c. **Annual mammogram**
   d. Chest radiographs, CT scans, and tumor markers are not needed unless clinical suspicion arises.

2. **Edema of the arm**
   a. Ten percent of women who have had axillary lymphadenectomy or modified radical mastectomy develop edema of the arm (acute or chronic).
   b. Edema is worsened by radiation therapy to the axilla.
   c. **All minor trauma to the affected arm must be avoided.**
   d. **Treatment**
      (1) Because each infection increases lymphatic obstruction by obliterating the remaining open channels with fibrosis in reaction to the bacteria, even **minor skin infections** should receive early treatment with antibiotics.
      (2) Chronic edema can be treated with an elastic sleeve or a pneumatic compression device.

3. **Complications.** Chronic edema lasting 10 years or longer can lead (although rarely) to the development of lymphangiosarcoma in the affected arm.

I Recurrent disease

1. Patients with a recurrence in the first 2 years after treatment have a worse prognosis than do patients who have a recurrence after 5 years.

2. Most recurrences occur in the same quadrant as the original lesion.

3. Metastatic disease is present in 10% of patients with recurrence.

4. The treatment of an isolated breast recurrence after primary radiation therapy is mastectomy.

5. Radiation therapy can be a very effective form of palliative therapy in patients with bone or central nervous system metastases, resulting in relief of pain and control of local disease.

6. A local or regional recurrence can involve the operative field of a mastectomy, the breast after primary radiation therapy, or the axilla. Larger tumor size, receptor-negative status, and involved axillary nodes are all risk factors for the development of local or regional recurrences.

7. **Chest wall recurrences**
   a. After mastectomy, chest wall recurrences are treated with radiation therapy.
   b. Breast recurrences after radiation are treated with mastectomy.
   c. Systemic therapy may also have a role in some cases.

8. **Distant metastasis**
   a. **Hormone therapy.** Patients who respond to one hormone treatment modality generally continue to respond to sequential hormone therapy, whereas nonresponders do not. Few patients are cured once metastasis occurs, but hormone therapy is very effective in prolonging survival and in reducing the size of the tumor.
   b. **Chemotherapy** is used for patients with recurrent disease who are estrogen-receptor negative or who do not respond to hormone therapy. Combinations of cyclophosphamide, methotrexate, fluorouracil, and doxorubicin are usually used in these cases. Temporary favorable responses, which are determined by a measurable decrease in tumor size or the relief of pain, are obtained in 60%–80% of patients with stage IV disease when this therapy is initiated.

J **Special cases**

1. **Breast cancer in pregnancy**
   a. Breast cancer occurs in 1.5% of women during their childbearing years.
   b. Diagnosis is usually delayed secondary to normal nodularity that forms in breasts during pregnancy.
   c. A suspicious mass should be evaluated with mammogram and ultrasound.
   d. Core or excisional biopsy should be performed for any suspicious mass.
   e. Excisional biopsy can be performed safely under sedation with local anesthesia.

2. **The male breast**
   a. **Gynecomastia**
      (1) **Prepubertal gynecomastia** is rare and is caused by adrenal and testicular carcinoma.
      (2) **Pubertal gynecomastia** occurs in 60%–70% of prepubertal boys (12–15 years of age). Breast enlargement in the healthy male adolescent does not require treatment. In nearly all cases, the enlargement will regress with age. If enlargement is significant, unilateral, or distressing the patient, treatment is simple mastectomy.
      (3) **Senescent gynecomastia**
         (a) Forty percent of aging men have decreased testosterone, increased estradiol, and increased luteinizing hormone.
         (b) Unilateral or bilateral enlargement of the breast tissue directly behind the nipple
         (c) **Causes of gynecomastia**
            (i) Idiopathic
            (ii) Drug therapies such as thiazide diuretics, digoxin, theophylline, antidepressants, and hormones
            (iii) Alcohol and marijuana abuse
            (iv) Disease conditions such as cirrhosis, renal failure, and malnutrition
         (d) **Treatment**
            (i) Evaluate for mass with mammography and physical exam
            (ii) If a dominant mass is present, a biopsy must be performed to rule out cancer. Then, if no cancer is present, withdraw the offending agent, treat the underlying medical condition, perform a hormonal workup, and provide reassurance.
   b. **Cancer of the male breast**
      (1) This type occurs in 0.7% of all breast cancers and in less than 1% of male cancers.
      (2) The average age is 63–70 years, which is older than in women.
      (3) **Klinefelter's syndrome** has been associated with male breast cancer (testicular hormone factors).
      (4) Many risk factors associated with male breast cancer can be linked to elevated estrogen levels.
      (5) Most patients present with a painless unilateral mass that is usually subareolar with skin fixation, chest wall fixation, and ulceration.
      (6) The workup is identical to that used for a woman. Gynecomastia is the primary differential diagnosis. Bilaterality and tenderness favor gynecomastia.
         (a) A thorough history of drug and hormone use along with alcohol intake is necessary.
         (b) Mammography may distinguish between the two.
      (7) This type originates as a **ductal cancer.**
      (8) **Treatment** is similar to that for carcinoma of the female breast.
         (a) **Radical mastectomy** has been the standard treatment.
         (b) **Modified radical mastectomy** is done if the pectoralis major muscle is not involved.
         (c) **Breast conservation** is done with radiation therapy if the primary tumor is small and does not involve the nipple-areola complex.
         (d) **Hormonal manipulation** involves castration or tamoxifen therapy.
      (9) **Survival** is similar to the rates for female breast cancer when compared stage for stage. Male patients tend to present at later stages.

chapter 24

Organ Transplantation

MICHAEL J. MORITZ • VINCENT T. ARMENTI • BENJAMIN PHILOSOPHE

I OVERVIEW

A Candidate evaluation

1. **Potential recipients** are carefully evaluated. The diseased organ and associated problems are carefully reviewed. For example, the physician should ensure that a patient with renal failure due to posterior urethral valves has had the valves corrected so that the bladder's reservoir and voiding functions are intact.

2. **Other related organ systems are evaluated.** For example, an evaluation of a liver transplant candidate with alcoholic cirrhosis looks for cardiomyopathy or cerebral atrophy. Another example is an evaluation of whether a patient with renal failure from diabetic nephropathy has significant coronary artery disease.

3. **General health issues** are evaluated. The following typical studies may be needed for each organ system
   a. **Pulmonary:** chest radiograph, pulmonary function tests
   b. **Cardiac:** electrocardiogram (ECG), echocardiogram, stress test, cardiac catheterization
   c. **Gastrointestinal:** upper gastrointestinal series, barium enema, endoscopy, liver function tests, ultrasound
   d. **Renal/urologic:** creatinine clearance, cystourethrogram
   e. **Immunologic:** purified protein derivative (PPD); rapid plasmin reagin (RPR) test; serology for hepatitis B and C, cytomegalovirus (CMV), Epstein-Barr virus (EBV), and human immunodeficiency virus (HIV); vaccination status
   f. **Cancer screening:** mammography, prostate-specific antigen, Papanicolaou test

4. **Specific issues** are also typically addressed for the following transplant recipients:
   a. **Renal transplant.** Renin levels should be checked if the patient has refractory hypertension. Parathyroid metabolism should be evaluated. Calcium and phosphate should be controlled. The lower urinary tract must be sterile; a urine culture and urinalysis should be performed.
   b. **Liver transplant.** Liver biopsy should be performed. Patency of the portal system should be checked. The α-fetoprotein level should be measured.
   c. **Pancreas transplant.** The C peptide level must be checked (must be low to prove that the patient has type I diabetes).
   d. **Heart transplant.** Pulmonary vascular resistance must be measured.
   e. **Lung transplant.** Right and left heart function should be evaluated.

B Terms

1. **Genetic relationship between the donor and the recipient.** Physicians should remember that **allografts and xenografts require immunosuppression; otherwise, they will fail because of rejection.**
   a. **Autograft** describes tissue transfer within the same individual (e.g., skin graft).
   b. **Isograft** describes tissue transfer between genetically identical individuals (e.g., identical twins).
   c. **Allograft** describes tissue transfer between genetically nonidentical members of the same species (includes living related donor and cadaver donor human transplants). Immunosuppression is required.

   d. Xenograft describes tissue transfer between different species. Immunosuppression is required.

   2. Surgical position

   a. Orthotopic. The old organ is removed, and the new one is placed in the same position.

   b. Heterotopic. The new organ is placed in a different position.

C **Donors**

   1. Cadaver donors are individuals with severe brain injury resulting in brain death, which is defined as complete irreversible cessation of all brain function, including the brain stem.

   a. Diagnosis. The mainstay of diagnosis is the neurologic examination, which must demonstrate unresponsiveness, absence of spontaneous movement, and absence of reflexes from the brain stem and higher. Also:

   (1) The patient must be normothermic.

   (2) Depressant drugs (especially barbiturates) must not be present.

   (3) An apnea test result must be negative (i.e., no respiratory effort despite a high arterial carbon dioxide level).

   (4) Electroencephalogram (EEG) and cerebral blood flow studies are optional.

   b. Causes. Cerebrovascular disease is most common, followed by trauma.

   c. Exclusions. Disseminated or uncured extracranial cancers, sepsis, or poor organ function.

   2. Living donors are individuals motivated by altruism.

   a. Types of living donors

   (1) Living unrelated donors on average share no more genes with a recipient than a cadaver donor. An example is the patient's spouse.

   (2) Living related donors share a substantial portion of their genomes with the recipient.

   b. Requirements. Living donors must be in almost perfect health, have normal function of the organ under consideration, and be good candidates for anesthesia and the operative procedure. The workup includes:

   (1) ABO typing, tissue typing, and cross matching (see I F)

   (2) Complete history and physical examination; chest radiography; ECG; complete blood count; sequential multiple analysis (SMA) for 6 and 12 serum tests (SMA-6, SMA-12); 24-hour creatinine clearance and protein; RPR test; serology for hepatitis B and C, CMV, and HIV; urinalysis; PPD

   (3) For renal donors, arteriography and intravenous pyelogram (now combined as a helical computed tomography [CT] scan).

   c. Risks. Perioperative mortality for living kidney donors is 0.03% (3 per 10,000). A living donor provides one kidney, and the remaining kidney hypertrophies and achieves 80% of creatinine clearance before donation. Newer procedures include donation of the left lateral segment or a lobe of the liver and segment(s) or lobe(s) of the lung. In these procedures, the safety of the donor is not assured. Although, traditionally, most living kidney donations are performed as an open surgical procedure, there is increasing experience with laparoscopically performed nephrectomy. This method potentially offers the advantage of minimally invasive surgery while still producing an excellent kidney.

D **Removal of the donor organ** The donor organ is removed in a formal surgical procedure, wherein the blood supply of the organ is controlled and then the organ is rapidly flushed with a cold (4°C) solution to render it cold and ischemic. All organs are more tolerant of cold ischemia than warm (normothermic) ischemia.

E The **practical** limit of cold ischemia with current preservation methods is 4 hours for the heart, 6 hours for a lung, 12 hours for the liver, 36 hours for the pancreas, and 40–48 hours for a kidney. As the limit is approached or passed, the risk increases for delayed function, damage, or nonfunction of the organ.

F The **immunologic compatibility** of the donor and recipient influences the outcome for any type of organ transplant (Table 24-1).

TABLE 24-1 Effects of Immunologic Compatibility on Transplant Outcome

Organ	HLA Matching	Cross Match	Effect of High PRA
Heart	Not important	Only done for high-PRA patients	Increased risk of early graft failure
Liver	Not important	Not done pretransplant, but positive cross-match recipients have the same risks as high-PRA patients	Increased intraoperative blood loss; increased platelet transfusion requirements; and increased risk of early graft failure.
Kidney	Important for both living and cadaver donors	Mandatory pretransplant and must be negative	Increased risk of delayed graft function, early graft failure
Pancreas	Very important for pancreas transplant done alone	Mandatory as for kidney recipients	

HLA, human leukocyte antigen; PRA, panel-reactive antibody.

1. **ABO blood group compatibility.** The same rules apply as for red blood cell transfusions.
2. **Cross-match compatibility must be present for kidney, pancreas, and some heart transplants.** The recipient's serum is tested for the presence of cytotoxic antibodies directed against surface antigens (usually antihuman leukocyte antigen [HLA]) on the T lymphocytes of the donor. If antidonor cytotoxic antibodies are present, the donor is unacceptable because the recipient's antibodies will immediately attack the new kidney and rapidly destroy it (hyperacute rejection; see I G 1).
   a. A **positive cross match** is positive for the presence of preformed antidonor antibodies in the serum of the prospective recipient and precludes transplantation between that donor and the recipient.
   b. A **negative cross match** (i.e., absence of antidonor antibodies) is mandatory before the transplant.
   c. A few patients have antibodies against most other humans (so-called high panel-reactive antibody [PRA] patients). High-PRA patients have formed antibodies against a high proportion of a **panel of human cells,** which is used to screen for reactivity; therefore, acceptable donors are difficult to find. Also, high-PRA patients are at higher risk for early graft failure.
3. **Human leukocyte antigen (HLA).** These are the histocompatibility antigens and are defined by **tissue typing.**
   a. Six human HLA genes (HLA-A, -B, -C, -DR, -DP, and -DQ) are located on chromosome 6.
   b. HLA-C, -DP, and -DQ are not believed to be important in clinical transplantation.
   c. The contents of each chromosome 6 is a haplotype, and all humans have two of these chromosomes—one from the mother and one from the father. Therefore, **six HLA antigens are defined by tissue typing** (i.e., two each for HLA-A, -B, and -DR).
   d. HLA-A and -B have more than 40 defined types, which are designated numerically. HLA-DR has more than 10 defined types. An example of an HLA type is HLA-A2, 27; B1, 44; DR 3, 7. An example of a haplotype is HLA-A2; B1; DR7.

G **Rejection**   The **three types** of rejection are hyperacute, acute, and chronic.

1. **Hyperacute rejection** occurs when the serum of the recipient has preformed antidonor antibodies. These antibodies adhere to and kill endothelium, which results in rapid graft infarction (within 24 hours). Because hyperacute rejection can be predicted by a positive cross match (see I F 2 a), it is **avoidable.** However, once hyperacute rejection begins, it **cannot be treated.**
2. **Acute rejection** is a cell-mediated immune response initiated by helper T cells. The pace of proliferation of alloreactive T cell clones dictates that acute rejection usually occurs after the sixth

post-transplant day. In some cases, a memory immune response can trigger cellular rejection sooner.

   a. The diagnosis is usually made via the detection and workup of graft dysfunction, culminating in a **biopsy.**

   b. Acute rejection is **treatable and reversible** by a short course of high-dose immunosuppressive drugs.

   c. When acute rejection is refractory to treatment or recurs, graft failure can result.

   d. Acute rejection usually takes place within 3 months of transplant and rarely occurs after 1 year, unless triggered by an event such as infection or lack of adequate immunosuppression.

3. Chronic rejection usually occurs late. It has an insidious onset and is multifactorial, with both the cell-mediated and humoral arms of the immune system involved. Chronic rejection is poorly understood and therefore **not treatable or reversible.**

H **Immunosuppression (Table 24-2).**   Almost all allografts require indefinite suppression of the recipient's immune system to prevent rejection. This is in contrast to tolerance, in which the recipient's immune system responds normally to all antigens except those of the donor (i.e., the donor antigens are "tolerated").

1. Immunosuppression attempts to disable or destroy components of the immune response (typically lymphocytes).

   a. Conventional immunosuppression is created by drug therapy; administration of biologic reagents (sera); and, rarely, radiation therapy.

   b. Multiple drug therapy is standard and aims for synergistic immunosuppression while minimizing the side effects.

2. Immunosuppression can be loosely classified into **three types:** induction regimens, antirejection regimens, and maintenance therapy.

   a. Induction regimens aim to avoid rejection and establish good graft function within the first two post-transplant weeks. Induction regimens use an antilymphocyte serum plus part of the maintenance regimen (see I H 2 c), withholding one drug to avoid unwanted side effects.

      (1) The nephrotoxicity of cyclosporine and tacrolimus is of particular concern after any transplant.

      (2) Impaired healing of the bronchial anastomosis from high-dose steroids is disadvantageous after lung transplantation.

   b. Antirejection regimens are high-dose, short-term (<3 weeks) treatments aimed at reversing acute rejection episodes. These regimens include high-dose (pulse) corticosteroids, typically methylprednisolone, antilymphocyte sera, or monoclonal antibodies.

   c. Maintenance therapy provides long-term immunosuppression to prevent rejection. These regimens usually include two or three drugs. The principal drugs are cyclosporine or tacrolimus. One of these is combined with a corticosteroid (e.g., prednisone), and a third drug may be added. More recently, coritcosteroids have been eliminated from maintenance regimens.

3. **Corticosteroids** have broad anti-inflammatory and immunosuppressive effects. Generally, they inhibit all types of leukocytes, in contrast to the other immunosuppressive drugs, which are more lymphocyte selective.

   a. Methylprednisolone is used intravenously for induction or antirejection therapy.

   b. Prednisone or **prednisolone** is given orally as maintenance **therapy.** With good bioavailability, drug levels are not needed.

   c. Side effects are common and include obesity, cushingoid facies, poor wound healing, atrophic skin, striae, and acne.

   d. In contrast to the prevalent side effects, **complications** include diabetes, hypertension, osteoporosis, aseptic necrosis (usually of the hips), cataracts, peptic ulcer disease, and psychiatric disturbances. These broad complications have led many centers to successfully eliminate steroids from maintenance protocols.

4. **Calcineurin inhibitors** have become the mainstays of most immunosuppressive regimens owing to their superior effectiveness. These drugs block the calcineurin-dependent pathway

TABLE 24-2 Immunosuppressive Drugs

Drugs	Uses	Effects	Side Effects	Comments
Cyclosporine	Maintenance	Profound inhibitor of helper T-cell function	Nephrotoxicity, hypertension, tremor, hirsutism	Relatively selective for alloimmune responses Cannot be used with tacrolimus (FK-506) due to synergistic nephrotoxicity
Tacrolimus (FK-506)	Maintenance, antirejection	Profound inhibitor of T-cell function	Nephrotoxicity, neurotoxicity, diabetes	
Corticosteroids (Prednisone po, Methylprednisolone IV)	Maintenance antirejection	Inhibits all leukocytes; high-dose causes lymphocytolysis	Cushingoid fascies, diabetes, excessive weight gain, aseptic necrosis of the hip	Innumerable troublesome side effects; nonspecific immunosuppressant
Azathioprine	Maintenance	Inhibits clonal proliferation of T cells	Leukopenia	Nonspecific
OKT3	Antirejection, induction	Disables or depletes all T cells	First-dose reaction due to cytokine release can cause fever, chills, bronchospasm	Low frequency of development of anti-OKT3 antibodies, maximum duration of therapy 2–3 weeks
Antithymocyte globulin	Antirejection, induction	Depletes T cells	Fevers, chills	Maximum duration of therapy 2–3 weeks
Mycophenolate mofetil	Maintenance	Akin to azathioprine	Diarrhea; leukopenia	More lymphocyte selective than azathioprine
Rapamycin (Sirolimus)	Maintenance	Inhibits helper T cells	Potential thrombocytopenia and hyperlipidemia	Some similarities to cyclosporine, FK-506 class of drugs; synergistic only with cyclosporine
Basiliximab (Simulet)	Antirejection prophylaxis	Inhibits interleukin-2–mediated (activation of lymphocytes	Possible anaphylactoid reaction	Immunosuppressive chimeric monoclonal antibody
Daclizumab (Zenapax)	Antirejection prophylaxis	Inhibits interleukin-2–medicated (activation of lymphocytes)	Possible anaphylactoid reaction	Immunosuppressive humanized monoclonal antibody

of helper T-cell activation, thus blocking transcription of cytokine genes that initiate and amplify the immune response. This mechanism is more specific for the alloimmune response to an organ allograft than the older drugs (e.g., corticosteroids, azathioprine). Therefore, lower doses of other immunosuppressive drugs can be used, the incidence and severity of rejection are decreased, and outcomes are improved. They are typically used for maintenance therapy.

    a. Cyclosporine dosing is adjusted to achieve a desired trough blood level because bioavailability is low and varies greatly.

        (1) Toxicity includes nephrotoxicity, hypertension, neurotoxicity, hirsutism, gingival hyperplasia, and hyperlipidemia.

        (2) At appropriate levels, cyclosporine does not cause progressive deterioration in renal function.

    b. Tacrolimus (FK-506) is more potent than cyclosporine. Dosing is done by trough levels. Toxicity is similar to cyclosporine without hirsutism, hyperlipidemia, and gingival hyperplasia but with headache, diarrhea, and an increased risk of diabetes.

5. Antimetabolites are drugs that inhibit purine or pyrimidine metabolism, thereby inhibiting rapidly dividing cells, including clonally proliferating alloreactive T cells. They are usually used as third maintenance immunosuppressants with corticosteroids and a calcineurin inhibitor.

    a. Azathioprine is a purine metabolism inhibitor. Toxicity causes leukopenia.

    b. Mycophenolate mofetil is a purine metabolism inhibitor that appears to be more lymphocyte specific than azathioprine. When used as a third drug, the incidence of acute rejection is significantly decreased. Toxicity includes reversible bone marrow suppression and gastrointestinal side effects.

6. Antilymphocyte sera are biologic agents derived from animals immunized against human determinants. Two agents that are used for either induction or antirejection therapy are muromonab CD3 (OKT3) and antithymocyte globulin (ATG). Muromonab CD3 is a murine monoclonal immunoglobulin (IgG) to an antibody that binds to the CD3 antigen on human T cells. Antithymocyte globulin is a polyclonal antilymphocyte serum harvested from horses or rabbits, which depletes T cells.

7. Interleukin-2 (IL-2) receptor blockers. Two IL-2 receptor blockers have been developed. Studies have suggested that when used as part of an immunosuppressive regimen including steroids and cyclosporine, these agents can reduce the frequency of acute rejection in kidney transplant recipients. IL-2 receptor blockers bind to the IL-2 receptor alpha chain on the surface of activated T lymphocytes. One agent is a humanized monoclonal antibody, dacliximab (Zenapax) and the other a mouse-human chimeric monoclonal antibody, basiliximab (Simulect). Simulect is given at transplant and is repeated 4 days later, whereas Zenapax is given within 24 hours of transplant and then at 14-day intervals for four doses. No significant adverse reactions or drug interactions have been reported with these agents. The long-term effects of these agents are not yet known.

8. Sirolimus (Rapamycin) is the newest drug. It binds to the same intracellular carrier site as does tacrolimus and may partially antagonize its effects. It is synergistic with cyclosporine. It acts at a separate, later site of T-cell activation than the calcineurin inhibitors. Side effects include hypercholesterolemia, hypertriglyceridemia, and mild bone marrow suppression.

I   General complications of immunosuppression

1. Infections. The nonspecificity of current immunosuppression also impairs host defenses against a diverse group of pathogens (e.g., opportunistic infections).

    a. A broad range of bacterial, fungal, and protozoal organisms are an uncommon cause of infections, but they require prompt diagnosis and treatment, as they can be lethal.

    b. CMV is a frequent infectious problem in the early months after a transplant. The risk is related to prior exposure (serostatus), and seronegative recipients of organs from seropositive donors are at highest risk. The agent for prophylaxis and treatment of CMV infection is ganciclovir.

2. **Neoplasia.** The three major areas of increased risk are skin cancer, post-transplant lymphoproliferative disorders (PTLDs), and oral squamous cell cancers or female genital tract cancers.

    a. **Skin cancer.** Squamous cell cancers of sun-exposed skin are very common in post-transplant patients.

    b. **PTLD** is a form of lymphoma, commonly arising from B cells and usually associated with EBV. Early stages may respond to acyclovir and profound reduction in immunosuppression. Later stages are treatable with chemotherapy, but the prognosis is poor.

    c. **Oral squamous cell cancers** and **female genital tract cancers** (e.g., cervical, vaginal, labial) occur with greater frequency in post-transplant patients.

3. **Parenthood after transplantation**

    a. Organ failure is generally associated with endocrine abnormalities that result in difficulties in fertility or the ability to conceive. The endocrine abnormalities are reversed after successful transplantation. With successful transplantation, recipients regain the capacity to become pregnant or to father a child.

    b. No obvious problems have been present in the offspring of male organ recipients.

    c. Female recipients often have premature deliveries or low birth weight infants. The severity of these outcomes seems to be related to the degree of graft problems and other comorbid conditions. Therefore, female recipients who are doing well with good graft function and who have good control of their medical problems can be expected to have reasonably good outcomes, although they must be treated as high-risk pregnancies.

II   HEART TRANSPLANTATION

A   **Candidates** have end-stage heart disease (New York Heart Association class III or IV) and are likely to die within 1–2 years without transplantation.

1. Two diagnoses, cardiomyopathy (40%) and coronary artery disease (40%), are most common. Congenital heart disease, valvular disease, and retransplantation comprise the remaining 20%.

2. The age of recipients ranges from newborns to adults in their mid-60s.

3. Increasingly, very ill heart transplant candidates are receiving a ventricular assist device (partial mechanical heart), with the diseased heart remaining in situ. This procedure is considered a "bridge to transplant."

B   **Contraindications** include severe pulmonary hypertension (although an absolute cutoff is difficult to define), tobacco use within 6 months, and poor renal or pulmonary function.

C   The **orthotopic procedure requires institution of cardiopulmonary bypass** (heart-lung machine; see Chapter 6) followed by partial excision of the heart, preserving the posterior half of the atria and the interatrial septum. The donor heart is then implanted with two atrial suture lines, the pulmonary artery anastomosis, and the aortic anastomosis.

D   **Postoperatively,** the heart provides normal cardiac output. As the heart is denervated, bradycardia is treated with pacing via temporary pacing wires implanted at surgery or via chronotropic drugs (e.g., isoproteronol). Atropine, which is a vagolytic drug, will not work.

1. **Initial immunosuppression** is usually with corticosteroids, a calcineurin inhibitor, and an antimetabolite, which are continued as maintenance therapy.

2. **Acute rejection** is difficult to diagnose clinically. Standard **surveillance for rejection** involves periodic **endomyocardial biopsy.** Under fluoroscopic guidance, a biopsy device is passed via the internal jugular vein into the right ventricle, where a biopsy is taken.

E   **Donors** An enormous gap exists between the number of cadaver donor hearts available and the number of candidates in need. Therefore, almost every cadaver donor is investigated as a possible heart donor. Coronary arteriography may be required as part of the workup of the potential cadaver donor. Donors are matched with recipients by blood type and size (i.e., weight, height).

F **Complications and results**

1. **Acute rejection** is common. Severity is determined histologically.

2. **Chronic rejection** is manifest as graft coronary artery disease. This process has a different distribution from atherosclerotic coronary disease because it favors smaller arteries. Accordingly, it is difficult to treat with angioplasty or bypass surgery and may require retransplantation.

3. **Hypertension** and **renal insufficiency** from cyclosporine or tacrolimus can be difficult to manage.

4. **Mortality.** Almost 10% of recipients die in the first month after transplantation. These deaths are often related to multiple organ failure or initial graft failure. Another 5% die during the next 11 months. Patient survival at 1 year is 85%.

5. **Long-term** patient survival is 70% at 5 years. Patient survival for heart and liver recipients is very similar.

III   LUNG TRANSPLANTATION

Lung transplantation can involve one or two lungs.

A **Candidates** have end-stage pulmonary parenchymal or vascular disease. They are New York Heart Association class III or IV, and they have an anticipated survival of less than 2 years without transplantation. Abstinence from tobacco for a minimum of 6 months is mandatory. **Three common indications** account for 70% of candidates: emphysema or chronic obstructive pulmonary disease, including α_1-antitrypsin deficiency (45%), primary pulmonary hypertension (12%), and cystic fibrosis (10%).

B **Specific assessment** of the following is critical.

1. **Cardiac function.** If left ventricular function is too poor, or if surgically uncorrectable congenital heart defects are present (usually Eisenmenger's syndrome), the patient is not a candidate for lung transplantation but may be considered for a heart-lung transplant.

2. If patients have **bilateral pulmonary infections** (e.g., from cystic fibrosis), they require double-lung transplants, because retention of an infected lung allows spread to the transplanted lung. Otherwise, single-lung transplants are used.

3. **Renal and hepatic function must be adequate.** Contraindications include current or recent tobacco or alcohol use and advanced pulmonary disease (e.g., ventilator-dependent conditions, intractable pulmonary infections, or excessive steroid requirements [for bronchospasm]).

C **Operative strategy**   Lung transplants are orthotopic, with excision of the diseased lung(s).

1. Lung transplantation has gained acceptance only recently. Many obstacles have appeared en route to success.
   a. The question of whether a single transplanted lung is adequate to treat patients has been resolved affirmatively, at least for restrictive lung diseases.
   b. Substantial difficulties with healing of the bronchial anastomosis have been improved.
   c. The lung represents a large immunologic target, requiring more immunosuppression than most other transplants.

2. **Single-lung transplants** are performed via lateral thoracotomy. Cardiopulmonary bypass is not usually required, unless pulmonary artery pressures rise excessively or blood gases deteriorate excessively when the pulmonary artery is clamped.
   a. Bronchial, pulmonary artery, and donor left atrial anastomoses (left atrial patch includes the pulmonary vein orifices) are performed.
   b. The bronchial anastomosis is performed by using a telescoping interrupted suture technique. Wrapping the bronchial anastomosis with a vascularized pedicle of omentum has also been used.
   c. Induction therapy with antilymphocyte sera and avoidance of high-dose steroids (which inhibit bronchial anastomotic healing) is often chosen.

3. **Double-lung transplants** are usually performed through a transverse anterior thoracotomy with or without cardiopulmonary bypass, and the procedure resembles two single-lung transplants. The two bronchial anastomoses are performed like single-lung transplants.

D **Postoperatively,** the new lung(s) rapidly accommodate, and prompt extubation is the rule. Both rejection and infection are monitored with serial chest radiographs, bronchoscopy with bronchoalveolar lavage or transbronchial biopsy, and measurements of forced expiratory volume in 1 second (FEV_1, only for rejection surveillance).

E **Donors** are scarce because prolonged intubation, chest contusions, aspiration injury, and pneumonia—any of which may contraindicate lung donation—are all common in brain-dead individuals. Bronchoscopy is required before donation and is often performed in the operating room just before the donor surgery.

F **Complications and results**

1. **Acute rejection** is characterized by fever, infiltrates on a chest radiograph, worsened blood gas exchange, and exclusion of infection by bronchoalveolar lavage. The incidence of acute rejection is 60%.

2. **Bronchial anastomotic complications** occur in approximately 15% of recipients and are treated with various methods from observation through surgical repair or stent placement. Complete breakdown or dehiscence of the bronchial anastomosis requires surgical repair or retransplantation.

3. **Pneumonia** is a common source of morbidity and potential mortality. The prevalence of bacterial pneumonia is 50%. The prevalence of CMV pneumonia varies with the serostatus (prior infection) of the donor and the recipient, but it can be fatal and prophylaxis is required. Fungal infection is uncommon (<10%) but is usually lethal.

4. **Survival** is similar for single-lung, double-lung, and heart-lung transplantation, with a 70% 1-year survival rate. Chronic rejection is a significant long-term problem. It is diagnosed histologically as bronchiolitis obliterans or clinically as bronchiolitis obliterans syndrome. Mortality with this diagnosis is high (40% within 2 years).

5. **Survival by diagnosis,** from best to worst, is as follows:
   a. Obstructive lung disease
   b. Cystic fibrosis
   c. Restrictive lung disease
   d. Pulmonary hypertension

IV HEPATIC TRANSPLANTATION

Hepatic transplantation is technically difficult because portal hypertension, portosystemic venous collaterals, and coagulopathy are usually present. The postoperative course depends on the initial condition of the patient, the function of the new liver, and technical problems in the perioperative period.

A **Candidates** have end-stage liver disease and are likely to die within 1–2 years without transplantation. Most candidates are between 6 months and 70 years of age. Careful evaluation of cardiopulmonary and renal function is essential. Once listed, priority is based on their MELD (Model for End-stage Liver Disease) score. The score is based on bilirubin, creatinine, and international normalized ratio (INR) and ranges from a minimum of 6 to a maximum of 40. The sicker the patient, the higher the values, and the higher the MELD score. Since priority is based on MELD, severity of disease is emphasized rather than waiting time.

B **Indications for liver transplantation** Approximately 95% of candidates have chronic disease; the remaining 5% have **fulminant hepatic failure,** which is a disorder that progresses rapidly.

1. Adults. In adults, the common chronic diseases that require liver transplantation include cirrhosis from **chronic hepatitis C** (40%), **alcoholic cirrhosis** (15%), **chronic hepatitis B** (<10%), **primary biliary cirrhosis** (<10%), and **primary sclerosing cholangitis** (<10%).

2. **Children.** In children who require liver transplantation, more than 50% have **biliary atresia** as the cause of liver failure.

3. **Three major complications herald end-stage liver disease** and indicate the need to consider liver transplantation.
   a. **Difficult-to-manage ascites** (refractory to treatment, associated with spontaneous bacterial peritonitis, or hydrothorax from peritoneal–pleural leaks)
   b. **Encephalopathy**
   c. **Esophageal variceal hemorrhage** (recurrent or associated with hepatic decompensation)

C **Four areas of controversy**

1. **Alcoholic patients with cirrhosis** have the same chance for successful transplantation as do patients with other diagnoses. However, they require screening to identify and exclude those who are likely to return to drinking. Most programs require a minimum of 6 months of abstinence. Alcoholic patients with cardiomyopathy and cerebral atrophy must be excluded.

2. **Patients with fulminant hepatic failure** can develop cerebral edema, herniation, and brain death. When fulminant hepatic failure results from a suicide attempt (classically from acetaminophen overdose), the patient can be excluded if the psychiatric history has documented multiple suicide attempts.

3. **Patients with primary hepatic malignancies** treated with transplantation have high recurrence rates and a poorer outcome. Therefore, their suitability as candidates is controversial. However, candidates with cirrhosis and a single, small (<5 cm) hepatocellular carcinoma that is not amenable to resection do not have a substantial risk of recurrence and are good candidates.

4. **Patients with cirrhosis from chronic viral hepatitis** face risks of recurrent hepatitis and the potential for recurrent cirrhosis. Treatment varies with the causative virus.

D **Donors** must match the recipient for size. For small children, the number of size-appropriate donors is insufficient. This problem has alternatives, including:

1. An adult cadaver liver is split, and the left lobe or lateral segment is transplanted to the child.

2. Adult living donors donate their left lateral segment to the child.

E **Operative strategy** The procedure generally requires 6–10 hours to perform.

1. **Removal of the diseased liver** requires dissection of the porta hepatitis, the inferior vena cava, and the diaphragmatic and retroperitoneal attachments of the liver. The blood flow to the diseased liver is interrupted, and the liver is removed. The patient is then **anhepatic** and requires intensive monitoring to maintain homeostasis. A segment of the retrohepatic vena cava may be removed with the liver, interrupting venous return.

2. **Implantation of the new liver**
   a. **External venovenous bypass** from the femoral and portal veins to the axillary vein may be used to bypass the inferior vena cava.
   b. **Venous anastomoses** are created for the suprahepatic vena cava, infrahepatic vena cava, and portal vein. These veins can then be opened, supplying the liver with warm, oxygenated blood and re-establishing caval flow. Alternatively, a piggyback method is used. The donor suprahepatic cava is anastomosed to the preserved recipient vena cava, and the donor infrahepatic cava is closed.
   c. **Hemostasis** is obtained, the hepatic artery is reconstructed, and the biliary tract is reconstituted to complete the procedure. The donor bile duct is anastomosed either to the recipient's bile duct or a Roux-en-Y segment of jejunum (see Chapter 11).

F **Postoperatively,** the function of the new liver can be ascertained by production of bile, uptake of potassium by hepatocytes (hypokalemia), correction of coagulopathy, and metabolism of the citrate anticoagulant of blood products (alkalosis).

1. **Nonfunction** of the liver graft is manifest by the absence of bile, persistent coagulopathy, and the inability to fully awaken. This uncommon complication (<10%) requires urgent retransplantation.

2. **Immunosuppression** is achieved by either cyclosporine or tacrolimus with steroids and often an antimetabolite.

G Complications and results

1. **Surgical complications** requiring reoperation are common, and they relate to any of the five anastomoses between the donor and the recipient. **Hepatic artery thrombosis** is especially common in children (5%–10%) and often requires retransplantation. **Biliary** complications are also fairly common. Anastomotic strictures are more common than leaks, and these usually happen early. Late strictures can be related to rejection.

2. **Acute rejection** usually manifests as increased liver function tests and occurs in about 40% of recipients. Fever or jaundice can occur with rejection. Diagnosis is made by liver biopsy. Rejection is almost always reversible.

3. **Chronic rejection,** also called vanishing bile duct syndrome, represents immunologic attack on the bile ducts and the small arteries that nourish them. This is uncommon but may require retransplantation because it is generally untreatable.

4. **Post-transplant death** is usually related to multiple organ failure. It is usually brought on by a combination of infection or rejection plus nephrotoxicity from cyclosporine or tacrolimus.

5. **Recurrence of hepatitis. Hepatitis B** recurrence can be treated with lamivudine. Recurrence of hepatitis C is universal and usually takes an insidious course. The long-term outcome of recurrent hepatitis C is mild or no hepatitis in 40%, moderate hepatitis in 45%, and recurrent cirrhosis in 15% (at 5 years).

6. **Survival of pediatric patients** after liver transplantation is slightly better than that of adults.

7. **Survival of adult patients** is more variable than survival of children (Table 24-3). Again, two factors have strong statistical influence.
   a. **Diagnosis.** The diagnoses of cancer and fulminant hepatic failure are associated with poorer outcomes.
   b. Patients who are more ill at the time of transplantation do not fare as well as those who are less ill.

TABLE 24-3   Patient Survival after Liver Transplantation

Pre-operative Status	Patient Survival (%) (1 year)	Patient Survival (%) (5 years)
Pediatric recipients (all)	80	74
Age <1 Year	74	67
Age <10 years	84	77
Patient status		
Life support	61	58
ICU	80	71
Hospitalized	77	71
At home	86	80
Adult recipients (all)	81	67
Patient status		
Life support	64	55
ICU	74	60
Hospitalized	79	62
At home	86	72
Diagnosis		
Hepatitis C	82	65
Hepatitis B	78	59
Cancer	67	32
Fulminant hepatic failure	71	63

ICU, intensive care unit.

V **RENAL TRANSPLANTATION**

When renal transplantation is successful, patients return to normal lives unencumbered by dialysis.

A **Candidates** Patients from newborn to 70 years of age with end-stage renal disease and on maintenance dialysis are typical candidates. Patients with declining renal function who are almost at the stage of requiring dialysis are also candidates.

1. Renal transplantation is **elective** in the sense that dialysis is always an option. Therefore, candidates should be stable before transplantation.

2. **Common indications for renal transplant** in adults include glomerulonephritis (41%), diabetes mellitus (16%), polycystic disease (13%), hypertension (12%), and pyelonephritis or interstitial nephritis (6%). In children, approximately 50% of candidates have congenital or hereditary renal disease, and the remaining 50% have acquired renal disease.

B **Donors**

1. **Living related donors** represent 30% of kidney transplants. A related donor and recipient share more genes than do unrelated pairs. **Three types of histocompatibility match** occur between related individuals.
   a. A **perfect match** (two haplotypes). Two siblings share the same HLA haplotype from both their mother and father. Siblings have a 25% chance of being a perfect match.
   b. A **half match** (one haplotype). The donor and recipient share one of two HLA haplotypes. Siblings have a 50% chance of being a half match; all parent–child pairs are a half match.
   c. A **zero match** (no haplotypes). Two siblings share neither haplotype. This situation occurs in 25% of sibling pairs.

2. **Cadaver donors** represent 70% of kidney transplant donors. The donor and the recipient can match from zero to six of their HLA antigens (see I F 3 c).

3. **Living unrelated donors** represent 3%–4% of kidney transplants and have the same types of matches as cadaver donors.

C **Graft survival** Graft survival rates vary from one center to another. Regardless, all four types of living donor kidneys have better results than do cadaver donor kidneys (Table 24-4).

1. **Factors that adversely affect graft survival**
   a. Retransplantation
   b. High-PRA patients
   c. Poor-quality donors
   d. Delayed graft function

TABLE 24-4 Results of Kidney Transplantation Related to Donor Source

	1-Year Graft Survival (%)	Half-life (years)
Living related donor		
Perfect match	95	27
Half match	92	13
Zero match	92	13
Living unrelated donor	92	13
Cadaver donor		
6-antigen match	90	13
All other matches	85	9
Second cadaver transplants (retransplants)	80	8

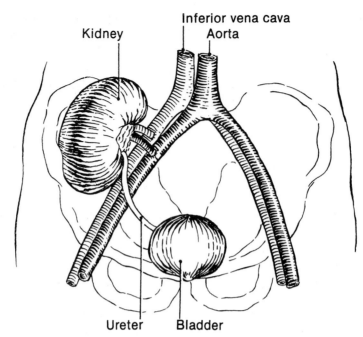

FIGURE 24-1 Placement of the renal transplant.

2. **Outcome** of renal transplantation is best expressed as the annual rate of graft loss (%/year) or as the half-life (i.e., the period of time by which half of the kidneys transplanted have failed).
   a. Patient survival and graft survival are separate outcomes. If the graft fails, the patient returns to dialysis.
   b. The **1-year graft survival** reflects avoidance of acute rejection and related graft loss. After the first year, the rate of graft loss is much slower and is caused by chronic rejection. The rate of late graft loss is relatively constant over time.
   c. **Patient survival rates** are relatively high. Living related recipients have a 5-year patient survival rate of 90%–95%. Patients who received donor kidneys from a cadaver have a 5-year patient survival rate of 75%–85%.

D **Operative strategy**

1. The urinary tract must be free of obstructions, stones, and infection. Nephrectomy is indicated for chronic persistent pyelonephritis, persistent upper tract stones, vesicoureteral reflux, severe unmanageable high-renin hypertension, and severe cyst complications with polycystic disease.

2. The **surgical procedure** involves placing the kidney in the retroperitoneum, a heterotropic location. The renal vessels are anastomosed to the iliac artery and vein in adults and occasionally to the aorta and inferior vena cava in small children. The ureter is directly implanted into the bladder (Fig. 24-1). The native kidneys are usually not removed.

E **Postoperatively,** 70%–90% of cadaver donor kidneys and all living donor kidneys function immediately, with a brisk diuresis and rapid drop in serum creatinine. Between 10% and 30% of cadaver donor kidneys do not function immediately (i.e., delayed graft function, acute tubular necrosis). This condition is usually temporary (7–14 days); then, the kidney gradually attains normal function.

F **Complications**

1. **Acute rejection** occurs in approximately 40% of recipients who receive prednisone, cyclosporine, ± azathioprine. The incidence of acute rejection is lowered with the addition of either an anti–IL-2 receptor antibody (see I H 7) or replacing azathioprine with mycophenolate mofetil. Only 20% of perfect-match living related recipients will experience acute rejection.

Treatment is pulse corticosteroids or antilymphocyte sera. Approximately 80% of episodes of acute rejection are reversible. If the episode is irreversible, the graft fails and the patient returns to dialysis.

2. **Chronic rejection** is reflected in the half-life (Table 24-4). A prior episode of acute rejection is the strongest predictor of increased risk of chronic rejection. Chronic rejection results in graft failure and return to dialysis.

3. **Surgical complications** are not uncommon, and they can usually be treated if they are recognized at an early stage.

   a. **Vascular complications** include renal artery stenosis or thrombosis and renal vein thrombosis and occur in 3%–5% of recipients. Patients may present with sudden anuria or hypertension.

   b. **Lymphatic complications** occur in less than 5% of recipients and appear as a perinephric lymph collection (lymphocele). The diagnosis is made by decreased urine output or an elevated creatinine level, which prompts a diagnostic ultrasound. The lymphocele is drained by percutaneous aspiration or, optimally, by (laparoscopic) drainage into the peritoneal cavity.

   c. **Urologic complications** occur in less than 10% of renal transplant patients and include urine leakage at the ureter-bladder anastomosis and ureter obstruction or infarction caused by compromise of the ureteral blood supply, which may occur during donor nephrectomy. Arteries leading to the lower pole of the kidney usually vascularize the upper ureter and must be preserved. The diagnosis of urologic complications can be confirmed by means of radioisotope scanning, ultrasound examination, or cystography.

VI PANCREAS TRANSPLANTATION

Pancreas transplantation provides an entire cadaver donor pancreas as an endogenous source of insulin to replace exogenous insulin for patients with **type I** insulin-dependent diabetes mellitus. With long-term euglycemia, improvement or stabilization of diabetic complications of the eyes, kidneys, and diabetic neuropathy can be demonstrated. Transplantation of the islets of Langerhans without the exocrine pancreatic tissue (islet transplants) is now performed under experimental protocols with excellent short-term results. As of yet, the longevity of islet transplants has not equalled that of whole pancreas transplants.

A **Candidates** are usually 25–55 years of age, as it takes 10–20 years of diabetes to develop diabetic complications, particularly nephropathy.

1. Candidates can be considered in **three groups.**
   a. **Diabetic patients with end-stage renal disease** are candidates for a simultaneous pancreas-kidney (SPK) transplant.
   b. **Diabetic patients with renal failure** may opt for a kidney transplant first (particularly if they have a good living donor) and later undergo pancreas after kidney (PAK) transplantation.
   c. Recipients without nephropathy but with other severe complications (e.g., retinopathy, severe neuropathy, hypoglycemic unawareness) are candidates for pancreas transplantation alone (PTA).

2. The high prevalence of coexistent coronary artery disease mandates **cardiac evaluation,** including stress testing.

3. **Contraindications** to pancreas transplantation include age higher than 60 years, severe peripheral vascular or coronary artery disease, obesity, and type II diabetes.

B **Donors** are younger than 60 years. Contraindications to donation include current or prior pancreatitis, pancreatic damage from trauma, diabetes (any type), and alcoholism.

1. Operatively, the blood supply of the liver and pancreas of the donor must be identified and shared when both organs will be used.

2. Pancreas donors also donate the **iliac artery bifurcation** for arterial reconstruction.

3. The **spleen** is removed with the pancreas and is separated after revascularization.

C Types of operations

1. **SPK transplantation.** Rejection is the most common cause of pancreas graft loss. Unfortunately, it is difficult to diagnose and often is irreversible. An important advantage to SPK transplantation is that the kidney serves as a marker for rejection of the pancreas.
    a. **Advantages.** Other advantages to SPK transplantation include the following:
       (1) Only one surgery is needed.
       (2) High doses of induction immunosuppression drugs are needed only once.
    b. **Disadvantages** to SPK transplantation are the extended procedure for some patients and, until recently, the inability to use potential living kidney donors. A newer procedure, the simultaneous cadaver pancreas and living donor kidney transplantation (the SPLK), is currently used in select centers. This procedure avoids the necessity of two separate operations.

2. **PAK transplantation**
    a. **Advantage.** The advantage to the PAK approach is that this group is selected by their good response to a kidney transplant. It is hoped that these patients have a relatively low risk of rejection.
    b. **Disadvantages** include two separate procedures: a repeat course of induction immunosuppression drugs, and the kidney not serving as a marker for rejection because the pancreas is from a different donor.

D Operative strategy

1. **Anatomy.** Embryologically, the pancreas is derived at the foregut-midgut junction and therefore receives blood supply from the celiac axis and the superior mesenteric artery. The splenic artery from the celiac axis supplies the tail, whereas the inferior pancreaticoduodenal arteries from the superior mesenteric artery supply the head.
2. Recipients receive the **whole pancreas** along with a segment of duodenum.
    a. The exocrine secretions pass via the ampulla of Vater into the duodenum, which is anastomosed either to the bladder or to the small bowel.
    b. The two arterial blood supplies to the pancreas are joined by an arterial Y graft (the bifurcation of the donor common iliac artery is anastomosed to the splenic artery and the superior mesenteric artery).
3. **Procedure.** Through a lower midline incision, the pancreas is placed in the right iliac fossa. Anastomoses (donor to recipient) include portal vein to iliac vein, common iliac artery Y graft to iliac artery, and duodenum to bladder or small intestine. For SPK transplantation, the kidney is placed in the left iliac fossa through the same incision. An alternative for venous drainage of the pancreas is to the recipient superior mesenteric vein (portal drainage) in conjuction with enteric exocrine drainage. Portal drainage may have immunological advantages.

E Complications and results

1. **Postoperatively,** the patients quickly become insulin independent. Induction immunosuppression drugs generally include an antilymphocyte serum. Maintenance immunosuppression usually consists of corticosteroids, a calcineurin inhibitor, and mycophenolate mofetil.
2. **Surveillance for rejection**
    a. **SPK transplant patients** are monitored indirectly via the kidney (i.e., creatinine).
    b. **Pancreas transplants** with bladder drainage are followed by urinary amylase, although this marker is not very reliable.
    c. In the absence of a clinical marker, enteric-drained pancreas transplants and PAK and PTA transplants are monitored by plasma amylase and/or lipase and periodic (protocol) pancreas biopsies to search for rejection.
    d. **Elevated blood glucose levels** usually indicate substantial and often irreversible loss of islet function.
3. **Patient survival.** The 1-year patient survival rate for all three pancreas procedures (SPK, PAK, and PTA) is 94%, which is similar to the 1-year patient survival rate after kidney transplant for diabetic recipients.

4. **Graft survival.** The graft survival rate most strongly reflects the type of procedure that was performed. The 1-year pancreas graft survival rates are 80% for SPK transplantation, 75% for PAK, and 80% for PTA transplantation.

5. **Rejection** is common. Up to 40% of SPK patients have at least one episode of acute rejection.

6. **Complications** include graft pancreatitis, pancreatic leaks and fistulas, graft thrombosis, and bladder complications related to pancreatic enzymes (e.g., cystitis, hemorrhagic cystitis, urethritis).

VII SMALL BOWEL TRANSPLANTATION

Experience with small bowel transplantation is more limited than with the previous organs discussed.

A **Candidates** for small bowel transplantation have irreversible intestinal failure and are permanently dependent on total parenteral nutrition (TPN). With long-term TPN, patients may develop TPN-induced hepatic failure, which may necessitate a combined liver and small bowel transplant

B **Causes**   Short bowel is the primary reason for small bowel transplantation. Patients with adequate length of bowel but poor bowel function (e.g., Crohn's disease, visceral myopathies) may be candidates.

1. In **children,** causes include congenital atresias, volvulus, necrotizing enterocolitis, and gastroschisis.

2. In **adults,** causes include Crohn's disease, volvulus, trauma, and vascular accidents, such as superior mesenteric artery occlusion.

C **Operative strategy**   Venous outflow can be to the portal or systemic veins. Options for gastrointestinal continuity include no bowel anastomoses and two stomas, two bowel anastomoses and no stomas, or one bowel anastomosis and one stoma. The last option is preferred because it provides proximal bowel continuity plus a distal stoma for easy biopsy access.

D **Postoperative immunosuppression** is usually with tacrolimus plus other drugs.

E **Complications** include sepsis, stomal complications (including retraction and ischemia), and graft failure resulting from vascular thrombosis or hemorrhage. Lymphatic drainage problems are usually short term but may affect long-chain fatty acid absorption.

1. Because the small bowel is rich in lymphoid tissue, **graft-versus-host disease** has been a problem more prevalent in small bowel transplantation than in other organ transplants. This cascade of events is caused by the proliferation of donor-derived immunocompetent cells manifested as skin rash, diarrhea, altered liver functions, and anemia and can appear in the intestine as sloughing, shortening, and blunting of the villi.

2. **Graft function is monitored** by looking at various absorption studies (including ethylenediaminetetraacetic acid [EDTA] and maltose) and direct biopsy techniques.

3. The **histologic appearance** of the gut during rejection includes blunting of microvilli, mononuclear infiltration of the intestinal wall, and epithelial cell attenuation.

F **Graft survival rates** have been reported to be approximately 70% at 1 year for small bowel only and approximately 60% for liver and small bowel. Experience is still limited, and surgical and immunologic challenges lie ahead.

chapter 25

Urologic Surgery

HUNTER WESSELLS · BRUCE L. DALKIN

I   URINARY TRACT INFECTIONS

A   Definitions

1. **Bacteriuria** is the presence of bacteria in the bladder. It can occur with or without pyuria and can be symptomatic or asymptomatic.

2. **Pyelonephritis** is a clinical syndrome with fever, chills, and flank pain accompanied by bacteriuria and pyuria.

3. **Cystitis** is an inflammatory condition of the bladder. It can be bacterial or nonbacterial (e.g., radiation, interstitial, fungal causes).

4. **Reinfection** signifies recurrent infection with different bacteria from outside the urinary tract.

5. **Relapse** indicates recurrent infection caused by the same bacterial strain from a focus within the urinary tract.

6. **Prophylactic antimicrobial therapy** refers to prevention of reinfection of the urinary tract by administration of antimicrobial therapy.

7. **Suppressive antimicrobial therapy** is used to suppress an existing urinary tract infection (UTI) that cannot be eradicated.

B   Etiology

1. **Ascending infection.** Most UTIs are thought to result from ascending colonization from the introitus in women or from the periurethral area in men. **Fecal flora** are the most common pathogens, including *Escherichia coli*, other gram-negative rods, and entercocci. Other pathogens include staphycoccal species.

2. **Incidence.** UTIs are more common in women than in men, possibly because women have a shorter urethra. There may also be a protective effect of the prostatic urethra in men. Newer concepts of bacterial adherence factors in the bladder are being investigated.

C   Clinical presentation

1. **Cystitis** symptoms include:
   a. Urinary frequency
   b. Urgency
   c. Dysuria
   d. Cloudy or foul-smelling urine
   e. Hematuria

2. **Pyelonephritis** symptoms include all of the symptoms of cystitis plus fever, chills, and flank pain.

D   Diagnosis

1. **Urinalysis**
   a. **Pyuria.** The presence of white blood cells in the urine indicates inflammation.
   b. **Bacteriuria.** The detection of bacteria in the urine may require a Gram stain.
   c. **Nitrate reduction.** Nitrate in the urine is reduced to nitrite in the presence of bacteria.
   d. **Leukocyte esterase.** White blood cells contain esterases that can be detected in the urine.

2. **Urine culture** is performed on a split agar disposable plate and determines the presence of bacteria in the urine. The common quantization for infection is $\geq 10^{-5}$ bacteria. However, lower numbers present in symptomatic patients may signify infection.

E **Treatment**

1. **Choice of antimicrobial agent**
   a. **Uncomplicated cystitis.** Good results have been obtained with ampicillin, amoxicillin, first-generation cephalosporins, fluoroquinolones, nitrofurantoin, and trimethoprim-sulfamethoxazole. Regional differences in antibiotic resistance exist and should dictate choice of antimicrobial agent.
   b. **Complicated UTI.** Fluoroquinolones or parenteral regimens are recommended for initial empirical therapy of a UTI associated with significant anatomic or structural abnormality of the urinary tract or with acute pyelonephritis or prostatitis.

2. **Duration of therapy**
   a. Uncomplicated cystitis therapy lasts for 1–3 days.
   b. Complicated UTI therapy lasts for 7–14 days.
   c. Acute prostatitis therapy is given over 14–28 days.
   d. Pyelonephritis therapy lasts for 14–21 days.

F **Serious complications of a UTI**

1. **Renal papillary necrosis.** Sloughing of the renal papillae is frequently seen in diabetic patients. This sloughing can cause ureteral obstruction and hydronephrosis.

2. **Pyonephrosis** is infected hydronephrosis associated with infectious destruction of renal parenchyma. Usually, the patient is very ill and has a fever and chills.
   a. **Cause.** Obstruction (e.g., ureteral calculus) with infection
   b. **Treatment**
      (1) Ureteral catheter drainage
      (2) Percutaneous nephrostomy tube, if a ureteral catheter is not possible

3. **Perinephric abscess** is thought to occur usually from renal extension of ascending infection.
   a. **Clinical presentation** varies among patients.
      (1) Fever, chills, and flank pain are common.
      (2) Symptoms may persist after appropriate antimicrobial therapy.
   b. **Diagnosis.** Ultrasound and computed tomography (CT) scan are the best methods.
   c. **Treatment** can include the following:
      (1) Percutaneous aspiration and drainage
      (2) Relieving obstruction if present (e.g., removal of a ureteral catheter)
      (3) Antimicrobial therapy

G **Prostatitis/Chronic pelvic pain syndrome is a spectrum of infectious and noninfectious diseases of the prostate gland.**

1. **Clinical presentation** includes urinary frequency, urgency, perineal pain or fullness, and dysuria.

2. **Subsets** include acute bacterial prostatitis, chronic bacterial prostatitis, nonbacterial prostatitis, and prostatodynia (Table 25-1).

3. **Diagnosis**
   a. Acute bacterial prostatitis presents with most of the aforementioned symptoms plus a fever. Prostatic massage should not be performed to avoid bacteremia.
   b. **Urinalysis.** Patients with acute bacterial prostatitis usually have inflammatory findings on urinalysis.
   c. **Expressed prostatic secretions (EPS),** which are fluid obtained by digital massage of the prostate, are tested for leukocytes in chronic inflammatory conditions.

4. **Bacteriologic etiology**
   a. **Young men** (younger than 50 years of age). *Chlamydia* and gram-negative organisms predominate.

TABLE 25-1 Diagnostic Features of Prostatitis/Chronic Pelvic Pain Syndrome

Type of Prostatitis	Symptoms	Systemic Signs	Increased WBC in EPS	Positive Culture
Acute bacterial prostatitis	Yes	Yes	Yes	Yes
Chronic bacterial prostatitis	Yes	No	Yes	Yes
Nonbacterial prostatitis	Yes	No	Yes	No
Prostatodynia	Yes	No	No	No

WBC, white blood cell count; EPS, expressed prostatic secretions.

    b. Elderly men (older than 50 years of age). Gram-negative organisms are the most common pathogens.

  5. Treatment
    a. Acute bacterial prostatitis
      (1) Trimethoprim-sulfamethoxazole for 30 days
      (2) Fluoroquinolone for 30 days
      (3) Parenteral therapy with ampicillin and gentamicin or vancomycin, if the patient is systemically ill or has a complicated UTI
    b. Chronic bacterial prostatitis. Treatment is based on culture and sensitivity.
      (1) Trimethoprim-sulfamethoxazole for 6 weeks
      (2) Fluoroquinolone for 6 weeks
      (3) To treat symptomatic episodes or to consider suppression if therapy is ineffective (which it commonly is)
    c. Nonbacterial prostatitis
      (1) Doxycycline for 4–6 weeks
      (2) Symptomatic control, including sitz baths
    d. Prostatodynia. Because the cause may be multifactorial and include poorly understood, treatment is evolving.
      (1) Symptomatic control with empirical antimicrobial therapy
      (2) α-Adrenergic antagonists
      (3) Trycyclic antidepressents or membrane stabilizing agent (e.g. gabapentin)
      (4) Muscle relaxants (e.g., diazepam)
      (5) Biofeedback
      (6) Stress reduction techniques
      (7) Saw Palmetto and Pygeum extracts; anti-irritants to the prostate

II URINARY CALCULI

A Etiologic theories

  1. Supersaturation and crystallization
    a. Uric acid and cystine calculi form when urine with an acid pH less than 6.0 becomes oversaturated with uric acid or cystine.
    b. Struvite (magnesium ammonium phosphate) **calculi** form when the magnesium ammonium phosphate ions exist in an alkaline urine.
  2. Inhibitor deficiency. Inhibitors (e.g., high molecular weight glycoproteins, citrate, magnesium, phosphates [pyrophosphate], zinc) that exist in the urine and can retard stone formation may be lacking.

B Types of urinary calculi

  1. Calcium oxalate calculi are the most common stones. They are radiopaque owing to the calcium ion. They exist in monohydrate (more radiodense) and dihydrate forms.
  2. Uric acid calculi are radiolucent stones that are formed from excess urinary uric acid levels.

3. **Cystine calculi** are faintly radiopaque because of the sulfur ion.
   a. **Cause. Cystinuria** is an autosomal recessive disorder that results in a defect in renal tubular reabsorption of four amino acids: cystine, ornithine, arginine, and lysine. Only cystine forms calculi.
      (1) Heterozygotes will most likely not form calculi; homozygotes invariably form multiple calculi.
      (2) Cystine calculi form because of the low solubility of cystine in urine with a pH less than 7.0.
   b. **Prevention.** Overhydration and urine alkalinization to pH 7.5 are the most effective preventive measures. Oral cystine-binding drugs, such as D-penicillamine or α-mercaptopropionylglycine, also help to prevent stone formation.
   c. **Treatment** of existing stones is usually multimodal with percutaneous procedures, extracorporeal shock-wave lithotripsy (ESWL), and dissolution therapy (percutaneous). Dissolution solutions include *N*-acetylcysteine or bicarbonate.

4. **Struvite calculi** are also radiopaque. They are usually related to chronic UTIs with urea-splitting bacteria, which maintain an alkaline urine:
   a. Proteus, which is most common
   b. Providencia
   c. Pseudomonas
   d. Klebsiella

C **Clinical presentation** The most frequent symptom is **pain,** which is caused by ureteral obstruction. The site of pain is related to the location of the obstructing calculus (e.g., flank pain, lower abdominal pain, testicular pain, or vulvar pain). Other symptoms that can occur include:

1. Hematuria (visible or microscopic)
2. Nausea and vomiting
3. Irritative bladder symptoms (e.g., from a ureterovesical junction calculus)

D **Diagnosis**

1. **Physical examination.** Patients are usually in distress and have costovertebral angle tenderness. Occasionally, an associated paralytic ileus can occur, which must be differentiated from an acute abdomen.
2. **Urinalysis**
   a. **Hematuria** is usually present.
   b. A uric acid stone is unlikely to be found in a patient with a urine pH of 6.5 or higher.
3. **Noncontrast spiral computed tomography (CT)** is now the diagnostic test of choice. This procedure is less costly, less time consuming, without contrast and is very accurate; however, although improvements are being made, it is not yet as informative as intravenous pyelography (IVP).
4. **Excretory urography (IVP)** can be useful to delineate complex anatomy or as alternative to CT (Fig. 25-1).
   a. Renal function should be assessed before IVP to avoid contrast nephrotoxicity.
   b. IVP should define stone size, location, and degree of obstruction.
5. **Ultrasonography** is best used in patients with elevated serum creatinine or with a severe allergy to contrast media. It defines hydronephrosis or an acoustic shadow from a calculus. Ultrasonography is often used in conjunction with a plain abdominal radiograph.
6. **Cystourethroscopy** and **retrograde pyelography** may need to be used to confirm the presence of a calculus and reveal its location if it is difficult to identify the calculus on imaging studies.

E **Treatment**

1. **Indications for emergency surgery** include:
   a. **Fever.** Obstructive calculi in a patient with a fever requires emergent decompression of the obstructed system. This is best accomplished through cystoscopy and retrograde placement of a ureteral catheter or stent. No further manipulation of the calculus should be performed

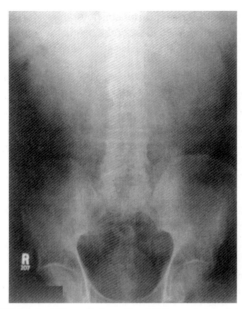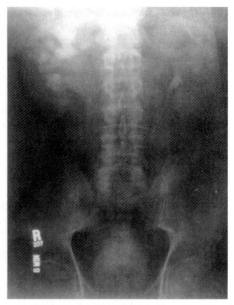

FIGURE 25-1 IVP; preliminary film **(left)** reveals a radiointensity **(right)** between L2 and L3. After injection of intravenous contrast, the density is seen obviously in the proximal ureter with resultant hydrouteronephrosis.

at that time because of the risk of sepsis. If the obstructed system is unable to be decompressed in this manner, a percutaneous nephrostomy tube should be placed.

b. Renal insufficiency. An elevated serum creatinine level or ureteral calculi requires urgent ultrasonography. Similarly, cystoscopy with retrograde pyelography can further delineate an anatomic problem, and stent placement may be necessary. A classic situation is the solitary kidney with an obstructing calculus.

2. **Observation** for spontaneous stone passage
   a. The patient must have adequate pain control (orally), an ability to take liquids by mouth, and a stone that has a favorable chance of passing.
   b. The likelihood of spontaneous passage is related to the size of the stone and the site of obstruction. Most distal ureteral calculi of 5 mm or less will pass spontaneously.

3. **Surgical procedures.** Advances in endoscopic techniques, ESWL, and endourology successfully allow most calculi to be removed without open surgical procedures.
   a. **Indications for intervention** include:
      (1) Severe pain
      (2) Nonprogression of calculus passage
      (3) Infection (emergent)
      (4) Prolonged obstruction
      (5) Interference with lifestyle
   b. **Percutaneous nephrostomy procedures** allow renal calculi to be approached through a nephrostomy tube tract in the flank. This is best suited for large calculi that can be fragmented and removed using ultrasonic, electrohydraulic, or laser lithotriptors.
   c. **Ureteroscopic procedures.** A transurethral approach into the ureter is best for calculi in the distal half of the ureter but may also be used for upper ureteral and renal calculi.
      (1) Calculi can be "grabbed" in a wire basket and removed intact, or laser, electrohydraulic, or ultrasonic lithotriptors may be used to fragment calculi.
      (2) A **stent** is often left in the ureter after manipulation to alleviate obstruction from edema.
   d. **ESWL** can be used for renal or ureteral calculi. It consists of an external energy source, which is focused by fluoroscopic or ultrasound guidance on a calculus to provide a high-pressure zone that can fragment the calculus. The gravel-like fragments pass through the ureter.
      (1) **Complications** include bleeding, perinephric hematoma, "steinstrasse" (gravel causing ureteral obstruction), and hypertension.

(2) Contraindications include coagulopathy, antiplatelet medications, or infection. Simultaneous bilateral treatment is contraindicated.

F **Metabolic evaluation and prophylaxis**   Patients who require a metabolic evaluation to determine the etiology of their calculus formation include young people (younger than 40 years of age) experiencing their first calculus event, people with multiple calculi, and people with recurrent stone formation. Most of these patients will have a metabolic abnormality that can be benefited by medical therapy. All patients require radiographic assessment to rule out anatomic causes for calculi formation, such as obstruction with urinary stasis.

G **Analysis of calculi**   The retrieved calculus or fragments should be analyzed to determine their composition.

1. **Calcium-containing calculi** consist mainly of calcium oxalate or calcium phosphate.
   a. Serum chemistry, urinalysis, and 24-hour urine collection for calcium, oxalate, phosphate, uric acid, citrate, and creatinine are performed.
   b. The goal is to differentiate the various **causes of calcium stone formation,** such as:
      (1) Renal hypercalciuria (leak of renal calcium)
      (2) Absorptive hypercalcuria (excessive gastrointestinal absorption of calcium)
      (3) Hyperparathyroidism
      (4) Normocalciuria
      (5) Renal tubular acidosis (in association with sarcoidosis, hypercalcemia, vitamin D intoxication, immobilization syndrome)
   c. **Treatment** for calcium-containing calculi includes:
      (1) Hydration to maintain a urine output greater than 2 L/day
      (2) Thiazide diuretics for renal hypercalcuria
      (3) Orthophosphates (absorptive hypercalcemics) to bind calcium in the gastrointestinal tract
      (4) Citrate to increase urinary citrate, which is an inhibitor of calculus formation
      (5) Low-calcium diet

2. **Struvite calculi** require the presence of urea-splitting bacteria, which maintain an alkaline urine environment.
   a. *Proteus* is the most common pathogen.
   b. **Treatment.** Removal of all stone fragments plus eradication of infection is imperative. Frequently, the patient requires a combination of percutaneous and ESWL treatment. Percutaneous dissolution therapy is sometimes used on remaining small fragments.

3. **Uric acid calculi** are radiolucent on plain radiographs and dense (white) on a CT scan. They form in acid urine pH (i.e., pH <6.0). Alkalinization of urine to pH 7.0 will dissolve uric acid calculi. Potassium citrate or sodium bicarbonate is also effective. If hyperuricemia is present, allopurinol should be added for prevention of future calculi.

4. **Cystine calculi** (see II B 3)

III   BENIGN PROSTATIC HYPERPLASIA

Benign prostatic hyperplasia (BPH) is a benign enlargement of the prostate gland that occurs commonly in aging men. Histologic changes include stromal and epithelial hyperplasia in the transition (periurethral) zone, which can compress the prostatic urethra and obstruct urinary flow. This process depends on testosterone, but the exact etiology remains unknown. The clinical sequela of BPH, **lower urinary tract symptom (LUTS),** occur in only a subset of patients with histologic BPH. Obstruction is thought to have a **static component** (mechanical) and a **dynamic component** (bladder neck, prostatic capsule, and urethral tone).

A **Diagnosis** is based on the patient's symptoms and findings on digital rectal examination (DRE). Cold weather, ingestion of alcohol, narcotics, antihistamines, anticholinergics, and holding urine for prolonged periods may exacerbate symptoms or precipitate urinary retention.

1. **Symptoms**
   a. **Obstructive voiding symptoms of BPH.** These symptoms tend to respond best to treatment.
      (1) Diminished force of urinary stream despite a full bladder
      (2) Hesitancy in initiating flow
      (3) Sense of incomplete emptying
      (4) Intermittency or "double voiding"
      (5) Urinary retention
   b. **Irritative voiding symptoms.** These are thought to be caused by detrusor instability from chronic obstruction.
      (1) Frequency
      (2) Urgency, possibly urge incontinence
      (3) Nocturia
      (4) Dysuria
   c. **The International Prostate Symptom Score is a seven-item validated questionnaire that is useful to quantify severity of LUTS. Scores range from 0 to 35 and are subdivided into Mild (0–7), Moderate (8–19), and Severe (19–35).**

2. **Physical examination and diagnostic testing** include:
   a. Palpation of the gland to assess size, consistency, and presence or absence of induration (risk of cancer)
   b. Palpation of a suprapubic mass consistent with a full bladder
   c. Hematuria (microscopic or gross)
   d. Prostatic-specific antigen (PSA) (optimal)
   e. Assessment of residual urine volume via transabdominal ultrasonography or direct catheterization
   f. Uroflowmetric findings of diminished flow rate and prolonged voiding, or urodynamic evidence of low flow rate despite high intravesical pressure
   Optional Additional Tests
   g. Cystourethroscopy to assess visual obstruction, bladder trabeculation, cellule or diverticuli formation, or bladder calculi. (None of these findings is specific for BPH, and each can be present in the absence of significant symptoms.)
   h. Transrectal ultrasonography (TRUS) to demonstrate enlargement and allow estimation of the volume of prostatic tissue, and biopsy if a significant risk of cancer exists
   i. IVP to demonstrate an enlarged prostatic impression on the inferior bladder, bladder wall thickening, hydroureteronephrosis, "J hooking" of the distal ureters, or bladder calculi. (IVP is no longer a standard part of the evaluation but may be included if infection or hematuria is present.)

B **Treatment**

1. **Indications for treatment.** Absolute indications for intervention include:
   a. Urinary retention
   b. Significant or recurrent gross hematuria not due to other causes.
   c. Bladder calculi
   d. Bilateral hydroureteronephrosis with renal insufficiency secondary to bladder outlet obstruction
   e. Repeated UTIs caused by urinary stasis
   f. Most men initiating treatment do so for relief of symptoms rather than any absolute indication.

2. **Goals of treatment** include:
   a. Symptomatic improvement
   b. Enhancement of bladder emptying and flow dynamics
   c. Preservation of bladder and upper urinary tract function
   d. Resolution of hematuria, if present

3. **Therapies.** Surgical treatment remains the gold standard for removing the transition zone tissue of the prostate. However, there is an increasing demand for conservative therapy driven by cost considerations and by pharmacologic and technical advances.
   a. **Surgical therapy**
      (1) **Transurethral resection (transurethral prostatectomy; TURP)** provides reliable and immediate improvement in both symptoms and voiding dynamics. A wire loop attached

to an electrocautery unit is used to resect tissue under direct cystoscopic vision. Complications include bleeding, infection, retrograde ejaculation, bladder neck contracture, urethral stricture, and impotence (rarely). Regional anesthesia is commonly utilized. **Transurethral incision (TUI)** may be appropriate for patients who have small (<20 g) glands. TUI is associated with a lower incidence of bladder neck contracture and retrograde ejaculation.

(2) **Open prostatectomy, or enucleation,** is usually reserved for patients with glands larger than 60 g or in whom other pathology exists (e.g., vesical calculus or bladder diverticulum requiring repair).

(3) **Laser ablation techniques** cause delayed sloughing or more immediate evaporation of obstructing tissue. Numerous laser techniques exist; the results are reasonable with the newest vaporization lasers comparable at 3 years to TURP, unlike other laser techniques. Anticoagulated patients currently represent the most appropriate candidates for this technique because bleeding complications are minimal.

(4) **Microwave therapy** is a technique for men with mild to moderate symptoms with marginal efficacy.

(5) **Intraprostatic stents** are available to mechanically relieve bladder outlet obstruction but have seen a declining role. Risks of infection, erosion, migration, encrustation, and severe irritative symptoms limit use to rare patients who are too ill to undergo a more definitive procedure.

b. Medical therapy is used to relieve symptoms in men with mild to moderate disease. Although objective improvement may be minimal, if symptomatic improvement occurs, treatment is successful.

(1) **Selective α_1-sympatholytics** block α_1-receptors in the prostatic capsule and bladder neck area, reducing outlet resistance and improving symptoms. In men with mild to moderate symptoms of prostatism, these agents represent the most commonly used first-line treatment with fairly good symptomatic improvement. Principal side effects include orthostatic hypotension and asthenia.

(2) **5 α-Reductase inhibitors** block intraprostatic conversion of testosterone to dihydrotestosterone (DHT), reducing prostatic size and improving symptoms with minimal side effects. Objective symptom improvements have been modest, and a trial of 3–6 months may slightly be required to determine efficacy. These agents reduce the risk of acute urinary retention and the need for TURP.

(3) **Combination Therapy** (e.g. 5 α-reductase inhibitor plus α-sympatholytics) has been shown in a RCT to be superior to single-agent therapy for the prevention of disease progression.

IV CARCINOMA

A Prostate tumors

1. **Epidemiology.** There is an increasing number of new cases; in the United States, blacks have a higher mortality rate compared with whites, even when the rate is adjusted for age and socioeconomic status, likely due to later presentation.

2. **Etiology.** There appears to be an increased risk in men with one or more relatives diagnosed before 70 years of age. A hormonal dependence exists but is not clarified.

3. **Pathology.** Approximately 95% of prostatic carcinomas are adenocarcinomas. Transitional cell carcinoma of the prostatic urethra, small cell carcinomas, and sarcomas are uncommon lesions.

a. The **anatomic site of origin** is most commonly the peripheral zone, which is felt on DRE. The transition zone, or periurethral zone (area removed at transurethral resection for benign disease), is the other common site of cancer.

b. Premalignant change. Prostatic–intraepithelial neoplasia (PIN), when high grade, is frequently associated with concomitant adenocarcinoma. Whether it is a true precursor is unknown.

c. Tumor grading

(1) Grading is the histologic assessment of the metastatic potential of a tumor.

(2) The **Gleason grading system** is most commonly used: Gleason grade ranges from 1 (low) to 5 (high). The Gleason sum total is derived by adding the most common and the

second most common grades seen in the specimen; that is: 3 + 2. The sum total is subdivided as low (2–4), moderate, (5–6), and high (7–10).

4. **Diagnosis**
   a. **Present diagnostic modalities** include DRE, PSA serum level, and TRUS.
      (1) **DRE** is a traditional method of cancer detection, assessing for induction, or a "module," in the prostate and is a means to diagnose some cancers missed by other modalities (e.g., PSA, TRUS).
      (2) **PSA level.** PSA is a serine protease that serves to liquefy semen after ejaculation. It has a diagnostic role as well as a role in following response to cancer treatment. When combined with DRE, determination of the PSA level improves the ability to detect cancers. Free PSA: a subset of total TSA also providing assistance in diagnosis. A low level, <15% of total PSA, correlates with a higher risk of cancer.
      (3) **TRUS** is an operator-dependent technique that is marginally helpful at identifying lesions. TRUS is excellent in aiding or directing biopsies of the prostate.
   b. **Screening.** Cancer detection devices are most often used on men who would require aggressive treatment if a tumor is identified, , generally in men with a >7–10 year projected survival.
   c. **Prostate biopsy** is an office-based procedure performed with TRUS guidance in men who have a suspicious DRE and/or an elevated level of PSA. Risks include bleeding (urinary tract or rectal), infection (biopsy is usually done transrectally), and bloody ejaculate. Significant complications occur in fewer than 1 in 500 men.
   d. **Staging** is the clinical evaluation of the metastatic status of a tumor.
      (1) **DRE.** A nodular extension outside the margins of the prostate indicates periprostatic extension.
      (2) **TRUS** may similarly identify the periprostatic spread of a tumor.
      (3) **PSA.** There is a reasonable correlation between PSA and risk of extraprostatic disease as well as the long-term benefit from treatment for localized cancer.
      (4) **CT scan of the abdomen and pelvis.** Evaluation for pelvic or retroperitoneal lymph node metastases and local extraprostatic extension is probably only cost-effective in men with a markedly elevated level of PSA, and/or high-grade disease who are at risk for these abnormalities.
      (5) **Magnetic resonance imaging (MRI) of the prostate** is an expensive procedure to identify local extraprostatic spread of disease. It is unclear whether MRI offers additional information to the combination of DRE, TRUS, and PSA.
      (6) **Radionuclide bone scan.** Bone metastases are common with prostate cancer. Recent evidence supports not ordering bone scans in men with a low PSA (<15 ng/mL) and low volume disease on biopsy. Higher-risk individuals should be studied (Fig. 25-2).

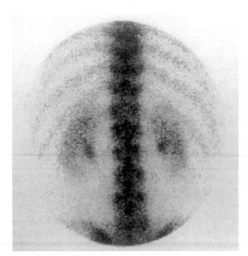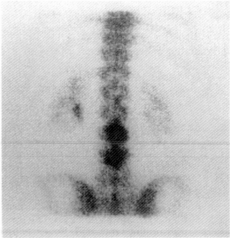

FIGURE 25-2 Radionuclide bone scan in the same patient as in Figure 25-1 revealing a normal examination **(left)** and, later, new areas of increased tracer uptake representing metastatic disease at the L3 and L4 vertebral bodies **(right).**

TABLE 25-2   TNM Staging Classification of Prostate Carcinoma

T (Tumor)

T1	Incidental histologic finding
T1a	<5% of tissue removed and low grade
T1b	>5% of tissue removed or moderate or high grade
T1c	Discovered at biopsy for an elevated prostate-specific antigen only
T2	Clinically palpable tumor
T2a	<1.5 cm of tumor
T2b	>1.5 cm of tumor confined to prostate
T3	Tumor invades capsule or beyond into bladder neck or seminal vesical and is not fixed
T4	Tumor is fixed or invades adjacent structures other than T3

N (Nodes)

N0	No regional lymph node metastases
N1	Single node, under 2 cm
N2	Single node 2–5 cm or multiple nodes <5 cm
N3	One or more nodes >5 cm

M (Distant metastases)

M0	No distant metastases
M1	Distant metastases, bone or viscera

(7) **Pelvic lymph node dissection.** A routine part of radical prostatectomy to remove the obturator/iliac lymph node packet. Reasonable staging procedure (open or laparoscopically) in high-risk men, based on grade, PSA, and clinical stage, if it will alter recommended treatments.

(8) **Prostascint scan and nuclear imaging study** to attempt to identify a low-volume recurrence of cancer in men previously treated. Accuracy and clinical role are still unclear.

5. **Treatment by stage** (Table 25-2)

a. **Clinically localized disease** (T1-T2, N0, M0)

(1) Based on the natural history of untreated disease, men with a **projected survival of longer than 7–10 years** should be considered for aggressive treatment with radiation therapy or radical prostatectomy.

(2) **Radiation therapy** can be delivered via external beam or radioactive seed implantation. Complications frequently include urinary urgency and frequency, hematuria, strictures, impotence, incontinence, and rectal complaints.

(3) **Radical prostatectomy** via a retropubic or perineal approach is removal of the prostate, the ampullae of the vas deferens, and the seminal vesicles. The urinary bladder is reanastomosed to the membranous urethra. Complications include bleeding, impotence (30%–100%), incontinence (2%–5%), and rectal injury.

(4) **Clinical observation.** Serial PSA and DRE monitoring with the use of androgen ablation therapy when disease progression occurs is best utilized in men with a lower than 7- to 10-year projected survival, or possibly in healthy men with T1 lesions.

b. **Locally extraprostatic disease (stage T3).** There is no consensus treatment at present. Newer combination modalities include neoadjuvant androgen ablation with surgery or radiation.

c. **Pelvic lymph node metastases.** Most patients are treated by androgen ablation therapy without radiation treatment to the prostate. The possibility of removing the prostate in conjunction with androgen ablation therapy does not clearly improve survival, although it is done in some clinical centers.

d. **Distant metastatic disease** (bone, retroperitoneal lymph nodes, or other soft tissue metastases)

(1) **The standard treatment** is androgen ablation therapy to lower serum testosterone. Methods of lowering testosterone include:

(a) **Bilateral scrotal orchiectomy**

(b) **LHRH agonist.** Injections downregulate pituitary LH production, thus lowering serum testosterone.

(c) **Estrogens** (e.g., diethylstilbestrol) create negative feedback to the pituitary to inhibit LH secretions (no longer available).

(2) **Side effects** include impotence, breast enlargement and tenderness (estrogens), hot flashes, fatigue, osteoporosis, and weight gain.

(3) **Total androgen blockade**

(a) Orchiectomy or an LHRH agonist plus antiandrogen supplement

(b) Antiandrogens are competitive inhibitors at the androgen receptor level.

(c) Numerous studies have been done comparing standard androgen ablation with total androgen blockade, with an unclear possible survival advantage to total blockade.

(4) **Survival.** Median survival with metastatic disease is 2–2.5 years. Men who have a good biochemical response (PSA nadir <4 ng/mL) have a longer survival than do men who have a poor biochemical response (PSA nadir >4 ng/mL).

e. **Hormone refractory disease** is the progression of disease after androgen ablation therapy. Survival averages 12–18 months. To date, no therapies are consistently effective, but several chemotherapy agents are approved with modest efficacy (mitoxantrone, paclitaxel [Taxol]).

B **Bladder carcinoma**

1. **Epidemiology**

a. In the United States, more than 45,000 new cases per year of bladder carcinoma were diagnosed recently, and men were more commonly affected than women.

b. Generally, carcinoma of the bladder is a disease of the elderly, with a median age of 67–70 years.

2. **Etiology.** Likely contributors to development of bladder carcinoma include:

a. **Occupational exposure** to aniline dyes, aromatic amines, and β-naphthylamine

b. **Cigarette smoking**

c. **Phenacetin** (analgesic) abuse

d. **Chronic inflammation** from indwelling urethral catheters, suprapubic tubes, or calculi, which can predispose to squamous cell carcinoma

e. *Schistosoma haematobium* **cystitis,** which also is associated with a high risk for squamous cell carcinoma

f. History of **cyclophosphamide** treatment

g. History of **pelvic irradiation**

3. **Clinical presentation.** Painless hematuria is the most common (85%) presenting symptom. Bladder irritability with urinary frequency, urgency, and dysuria is frequently associated with diffuse carcinoma in situ or invasive cancer.

4. **Diagnosis**

a. **Urinalysis** may show microscopic hematuria.

b. **Intravenous urogram** is used to evaluate the kidneys and ureters but may miss many smaller bladder lesions.

c. **Cystourethroscopy.** A thorough inspection of the bladder is required to identify the number and location of the lesions (frequently multifocal) as well as their appearance (papillary or nodular). A saline washing (bladder barbotage) can be performed, and the washings can be evaluated to identify malignant cells.

d. **Molecular diagnostic tests** exist, but sensitivity and specificity vary, making them ineffective screening tests (BTA, NMP-22).

5. **Pathology.** Types of bladder carcinoma include:

a. **Transitional cell carcinoma,** which accounts for more than 90% of tumors in the bladder

b. **Carcinoma in situ (CIS).** Poorly differentiated transitional cell carcinoma confined to the urothelium.

c. **Squamous cell carcinoma,** which is associated with *Schistosoma haematobium* infection (mainly in Egypt) and in patients with chronic cystitis due to foreign bodies

d. **Adenocarcinoma** is a rare tumor that usually occurs in the dome of the bladder (urachal remnant). Rarely, it is seen in people born with exstrophy of the bladder.

6. **Staging** is determined based on the following:
   a. **Endoscopic resection.** The tumor is resected in superficial and deep components. Deep resection is performed to define muscle-invasive disease. All visible tumors should be resected. Random bladder and prostatic urethral biopsies may be performed to determine the multifocal extent of disease. Pathologic evaluation includes grade of lesion, evidence of invasion into the lamina propria or muscle, and presence of CIS in random bladder biopsies.
   b. **Bimanual examination under anesthesia** is performed after transurethral resection to evaluate extravesical spread and manual mobility of the primary lesion (e.g., pelvic side wall fixation).
   c. The presence of **muscle-invasive disease mandates metastatic evaluation** and includes:
      (1) CT scan of the abdomen and pelvis to evaluate disease spread to the pelvic or para-aortic lymph chain, liver, or adrenal glands.
      (2) **Chest radiograph and chest CT scan**
         (a) A chest radiograph is usually adequate; indeterminate results can be evaluated by CT scan.
         (b) CT scan may be best used in patients with known intra-abdominal metastases to define possible pulmonary metastases.
      (3) **Bone scans** should be performed routinely to evaluate bone metastases. Serum alkaline phosphatase is a helpful marker for bony metastases but should not be used exclusively.
   d. **Staging system** (Table 25-3)
7. **Treatment**
   a. **Superficial transitional cell tumor (Ta, T1 lesions)**
      (1) These tumors are treated primarily by **complete transurethral resection.** Serial endoscopic and cytologic follow-up evaluation should be done at regular intervals. Approximately 70% of patients develop recurrences.
      (2) **Intravesical adjuvant therapy** may reduce the recurrence rate to 30%–45%.
         (a) **Thiotepa** (an alkylating agent)
         (b) **Mitomycin C,** which inhibits DNA synthesis
         (c) **Doxorubicin,** which inhibits DNA synthesis

TABLE 25-3   Staging Classifications of Urinary Bladder Cancer

T (Primary tumor)	
TX	Primary tumor cannot be assessed
T0	No evidence of primary tumor
Tis	Carcinoma in situ
Ta	Noninvasive papillary carcinoma
T1	Tumor invades submucosa/lamina propria
T2a	Tumor invades superficial muscle
T2b	Tumor invades deep muscle
T3	Tumor invades perivesical fat
T4	Tumor invades adjacent organs
N (Regional lymph nodes below aortic bifurcation)	
NX	Regional lymph nodes cannot be assessed
N0	No regional lymph node metastases
N1	Metastases in single node <2 cm
N2	Metastases in single node >2 cm but <5 cm or multiple nodes <5 cm
N3	Metastases in nodes >5 cm
M (Distant metastases)	
MX	Presence of distant metastases cannot be assessed
M0	No distant metastases
M1	Distant metastases

(3) **Bacillus Calmette-Guerin (BCG),** which is an attenuated strain of *Mycobacterium bovis* that has a stimulatory effect on immune responses (probably the most effective agent for preventing a recurrence or for treating carcinoma in situ)

(4) **α-Interferon,** an immune modulator

b. **Carcinoma in situ (Tis).** Intravesical BCG is the most effective agent. It is usually given in six weekly instillations, with a repeat course if a complete response (normal follow-up cystoscopy, biopsies, and cytology) is not attained.

c. **Muscle-invasive localized disease** (T2, T3, T4). The 5-year survival for organ-confined lesions is 70%–75%.

(1) **Radiation therapy** is relatively ineffective, with a 20% long-term survival. Newer investigational uses of radiation therapy involve attempts at bladder preservation through combination protocols using systemic chemotherapy plus radiation therapy. Radiation therapy prior to radical cystectomy has not improved survival or decreased the incidence of local recurrence.

(2) **Radical cystectomy**

(a) In men, pelvic lymphadenectomy with cystoprostatectomy is performed. Urethrectomy is performed if there is tumor involvement of the prostatic urethra.

(b) In women, anterior pelvic exenteration is performed, in which the bladder, urethra, uterus, fallopian tubes, ovaries, and anterior vaginal wall are removed.

(3) **Chemotherapy prior to cystectomy** is a newer combination approach with debatable improvements in survival.

(4) **Urinary diversion**

(a) **Conduits** can be created using ileum or transverse colon. These allow urine to traverse into an external collection device on the abdominal wall.

(b) **Continent diversion** involves the creation of an intra-abdominal reservoir for urine, which is drained by passing a catheter through a stoma on the abdominal wall.

(c) **Neobladder formation** using the small bowel (ileum) or colon allows men to void via urethra. Preliminary results among women are fair, with high rates on inconsistence.

d. **Metastatic transitional cell carcinoma**

(1) Combination regimens of methotrexate, vinblastine, adriamycin, and cisplatin are most effective. Newer paclitaxel-based regimes may have lower rates of toxicity and equal efficacy.

(2) Between 50% and 70% of patients have a partial or complete response. Only approximately 10% are durable responses (>3 years).

C **Transitional cell carcinoma of the renal pelvis and ureter**

1. **Epidemiology**

a. Uncommon tumor

b. Risk factors similar to bladder lesions, with addition of Balkan nephropathy and analgesic abuse

c. Usually unilateral; bilateral in 2%–5%

d. Only 2%–4% of people with bladder transitional tumors will develop upper tract lesions.

e. At least 50% of people presenting with an upper tract transitional tumor will develop a bladder lesion.

2. **Signs and symptoms** include gross hematuria, microscopic hematuria, and flank pain caused by an obstruction.

3. **Diagnosis**

a. **IVP** reveals a radiolucent filling defect.

b. **Retrograde pyelography via cystoscopy** provides better visualization.

c. **Ureteroscopy** can confirm a lesion, and biopsy or brushings for cytology may be obtained (Figs. 25-3 and 25-4).

d. **Metastatic evaluation** is similar to that for bladder lesions, except that lymph node spread is to para-aortic, paracaval, or pelvic nodes, depending on the location of the tumor.

4. **Treatment**

a. **Nephroureterectomy**

(1) The **traditional radical treatment** is removal of the kidney, entire ureter, and a cuff of bladder at the ureteral orifice.

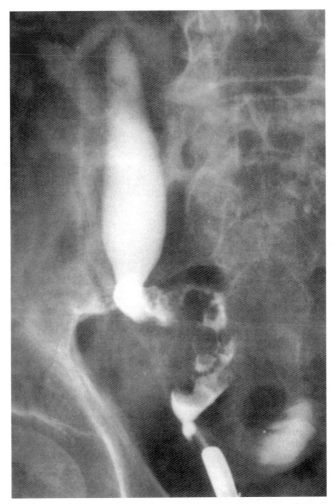

FIGURE 25-3 A retrograde pyelogram reveals a large radiolucent irregular filling defect in the distal ureter with proximal hydroureteronephrosis. Ureteroscopy with biopsy confirmed a transitional cell carcinoma.

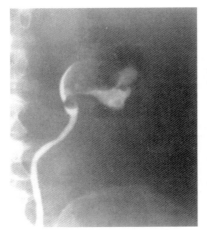 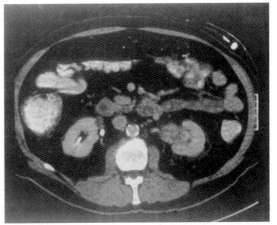

FIGURE 25-4 **Left:** A retrograde pyelogram reveals a large radiolucent filling defect that involves most of the renal pelvis. A computed tomography (CT) scan **(right)** shows this mass to be soft tissue density (not a calculus). Ureteroscopy and biopsy confirmed a transitional cell carcinoma.

(2) Conservative excision may be appropriate for low-grade, low-stage ureteral tumors. This involves tumor excision with primary ureteroureterostomy or ureteral reimplantation (into the bladder) for distal ureteral lesions.

b. **Endoscopic treatment.** Newer equipment has allowed for endoscopic ureteral resection of low-grade and low-stage tumors. The role is still evolving but is currently reserved for patients with low-grade, papillary tumors in solitary renal units or for patients whose health precludes major surgical intervention.

D Renal cell carcinoma

1. **Epidemiology.** There are approximately 30,000 new cases of renal cell carcinoma per year. The disease is more common in men than in women and has a peak incidence in the fifth to seventh decades of life. Renal cell carcinoma is associated with von Hippel–Lindau disease (VHL).

2. **Etiology.** There is no known specific causative agent, but smoking may be a risk factor. Cytogenetic studies most commonly show defects in chromosome 3, the locus of the VHL gene, a tumor suppressor gene.

3. **Clinical presentation.** Renal cell carcinoma is commonly discovered during radiographic studies for other complaints (incidental). The classic triad of pain, hematuria, and flank mass is very uncommon. **Paraneoplastic syndromes** are uncommon but include:

   a. **Stouffer's syndrome** (nonmetastatic hepatic dysfunction), which is a poor prognostic sign

   b. **Hypercalcemia,** which has an unclear etiology

   c. **Hypertension,** due to a local vascular phenomenon or renin secretion

   d. **Erythrocytosis,** due to erythropoietin production

   e. **Endogenous pyrogen production** and **fevers,** the cause of which are unknown

4. **Diagnosis**

   a. **Excretory urography with nephrotomography** allows abnormal renal contours or extrinsic compression of the renal collecting system to be seen.

   b. **Ultrasonography** is useful for differentiating a simple renal cyst from a complex or solid lesion. Criteria for a simple cyst are absence of internal echoes; a smooth, thin wall; and an acoustic shadow arising from the edges of the cyst. Any lesion that is *not* a simple cyst on ultrasound requires a CT evaluation.

   c. **CT scan with intravenous and oral contrast** is the most cost-effective diagnostic and staging modality. It evaluates local tumor, venous extension, regional lymph nodes, and liver metastases.

   d. **MRI** may be better at defining venous extension than CT scan. Its cost-effectiveness is not clear.

   e. **Renal arteriography** is rarely used, being reserved for renal-sparing surgery (i.e., partial nephrectomy). Its diagnostic role has been replaced by the CT scan.

   f. **Venacavography** is used for delineating the renal vein or caval tumor thrombus but has been replaced by MRI.

   g. **Percutaneous aspiration and biopsy** is usually unnecessary. Biopsy is a reasonable method of diagnosis for patients with metastatic disease for tissue confirmation.

5. **Solid renal tumor.** The differential diagnosis for a solid renal tumor includes:

   a. Renal cell carcinoma

   b. Renal oncocytoma, which comprises approximately 3%–5% of solid renal tumors and has a benign natural history

   c. Renal angiomyolipoma, which is a benign tumor that contains smooth muscle, blood vessels, and adipocytes. A CT scan can distinguish this tumor based on the presence of fat. This type of tumor is associated with tuberous sclerosis.

   d. Fibroma, lipoma (rare)

   e. Renal adenoma, which is thought historically to be benign. It is often found at autopsy and is less than 3 cm in size. Histologically, it is identical to renal cell carcinoma. It is now considered to be a small renal cell carcinoma.

TABLE 25-4 TNM Staging Classification of Renal Cell Carcinoma

T (Primary tumor)

T0	No evidence of tumor
T1	Tumor <7 cm and confined to the kidney
T2	Tumor >7 cm and confined to the kidney
T3a	Extends to perinephric tissue or adrenal gland
T3b	Involves the renal vein or vena cava below the diaphragm
T3c	Involves vena cava above the diaphragm
T4	Invades adjacent tissues beyond Gerota's fascia

N (Regional lymph nodes)

N0	No lymph node metastases
N1	A single node
N2	More than one lymph node

M (Distant metastases)

M0	No distant metastases
M1	Distant metastases present

Reprinted with permission from Lawrence PF, Bell RM, Dayton MT. *Essentials of Surgical Specialties*, 2nd ed. Baltimore: Williams & Wilkins; 1993:393.

6. **Staging and prognosis**
   a. **Staging classification** (Table 25-4)
   b. **Prognosis**
      (1) Patients with lymph node metastases have a 5-year survival rate between 10% and 50%.
      (2) Patients with stage I lesions have a 5-year survival rate of approximately 75%.
      (3) Patients with stage II or IIIa lesions have a 5-year survival rate of approximately 50%.

7. **Treatment**
   a. **Stage I and stage II lesions**
      (1) **Radical nephrectomy (open or laparoscopic)** is surgical removal of the ipsilateral adrenal gland, kidney, and investing adipose tissue and fascia. Regional lymphadenectomy may also performed.
      (2) **Lymphadenectomy.** For left-sided lesions, the para-aortic nodes are removed. For right-sided lesions, paracaval are removed.
   b. **Stages IIIa and IV.** Treatment involves the concomitant excision of the renal vein or caval thrombus. The surgical approach is based on the extent of caval disease.
   c. **Stage IIIb**
      (1) **Minimal disease.** Complete excision may be warranted, but the prognosis is poor.
      (2) **Bulky disease or stage IV lesions** may require nephrectomy for palliation of symptoms or for research and study purposes.
   d. **Metastatic renal cell carcinoma**
      (1) **Chemotherapy** is essentially ineffective, possibly because of the frequent expression of the multidrug resistance (MDR) gene or P-glycoprotein.
      (2) **Hormonal therapy** is ineffective.
      (3) **Immunotherapy.** Ongoing investigations using interferon, interleukin, lymphokine-activated killer (LAK) cells, and tumor-infiltrating lymphocytes (TIL) have shown objective responses in 15%–30% of patients. Interferon plus nephrectomy has a median survival of less than 12 months.

E Testicular tumors

1. **Pathology**
   a. The major **germ cell tumors** of the testis are **seminomatous** and **nonseminomatous** tumors. Nonseminomatous germ cell tumors (NSGCT) include embryonal carcinoma, teratoma,

choriocarcinoma, and yolk sac tumors, alone or in combination. Secondary tumors include lymphomas.

   b. **Cryptorchidism** (undescended testis) increases the risk of testicular malignancy.

2. **Epidemiology**

   a. Although testis tumors are generally uncommon, they are the most common malignancy in men between the ages of 20 and 34 years.

   b. **Age.** The **tumor type** is age dependent: Yolk sac tumors and teratomas are common in infants. All cell types may be seen in young adults: Seminoma is more common in men between the ages of 35 and 60 years, and lymphomas predominate in men older than 60 years.

   c. **Race.** Testicular cancer occurs infrequently in blacks compared with whites.

3. **Clinical presentation.** Despite efforts to educate physicians and patients about routine testicular self-examination, a significant delay is common before diagnosis. Approximately 33%–50% of patients have identifiable metastatic disease at initial presentation.

   a. **Local signs and symptoms**

      (1) Painless swelling or enlargement of the testicle occurs in 65% of patients. Pain (13%–49%) suggests hemorrhage or infarction and may be confused with epididymitis.

      (2) "Heaviness" may be experienced on the affected side.

      (3) Failure of epididymitis to resolve as expected with appropriate antimicrobial agents should alert the physician to the possibility of occult malignancy.

      (4) Excessive pain or injury from minimal testicular trauma may indicate an underlying malignancy.

   b. **Signs and symptoms of metastatic disease** prompt evaluation in 10% of patients and may include abdominal or back pain, nausea, anorexia, weight loss, gynecomastia, abdominal mass, cough, dyspnea, and hemoptysis.

4. **Diagnosis**

   a. Physical examination may reveal a firm, nontender, or mildly tender distinct mass or diffuse testicular swelling.

   b. A reactive hydrocele occurs in 5%–10% of cases.

   c. Findings of gynecomastia or an abdominal mass suggest an advanced testicular malignancy.

   d. Ultrasonography is very sensitive in determining the size, location, and echogenicity of palpable testicular abnormalities, particularly if a hydrocele limits the physical examination.

   e. Serum marker levels of **α-fetoprotein (AFP)** and **β-human chorionic gonadotropin (HCG)** are useful for diagnosis, for following the response to treatment, and for identifying recurrent disease. AFP may be elevated in patients with yolk sac tumors, embryonal carcinoma, and teratocarcinoma. β-HCG elevation may accompany choriocarcinoma and seminomas. Seminomas do not elaborate AFP; thus, an elevation in this marker confirms a nonseminomatous component.

   f. **Definitive diagnosis** requires **surgical exploration** via an inguinal approach to avoid potential "contamination" of scrotal lymphatic draining during tumor manipulation. Similarly, trans-scrotal biopsies should be avoided.

5. **Staging** is shown in Table 25-5.

   a. Metastatic evaluation should include a CT scan of the abdomen and pelvis and either a chest radiograph or a chest CT scan.

   b. Postorchiectomy serum markers should normalize within predictable time periods based on their half-lives (AFP, T1-T2 = 5 days; β-HCG, T1-T2 = 1 day). Failure to normalize virtually confirms disseminated disease.

6. **Treatment** of testicular tumors varies with the cell type and stage of disease.

   a. **Seminoma** is uniquely radiosensitive and chemosensitive.

      (1) **Stage I seminoma.** Postorchiectomy treatment options include close observation or radiotherapy (2,500 rad) to para-aortic with or without the ipsilateral pelvic nodes. Survival is approximately 100%.

      (2) **Stage II seminomas**

         (a) Receive retropetal radiation α

         (b) Stage IIb and c are best treated by systemic chemotherapy.

         (c) Survival approaches 95%.

TABLE 25-5 Staging of Germ Cell Tumors

Stage I	Metastatic workup is negative; preoperative markers, if positive, normalize. Tumor is isolated to the testicle.
Stage IIA	Microscopic retroperitoneal disease.
Stage IIB	Minimal retroperitoneal disease on radiographic studies (<5 mL).
Stage IIC	Bulky retroperitoneal disease (>5 mL).
Stage III	Disease beyond retroperitoneal lymph drainage, or positive markers after retroperitoneal lymph node dissection.

Reprinted with permission from Lawrence PF, Bell RM Dayton MT: *Essentials of Surgical Specialties,* 2nd ed. Baltimore, Williams & Wilkins, 1993:393.

    (3) Stage III. Current recommendations include up to four courses of chemotherapy with cisplatin, etoposide, and bleomycin. Postchemotherapy radiation is considered occasionally for patients with a residual retroperitoneal mass. An 85% complete response rate to chemotherapy and an overall survival rate of 92% can be expected.

  b. NSGCT

    (1) Stage I NSGCT. Treatment involves inguinal orchiectomy followed by either modified retroperitoneal lymphadenectomy (RPLND) or by an intense surveillance protocol.

      (a) Surveillance is generally reserved for compliant patients who are at low risk of micrometastatic disease. Risk factors of the primary testis tumor favoring RPLND include an embryonal carcinoma component, vascular or lymphatic invasion, and extension into peritesticular structures.

      (b) RPLND involves surgical removal of specific high-risk lymphatic tissue. Approximately 30% of stage I patients have nodal disease at RPLND. Most patients with micrometastases receive two cycles of adjuvant platinum-based chemotherapy.

      (c) Survival for both groups approaches 100%.

    (2) Stage II NSGCT. Patients with minimal nodal involvement radiographically or failure to normalize markers postorchiectomy should undergo either RPLND or chemotherapy alone. Survival is approximately 98%.

    (3) Stage III NSGCT require induction chemotherapy employing platinum-based combinations for three to four cycles, with follow-up serum markers and radiographic re-evaluation. Markers and radiographs normalize in 70%–80% of patients, who can be followed without additional surgery. Those patients whose markers normalize but who have residual pulmonary, mediastinal, or retroperitoneal masses should undergo complete surgical resection of these masses. There is pathologic confirmation of carcinoma in approximately 20% of patients undergoing postchemotherapy surgery, and it dictates additional chemotherapy. Failure to normalize markers after chemotherapy portends a poor prognosis with or without additional surgery. Salvage chemotherapy or high-dose chemotherapy and autologous bone marrow transplantation may be considered in these cases.

7. Infertility issues in patients with testis cancer. Because testis cancer affects a population that is often interested in future fertility, counseling on this issue should be considered part of the treatment. Testis cancer itself adversely affects fertility, and the additional insults of surgical stress, orchiectomy, chemotherapy, and RPLND may further depress fertility. Men interested in future fertility should undergo preoperative semen analysis; if adequate parameters exist, sperm banking should be considered.

V MALE ERECTILE DYSFUNCTION

A The penis

  1. Anatomy

    a. Penile **erectile tissue** is contained within three **erectile bodies**—two dorsally situated **corpora cavernosa** and one ventrally located **corpus spongiosum.**

      b. The **urethra** lies within the corpus spongiosum, which consists of cavernous, expansible spaces. Each of the three corpora is surrounded by the **tunica albuginea,** a thick, fibrous tissue layer. The thickness of the tunica around the cavernosa is much thicker, which is consistent with the increased pressure in these spaces.

    2. Arterial supply is derived bilaterally from the internal pudendal artery, which is a terminal branch of the internal iliac artery. Branches to the penis are the bulbar artery, urethral artery, dorsal artery, and deep penile artery. The latter is the main blood supply to the corpora cavernosa.

    3. Venous drainage is complex. A deep dorsal vein and a superficial dorsal vein exist as well as deep veins within the corpora cavernosa and the circumflex veins.

    4. Innervation

        a. Sympathetic innervation. The lower thoracic and upper lumbar regions of the spinal cord innervate the superior hypogastric plexus, which innervates the hypogastric nerve, which innervates the pelvic plexus.

        b. Parasympathetic innervation. The sacral nerve roots (S2-S4) innervate the pelvic nerve, which innervates the pelvic plexus. The pelvic plexus sends nerve fibers to the penis via the cavernous nerve.

        c. Somatic innervation of the penis is carried in the pudendal nerve (S2-S4).

B **Penile erection and detumescence** are primarily hemodynamic events.

    1. Arterial flow increases, and increased venous resistance also contributes.

    2. The exact mechanism of neurovascular interaction is mediated by the cavernous nerves.

    3. Neurophysiology

        a. Erections with genital stimulation require only an intact sacral reflex.

        b. The parasympathetic nervous system is of primary importance in penile erection. Nitric oxide released from nonadrenergic, noncholinergic neurons and the endothelium leads to vascular and corporal smooth muscle relaxation.

    4. Hormonal factors are involved in both erectile function and sexual desire (libido). The exact nature of these factors is not fully understood.

C **Diagnosis**

    1. Taking the patient's **history** is very important when evaluating the cause of erectile dysfunction.

        a. The nature of onset and the duration of the problem are important. Psychogenic impotence may be abrupt in onset with a life stress.

        b. An interview with the patient's sexual partner may prove beneficial.

        c. The presence of nocturnal or early morning erections may suggest a psychogenic cause.

        d. History of pelvic trauma, including vascular or neurogenic injury, is important to discern.

        e. Risk factors include diabetes, hypertension, smoking, heart disease, and hypercholesterolemia.

    2. Physical examination. There is a special emphasis on the neurologic and vascular examination. A DRE is performed to evaluate for prostate cancer with general evaluation of the genitalia. The penis should be examined for plaques and the testes for size and consistency.

    3. Laboratory tests include:

        a. Testosterone level

        b. Serologic tests for systemic disease (e.g., anemia, renal insufficiency)

    4. Diagnostic tests are not indicated in every patient. They include:

        a. Nocturnal penile tumescence. Measurements are taken of nocturnal erections occurring during rapid eye movement sleep. Gauges are placed on the flaccid penis at bedtime and attached to a monitor overnight that evaluates the number, duration, and rigidity of erections.

        b. Intracorporeal injections of vasoactive substances, such as papaverine, phentolamine, and prostaglandin E, have been used to elicit an erection. Response with a normal erection eliminates a significant "venous leak" etiology for erectile dysfunction.

        c. Duplex sonography evaluation can provide an objective measure of arterial penile blood flow as well as a relative assessment of venous drainage. Cavernosal arteries are evaluated for increased width and flow after intracorporeal vasoactive injection. Venous outflow during erections should diminish; if venous outflow is still high on duplex study, a venous leak phenomenon may be present.

    d. Cavernosometry and cavernosography

       (1) Cavernosometry is a pressure flow evaluation of the penis during erection. After vasoactive injection, an erect penis requires little inflow infusion to maintain rigidity and high intracorporeal pressures. Cavernosometry evaluates the intracorporeal pressure and volume of necessary infusion to obtain and maintain an erection after a vasoactive injection.

       (2) Cavernosography is the injection of contrast material into the corpora to anatomically identify an abnormally excessive loss of venous blood during an erection.

    e. Pudendal arteriography can identify isolated correctable lesions in a select population of postpelvic trauma patients.

5. Treatment

    a. Counseling is required for men found to have a significant psychogenic component.

    b. Oral therapy has revolutionized treatment. Selective phosphodiesterase type 5 inhibitors enhance erection through the nitric oxide/cyclic guanosine monophosphate (GMP) pathway. Three agents have been approved by the Food and Drug Administration (FDA).

    c. A vacuum erection device is an external device that, under a pump mechanism, can draw blood into the penis to obtain an erection. The blood is retained by the placement of a constricting rubber ring at the base of the penis.

    d. Vasoactive intracorporeal injections are self-administered, with risks comprised of bruising, mild scar formation, or priapism (erections lasting >4 hours).

    e. A penile implant is a paired device that is surgically implanted into the corpora cavernosum. Several styles exist that are either malleable or inflatable. The main risk is infection associated with the prosthetic material.

VI   NEUROGENIC BLADDER

Voiding is a complex act involving detrusor contraction with sphincteric relaxation (the micturition reflex), which is coordinated in the pontine misturition center and controlled by cerebral input. Lesions occurring throughout the nervous system often profoundly affect voiding. As elsewhere, upper motor neuron lesions (suprasacral) tend to produce hyperreflexia (bladder overactivity), whereas lower motor neuron lesions (sacral nerve roots or cauda equina) cause areflexia (bladder flaccidity).

A Diagnosis

    1. History. Detailed historical information regarding frequency, urgency, nocturia, sensation of fullness, straining, incontinence, erectile function, bowel habits, paralysis, paresthesias, history of neurologic and vertebral disease, pelvic surgery, and trauma as well as a review of medications are vital parts of diagnosis.

    2. Physical examination includes an assessment of sensation, motor function, and reflexes of the lower extremities, perineum, and rectal areas. Anal sphincter tone should be assessed, as should the **bulbocavernosal reflex** (contraction of the anal sphincter with compression of the glans or clitoris or with traction on an indwelling urethral catheter).

    3. Urodynamic studies (Fig. 25-5)

       a. Filling cystometry involves the creation of a pressure versus volume curve during bladder filling. Normal bladder sensation, high compliance (accommodation to increasing volumes with minimal increase in pressure), and the absence of uninhibited contractions during filling comprise a normal study.

       b. The **voiding phase** assesses flow rate, contractility, and vesical pressure during voiding. Postvoid residual urine is recorded.

       c. Electromyelography (EMG) of the striated sphincter can be used to demonstrate sphincteric function and to determine if appropriate sphincter relaxation occurs with voiding. Denervation of the sphincter may be elicited.

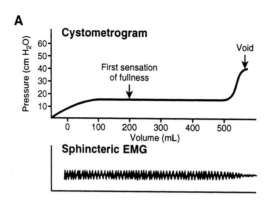

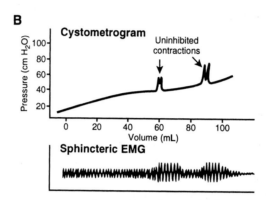

FIGURE 25-5 **A:** A normal cystometrogram. Note the normal compliance with filling and sphincteric relaxation during voiding. **B:** A cystometrogram study in a patient with a myelomeningocele. Note the poorly compliant bladder, uninhibited bladder contractions, and detrusor sphincter dyssynergia. EMG, electromyogram.

B Patterns of voiding dysfunction

1. **Detrusor hyperreflexia** (hypertonic neurogenic bladder) occurs with suprasacral lesions and is characterized by diminished bladder capacity and uninhibitable detrusor contractions.
    a. **Presenting symptoms** are irritative, such as urgency and frequency. If intravesical pressures become elevated, vesicoureteral reflux and upper tract deterioration may occur.
    b. **Treatment** includes anticholinergics; intermittent bladder catheterization; and, sometimes, surgical bladder augmentation.

2. **Detrusor-areflexia** (atonic bladder) occurs with lesions of the sacral cord, nerve roots, or cauda equina, resulting in loss of the sacral reflex arc. Increased capacity, decreased intravesical pressure, absence of efficient bladder contractions, and urinary retention with overflow incontinence may result. Medical therapy is generally ineffective. Catheterization (indwelling or intermittent) and urinary diversion are often used.

3. **Detrusor external sphincter dyssynergia (DSD)** involves contraction of the external sphincter during bladder contraction, causing a "functional" outlet obstruction. This condition results from lesions of the spinal cord and may occur alone or may complicate a hyperreflexic or atonic picture. Treatment involves medication to promote urinary retention (anticholinergics) and intermittent catheterization to overcome DSD.

C Voiding dysfunction in specific diseases

1. **Spinal cord injury** associated with suprasacral lesions usually causes hyperreflexia with DSD, and injury with sacral lesions usually causes areflexia.

2. **Cerebrovascular accidents** result in loss of cortical inhibition with detrusor hyperreflexia, manifested by urgency with urge incontinence. DSD is not featured, and patients often contract the sphincter voluntarily.

3. **Parkinsonism** causes detrusor hyperreflexia, resulting in urgency, frequency, incontinence, and failure of the external sphincter to relax, which may complicate the picture.

4. **Multiple sclerosis** leads to voiding dysfunction in 50%–80% of those affected, most commonly, urgency; frequency; incontinence; and, occasionally, retention. Urodynamic studies reveal detrusor hyperreflexia in most cases. Approximately 70%–80% exhibit features of DSD.

5. **Myelodysplasia** describes various abnormal conditions of vertebral development that affect spinal cord function. Myelomeningocele is the most common. Findings may include a poorly compliant bladder with high intravesical pressure, weak detrusor contractions, and DSD. Management includes use of anticholinergic agents to diminish bladder pressures and intermittent catheterization to overcome failure of the bladder to empty.

6. **Lumbar disc disease** causes detrusor acontractility and decreased sphincteric activity; obstructive voiding symptoms predominate. Urinary retention may occur.

7. **Diabetic cystopathy** is an autonomic neuropathy manifested by diminished bladder sensation, increased capacity, decreased contractility, and elevated postvoid residual.

D Treatment

1. **Pharmacologic treatment** allows manipulation of bladder contractility (by way of cholinergic receptors in the bladder) and allows changes in outlet resistance (via α-adrenergic receptors in the bladder neck, prostatic capsule, and urethra).

2. **Catheterization.** An **indwelling** catheter can be used. **Intermittent catheterization** frees the patient from continuous appliance usage and lowers the incidence of UTIs, meatal erosion, urethral stricture, and epididymitis. Patients develop **bacterial colonization,** which requires no treatment unless symptoms of infection occur.

3. **Urinary diversion** away from the bladder by formation of an ileal conduit or catheterizable reservoir may be necessary in patients with recurrent urosepsis or renal insufficiency caused by a detrusor problem.

4. **Bladder augmentation** to increase capacity and decrease intravesical pressure may be required in patients with hyperreflexia or in those with contracted, poorly compliant bladders secondary to long-standing neurologic disease (e.g., myelomeningocele), radiation cystitis, or chemically induced bladder fibrosis. Intermittent catheterization is usually required.

E Autonomic dysreflexia is an outpouring of sympathetic activity in response to afferent visceral stimulation in patients with spinal cord injuries with lesions above T6. Bladder, urethral, or rectal stimulation may produce profound hypertension, bradycardia, diaphoresis, headache, and piloerection in these patients. Treatment consists of withdrawing the stimulant and medication directed at the hypertensive crisis. Prophylaxis with various medications (e.g., chlorpromazine, nifedipine) is sometimes useful in affected patients who require urologic manipulation.

VII   UROLOGIC TRAUMA

A Evaluation   The need for radiographic assessment in patients with urologic trauma is based on the mechanism of injury, vital signs, physical examination, and urinalysis.

1. **Blunt trauma**
   a. Patients with **gross hematuria** or microhematuria and a systolic blood pressure (SBP) <90 mm Hg require radiographic evaluation of the kidneys.
   b. Patients with **microhematuria** who have always had an SBP <90 mm Hg do not require a radiographic evaluation unless clinical suspicion is high based on the mechanism of injury (e.g., fall from a height, direct blows, high-speed motor vehicle crashes).

2. All patients with **penetrating trauma,** regardless of the degree of hematuria, require an evaluation.

3. Possible **radiographic tests** include an IVP, CT scan of the abdomen and pelvis, cystogram, retrograde urethrogram, and renal angiography.

B Renal injuries

1. **Classification:** American Association for the Surgery of Trauma Organ Injury Scale
   a. **Contusion.** There is no obvious parenchymal injury, but there may be a subcapsular hematoma.
   b. **Minor lacerations** are superficial cortical disruptions that do not involve the collecting system.
   c. **Major lacerations** are deep corticomedullary lacerations that do not involve the collecting system.
   d. **Deep lacerations** of collecting system or injury to the renal artery or vein may be involved.
   e. Avulsion of the renal vessels may occur, or the kidney may be shattered and destroyed.

2. **Radiographic assessment** includes:
   a. **CT scan of the abdomen and pelvis.** It is the first-line test performed to rule out renal injury. Early venous phase and 10-minute delayed images are required.
   b. **Renal arteriography** is generally reserved for patients with possible vascular injuries that are not elucidated on the CT scan and may require embolization.

3. **Treatment**
   a. Contusions, minor lacerations, and some major lacerations can be managed nonoperatively with **bed rest, serial hematocrit evaluation,** and **hydration.** Ureteral stenting may be required in cases of ongoing urinary extravasation.
   b. Angiography and embolization can control most renal bleeding.
   c. Major lacerations or vascular injuries usually require **surgical staging** and **therapy.**
   d. Penetrating renal injuries usually require **exploration,** and in addition, they have a high risk of associated intra-abdominal injuries.
   e. Surgical exploration includes debridement of nonviable renal tissue, closure of the collecting system, coverage of the injury with perinephric adipose tissue, and drainage of the retroperitoneum. Stents are usually not needed.
   f. **Repair of vascular injuries** can frequently be problematic. Branch renal veins may be ligated, whereas arterial injuries with viable renal parenchyma require meticulous vascular repair. Prolonged ischemic time with arterial injuries usually mandates **nephrectomy.**

4. **Complications of renal trauma**
   a. **Post-traumatic hypertension** appears to be uncommon but may occur in 5%–10% of patients and is mediated by renin owing to ischemic tissue.
   b. **Associated injuries** are more common in patients with penetrating rather than blunt trauma. Right renal injuries are associated with liver trauma, and left renal injuries are associated with splenic injuries in blunt trauma. Bowel lacerations, pancreatic injury, and other vascular injuries occur with penetrating trauma. An initial identification of associated injuries with appropriate treatment will prevent many complications of renal trauma.

C Ureteral injuries

1. **Etiology.** Ureteral injuries are caused mainly by penetrating trauma or iatrogenic injury. Deceleration injuries may result in avulsion of the ureteropelvic junction, especially in children.

2. **Radiographic assessment.** The site of injury can usually be identified on **IVP** or **CT.**
   a. An **intraoperative retrograde pyelogram** can further delineate the injury.

3. **Treatment.** All ureteral injuries should be explored and repaired.
   a. **Upper and midureteral injuries** are debrided, primarily repaired, drained, and stented.
   b. **Lower ureteral injuries** usually require debridement, drainage, repair by ureteroneocystotomy, and stenting.
   c. **Iatrogenic crush injuries,** if identified at the time of injury, can usually be managed by ureteral stenting alone.
   d. **Unrecognized injuries** frequently present later as fistulas or urinomas, with fever and pain. Treatment of fistulas or obstruction may require stenting with or without percutaneous drainage. Primary open repair, after more than 3–5 days, risks renal loss.

D Bladder trauma (lower urinary tract)

1. **Etiology.** Blunt bladder trauma is frequently associated with pelvic fractures. Rupture can be extraperitoneal or intraperitoneal, depending on the location of the tear. Associated urethral injuries should always be considered as a possibility.

2. **Evaluation.** Blood at the urethral meatus, an elevated prostate gland on DRE, or a mechanism of injury possibly causing a urethral tear should prompt a **retrograde urethrogram** before catheterization of the bladder. A 20–24 French urethral catheter should be passed into the bladder. Drainage and oblique films are necessary with plain film cystography. A **cystogram** involves maximally (400–500 mL) filling the bladder to determine extravasation of contrast medium (e.g., **CT** or **plain film**).

3. **Treatment.** Many small extraperitoneal tears heal with a urethral catheter change alone. Extraperitoneal tears complicated by rectal or urethral trauma, any intraperitoneal tears, and exploration for other reasons require closure of the laceration and placement of a Foley catheter.

E **Urethral injuries**

1. **Evaluation.** The examination and radiographic assessment are described earlier (Chapter 21 C 7-D 1 a). A high index of suspicion should be maintained, because passage of a urethral catheter may significantly worsen a mild urethral injury.

2. **Treatment**
   a. All **penetrating** anterior urethral injuries should be explored, debrided, and repaired primarily. A urethral catheter should be left in place after repair.
   b. Complete prostatomembranous urethral disruptions from **blunt trauma** require open suprapubic tube placement.
      (1) Attempts at primary repair are not warranted.
      (2) Attempts at "realignment" over a urethral catheter or with flexible cystoscopes may be indicated.
      (3) Follow-up open repair of post-traumatic strictures should occur 3–6 months after the injury.

F **Penile injuries**

1. **Fracture** of the erect penis caused by direct blunt trauma that significantly bends the organ can result in a tear of the tunica albuginea of the corpora cavernosa. Urethral tears are associated injuries (20%).
   a. **Physical findings** include ecchymosis, swelling, and deviation of the penis.
   b. **Diagnosis** can usually be made based on the patient's history and physical examination.
   c. **Treatment** involves operative repair via a circumcising incision and closure of any cavernosal tear. An evaluation via a urethrogram with repair of the urethral injury may be necessary.

2. **Penetrating penile trauma** is evaluated and treated similarly to a fractured penis. All such injuries should be explored and repaired.

G **Testicular trauma**

1. **Blunt trauma.** The physical examination is an integral part of the evaluation. **Testicular rupture** is the primary injury that requires **surgical repair,** and testicular ultrasound is frequently beneficial when making this diagnosis. A large hematocele is an additional indication for surgical exploration.

2. **Penetrating trauma.** The physical examination and ultrasound may prove helpful. All suspected testicular or spermatic cord injuries should be explored.

chapter 26

Plastic Surgery and Skin and Soft Tissue Surgery

NICK TAROLA • JOHN H. MOORE JR.

I · PLASTIC SURGERY

Plastic surgery as an art and science deals with the reconstruction of body parts altered by trauma, birth defects, or advanced age. It is one of the oldest fields of surgery, having first been described in 700 B.C., in India. In 1818, von Graefe used the term *plastic* in his monograph on nasal reconstruction; and throughout the years since then, this term has been associated with surgery that is concerned with form and function. An understanding of the skin layers and of suturing techniques is essential to plastic surgery (see Chapter 2).

A **Skin,** or the **integumentary system,** is the largest organ in the body. **Three properties** of skin are essential for understanding reconstruction—elasticity, extensibility, and resilience.

1. **Elasticity** keeps skin in constant tension, owing to underlying collagen fibers. The function of elasticity becomes apparent when facial wrinkles form in its absence.

2. **Extensibility** refers to the skin's ability to stretch, which can be seen on abdominal skin during pregnancy.

3. **Resilience** is noted by the skin's resistance to infection and puncture.

B **Skin grafts** are segments of epidermis and dermis that have been detached from their native blood supply to be transplanted to another area of the body. A skin graft may be an **autograft** (i.e., from the same person), an **allograft** (i.e., from a genetically dissimilar individual of the same species, usually a cadaver), or a **xenograft** (i.e., from a different species, usually pigs) (see Chapter 24, I B 1). **Cultured skin** can be grown from human epidermal cells; this skin is most useful for extensively burned patients because more surface area can be covered; however, the cultured skin tends to be very thin.

1. **Types.** Skin grafts are classified according to thickness.
   a. **Split-thickness skin grafts** contain the epidermis and a portion of the dermis. They are further divided into thin, medium, and thick, based on the amount of dermis included in the graft (0.010–0.025 inch). The abdomen, buttocks, and thighs are common donor sites.
      (1) **Advantages** of split-thickness skin grafts include:
         (a) A large supply of donor areas
         (b) Ease of harvesting
         (c) Availability of donor site for reuse in 10–14 days
         (d) Decreased primary contracture
         (e) Coverage of large surface areas
         (f) Ability to be stored for later use
      (2) **Disadvantages** of split-thickness skin grafts include:
         (a) Cosmetic inferiority to full-thickness skin grafts
         (b) Decreased durability
         (c) Hyperpigmentation
         (d) Increased secondary contracture
   b. **Full-thickness skin grafts** contain the epidermis and the full thickness of dermis without subcutaneous fat. They are most useful for covering defects on the face or hand that are not

480

amenable to coverage with a skin flap (see I C). A good match of skin color can be obtained from donor sites in the postauricular or supraclavicular areas. Preauricular grafts provide the best color match for the face. The forearm and groin can also serve as donor sites for defects below the clavicle.

(1) **Advantages** of full-thickness skin grafts include:
   (a) Cosmetic superiority to split-thickness skin grafts
   (b) Decreased secondary contractures (grafts may be cut as required to fill the defect)
   (c) Increased durability
(2) **Disadvantages** of full-thickness skin grafts include:
   (a) Limited donor sites
   (b) Increased primary contracture

c. **Composite grafts** are those that are formed of multiple tissues (e.g., a fingertip containing skin, subcutaneous fat, and bone or a segment of ear containing skin and cartilage). These grafts may be effective in young patients or in situations where the distal portion of the graft is less than 1 cm from the blood supply.

2. **Grafting procedures**
   a. **Split-thickness skin grafts** are best obtained with specifically designed instruments rather than being taken freehand.
      (1) **Methods of obtaining the graft** include the following:
         (a) **Knives,** such as the Humby or Weck, are fitted with an adjustable roller or gauge to determine thickness. The knife is slowly advanced as cutting proceeds in a back-and-forth direction.
         (b) The **drum** (Reese) **dermatome** fixes the epidermis to the drum with glue, which allows the graft to be cut as the drum is rolled back. The cut grafts have a uniform thickness.
         (c) The **electrical dermatome,** such as the Brown or Padgett, has a rapidly oscillating knife and a gauge to adjust depth. Long strips of skin can be removed with this instrument.
      (2) **Care of the donor site** following the cessation of capillary oozing will aid in re-epithelialization.
         (a) **Meshed, nonadherent gauze** allows the scab to be incorporated into the dressing. In 2 days, the dressing is dry; the covering, with the incorporated scab, falls from the wound in 2 weeks.
         (b) **Semipermeable membranes** trap leukocyte-rich fluid to form an artificial blister, which hastens epithelialization. Patients note diminished pain at the donor site.
      (3) **Care of the recipient (grafted) site** (see I B 3)
         (a) Hemostasis is necessary to ensure adequate tissue contact.
         (b) When excessive wound drainage or potential infection may be a problem, the graft can be cut and a meshing device can be used to ensure adequate drainage. This technique is also useful for expanding the surface area of a graft. Epithelialization quickly occurs in the meshed interstices following graft "take." Meshing of the graft can sometimes lead to a "cobblestone" effect in the final result of the graft. This effect can be minimized with a pressure garment (e.g., Ace bandage, Jobst garment) in the first few months after the grafting procedure.
         (c) The graft may be fixed to the recipient site by sutures or tapes. An external fixation with a "tie-over bolus" dressing (i.e., a large dressing made of gauze or cotton) may be required in areas where immobilization is difficult or where shear forces are expected. The open method, in which the graft is left exposed, may be useful for large surface areas in burn patients; daily inspection for infection is important.
   b. **Full-thickness skin grafts**
      (1) **Method of obtaining the graft.** The grafts are "harvested" with a freehand technique using a no. 10 or no. 15 knife blade. A portion of subcutaneous fat is also harvested and must be excised carefully before grafting.
      (2) **Care of the donor site** involves primary skin closure in most instances. Split-thickness skin grafts may be necessary in some cases.

(3) Care of the recipient site is similar to care in split-thickness skin grafts. Tie-over bolus dressings are frequently used.

3. **Survival of skin grafts**
   a. **Vascular recipient beds** are necessary to provide nourishment for the transplant tissues.
      (1) Imbibition of plasma supports survival during the first 48 hours. **Fibrin** is laid down and helps to hold the graft in place.
      (2) **Inosculation** (vascular budding) occurs, and the graft is usually supported by a true circulation by the fourth to seventh day. Generally, a graft begins to turn pink at this time. Lymphatic connections are formed by the fifth day.
   b. **Contact of the skin graft** is essential for inosculation to take place. Factors that can lead to **loss of contact** include:
      (1) Tension on the graft
      (2) **Fluid** (e.g., blood, serum, or pus) underneath the graft
      (3) **Movement** between the graft and its bed
   c. **Preparation of wound to be grafted**
      (1) Bone denuded of periosteum, cartilage denuded of perichondrium, and exposed tendon do not support skin grafts; these areas require a flap procedure.
      (2) **Infected wounds do not support skin grafts.** The critical bacterial concentration appears to be 10^5 organisms per gram of tissue, and quantitative bacterial counts are useful when determining a wound's suitability for grafting. Mechanical debridement with a scalpel and scissors is necessary to remove necrotic tissue. Frequent dressing changes with saline or dilute (0.1 strength) Dakin's solution (i.e., sodium hypochlorite) are also quite effective in debriding wounds. Once there is no further necrotic material in the wound, the use of a biologic dressing (i.e., an allograft or xenograft) helps to reduce the bacterial count.

C **Flaps** are segments of skin and subcutaneous tissues that are moved from one part of the body to another, either retaining or transplanting their vascular supply, which is via a segmental artery through a perforating artery to a cutaneous artery supplying the dermal–subdermal plexus. Because of their intrinsic blood supply, flaps are useful for healing and for covering defects that require padding.

1. **Types** (Fig. 26-1)
   a. **Skin flaps**
      (1) **Random flaps** receive their blood supply from the dermal–subdermal plexus. These flaps lack an anatomically recognized arterial and venous system. Examples include:
         (a) Z-plasty (Fig. 26-2)
         (b) V-Y advancement flaps
         (c) Rotation flaps (Fig. 26-3)
         (d) Transposition flaps (Fig. 26-4)
      (2) **Axial flaps** have a direct cutaneous artery and vein supplying their subdermal plexus. Therefore, the blood supply is more reliable than with random flaps, and flaps of greater length may be obtained. Axial flaps may be detached as free microvascular flaps and transplanted to other areas of the body, provided that the vessels are large enough. Examples of axial flaps include:
         (a) Forehead flaps
         (b) Groin flaps
         (c) Deltopectoral flaps
   b. **Muscle flaps** provide increased blood supply to an area. Generally, they are used to cover exposed bone and are usually skin grafted. When the overlying skin and subcutaneous tissue are included, they are called **myocutaneous (musculocutaneous) flaps.**
      (1) The blood supply is predictable, and the flaps can be outlined anatomically. The flaps contain muscle with a named artery, which must be identified and preserved (Fig. 26-5).
      (2) Muscle flaps have been most useful in reconstruction of the lower extremity and in areas of poor vascularity. Myocutaneous flaps have been useful for reconstruction of tissue that has been injured by radiation.

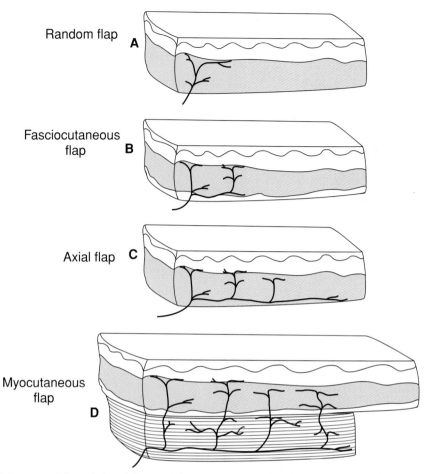

FIGURE 26-1 Types of flaps. (Adapted from Daniel RK, Kerrigan CL. Principles and physiology of skin flap surgery. In: McCarthy JG, ed. *Plastic Surgery*. Vol. 1. Philadelphia: WB Saunders; 1990:293.)

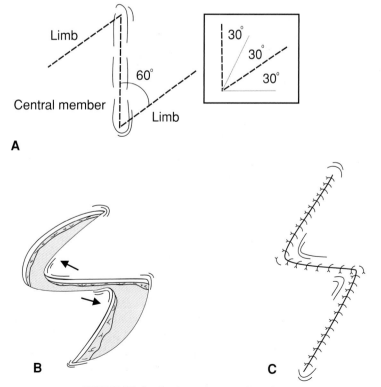

FIGURE 26-2 Classic 60-degree angle Z-plasty.

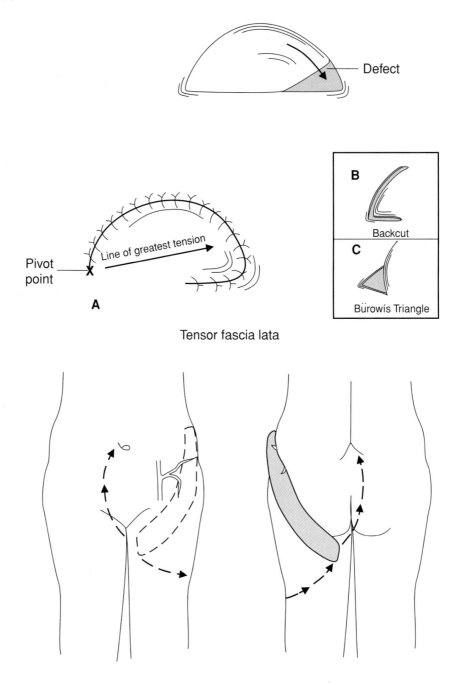

FIGURE 26-3 **A:** Technique for rotation of flap. **B:** Rotation of a myocutaneous flap used for reconstruction of posterior thigh defect with tensor fascia lata flap.

    c. Fasciocutaneous flaps involve the transfer of skin, subcutaneous tissue, and the underlying fascia with an anatomically distinct artery. Because there is no mobilization of underlying muscle, there is less functional debilitation. The donor site must be skin grafted, and these flaps are cosmetically inferior to muscle flaps.

    d. Free flaps (free tissue transfer) are those in which the native blood supply is completely severed, with transplantation of the flap to a separate body area. They can be muscle, myocutaneous, fasciocutaneous, or axial flaps. They can be used to provide function (free neurotized muscle transfer for correction of facial nerve palsy). Revascularization is accomplished by microvascular anastomosis.

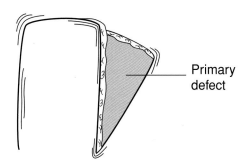

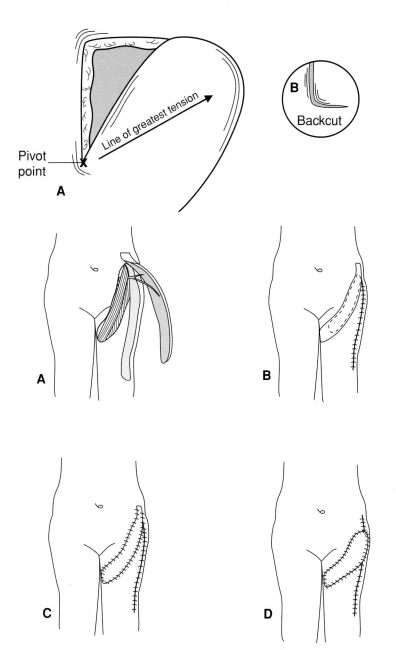

FIGURE 26-4 **A:** Diagram of technique for transposition flap. **B:** Transposition flap (tensor fascia lata) used for reconstruction of groin defect.

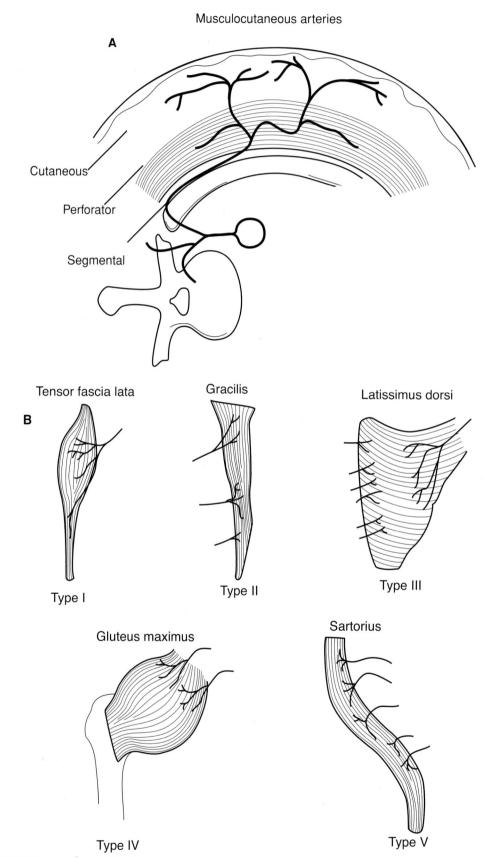

FIGURE 26-5 **A:** Arterial blood supply in musculocutaneous flaps. **B:** The five patterns of vascular anatomy of muscle. (Adapted from Mathes SJ, Nahai F. Classification of the vascular anatomy of the muscles: experimental and clinical correlation. *Plast Reconstr Surg.* 1981;67:177.)

2. **Uses of flaps include:**
   a. Wound closure in areas of poor vascularity (e.g., wounds overlying bare bone, cartilage, nerves, or tendons; radiation-injured tissue)
   b. Facial reconstruction (e.g., the nose or lips)
   c. Areas over bone where padding is needed (e.g., the ischial tuberosity in a patient with pressure sores)

3. **Vascular patency** may be assessed by color, temperature, Doppler flowmetry, fluoroscanning, and laser Doppler.

D **Reconstructive breast surgery** Techniques are available for treatment of micromastia (small breasts), macromastia (oversized breasts), and gynecomastia and for reconstruction following mastectomy. Because the breast is frequently viewed as a symbol of femininity, there is much emotional overlay in this type of surgery. Careful planning and realistic goals are necessary for patient satisfaction.

1. **Micromastia** is present when a patient feels that she lacks development of one or both breasts.
   a. **Treatment** is by augmentation with a prosthetic implant that can be placed either subglandularly (between the breast and the pectoralis major muscle) or submuscularly (underneath the pectoralis major muscle). The fill material for the prosthetic implant is either intraoperatively injected normal saline or factory-filled silicone. Silicone implants have the advantage of a more natural feel and shape. However, concerns about the potential health risks associated with silicone implants prompted the Food and Drug Administration (FDA) to ban their use in 1992 except in women who have undergone mastectomies or who are part of research studies. On October 16, 2003, an FDA advisory panel recommended that the government approve the use of silicone implants under certain conditions. On January 7, 2004, the FDA rejected the panel's recommendations pending further investigation. Studies by the Mayo Clinic, Harvard Medical School, and the National Academy of Sciences' Institute of Medicine panel found no evidence that leaked silicone from implants causes systemic disease.
   b. **Complications,** although rare, include infections and hematoma formation. A **capsular contracture** may form around the implant, which can lead to asymmetry and discomfort. This condition may require a subsequent surgical scar release and is more common when the implant is in the subglandular position.
   c. **Explantations,** or **removal of implants,** are becoming increasingly common. Rupture of the silicone gel implant is difficult to diagnose on mammograms, and either ultrasound or magnetic resonance imaging (MRI) is a better option. Frequently, there is no change in the breast of a woman with a ruptured silicone gel implant. If a saline implant ruptures, it generally deflates in a matter of days, making the diagnosis quite easy.

2. **Macromastia** is present when the patient feels that she has abnormally large breasts. Frequently, macromastia can be debilitating because of neck and back pain.
   a. **Treatment.** Various techniques have been described. All involve resecting breast tissue and the inferior breast skin, transposition of the nipple–areolar complex superiorly, and closure of the resultant flap defects. All resected specimens should be examined histologically because occult carcinoma may be present, although rarely is.
   b. **Complications** include hematoma formation, infection, change in nipple sensation, and necrosis.

3. **Mammary ptosis,** or drooping of the breast, is present when the nipple has extended below the inframammary fold. The breast skin envelope is larger than the underlying breast parenchyma. This condition usually occurs after significant weight loss, and it can occur after childbirth.
   a. **Treatment** involves skin excision similar to breast reduction incisions; however, very little or no breast tissue is removed.
   b. **Complications** include hematoma formation, infection, and skin loss.

4. **Gynecomastia** is enlargement of the male breast. In adolescents, the problem is often transient and regresses spontaneously. It can also occur in patients with various endocrine abnormalities and in patients with hepatic disease. Treatment by excision or suction-assisted lipectomy is aimed at restoring normal contour to the breast.

5. **Reconstruction of the breast following mastectomy** is an alternative to the use of external prosthetic devices. Reconstruction may be performed at the time of mastectomy or delayed for several months; however, the percentage of women who request reconstruction diminishes with increasing time following mastectomy.

   a. If there is adequate soft tissue and the pectoralis major muscle has been preserved, an implant can be used to reconstruct the breast mound. If the quality of the soft tissue is good but limited quantitatively, **tissue expansion** can be used. A tissue expander is a Silastic balloon, which is gradually inflated with saline over months to form a breast mound. It is generally replaced with a permanent prosthesis at a later date.

   b. If the soft tissue is inadequate either quantitatively or qualitatively, vascularized tissue may be transposed. The **latissimus dorsi myocutaneous flap** (with or without a prosthetic implant) and the transverse rectus abdominis myocutaneous (TRAM) flap are most commonly used. Figure 26-6 illustrates breast reconstruction by using a latissimus dorsi flap and a TRAM flap.

   c. Totally autogenous breast reconstruction with a **fleur-de-lys latissimus flap** or **TRAM** flap allows the reconstructive surgeon to create a breast mound without an implant. The reconstructed breast feels natural and fluctuates in size with the patient's weight change.

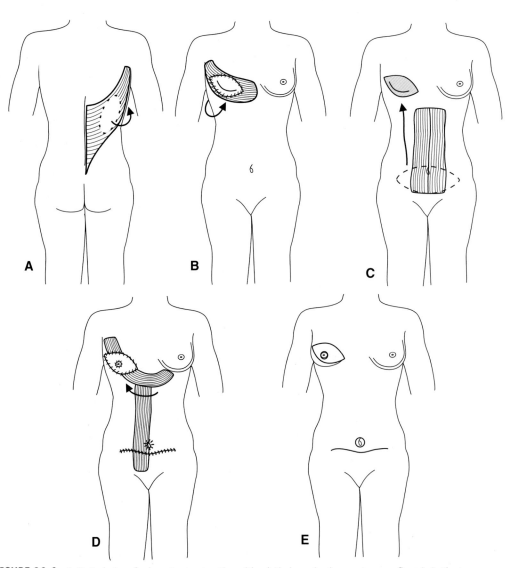

FIGURE 26-6   A, B: Technique for breast reconstruction with a latissimus dorsi myocutaneous flap. **C–E:** The transverse rectus abdominis myocutaneous (TRAM) flap is commonly used in breast reconstruction after a mastectomy.

d. Free flaps are occasionally indicated. The most common types are the **free TRAM** and **free gluteus maximus myocutaneous flaps** for breast reconstruction.

e. **Nipple–areola reconstruction** is usually done as a second stage. The nipple is reconstructed most commonly with local flaps and a skin graft to reconstruct the areola. If necessary, the nipple–areola complex can be tattooed to increase pigmentation.

f. Occasionally, a mastopexy or reduction mammoplasty is necessary for the opposite breast to achieve symmetry.

6. **Postoperative pain relief**

   a. **Regional anesthesia** includes peripheral nerve blocks, local wound infiltration, and epidural and spinal analgesia. Advantages of these types of anesthesia are reduced rates of blood loss, deep venous thrombosis (DVT), and adverse effects of general anesthesia as well as improved pain control. The **pain pump,** commonly used after breast reconstruction, breast augmentation, and abdominoplasty (procedures where there is a potential space) is a nonelectrical device that continuously delivers pain medication via very small catheters placed in the surgical site at the end of surgery. Commonly used medications are bupivacaine and lidocaine. The device delivers local anesthetic for approximately 48–72 hours, at which time the catheters can be removed by the patient at home.

   b. **Patient-controlled analgesia (PCA)** allows the patient to self-administer narcotics via an infusion pump of which the dose, dose interval, and infusion rate are preset by the physician. The pump helps to provide the patient with optimal pain relief. The patient has around-the-clock access to narcotics that can be delivered the moment she experiences pain or prior to expected activity. This tends to decrease the apprehension that patients often feel postoperatively about delays in medication administration. Prior to discharge from the hospital, the patient is weaned from the PCA and is given oral pain medication.

E **Reconstruction of congenital anomalies**   (see Chapter 29)

1. Congenital anomalies may result from genetic or environmental factors. In most cases, an initiating environmental factor acts on a genetically predisposed individual. The inheritance risk for most anomalies remains low. The repair and reconstruction of many congenital anomalies do not fall within the scope of plastic surgery; examples include the gastrointestinal anomalies discussed in Chapter 29.

2. **Maxillofacial deformities** can be reconstructed by craniofacial surgery.

   a. **Soft tissue and bony abnormalities** can be reconstructed by a specialized team approach. Examples include:

   (1) Hypertelorism

   (2) Orbital dystopia

   (3) Treacher Collins syndrome

   (4) Facial clefts

   (5) Crouzon's disease

   (6) Apert's syndrome

   b. **Cleft lip** may be unilateral, bilateral, or incomplete. It is seen in 1 in 1000 births and is more common in Asian children and male children. It is less common in blacks. Reconstruction is generally performed at approximately 3 months of age as determined by the **"rule of tens":** 10 lb, 10 weeks of age, and 10 g of hemoglobin. Some surgeons prefer to operate in the neonatal period.

   c. **Cleft palate** may occur as a defect in the primary or secondary palate or both. It occurs in 0.5 in 1000 births.

   (1) Reconstruction is performed before 2 years of age to aid in normal speech development. It commonly involves local flap advancement.

   (2) Secondary bone grafting is indicated before permanent teeth erupt if maxillary discontinuity exists.

   (3) Early attention to nutrition is important, because sucking is impaired.

F **Facial trauma** frequently accompanies other major trauma. After ensuring adequate ventilation and circulation, attention should be directed initially to areas where trauma is more life threatening (i.e., the chest and abdomen) (see Chapter 21 I). Once the patient is stabilized, the facial structures can be examined systematically.

1. **Soft tissue**
   a. **Lacerations of the face** bleed readily because of its rich blood supply. Bleeding is controlled by direct pressure and never by "blind" clamping. Control in the operating room may be necessary.
   b. Lacerations may involve deeper structures, such as the facial nerve and parotid duct.
   c. Most lacerations can be repaired by primary closure, following thorough debridement of all devitalized tissue.

2. **Blunt trauma** may result in **contusions** or **associated fractures.**
   a. Many injuries of this type can be diagnosed initially by inspection; facial asymmetry, if present, should be noted.
      (1) Dental malocclusion may signify a mandibular or maxillary fracture.
      (2) Instability of the upper jaw may signify a maxillary fracture or midface fracture.
      (3) Pain on palpation at the nose, depression, or asymmetry may signify a nasal fracture.
      (4) Diplopia, malar deformity, enophthalmos, or hypoesthesia of the cheek may signify an orbital blow-out fracture.
   b. Complete radiologic examination is essential. Operative stabilization is usually required.

G **Genitourinary anomalies** may interfere with normal urinary function and result in severe psychological problems if they are not corrected. These congenital anomalies are apparent at birth, and treatment should be initiated at an early age.

1. **Hypospadias** is a condition in which the urethral meatus opens on the ventral surface of the penis, scrotum, or perineum.
   a. It occurs in 1 in 300 live male births and is usually associated with downward curvature of the penis caused by fibrous tissue, a condition called **chordee.**
   b. Evaluation of the upper urinary tract is essential, because 10% of patients have associated abnormalities.
   c. If present, the chordee is resected, and reconstruction is completed by local skin-flap advancement, full-thickness skin grafts to create a urethra, or both.

2. **Epispadias** is failure of closure of the dorsal surface of the penis. **Exstrophy of the bladder** occurs when the anterior bladder wall opens on the abdomen. Both represent degrees of the same abnormality.
   a. These unusual disorders occur in 1 in 40,000 births.
   b. Associated upper urinary tract abnormalities are rare.
   c. Treatment is aimed at preserving renal function, which may be accomplished by closure of the bladder defect or excision of the bladder and urinary diversion.

3. **Vaginal agenesis** is repaired by vaginal reconstruction, using split-thickness skin grafts. Myocutaneous flaps are used for reconstruction following ablative surgery (Fig. 26-7).

4. **Gender dysphoria** is treated surgically by altering sexual appearance to coincide with personality. After careful preoperative evaluation, ablative surgery is performed, followed by reconstruction with flaps and skin grafts.

H **Aesthetic surgery** is an attempt to improve on nature or to control the body's ageing process by surgical means. Changes that occur secondary to ageing are the result of decreased elasticity of the skin and loss of subcutaneous fat. Most commonly, procedures are performed on the more noticeable areas of the body (e.g., face, neck, abdomen, extremities, and breasts). The expectations of the patient must be realistic; he or she must understand that surgery will alter appearance but not the person.

1. **Rhytidectomy (face-lift)** is a procedure that undermines the skin of the face and neck. Excision of redundant pre- and postauricular skin completes the procedure. Occasionally, the **submuscular aponeurotic system (SMAS)** of the face is plicated at the same operative setting. With this procedure, the skin of the face and neck is tightened to give a more youthful appearance.

2. A **brow-lift** corrects ptosis, or droop, of the forehead and can be combined with a rhytidectomy. With the advent of endoscopic techniques, a brow-lift can be performed with minimal incisions.

3. **Dermabrasion** is the physical abrasion of skin. It is most commonly used to treat acne scarring.

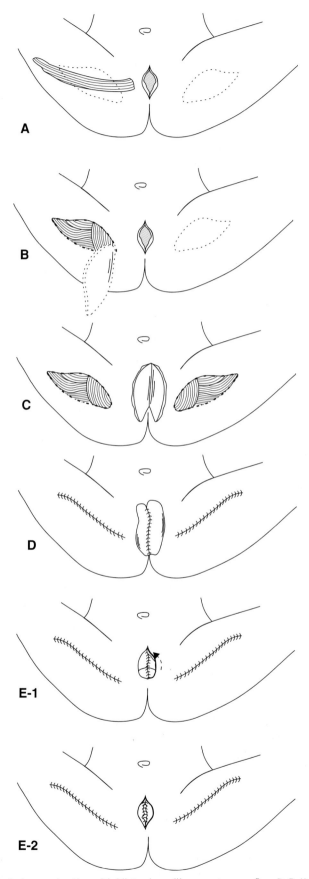

FIGURE 26-7 A–C: Vaginal reconstruction with bilateral gracilis myocutaneous flap. **D–E:** Vaginal reconstruction with bilateral gracilis myocutaneous flap.

4. **Laser treatments** to facial areas (most commonly, CO_2 and erbium lasers) are used to treat photoaging of the skin. Other lasers are useful for treating spider veins, benign skin discoloration, and hair removal.

5. **Chemical face peel** is an induced mild chemical burn to the superficial skin and is used most commonly to treat fine facial wrinkles. Phenol, trichloroacetic acid, and glycolic acid are commonly used agents.

6. **Blepharoplasty** is used to treat **baggy eyelids.** This surgery may be functional in the upper lids because redundant skin may obscure lateral gaze fields. It is accompanied by excision of varying amounts of skin and fat to give a more youthful or "less tired" look to the eyes.

7. **Rhinoplasty** is performed to correct congenital or acquired nasal defects. This surgery may be done for esthetic or functional reasons. The procedure involves a controlled nasal fracture with excision of varying amounts of bone and cartilage.

8. **Abdominoplasty** is the excision of excess abdominal fat and skin. In many cases, repair of diastasis recti brought on by pregnancy or prior obesity is performed to tighten the abdominal wall.

9. **Liposuction** (suction-assisted lipectomy) is a procedure commonly used to remove localized deposits of fat. Subcutaneous fat is aspirated by high-vacuum suction or syringe to restore body contour. Blood loss can be minimized with the preoperative subcutaneous infusion of a dilute epinephrine solution. Liposuction is not a weight-reduction procedure.

10. **Skin filler** injections are useful for correcting localized contour irregularities (usually on the face) such as acne scars, wrinkles, lines, and traumatic scars. The depth of the defect should determine the type of filler used to correct it. Collagen and hyaluronic acid polymers are examples of injectable fillers that are used to temporarily fill superficial defects. Collagen, usually of bovine origin, lasts 3–6 months, necessitating subsequent injections. Correction of deeper defects may be accomplished with Alloderm, synthetic products (implants or permanent fillers), or fat autotransplantation. At this time, fat autotransplantation is somewhat experimental because the amount of viable fat harvested by liposuction cannot be easily assessed clinically. The ideal filling agent, an injectable, nondegradable material that incorporates itself with the body's tissues without adverse effects, has not yet been discovered.

11. **Endoscopic surgery** is relatively new to plastic surgery. Techniques that have found application include brow-lift, rhytidectomy, breast augmentation, and abdominoplasty.

12. **Breast surgery** is discussed in I D.

13. **Botulinum toxin (Botox)** injections, originally used in the treatment of strabismus and other muscle conditions, produce excellent cosmetic results for facial rejuvenation. Botulinum toxin type A induces a temporary chemical paresis in the facial muscles that cause hyperfunctional lines and wrinkles with repeated use over years. The most commonly treated facial lines are the horizontal forehead, glabellar forehead, perioral, and lateral canthal lines.

II SKIN LESIONS

A **Overview** Many skin tumors can be **diagnosed at an early stage** because of their obvious difference from adjacent skin. They frequently have a **characteristic appearance,** which can aid in planning appropriate therapy.

1. **Examination should be systematic** and based on the gross appearance of the lesion. Inspection can reveal color changes and ulceration. Palpation can reveal fixation to underlying tissues or the involvement of adjacent lymph nodes.

2. **Biopsy** is usually required for accurate diagnosis and can be either **excisional** for smaller lesions or **incisional** for larger ones. In all instances, the biopsy should be carefully planned, because a more radical resection may be necessary. In addition, cosmetic considerations must be kept in mind.

B **Benign conditions**   are common, and frequently, the patient seeks medical attention for cosmetic reasons or from fear of cancer. Only the more common lesions are discussed in this chapter.

1. **Common warts (verrucae vulgaris)** occur most frequently in the second decade of life and may be transmitted by direct or indirect contact.
   a. **Etiology.** They are caused by a member of the papovavirus family, which invades the stratum spinosum epidermidis, causing papillomatosis.
   b. **Clinical presentation.** The fingers are the most common location. The lesions have a characteristic rough and elevated surface and can become tender.
   c. **Treatment** involves minimal destruction of normal tissue. In many cases, the warts resolve spontaneously. Problematic lesions can be treated by:
      (1) Curettage and electrodesiccation
      (2) Freezing with liquid nitrogen
      (3) Chemotherapy with caustic agents

2. **Cysts** are fluid-filled cavities in the subcutaneous tissues; they may resemble solid tumors.
   a. **Epidermal inclusion cysts** develop when epidermal cells are trapped in the subcutaneous tissue. Desquamation leads to the creation of a cavity. Excision is curative.
   b. **Sebaceous cysts** result from blockage of a sweat gland, which causes the accumulation of sebum and the creation of a cyst. Excision is curative and prevents a recurrence. If infection is present, the cyst should be incised and drained before excision.
   c. **Dermoid cysts** are congenital lesions that may occur later in life. If they occur in the midline (glabellar, nasal), a computed tomography (CT) scan is indicated because there may be intracranial communication. Treatment is by excision.
   d. **Ganglia** can occur in areas of weakened retinaculum, with outpouching of underlying synovial structures. They occur most commonly on the hands and feet in areas subjected to trauma or inflammation. Excision is curative, but there can be recurrences, which are probably caused by inadequate resection of the ganglion's stalk and base.

3. **Vascular birthmarks** are frequently disturbing to the patient and family because they are cosmetically deforming. They are classified on the basis of their clinical and cellular characteristics.
   a. **Hemangiomas (strawberry marks)** are characterized by increased number of mast cells during the proliferative phase and rapid postnatal growth. These elevated, red, soft, compressible lesions grow rapidly during the first year of life and are most commonly located on the head and neck area and extremities. Spontaneous regression is characteristic. Surgery or steroid therapy is indicated for lesions causing functional impairment (e.g., to the eyes, ears, throat). Rarely, platelet consumption occurs. Hemorrhage is uncommon, and there is usually minimal residual scarring.
   b. **Vascular malformations** grow at the same rate as the patient; thus, they may not be obvious at birth. They have a normal number of mast cells and may be divided according to the predominant vascular tissue: capillary, venous, lymphatic.
      (1) **Capillary malformations (capillary hemangioma, port-wine stains)** are found on the face, chest, and extremities. They may be associated with Sturge-Weber and Klippel-Trenaunay-Weber syndromes. There is dilatation of the capillaries in the subpapillary, dermal, or subdermal layer. If the tumor is small, excision is curative. Treatment of larger lesions requires careful planning for optimal results. The laser has recently proved to be helpful in treatment.
      (2) **Venous malformations (cavernous hemangiomas)** involve a matrix of mature vessels in the subcutaneous tissues; frequently, they involve deeper structures, including muscle. These lesions may sequester platelets. After careful preoperative planning, treatment involves wide excision with attention to the involved structures. Occasionally, a direct sclerosant injection may be helpful.
      (3) **Lymphatic malformations (lymphangioma, cystic hygroma)** commonly cause hypertrophy of involved soft tissues. Surgical treatment is excision, and seroma is a common complication.
      (4) **Arteriovenous malformations** frequently remain stable in size and then expand. Treatment is by surgical excision.

4. **Vascular tumors** are frequently benign; they may cause concern because of their prominence.
   a. **Pyogenic granulomas** are papular lesions that are commonly located on the face, chest, and fingers; the lesions develop rapidly and then stop enlarging after variable periods of growth. They tend to bleed freely. Surgical excision is usually curative.

    b. Spider nevi (telangiectasias) occur in all age groups and are commonly located on the face, chest, and extremities. They may arise during pregnancy and with cirrhosis. The lesion consists of a central arteriole with vessels resembling venules that radiate from the center. They rarely bleed, and treatment (i.e., laser therapy, electrodesiccation, or cryotherapy) is undertaken primarily for cosmetic reasons.

    c. Glomus tumors, which are extremely painful, are located most frequently in the nail beds. Treatment is by excision.

5. Lipomas (fat tumors) can be found in any area of the body where fat is normally found, but they are most common on the neck, shoulders, back, and thighs. Malignant transformation is uncommon, and excision is curative.

6. Nerve tumors (see Chapter 18, IV F 1, 3) come in two varieties.

    a. Neurilemomas arise from the Schwann cell sheath. They do not cause much pain, and they are treated by excision.

    b. Neurofibromas involve masses of nerve and fibrous tissue and are related to **von Recklinghausen's disease.** They may undergo malignant degeneration.

7. Seborrheic keratosis is a light- to dark-brown raised papular lesion, which must be differentiated from malignant skin lesions. Treatment is by biopsy followed by curettage and electrodesiccation.

8. Keloids are abnormal accumulations of fibrous tissue, which extend above and beyond an area that was previously traumatized (as opposed to hypertrophic scars that remain within those confines). They occur more commonly in blacks. Treatment is by excision and pressure. Occasionally, adjuvant corticosteroid therapy is necessary.

9. Hidradenitis suppurativa may be confused with a tumor, but it is an **infection** of the apocrine sweat glands and subcutaneous tissue that occurs most frequently in the axilla or groin. Treatment involves controlling the infection with antibiotics and (if indicated) incision and drainage, followed by excision with either primary closure or a split-thickness skin graft.

C **Premalignant skin lesions** are benign lesions with a high likelihood of progressing to invasive squamous cell carcinoma.

1. Actinic keratosis is a rough, scaly epidermal lesion that occurs in areas of the body subjected to chronic sun exposure.

    a. It may appear in the third or fourth decade of life, and approximately 10%–20% of the lesions undergo malignant transformation.

    b. If biopsy proves the lesion to be benign, it is treated by excision or cryotherapy. Topical chemotherapy with 5-fluorouracil has been useful in patients with many keratoses.

2. Bowen's disease is intraepidermal squamous cell carcinoma or carcinoma in situ of the skin. It appears as a well-defined, erythematous plaque covered by an adherent scaly yellow crust.

    a. There are no lymphatics in the layer affected, and there is no potential for metastasis.

    b. Bowen's disease occurs mainly in the fourth to sixth decade of life, and ingestion of arsenic and viruses have been implicated as etiologic agents. Treatment is similar to that for actinic keratosis.

3. Keratoacanthoma is a locally destructive skin lesion that is found most commonly on the head, neck, and upper extremities.

    a. Rapid progression of the tumor occurs within 2–8 weeks, followed by spontaneous resolution.

    b. Treatment is by excision and biopsy of the lesion; squamous cell carcinoma is found in approximately one quarter of the lesions biopsied.

D **Nevi (moles)**

1. Overview

    a. Nevi are pigmented lesions of the skin that frequently concern the patient because of the fear of malignancy. Because the average white man has 15–20 nevi, total excision is unreasonable.

    b. Clinical diagnosis is important, because **malignant transformation** can occur. In general, however, malignant transformation is rare in children. Also, well-circumscribed lesions and lesions with a uniform color rarely progress to malignancy.

   c. Suspicious-looking lesions should be biopsied by excision with a margin of normal skin.

2. Benign pigmented lesions

  a. Junctional nevi are dark, flat, smooth lesions, which range generally from 1–2 cm in diameter. They are occasionally hairy and develop from the basal layer of epidermis. Nevi that are located on the palms and soles are usually junctional. They can develop into malignant melanoma, but this rarely occurs before puberty.

  b. Compound nevi are brown-to-black, well-circumscribed lesions that are usually less than 1 cm in diameter. They may be elevated and are frequently hairy, arising from the epidermal–dermal interface and from within the dermis. Malignant transformation is rare.

  c. Intradermal nevi are light-colored, well-circumscribed lesions less than 1 cm in diameter. Hairs are usually present, and the cell distribution occurs in the dermis. Malignant transformation is rare.

  d. Giant pigmented nevi

    (1) These brown-to-black, hairy lesions have an irregular nodular surface. They frequently involve more than 1 ft² of body surface and arise from the dermis and junctional areas. The lesions are frequently described, in terms of distribution, as "bathing trunk," "vest," "sleeve," or "stocking."

    (2) Malignant degeneration has been estimated at approximately 10%.

    (3) Excision with a margin of normal tissue is indicated, either in stages or with flap reconstruction.

  e. Blue nevi are smooth, hairless lesions measuring less than 1 cm in diameter. They arise in the dermis, and malignant degeneration is rare.

  f. Spitz nevi (benign juvenile melanomas) are smooth, round, pink-to-black lesions measuring 1–2 cm in diameter. They have increased cellularity and occur in nests within the upper dermis. Malignant degeneration is rare.

  g. Nevi must be distinguished from **freckles (ephelides).** These pigmented lesions occur in the basal and upper dermis and have no malignant potential.

3. Treatment

  a. Treatment is indicated for **junctional** and **giant pigmented nevi** because of their malignant potential.

  b. Indications for excision of any pigmented lesion include:

    (1) Changes in color, size, shape, or consistency

    (2) Pain

    (3) Satellite nodules

    (4) Regional adenopathy

  c. Except for large lesions, **excisional biopsy,** with a margin of normal skin, should be performed. Further therapy may be indicated, depending on the histologic diagnosis and location of the lesion.

  d. For large lesions, a full-thickness wedge biopsy, including a small area of normal skin, should be taken.

E **Malignant melanoma** (see Chapter 19, X B) is a melanoblastic tumor that may develop in the skin or eye.

1. Epidemiology. The incidence is approximately 13 new cases per 100,000 population a year, representing an increase of 50% in the past decade. The tumor occurs most commonly in the fifth decade of life, and the incidence is approximately equal in men and women.

2. Etiology. Exposure to sunlight appears to be an initiating event in the development of melanoma, and fair-skinned white people with frequent direct (overhead) exposure to the sun are most often affected.

3. Detection of melanoma is determined by changes in the color, size, or shape of a nevus.

  a. Men are most frequently affected on the back, chest, and upper extremities.

  b. Women are most frequently affected on the back, lower extremities, and upper extremities.

4. Classification of melanomas is based on their gross and histologic appearance.

  a. Superficial spreading melanoma accounts for 70% of all melanomas. It can be present on any area of the body but is found most frequently on the back and legs. The median age at diagnosis is the fifth decade. The tumor has irregular borders with a varied color pattern. Cell distribution is in the upper dermis with lateral junctional spread. Generally, the prognosis is good.

b. Nodular melanoma accounts for 15% of melanomas and occurs most commonly in the sixth decade of life. The tumor is blue-black and may be found on any area of the body. Spread is primarily vertical with rapid dermal invasion, and the prognosis is poor.

c. Acrolentiginous and mucosal melanomas make up 10% of all melanomas. They occur most commonly in the fifth decade of life and are distributed on the mucous membranes, palms, and soles. Irregular borders are common; lesions are generally black but may be amelanotic. Growth occurs slowly in a radial direction; cells are mainly in the upper dermis with occasional deep invasion. The prognosis depends on the depth of invasion and is between that of superficial spreading and nodular melanomas.

d. Lentigo maligna (melanotic freckle of Hutchinson) is the least common of the melanomas, and it appears most frequently in the seventh decade of life. The lesions are brown-black and contain elevated nodules within a smooth freckle. They occur most frequently on the head, neck, and hand. Growth is slow and in a radial direction, with cells in the upper dermis; vertical extension is infrequent. The prognosis is excellent.

5. Staging. Classification of the lesion is imperative for optimal treatment. Histologic evaluation with regard to the depth of invasion as well as the type of tumor is important for determining prognosis. To complete the staging, a thorough history and physical examination are necessary, including a complete blood count, 12-test sequential multiple analysis (SMA-12), urinalysis, and chest radiograph.

a. Clark's classification assesses the **level of invasion** and has been adopted by the American Joint Committee for Cancer Staging and End Results.

(1) Level I: The tumor is confined to the epidermis.

(2) Level II: The tumor invades the papillary dermis.

(3) Level III: The tumor fills the papillary dermis but does not invade the reticular dermis.

(4) Level IV: The tumor invades the reticular dermis.

(5) Level V: The tumor invades the subcutaneous fat.

b. Breslow's method is an additional method that is sometimes used. It involves measuring the depth of invasion precisely in millimeters. However, erroneous estimates of the depth of invasion can occur if ulceration is present.

(1) Patients with Clark's level I, II, or III lesion and with a depth of invasion that is less than 0.76 mm are at low risk for metastasis.

(2) Patients with lesions at level IV or V and with a depth of invasion greater than 1.5 mm are at high risk for distant spread.

6. Treatment depends on the depth of invasion. Biopsy is by total excision when feasible; otherwise, incisional biopsy is performed. Frozen section is inaccurate in determining the depth of invasion.

a. Excision. There is debate over the previously accepted 5-cm margin.

(1) For melanoma in situ, 0.5 cm margins are indicated.

(2) For lesions less than 1.0 mm in thickness, a 1-cm margin is generally sufficient.

(3) For lesions 1–4 mm in thickness, 2-cm margins are indicated. The need to excise the underlying fascia is debatable.

(4) For lesions more than 4 mm in thickness, 3-cm margins are indicated.

b. Lymph node removal

(1) Clinically involved regional lymph nodes with level II, III, IV, or V disease should be resected with an elective lymph node dissection (ELND), which in the case of melanoma entails resection of level I, II, and III lymph nodes.

(2) Sentinel node biopsy is a minimally invasive way of staging clinically occult regional lymph node metastases. Several hours prior to surgery, the area adjacent to the primary lesion is injected with a radiotracer (technetium sulfur colloid) for lymphoscintigraphy in the radiology department for lymph node localization intraoperatively. A visible (isosulfan blue) dye is also injected perioperatively near the lesion. The lymph node(s) in the regional node basin that first takes up these tracers is considered the sentinel node. It is excised and examined for disease. The sentinal node biopsy is useful in that it prevents unnecessary ELND and the associated morbidity. If the sentinal node if free of disease, the patient is spared an ELND.

(3) Postoperative morbidity from lymph node resection needs to be considered when lesions involve the face or lower extremities.

c. **Adjuvant therapy** is recommended by some authors to prolong the diseasefree interval.

(1) **Regional hyperthermic perfusion** involves isolating the blood supply of a limb with a pump oxygenator, enabling high doses of chemotherapy to be delivered to the limb at elevated temperatures (40°C) without the side effects of systemic toxicity. The role of this treatment has yet to be clarified.

(2) **Chemotherapy** with dacarbazine (DTIC), carmustine (BiCNU), and lomustine (CeeNU) has not significantly altered the course of disease.

(3) **Immunotherapy** is useful for the control of cutaneous metastases, but visceral metastases have not responded to any significant degree.

(4) **Radiotherapy** is strictly palliative and has been used for brain and bone metastases.

7. **Prognosis** is related to the status of the regional lymph nodes. When disease is confined at the primary site, the 5-year survival rate is approximately 80%–90%. If regional lymph nodes are involved, this figure drops to 30%–50%. Patients with distant or visceral metastases usually die within 12 months.

F **Other malignant tumors of the skin** commonly occur in exposed areas. Generally, they are low-grade tumors and metastasize late. For this reason, they are highly curable.

1. **Basal cell carcinoma** (see Chapter 19, X A) is the most common skin tumor seen. It is localized and grows slowly, and it generally occurs in the head and neck. It is found most commonly in individuals of northern European descent.

a. **Etiology.** Basal cell carcinoma has also been associated with xeroderma pigmentosum, basal cell nevus syndrome, nevus sebaceus, and unstable burn scars. With the advent of radiation therapy, basal cell carcinomas are being seen with increasing frequency in areas of dermatitis.

b. **Clinical presentation.** The lesion has pearly, translucent edges, which may become erythematous or pigmented. Frequently, a visible telangiectasia is present. As the lesion grows, it may ulcerate and eventually invade underlying structures. Morphologic types of basal cell cancer include superficial, nodular, pigmented, and morphealike (sclerosing). Metastatic disease is rare.

c. **Treatment** involves the complete removal of the tumor to achieve a cure. **Biopsy is mandatory** to establish a pathologic diagnosis.

(1) **Curettage and electrodesiccation** result in a 95% cure rate, and the technique is acceptable for lesions less than 2 cm in diameter. The disadvantage is the lack of a specimen for determining the adequacy of resection.

(2) **Radiation therapy** can be used in areas where tissue preservation is important (e.g., the eyelids). The cure rate is approximately 90%. The disadvantages are that depigmentation and skin atrophy can occur with time.

(3) **Excision with primary closure** results in a cure rate of approximately 95% and allows inspection of the specimen for adequate margins. If necessary, reconstruction can be performed at the same sitting.

(4) **Mohs' micrographic surgery** involves tumor mapping to determine the adequacy of resection. Generally, it is most applicable to recurrent tumors, morphealike tumors, and those of the nose or perinasal areas. As cure rates approach 99%, immediate reconstruction can achieve excellent esthetic results.

(5) **Cryotherapy** is acceptable in certain cases. It has a higher morbidity, and scarring is less predictable than with other techniques.

(6) **Topical chemotherapy** results in unacceptable cure rates.

d. **Recurrent disease** requires wide re-excision.

2. **Squamous cell carcinoma** (see Chapter 19, X A) is second to basal cell carcinoma in occurrence. It may grow rapidly and has the capacity to metastasize via the blood and lymphatic system.

a. **Etiology. Exposure to sunlight** appears to be a causative factor, because the tumor is more common on the head and hands. Squamous cell carcinoma may develop from the premalignant lesions already mentioned (see II C) or from old burn scars; it may also occur in people exposed to arsenicals, nitrates, or hydrocarbons.

b. **Clinical presentation.** The lesion may have satellite nodules or a central area of ulceration that may become encrusted, obscuring deeper invasion. The tumor is common on the lips, in the paranasal folds, and on the axilla. It can be classified as well-differentiated or poorly differentiated squamous cell carcinoma, based on the histologic examination.

c. **Treatment**

  (1) Treatment is based on examination of the biopsy specimen.

    (a) **Excisional biopsy** with a cuff of normal tissue is preferred for lesions less than 1 cm in diameter.

    (b) **Incisional biopsy** can be performed for larger lesions or for those on the face.

  (2) **Treatment methods**

    (a) **Electrodesiccation** can be used to treat lesions less than 1 cm in diameter. It can also be used in elderly individuals and in patients with a history of repeated tumors.

    (b) **Excision with primary closure** offers the advantage of histologic examination of the specimen. Reconstruction following the excision of large lesions may be required.

      (i) Regional lymph node dissection should be performed only if there is clinical evidence of nodal disease.

      (ii) Frequently, regional adenopathy may accompany ulcerated lesions. In this case, the lymph nodes should not be excised at the same sitting as the primary tumor, because the nodes will resolve with time if the adenopathy is inflammatory in nature.

    (c) **Radiation therapy** can result in a cure, with improved cosmetic results in certain cases.

    (d) **Mohs' surgery** (see Chapter 19, X A 3 c) also has been successful in treatment.

3. **Sweat gland tumors** are rare lesions arising from the eccrine or apocrine glands. They occur in later life and present as a soft tissue mass that has been present for years. Metastases to regional lymph nodes are common, and consideration should be given to regional node dissection at the time of initial excision. The overall 5-year survival rate is approximately 40%.

G **Sarcomas of the soft tissue**

1. **Overview.** Sarcomas of the soft tissue constitute only 1% of malignant tumors, and they may occur at any location in the body. Approximately 20 different types have been described, each with a slightly different tendency to metastasize or to invade locally.

a. **Clinical presentation.** These tumors usually present as an enlarging mass, which is frequently painless. If they occur in deep locations, such as the retroperitoneum, they are often quite large at the time of diagnosis.

b. **Diagnosis** is made on permanent sections of a representative biopsy. MRI is helpful in determining the extent of the tumor. The biopsy should be planned with the future surgical procedure in mind. Excisional biopsy is indicated for lesions less than 3 cm in diameter; otherwise, incisional biopsy is indicated.

c. **Treatment.** These tumors are frequently treated inadequately because they have a pseudo-capsule, which may lead the surgeon to assume falsely that all of the tumor has been removed. In reality, these tumors extend along tissue planes well beyond their apparent margins.

  (1) **Wide local excision or amputation** is the current accepted treatment. Chemotherapy and postoperative radiotherapy are frequently indicated.

  (2) **Limb-sparing surgery** is indicated when wide local excision can be accomplished without jeopardizing the function of the extremity (i.e., involvement of major nerves or vessels).

  (3) **Limited surgery with high-dose radiotherapy** yields a local recurrence rate similar to that for radical surgery (20%–50%).

d. The **route of metastasis** is usually **hematogenous,** and the lungs are the most frequent site of involvement. Lymphatic spread occurs less often and usually late in the course of the disease. Metastatic lesions in the lungs should be resected if the primary tumor is under good control and there is no evidence of other sites of involvement.

2. **Major soft tissue sarcomas**
   a. **Liposarcoma** is the most common of the soft tissue sarcomas in the adult.
      (1) Only 1% arise from pre-existing benign lipomas.
      (2) Liposarcomas can occur in any area, including the retroperitoneum.
      (3) They are **treated** by wide excision. The tumors are radiosensitive, and radiotherapy may be helpful in locations where wide excision is not possible.
      (4) Well-differentiated lesions have a 70% 5-year survival rate, whereas poorly differentiated lesions have only a 20% survival rate at 5 years.
   b. **Fibrosarcoma** is the second most common soft tissue sarcoma in the adult.
      (1) These lesions are usually found in an extremity, where they present as a hard, round mass. They are more common in men than in women and are the most common sarcoma found in black persons.
      (2) They are radioresistant, and the **treatment** is wide excision. Fibrosarcomas are very susceptible to local recurrence and must be treated aggressively at the time of presentation.
      (3) Adequately treated fibrosarcomas have a 5-year survival rate of 77%.
   c. **Rhabdomyosarcoma** arises from skeletal muscle and occurs in both a juvenile and an adult form.
      (1) **Embryonal rhabdomyosarcoma** usually occurs in children younger than 15 years of age.
         (a) The head, neck, and genitourinary system are most frequently involved.
         (b) This tumor has recently enjoyed a spectacular increase in the 5-year survival rate. The combination of surgery, radiotherapy, and multidrug chemotherapy now achieves a 70% 5-year survival rate for patients with isolated lesions. If metastases are present, the survival rate is lower but is still approximately 40%.
      (2) **Pleomorphic rhabdomyosarcoma** is the histologic type that is usually found in adults.
         (a) **Wide excision** (including amputation, if necessary) is the **treatment of choice.** Chemotherapy is much less effective in this form of the tumor.
         (b) Although lymph node dissections are not done in most cases of sarcoma, they should be done for pleomorphic rhabdomyosarcoma because 25% of patients have regional nodal metastasis.
         (c) The 5-year survival rate is 30%.
   d. **Kaposi's sarcoma,** which has attracted attention recently in connection with acquired immunodeficiency syndrome (AIDS), is a malignant lesion of vascular origin.
      (1) Until recently, it was usually seen in the lower extremities of older men. Now, it is often seen in the perianal area in connection with AIDS.
      (2) It usually begins as a single bluish-red macule, and gradually, multiple nodules appear and may ulcerate.
      (3) A solitary nodule should be excised, and widespread disease should be treated with radiotherapy. Although there is no cure for systemic Kaposi's sarcoma, patients may live for many years.
   e. **Lymphangiosarcoma** is a peculiar tumor that develops in areas of chronic lymphedema (e.g., in the arm of women with postmastectomy edema, particularly if radiotherapy has also been used). The prognosis is dismal, and there is no effective treatment.
   f. **Benign sarcomas**
      (1) **Desmoid tumors** are classified as benign fibromatoses that have the capacity to grow to a large size with a high rate of recurrence after excision. They are associated with **Gardner's syndrome.** They usually affect the shoulder and trunk and may affect the abdominal wall in parous women.
      (2) **Dermatofibrosarcoma protuberans** is a slow-growing nodular tumor with a high recurrence rate after excision. Histologically, it exhibits a "cartwheel" pattern of fibroblasts.
      (3) **Paraganglioma (chemodectoma, carotid body tumor)** presents as a painless mass in the neck overlying the carotid bifurcation. Most tumors are benign. Excision is curative.

chapter 27

Neurosurgery

ALLAN J. HAMILTON • MARTIN WEINAND

I   INTRODUCTION

Neurosurgery is surgical management of nervous system disease. The 1990s have seen rapid expansion and application of innovative technologies, including magnetic resonance imaging (MRI) and angiography for detecting lesions of the brain and spinal cord; positron emission tomography (PET) for evaluation of metabolic defects in the brain; and minimally invasive techniques such as implantable deep brain stimulators, interventional radiology for aneurysms, and radiosurgery. There have also been refinements of operative tools, including the computed/image-guided neuronavigation operating microscope, the ultrasonic aspirator, and the laser.

II   ANATOMY

The brain accounts for only 2% of the body weight but requires 18% of the **cardiac output** and 20% of the **oxygen** used by the body. The normal **cerebral blood flow** is about 50 mL/100 g of brain tissue per minute.

A **Arterial supply to the brain**

1. The **anterior circulation** is derived from the two **internal carotid arteries,** giving rise to the **middle cerebral** and the smaller **anterior cerebral** arteries. These vessels supply mainly the **frontal, temporal,** and **parietal lobes** as well as the **deep gray matter.**

2. The **posterior circulation** is comprised of the two vertebral arteries.
   a. At the caudal margin of the pons, the arteries unite to form the **basilar artery.**
   b. The basilar artery gives off branches supplying the **pons, cerebellum, thalamus,** and dividing into the posterior cerebral arteries, it supplies the **occipital lobes.**

3. The **circle of Willis,** an arterial circle, is formed by communicating arteries between the major branches of the anterior and posterior circulations. In the event of a trunk vessel occlusion, the blood supply to its territory may be supplied by another vessel via the circle of Willis.

B **Venous return to the brain**

1. **Superficial cerebral veins** drain the cortex and subcortical white matter and drain into the superior sagittal sinus or the basal sinuses (i.e., the transverse, petrosal, or cavernous sinuses).

2. **Deep cerebral veins** drain the deeper structures (nuclei). The deep veins consist of the paired **internal cerebral** and **basal (Rosenthal) veins,** which form the **great vein of Galen** before emptying into the **straight sinus.**
   a. All venous blood from the brain returns to the heart via the internal jugular veins.
   b. Sampling of blood from the jugular bulb provides an estimate of cerebral metabolism.

C **Arterial supply to the spinal cord**   The spinal cord is supplied by the **anterior spinal artery** and the paired **posterior spinal arteries,** reinforced by the **segmental radicular arteries.**

1. The **anterior spinal artery** branches into the **anterior sulcal artery** in the anterior sulcus, which supplies the anteromedial gray matter.

2. The **segmental arteries** are important because their interruption can lead to infarction of the spinal cord.

D **Venous return from the spinal cord** parallels the arterial supply.

1. **Anterior longitudinal venous trunks** drain corresponding areas of the cord and are drained, in turn, by 6–11 radicular veins into the epidural venous plexus.

2. **Posterior longitudinal venous trunks** drain the posterior funiculus, the posterior horns, and the white matter in the lateral funiculi. These trunks, in turn, are drained by 5–10 radicular veins into the epidural venous plexus.

3. The **epidural venous plexus** is located between the vertebral periosteum and the dura mater.
   a. The plexus consists of two or more anterior and posterior longitudinal veins interconnected at various levels.
   b. At each intervertebral space, there is an extensive anastomosis with intercostal, thoracic, and abdominal veins.
   c. None of these venous channels has valves, and thus, blood from these plexuses may directly enter the systemic circulation and vice versa.

E **Cerebrospinal fluid (CSF),** brain tissue, and blood are the major components of the intracranial space.

1. Normally, the total volume of the CSF is about 150 mL, with 25 mL located in the ventricles. The CSF is formed at a rate of 0.35 mL/minute (approximately 150 mL three times per day). Roughly 80% of the CSF is produced by the choroid plexus, and the rest is secreted in the interstitial spaces of the brain.

2. The **CSF flows** from the lateral **ventricles** to the third ventricle through the **foramina of Monro** and reaches the fourth ventricle via the **aqueduct of Sylvius** and **reaches the brain exterior** by the **foramina of Magendie** (midline) and **Luschka** (lateral).
   a. The CSF circulates around the spinal cord and the brain and is reabsorbed into the superior sagittal sinus via the arachnoid villi. Some of the CSF is absorbed around the spinal nerve roots.
   b. The **arachnoid villi** act as one-way valves, and they open at a pressure of 5 mm Hg.

F **Functional anatomy of the nervous system**   The following principles form the basis for evaluating and treating neurologic disease.

1. **Pathophysiologic processes** unique to the nervous system result from the:
   a. **Complexity of the functional organization** of the nervous system
   b. **Rigidity of the bony enclosures** of the brain and spinal cord
   c. **Responses of the nervous system** to injury

2. **Focal lesions** affect neurologic function by:
   a. Local destruction of brain tissue
   b. Tissue distortion with functional loss attributable to axonal stretching and subsequent synaptic damage
   c. Changes in **local blood flow,** causing ischemia or venous congestion
   d. Alterations in the **electrical or metabolic activity** of a local area, producing an epileptic focus

3. **Location of the lesion**
   a. A small focal lesion in the **brain stem** can produce devastating effects.
   b. A similar lesion in the **frontal (silent) area** may produce no significant neurologic deficit.

III PATHOPHYSIOLOGY

A **Cerebral edema**   The brain reacts to insults by developing edema. **Acute edema** causes more deterioration in neurologic function than does **chronic edema.** The **rate of edema formation** is directly proportional to the neurologic deficits.

1. **Types of cerebral edema**
   a. **Cytotoxic edema** is a result of depletion of neuronal glucose and oxygen stores. It is most commonly seen after cerebral infarction and may occur in association with Reye's syndrome. The blood–brain barrier is preserved.

b. **Vasogenic edema** (also called extracellular white matter edema) results from a breakdown of the blood–brain barrier and leakage of plasma into the extracellular spaces. This is the **most common type of edema seen clinically** and may be caused by trauma, brain tumor, infection, surgery, and systemic hypertonicity, such as that due to use of mannitol.

2. **Mechanisms by which edema alters neuronal and axonal function** include:
   a. Ischemia that occurs as increased intracranial pressure (ICP) compromises cerebral perfusion
   b. Decreased oxygen diffusion
   c. Lipid peroxidation in membranes

B ICP

1. The **skull,** a rigid box with a volume of approximately 1900 mL, harbors three major components:
   a. Approximately 85% is **brain** (5% is extracellular fluid, 45% is glial tissue, and 35% is neuronal tissue).
   b. Approximately 7% is **blood.**
   c. Approximately 7% is **CSF.**

2. **Monro-Kellie hypothesis.** Under normal conditions, these three components and the intracranial volume are in equilibrium, yielding normal ICP.
   a. To maintain a normal ICP, a change in one component must be offset by **compensatory changes** in the others.
   b. The **rate of volume change** is of great clinical significance.
      (1) A slow-growing tumor (e.g., a meningioma) can become quite large before there is any evidence of a change in ICP or in neurologic function.
      (2) A small but acute mass lesion (e.g., an acute epidural or subdural hematoma [SDH]) can cause a tremendous increase in ICP and severe neurologic deficits.

3. The **relationship between ICP and intracranial volume** is described by an exponential curve with an initial flat portion and a later steep portion (Fig. 27-1).
   a. Beyond a certain point (i.e., beyond the end of the flat portion of the curve), a slight increase in intracranial volume produces a very large increase in ICP (as evidenced by the steep portion of the curve).
   b. Equilibrium is maintained mainly by CSF buffering. With continued volume changes, CSF buffering becomes exhausted, and the elastic properties of the brain substance and the blood vessels play the major buffering role (represented by the steep portion of the pressure–volume curve in Fig. 27-1).
   c. The **upper limit** of normal ICP is considered to be **15 mm Hg.**

4. **Symptoms and signs of increased ICP (intracranial hypertension)** include:
   a. Headache
   b. Nausea

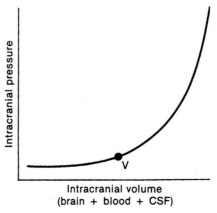

FIGURE 27-1 The pressure-volume relationship within the intracranial space can be represented by a pressure-volume curve. The ICP stays within normal limits until a critical volume (*V*) is reached, above which the pressure increases steeply. CSF, cerebrospinal fluid.

    c. Vomiting

    d. Clouding of mentation

    e. Papilledema

    f. Paralysis of upward gaze (Parinaud's syndrome)

    g. Sixth nerve palsy

    h. Bulging fontanelles and splitting sutures (in infants)

5. Measurement of ICP

    a. In clinical practice, ICP may be measured by ventriculostomy, intraparenchymal monitoring device, or subarachnoid bolt.

    b. An estimate of ICP may also be made by lumbar puncture in the absence of space-occupying intracranial lesions.

    c. Whereas intraparenchymal and subarachnoid bolt monitoring produce continuous ICP data, ventriculostomy monitoring produces both a continuous record of ICP *and* the therapeutic option of removing CSF to reduce ICP.

C **Herniation**   When all compensatory mechanisms have been exhausted and the ICP continues to increase, the brain "herniates" or shifts toward the low-pressure compartment (the falx and the tentorium divide the interior of the skull into compartments). Various **herniation syndromes** are recognized.

    1. Subfalcine herniation is a displacement from one supratentorial compartment to another underneath the falx. It may lead to loss of function in the opposite leg, loss of bladder control, or both.

    2. Transtentorial (uncal) herniation

        a. This is the **most common type of brain herniation seen clinically** and occurs when the medial temporal lobe of one or both hemispheres is forced down over the edge of the tentorium.

        b. Uncal herniation may occur as a result of diffuse brain swelling or of a supratentorial mass lesion.

        c. **Neurologic signs** are:

            (1) Progressive deterioration of consciousness

            (2) Ipsilateral pupillary dilatation from oculomotor nerve compression by the herniating gyri

            (3) Contralateral hemiparesis as a result of compression of the cerebral peduncles

        d. **Hemiparesis** is ipsilateral in 50% of the cases, whereas pupillary dilatation is ipsilateral in 80%. Thus, pupillary dilatation is more reliable in localizing the lesion. In 20% of the cases, the pupillary dilatation is opposite and hemiparesis is ipsilateral to the lesion—a false localizing sign known as the **Kernohan-Woltman notch phenomenon (Kernohan's notch).**

    3. Transforamen magnum herniation. The cerebellar tonsils herniate through the foramen magnum. The resulting medullary compression may elicit a Cushing's response (i.e., hypertension, bradycardia, and apnea) and ultimately leads to death.

D **Cerebral blood flow, autoregulation, and CPP**

    1. Overview (Fig. 27-2)

        a. The **average cerebral blood flow** normally ranges between **50 and 55 mL/100 g of brain tissue per minute,** with the gray matter having a higher flow (i.e., 75 mL/100 g/minute) than the white matter (25 mL/100 g/minute).

        b. The blood flow is coupled to the local metabolic demands and is highest where the density of synapses is greatest (termed **metabolic autoregulation**).

        c. The flow is directly proportional to the **mean arterial pressure** (MAP) and the vessel radius (r)(Q $\propto$ MAP $\times$ r^4, **Poiseuille's law**), and it is inversely proportional to the blood viscosity and vessel length. These factors can be manipulated to improve cerebral blood flow.

    2. Pressure autoregulation describes the observation that normally over a wide range of mean arterial pressure (50–150 mm Hg), the cerebral blood flow remains unchanged at 50 mL/100 g of brain tissue per minute (Fig. 27-2).

        a. This may change focally or globally as a result of head injury, subarachnoid hemorrhage (SAH), stroke, or a brain tumor.

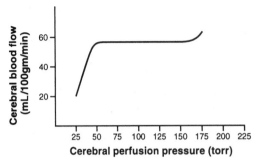

FIGURE 27-2 Cerebral blood flow versus cerebral perfusion pressure. Note that normal autoregulation that occurs for cerebral perfusion pressure is 50–150 mm Hg.

b. In the patient with intact autoregulation, ICP remains stable as blood pressure changes within the limits above.

c. However, if the ICP passively follows the arterial pressure, it is indicative of impaired autoregulation (vasoparalysis) and can often lead to irreversible and fatal cerebral edema.

d. The **cerebral perfusion pressure** (CPP) is equal to the mean arterial pressure (MAP) minus the ICP (CPP = MAP − ICP). Below 50 mm Hg, the cerebral blood flow becomes inadequate. The goal of neurosurgical intervention is to **maintain the CPP between 50 and 100 mm Hg,** particularly in patients suffering from altered autoregulation (e.g., brain trauma).

IV EVALUATING THE NEUROSURGICAL PATIENT

A Personal and family history

1. The **patient's history** is an important part of the diagnostic armamentarium.
   a. A good history may be the only clue to the diagnosis of either a transient ischemic attack or an SAH.
   b. It may help to ascertain the severity of head injury by identifying periods of anterograde and retrograde amnesia.

2. The **family history** helps to rule out congenital lesions, metabolic disorders, neurofibromatosis, Huntington's chorea, and various degenerative central nervous system (CNS) disorders.

B Physical examination

1. **Vital signs.** The vital signs are controlled by CNS mechanisms. Simple observation of blood pressure, pulse rate, and respiration can be helpful in localizing a lesion.

2. **Hypertension (Cushing's response).** Compression of the medullary centers by increased ICP results in hypertension; bradycardia; and short, shallow respirations. The Cushing's response is, however, generally considered to be a terminal response; when it is noted, irreversible neurologic changes have already taken place.

3. **Hypotension** in the neurosurgical patient may be due to loss of vascular tone secondary to loss of sympathetic control of peripheral vessels. This may be secondary to hypothalamic, medullary, or spinal cord injury (SCI).

4. **Patterns of respiration**
   a. **Lesions in the forebrain** can lead to **posthyperventilation apnea.**
      (1) In normal individuals, after a period of hyperventilation, there is a resumption of regular breathing without a delay, although there is a reduction of the tidal volume until normal carbon dioxide partial pressure (Pco_2) is restored.
      (2) Patients with **structural** or **metabolic forebrain damage** do not resume their regular breathing rhythm after hyperventilation, undergoing a period of apnea. Regular respirations are resumed after the Pco_2 returns to normal.
   b. **Lesions deep in the cerebral hemispheres** and involving the **basal ganglia** are associated with **Cheyne-Stokes respiration.**
      (1) Regular periods of hyperpnea alternating with apnea characterize this pattern.

(2) The breathing gradually rises in a smooth crescendo and then wanes in a smooth decrescendo.

c. **Lesions in the midbrain** can cause **central neurogenic hyperventilation** (deep breathing at a very fast rate) that may lead to severe **alkalosis.**

d. **Lesions in the lower pons** can cause **apneusis,** which is complete cessation of involuntary breathing, leading to respiratory arrest during sleep (**Ondine's curse**).

e. **Medullary lesions** can lead to various types of abnormal breathing patterns, which include:

(1) **Cluster breathing** (a disorderly sequence of clusters of breaths with irregular pauses)

(2) **Ataxic breathing** (Biot's breathing—periodic breathing in which apneic periods are punctuated by a few irregular deep breaths, lacking the waxing and waning pattern of Cheyne-Stokes respiration)

(3) **Cheyne-Stokes respiration** (see IV B 4 b)

(4) **Gasping** (breathing in which both deep and shallow breaths occur randomly with haphazard intervening pauses and a slow respiratory rate, which may finally lead to apnea)

f. **Kussmaul's respiration,** deep rapid breathing similar to central neurogenic hyperventilation, usually occurs as a result of diabetic or uremic acidosis.

C **Neurologic evaluation** A detailed neurologic evaluation may not be possible in some emergency situations, and a **brief examination** will have to suffice to assess the neurologic damage.

1. **The level of consciousness** should be determined first. Patients may present as:
   a. Alert, awake, and oriented
   b. Lethargic (i.e., sleepy but easily arousable)
   c. Stuporous (i.e., responsive only to noxious stimuli)
   d. Comatose (i.e., not responsive to noxious stimuli)

2. **Examination of the pupils.** The pupils are examined for their size and reaction to light, and the position and movement of the eyes are noted. A few general rules may be helpful in localizing a lesion.
   a. When a lesion in the cortex is present, the size of the pupil may be 6 mm or larger, and there may be wandering or roving eye movements.
   b. With a lesion in the **basal ganglia,** the pupils may range from 2–3 mm in size, and the eyes are deviated downward and inward.
   c. A lesion in the **midbrain** may be associated with pupils that are 4–5 mm in size (midrange), and convergent nystagmus or nystagmus retractorius may be present.
   d. A lesion in the **pons** may be associated with pinpoint pupils (1 mm) and with ocular bobbing.
   e. When a lesion in the medulla is present, the pupils may be slightly small (2 mm), and there is downbeat nystagmus.

3. **Brain stem reflexes,** such as the oculocephalic (doll's eye) reflex and the caloric (oculovestibular) responses, are checked to rule out irreversible brain stem damage.

4. **Motor examination** is then performed. In a comatose patient, it may only be possible to assess the response to painful stimuli.

5. **Sensory level determination** is important in patients with spinal cord lesions (see VI E 3).

6. **Deep tendon reflexes and plantar responses** are checked to distinguish a lower motor neuron lesion from an upper motor neuron lesion.

V   HEAD INJURIES

A **Incidence** Trauma is the leading cause of death in the United States in people between the ages of 1 and 44 years. In nearly 75% of all trauma-related fatalities, head injury contributes significantly to the outcome. Approximately 60,000 patients with severe head injuries reach a hospital alive each year; an equal number of patients die before receiving hospital care.

1. **Prevention** is the most important area of intervention in head trauma.

2. Drunk driving, as well as failure to use safety belts or motorcycle helmets, significantly contributes to the severity of head injury.

3. Care of the severely head-injured patient begins at the scene of the accident.

4. To prevent serious exacerbation of brain injury, it is essential to establish a secured airway, provide adequate ventilation, and support the circulation.

5. Hypoxia, hypercapnia, and hypotension must be corrected.

6. Hypotonic intravenous solutions (e.g., 5% dextrose in water) must be avoided because they promote an osmotic gradient between the intravascular compartment and brain interstitial space, causing traumatic cerebral edema. Colloid solutions, such as albumin and blood products, are preferred.

B **Classification**

1. **Brain injuries** occurring after trauma can be classified as:
  a. **Primary,** occurring instantaneously at the time of impact
  b. **Secondary,** resulting from a chain of events triggered by the initial injury. If not controlled, secondary injuries lead to further damage through ischemia, hypoxia, or both.

2. Primary and secondary injuries can be either:
  a. Nonhemorrhagic focal or diffuse **edema**
  b. **Hemorrhages**
    (1) **Intra-axial** (i.e., intracerebral; within the brain substance)
    (2) **Extra-axial** (i.e., extracerebral; outside the brain parenchyma, such as epidural and subdural hematomas)

C **Initial management and assessment**

1. **Immediate care** of a head trauma victim is not different from that of any other injured patient.
  a. **Priorities** (A, B, C)
    (1) **Establishment of adequate airway and ventilation** (A—airway)
    (2) **Control of hemorrhage** (B—bleeding)
    (3) **Maintenance of peripheral vascular circulation** (C—circulation)
  b. **Volume replacement** with colloids or blood products can be performed when necessary to reduce the risk that cerebral edema will develop or worsen.
  c. **Stabilization of the neck** with a hard cervical collar is necessary in all patients.
    (1) 10% of patients with severe head injuries have **associated spinal cord injuries;** thus, all patients with head injuries should be transported using SCI precautions.
    (2) **Precautions** include immobilization of the entire spine on a full spine board and use of a cervical collar.
  d. **Blood is drawn** for typing and cross matching and for other laboratory studies.

2. **Initial examination**
  a. **The type and magnitude of the injuries** can be determined by information gleaned from the initial examination. For example:
    (1) A **closed-head injury**—injury inflicted to the brain without any evidence of scalp laceration
    (2) An injury resulting from a **high-speed, nonimpact acceleration–deceleration**
    (3) **Blunt trauma** with or without a scalp laceration or contusion (all scalp lacerations should be checked manually for an underlying skull fracture)
    (4) A **penetrating wound** from a knife or a bullet (entrance and exit wounds must be sought)
  b. **Location of a fracture** can be determined by certain signs.
    (1) Fractures traversing the base of the skull (**basilar fractures**) often cause ecchymosis behind the ear (**Battle's sign**) and may be associated with otorrhea.
    (2) **Anterior basal fractures** often result in periorbital ecchymosis (**raccoon's eyes**) and subconjunctival hemorrhage and, if associated with **cribriform plate** fracture, may result in rhinorrhea.
    (3) Hematotympanum is associated with fracture of the **petrous ridge.**

3. **History.** After the initial management, and if the patient is awake, a quick history should be obtained. Severity of head injury and final outcome are directly related to the duration of unconsciousness, which the history may reveal.

4. **Neurologic evaluation.** A rapid assessment of the patient is performed.

a. The **Glasgow Coma Scale (GCS)** is now used almost universally in the assessment of the head-injury victim (see Table 21-2). Motor responses, eye responses, and verbal responses are measured.

b. The GCS **score** ranges from 3–15.

(1) The GCS score at 6 hours after trauma is a good predictor of the long-term outcome in head injury (i.e., recovery, disability, vegetative state, or death).

(2) Adult patients with a 6-hour GCS score below 7 are likely to have a poor outcome; the prognosis is much better in the pediatric population.

(3) Coma is defined as GCS score lower than 8.

c. Neurologic examinations are repeated periodically; a change of 2 or more in the GCS score is considered significant.

5. Radiographic studies

a. **Computed tomography (CT) scans** are preferable to skull radiographs in severely injured patients.

(1) **Diagnostic findings**

(a) **Hematomas** (see VII B 1–2) can be easily diagnosed because acute blood appears, relative to the brain:

(i) Hyperdense if hemoglobin >9 mg/dL

(ii) Isodense if hemoglobin = 9 mg/dL

(iii) Hypodense if hemoglobin <9 mg/dL

(b) **Epidural hematomas** appear as semilunar ("lenticular") dense collections with a convexity toward the brain.

(c) **Acute SDHs** have a concavity toward the brain and conform to the shape of the brain surface.

(d) **Cerebral edema** can be assessed by the size of the ventricles, basal subarachnoid cisterns, loss of gyral pattern, and degree of midline shift.

(2) If the CT scan is positive, the patient is taken immediately to the operating room for evacuation of hematomas or to the intensive care unit for ICP monitoring and management of brain swelling.

b. In a patient with significant neurologic deficits, **MRI brain scan** may show brain injury when a CT head scan result is normal.

(1) Locations of **shearing injuries** (white matter edema and disruption) are imaged better with MRI scan than CT scan.

(2) Diffuse shearing injuries are frequently located in the corpus callosum, subcortical white matter, thalamus, and brain stem.

c. **Radiographs** of the cervical spine are taken to rule out associated spinal injuries.

(1) The presence of cervical spine fracture or neurologic deficit referable to cervical spine is an **absolute contraindication** for removal of immobilization devices (cervical collar) or performance of flexion/extension views.

(2) **Cervical spine series** is incomplete until C-1 to T-1 levels are adequately visualized.

(3) In the absence of cervical fracture or cervical spinal cord deficit, **flexion/extension views** of the cervical spine are required to rule out ligamentous injury.

(4) In the patient who has been comatose for longer than 2 weeks, an MRI of the cervical spine can be useful to perform lateral or flexion/extension views to rule out occult ligamentous injury, disc herniation, or SCI.

D Management of increased ICP

1. Maintenance of an adequate CPP to prevent irreversible ischemic injury is the major goal of treatment of increased ICP. The patient's CPP is maintained above 50 mm Hg by manipulation of the ICP and the MAP.

2. Placement of an ICP monitor is necessary to evaluate status and ICP therapy in the unconscious patient.

a. **Criteria for placement of an ICP monitor** include one or all of the following:

(1) A **GCS score of less than 8.** In practical terms, for the intubated, unconscious patient, ICP monitoring is usually needed when the best motor response is decorticate or decerebrate posturing or flaccid.

(2) Associated systemic complications, such as severe hypotension or hypoxia

(3) CT evidence of diffuse cerebral swelling, especially with obliteration of perimesencephalic cisterns, indicating limited residual compliance and minimal tolerance to further brain swelling

b. ICP measuring devices (monitors) are of three types:

(1) Intraventricular catheter (ventriculostomy) gives the most accurate measurement and allows removal of CSF to lower the ICP in an emergency. Placement of an intraventricular catheter can be difficult in the presence of diffuse brain swelling with slitlike ventricles.

(2) Subarachnoid bolts (Richmond screw or Philly bolt) are easy to place, give accurate readings, and are associated with a low infection rate.

(3) Intraparenchymal monitors

(a) These devices are fiber-optic ICP probes and are useful when a ventriculostomy catheter cannot be placed.

(b) The intraparenchymal monitor is also useful for superficial cortical monitoring in patients with consumptive coagulopathy, thus reducing risk of hemorrhagic complication of a more deeply placed ICP monitoring probe.

3. Intracranial hypertension can be managed by a variety of methods. The following therapies can be used in sequence.

a. Elevation of the patient's head promotes venous drainage, thereby decreasing ICP.

b. Hyperventilation is used in patients with GCS score greater than 5. The cerebral vessels respond quickly to a change in the arterial Pco_2. A low Pco_2 causes vasoconstriction, thus reducing the blood component of the intracranial volume, whereas an elevated Pco_2 causes vasodilation.

(1) The Pco_2 is maintained between 22 and 28 mm Hg. Hyperventilation is not a long-term option for ICP control.

(2) If the ICP is not sufficiently lowered by hyperventilation, other therapies have to be used, such as:

(a) Hyperosmolar agents

(b) Loop diuretics

(c) Barbiturates

c. Increasing the serum osmolality (to approximately 300–310 mOsm)

(1) Hyperosmolar agents

(a) The diuretic most commonly used is **mannitol,** which is administered intravenously to adults in a bolus of 1.0 g/kg followed by infusion of 25–50 g every 4–6 hours. Its effect can be seen in **5–20 minutes.**

(b) A combination of albumin and loop diuretics (furosemide) has been shown in experimental studies to be superior to mannitol for achieving reduction of cerebral edema.

(2) Serum osmolality and electrolytes have to be measured every 6 hours.

(3) Mannitol should be held for serum osmolality greater than 310 mOsm/L, and systolic blood pressure less than 110 mm Hg.

d. Loop diuretics. Furosemide is the drug most commonly used and is administered intravenously. The effect of the drug is rapid.

e. Barbiturates may be used if all of the previously mentioned efforts fail to lower the ICP.

(1) An initial dose of 3 mg/kg of **sodium pentobarbital** is given intravenously, followed by a maintenance dose of 0.5–3 mg/kg/hour. The effect of the drug occurs within minutes. A burst suppression pattern on compressed spectral array electroencephalogram consisting of 3–6 bursts per minute suggests that a therapeutic response has been reached. It is not useful to monitor serum barbiturate levels.

(2) Barbiturates cause myocardial depression and loss of vascular tone, which lead to hypotension, and vasopressor agents may be necessary to elevate the MAP to maintain an adequate CPP.

(3) Although the exact mechanism of action is not known, barbiturates may act by:

(a) Decreasing cerebral blood flow

(b) Reducing the metabolic activity and nutritive demands of the brain

(c) Reducing synaptic transmission

(4) All patients undergoing barbiturate coma therapy should have a **Swan-Ganz catheter** placed to measure cardiac pressures and optimize cardiac output.

  f. Hypothermia may be used as an adjunct to other therapies. The core temperature of the body is lowered from normal to a temperature that ranges from 32°C–34¼°C. This method probably decreases the ICP by reducing cerebral metabolism.

    (1) Complications of hypothermia include cardiac depression below 32¼°C.

    (2) An increased incidence of infectious complications (e.g., pneumonia) has been reported with hypothermia therapy.

4. Consumptive coagulopathy

  a. Severe parenchymal brain injury causes release of tissue thromboplastin, which activates the extrinsic clotting pathway.

  b. Diffuse intravascular fibrinolysis ensues, completing disseminated intravascular coagulation and fibrinolysis, due to head injury.

  c. The **complete clinical syndrome** is diagnosed with extended prothrombin time (PT) and activated partial thromboplastin time (APTT) values, decreased fibrinogen level, elevated fibrin split products, and decreased platelet count.

  d. Extended PT and APTT are treated with fresh frozen plasma.

  e. Fibrinogen levels below 150 mg/dL require cryoprecipitate for treatment.

  f. Platelet packs should be given to treat head-injury patients with a platelet count less than 100,000/mL if the bleeding time is extended.

  g. Post-traumatic epilepsy. Risk of post-traumatic epilepsy correlates with severity and location of underlying brain injury. Failure of cerebral perfusion can occur when seizure activity is superimposed on the injured brain.

    (1) Patients who are at risk for early post-traumatic epilepsy include those with:

      (a) Intracranial hematoma

      (b) Supratentorial depressed skull fracture

      (c) Brain injury with focal neurologic signs or post-traumatic amnesia for more than 24 hours

      (d) Combat missile wounds

    (2) Prophylaxis for patients at risk, including those who have experienced more than one seizure due to head injury and patients in the high-risk categories mentioned above, is phenytoin (1.0 g intravenously [not to exceed 50 mg/minute] or by mouth as loading dose, followed by 300 mg per day, or as needed for therapeutic serum level). Dose for children is 10 mg/kg initially, followed by a maintenance of approximately 5 mg/kg per day.

E **Management of intracerebral hematomas and cerebral contusions**

1. Intracerebral hematomas result from the tearing of small vessels in the white matter and are due to penetrating trauma or acceleration–deceleration injuries.

2. Cerebral contusions. Superficial hemorrhages most commonly occur when the anterior temporal and frontal lobes strike the rough edges of the tentorium or skull.

  a. A **coup injury** occurs when the skull strikes the brain underlying the site of impact.

  b. A **contrecoup injury** occurs directly opposite to the impact site when the brain strikes the inner table of the skull on the opposite side along the force vector. Thus, if a person were struck on the back of the head, the coup injury would be to the occipital lobe and the frontotemporal tips would sustain the contrecoup injury.

3. Surgical decompression of intracerebral hematomas and cerebral contusions may be necessary when increased ICP (caused by a mass effect from the accumulated blood and the secondary edema) becomes refractory to medical management.

F **Management of scalp injuries**

1. The **scalp** is made up of **five layers:**

S—skin

C—dense subcutaneous tissue

A—aponeurosis

L—loose areolar tissue

P—pericranium

2. The scalp is **highly vascular,** and much blood can be lost from scalp lacerations before they are sutured.
   a. The scalp wound is thoroughly cleansed, debrided, and sutured as soon as possible.
   b. Any laceration larger than 6–8 inches should be closed in the operating room.

G Management of skull fractures

1. **Classification**
   a. **Linear, stellate,** or **comminuted** describe skull fractures, depending on the complexity of the fracture line.
   b. **Depressed fractures** are those in which a portion of the vault is displaced inward.
   c. **Compound fractures** are present if the overlying scalp is lacerated.
   d. **Basilar fractures** traverse the base of the skull.

2. **Operative intervention**
   a. **Depressed skull fractures** may be associated with dural tear and underlying brain damage. Depressed skull fractures larger than 1 cm or the width of the skull in depth are usually surgically elevated.
      (1) Epilepsy is due to the immediate neuronal injury that occurs at the time of the depressed skull fracture injury.
      (2) Elevation of depressed skull fracture does not affect the incidence of post-traumatic epilepsy.
   b. **Compound fractures** require a thorough debridement and closure to prevent subsequent infection.
      (1) Multiple skull fragments (comminuted) can frequently be reapproximated to reconstruct normal skull contour by use of nylon suture or small plating techniques.
      (2) Failure to remove all bone fragments and debride underlying brain of contaminated material (e.g., skin, hair, foreign bodies) may lead to subsequent development of brain abscess.

H Management of CSF

1. Leaks of CSF, if mixed with blood, can be **diagnosed** by the **ring (halo) sign:** If drops of CSF mixed with blood are placed on gauze, a lighter halo forms around a central bloodier area.

2. Most **post-traumatic CSF fistulas** close spontaneously with conservative management, which includes elevating the head to reduce both the ICP and the CSF leakage.
   a. **Post-traumatic rhinorrhea** frequently results from a fracture of the cribriform plate, with associated dural defect.
   b. **Post-traumatic otorrhea** is associated with fracture of the mastoid air cells and associated dural tear (Fig. 27-3).
   c. More than 95% of all patients with rhinorrhea or otorrhea due to basal skull fracture and dural tear will resolve with head of bed elevation at 45 degrees.
   d. In some cases, a lumbar CSF drain is placed for continuous CSF drainage to promote fistula healing.
   e. If lumbar drainage fails, craniotomy with closure of the dural defect may be necessary to resolve the leak.
   f. It is generally advised that prophylactic antibiotics not be used in the presence of CSF fistula because selection of resistant organisms may occur, which makes it more difficult to treat CSF infection.

VI SPINAL CORD INJURY

A Epidemiology   SCI is one of the leading causes of death and disability in the first decades of life.

1. There is a 4:1 preponderance of SCI among males to females.

2. Most SCIs occur as the result of motor vehicle accidents, sports accidents, and falls.

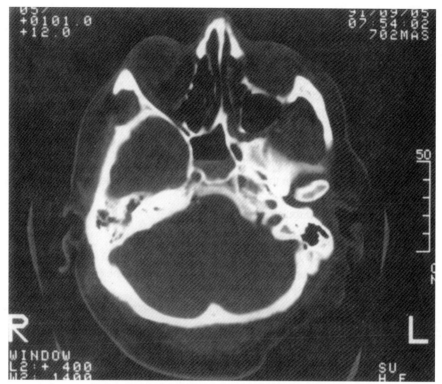

FIGURE 27-3 Basilar skull fracture with right mastoid air cell opacification due to fracture. As is typical, the mastoid fracture is not visualized on a CT scan. The air-fluid level in the sphenoid sinus suggests additional basilar skull fracture.

3. In the United States, 1 million people are hospitalized with traumatic SCI per year.

4. There are approximately 250,000 new quadriplegics and paraplegics in the United States every year.

B **Sites of SCI**   Common sites of injury to the spinal column are junctions between relatively fixed segments adjacent to relatively mobile segments, such as:

1. The cervicothoracic junction

2. The thoracolumbar junction

3. The lumbosacral junction

C The **extent of injury** to the spinal cord depends on multiple factors:

1. Speed of acceleration or deceleration

2. Hyperextension versus hyperflexion

3. Underlying abnormalities in the spinal column secondary to degenerative disease (e.g., disc disease)

4. The patient's age and associated systemic injuries

D **The aims of neurosurgical intervention**

1. **Primary** focus is on the ABCs of trauma resuscitation (see V C 1 a)
   a. SCI problems include hyperventilation secondary to SCI
   b. Hypotension secondary to neurogenic shock

2. **Additional** aims of specific neurosurgical intervention are:
   a. Restoration of bony alignment
   b. Preservation of neuronal function

E **Initial management**

1. **Immobilization of the spine** in the field before the patient is transferred to the hospital.
   a. An estimated 4%–25% of patients still suffer some improper manipulation of the spine before they arrive at a trauma center.
   b. Patients assumed to have cervical spine injury should be assumed to have more than one focus of spinal injury (i.e., use total spine precautions).
   c. Patients should be in a hard cervical collar and on a spine board.
   d. The use of transfer techniques such as log-rolling and scoop stretchers ensures that full spinal precautions are being maintained.

2. **Stabilization**
   a. A patient may have a complete SCI and not feel pain associated with a broken limb or with an internal hemorrhage.
   b. Vital signs and observation of the patient's overall hemodynamic status are very important in SCIs.
   c. Patients with high cervical or high thoracic SCIs may go into neurogenic shock secondary to interruption of the sympathetic pathways.
      (1) These patients will develop hypotension in association with bradycardia, secondary to unopposed vagal tone.
      (2) Patients often require volume resuscitation and may need pressor agents as well.
   d. **Methylprednisolone** is now shown in a national cooperative double-blind randomized study to be effective in the treatment of SCI.
      (1) Methylprednisolone in high doses should be administered shortly after the diagnosis of an SCI.
      (2) It must be administered within 8 hours of the time of SCI to be effective and must be given for 24 hours. Some data suggest that a 48-hour regimen may be beneficial if treatment is started with more than 8 hours' delay after the initial injury.
   e. Other agents currently under investigation for SCI resuscitation include G_{M1}-gangliosides, glutamate receptor inhibitors, and antioxidants.

3. **Neurologic evaluation**
   a. Information obtained from paramedics and emergency medical personnel is important to determine whether the patient ever exhibited motor function.
   b. Motor function must be assessed in all four extremities.
   c. A thorough sensory evaluation needs to be done and a determination made as to whether hemianesthesia exists.
      (1) It is important to determine whether hemianesthesia involves the face (not SCI) or just the arms and legs.
      (2) The sensory level should be measured, and a determination as to where the sensory level exists should be made rapidly.
      (3) The best way to determine a sensory level is to use a sharp pin and mark the level of a pinprick test result.
   d. **Reflexes**
      (1) It is important to make a quick determination of reflexes and to obtain truncal reflexes.
      (2) Abdominal reflexes, cremasteric reflexes, and sphincteric reflexes, such as the bulbocavernosus and anal twitch, must also be assessed.
      (3) Sacral reflexes are important because of sparing of the sacral segment of the cord. Prognosis for recovery is better if the patient exhibits sacral sparing.
   e. SCIs are classified as **complete** or **incomplete.**
      (1) **Complete SCIs** are those injuries with no motor or sensory function below the level of the injury. This is usually a dismal prognosis; 1% of patients exhibit significant recovery if the SCI remains complete for 24 hours.
      (2) **Incomplete SCIs** are important because rapid surgical intervention can help to restore function in these patients. **Examples** of incomplete SCIs include specific SCI syndromes:
         (a) **Central cord injury.** Results from a concussive blow to the cord. Deficits in the upper extremities are greater than in the lower extremities. Sensory function is usually

more affected than motor function, and peripheral musculature (e.g., the hands) is usually more severely affected than proximal musculature (e.g., the shoulders).

    (b) Anterior SCI usually involves damage to the anterior spinal artery, resulting in infarction or ischemia of the anterior two thirds of the cord. This results in significant muscle weakness. There is a loss of some spinothalamic function; the hallmark is preservation of the posterior column function with intact light touch, position sense, and vibration.

    (c) Brown-Séquard syndrome typically occurs from hemisection of the cord, which usually results from penetrating trauma to the spinal cord. The hallmark is ipsilateral loss of motor function, light touch, and vibration with a contralateral loss of pain and temperature.

  4. Radiographic studies. Any patient with an injury above the clavicle should be considered to have a cervical cord injury.

    a. Common practice in the emergency department is to obtain a lateral cervical spinal radiograph as a first assessment of spinal cord alignment. The film must permit evaluation of the C-7/T-1 junction.

    b. Evaluation of the entire cervical, thoracic, and lumbosacral spine may be required.

    c. Any patient with an SCI requires full radiographic assessment (often CT scan) through the area of abnormalities identified in spinal films.

    d. Once bony abnormalities have been identified with plain radiographs and CT scan (Fig. 27-4), an additional evaluation may be necessary. MRI is increasingly becoming the second study of choice. MRI can reveal intramedullary abnormalities (contusion or intramedullary hematoma) and extra-axial abnormalities (e.g., an epidural hematoma or ruptured intervertebral disc).

    e. In patients with contraindications to MRI (e.g., cardiac pacemaker, prosthetic metal devices), a full myelographic study of the spine may be necessary.

  5. Treatment

    a. Immobilization. The patient should not undergo any undue manipulation of the spine if an SCI is suspected.

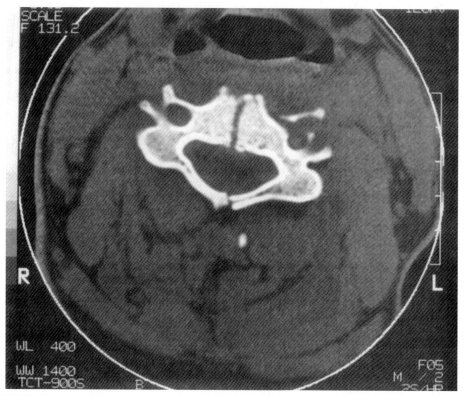

FIGURE 27-4 CT scan, axial view, C-5 level. Note the midline fracture through the C-5 body and spinous process base.

(1) The patient should be immobilized in a hard cervical collar as well as on a rigid spine board until the level of SCI has been fully revealed.

(2) If the patient requires closed reduction, traction is often successful.

(a) In the past, Gardner-Wells tongs were used almost exclusively for traction.

(b) More recently, lighter halo rings have been applied to the patient and used for traction.

(c) Patients who have highly unstable cervical cord injuries or cervical-thoracic cord injuries often will require immobilization in a halo device until definitive reduction can be accomplished.

b. **Open reduction and fixation.** In the last two decades, there has been an increasing trend toward aggressive surgical reduction and fixation for unstable vertebral injuries.

(1) Patients who undergo definitive surgical reduction and fixation can be more quickly mobilized and rehabilitated. This is translated into decreased mortality and morbidity from complications secondary to SCI.

(2) **Indications for acute surgical intervention.** Immediate surgical intervention is required in patients with incomplete SCI and in patients who exhibit progressive neurologic deterioration with myelographic evidence of a block or an MRI scan suggestive of external compression.

(3) For most SCI patients, surgery is required under more subacute conditions. These patients need extensive stabilization in the intensive care unit and then later undergo definitive reduction and fixation.

(4) For a complete SCI, common practice is not to proceed with acute surgical intervention because it has not yet been shown to be of any significant benefit versus subacute intervention.

6. **Complications of SCIs.** Patients with SCIs can suffer from several problems, such as:

a. **Hypotension** in the acute setting

b. **Ileus,** which can last 10–14 days

(1) For this reason, the patients require a nasogastric tube and will not tolerate tube feedings for an extensive period of time. Premature feeding of a patient with a cervical cord injury can result in respiratory compromise.

(2) Patients will often require extensive intravenous nutritional supplementation.

c. **Renal stones, pyelonephritis,** and **renal failure**

d. **Ectopic calcification**

e. **Deep venous thrombosis,** which can lead to pulmonary embolus.

(1) Deep venous thrombosis prophylaxis with sequential compression boots is imperative.

(2) Often, these patients are placed on a prophylactic regimen of subcutaneous heparin. Subcutaneous heparin should be given if not clearly contraindicated.

VII NEUROVASCULAR DISEASE

Neurovascular disorders requiring neurosurgical expertise usually involve intracranial hemorrhages, which generally fall into two broad categories: intra-axial and extra-axial (referring to whether the hemorrhage is within or outside of the brain itself).

A Intra-axial intracranial hemorrhages

1. **Hypertensive hemorrhages** occur within brain parenchyma, usually at the site of smaller, perforating arterioles.

a. **Sites** in descending order of frequency are basal ganglia, subcortical (temporal and frontal), cerebellum, and pons.

b. **Diagnosis.** Usually, a history of long-standing hypertension, relatively sudden onset of headache, and an examination notable for focal deficits, with or without decreased mentation or loss of consciousness, signifies a hypertensive intra-axial intracranial hemorrhage.

(1) An unenhanced CT scan is the study of choice.

(2) Blood counts and coagulation function should be checked.

c. **Treatment.** The best treatment is prevention by controlling hypertension and correcting any bleeding disorder.

(1) Most **supratentorial hemorrhages** are associated with significant deficits. Surgery is reserved only for those in reasonable clinical condition with surgically accessible lesions.

(2) **Infratentorial hemorrhages** require emergent neurosurgical evacuation before the patient loses consciousness to ensure a reasonable neurologic salvage.

2. **Vascular malformations** usually come to clinical attention because of intraparenchymal hemorrhage, which can often extend into the subarachnoid and intraventricular spaces.

   a. **Types** of vascular malformations:

   (1) **Arteriovenous malformations** are the most common type. They are composed of shunts between arteries and veins; usually, there is no normal brain in the arteriovenous malformation nidus.

   (2) **Telangiectasia.** Capillary tufts are separated by normal brain. This is most frequent in the pons and is unlikely to bleed.

   (3) **Cavernous angiomas** are packed sinusoidal vessels without normal brain in them. They can occur anywhere in the brain and are often multiple. Familial forms have been documented.

   (4) **Venous angioma** is an extensive venous network separated by normal brain.

   b. **Diagnosis.** Usually, there is a sudden onset of headache with focal deficit or loss of consciousness; often, photophobia and meningismus are present.

   (1) **Unenhanced CT scan** is the first study to order. If it is negative, a lumbar tap should be considered to document hemorrhage. The PT, APTT, and platelet levels should be checked prior to the lumbar tap to ensure that intraspinal hemorrhage will not be induced.

   (2) **MRI and angiography** are very helpful in delineating the site of bleeding and determining surgical accessibility.

   c. **Treatment**

   (1) The mass effect and increased ICP (which often requires ventriculostomy) should be controlled.

   (2) Any hypertension and bleeding tendency should be corrected.

   (3) The source of bleeding (e.g., MRI, MR angiography, and conventional cerebral angiography) should be identified.

   (4) Seizure activity should be controlled or treated prophylactically.

   (5) For most arteriovenous malformations, embolization with surgical removal or radiosurgical obliteration is the treatment of choice.

3. **Miscellaneous causes of intra-axial hemorrhages** can be associated with other less common etiologies of vascular malformations, such as a vascular brain tumor (e.g., renal cell carcinoma, melanoma), cerebral vasculitis, anticoagulation therapy, blood dyscrasias (e.g., thrombocytopenia, leukemia), systemic lupus erythematosus, or Sturge-Weber syndrome.

B **Extra-axial hemorrhages**

1. **Epidural hematoma** is a collection of blood between the bone and dura, usually of arterial origin, caused by laceration of the middle meningeal artery with an associated fracture of temporal bone. Less common etiologies include bleeding from the middle meningeal vein, venous sinus, or skull diploe.

   a. **Diagnosis**

   (1) Between 10% and 15% of patients present with a **lucid interval.** That is, the patient is knocked out immediately after injury (concussion effect), then quickly regains consciousness but has a headache, and then slowly loses consciousness (over minutes to hours) again as the epidural hematoma expands and creates mass effect and elevated ICP.

   (2) **Unenhanced CT** has a characteristic appearance of lenticular (or lens-shaped) high density adjacent to bone.

   b. **Treatment**

   (1) Very small epidural hematomas without evidence of significant mass effect and without clinical deficits can be followed up with serial CT scans and close clinical observation. If the hematomas do not expand or produce deficits, then they can be managed conservatively.

(2) Epidural hematomas that are associated with neurologic deficits or that produce significant mass effect must be evacuated, and the lacerated blood vessel must be identified and ligated.

2. **SDH** is a collection of acute or chronic blood that accumulates between the dura and the pia arachnoid.

    a. Usually, SDH is from disrupted **bridging veins** between the dura and the cortical surface. Often, the blood accumulates very slowly over days or even weeks after a trauma often perceived as trivial, especially in the elderly. Many times, a clot will begin lysing and become enveloped by a membrane of fibrous tissues and delicate capillaries, leading to what is called a **chronic SDH.**

    b. Diagnosis

        (1) **Acute SDH** presents as an evolving and expanding mass lesion. Often, there is deteriorating mental status with worsening focal deficits.

        (2) **Chronic SDH** is often a subtle, slow, progressive deterioration (e.g., headache, hemiparesis, hemianopsia) over weeks or months, which often presents as dementia, typically in the elderly patient. Chronic SDH is called the "great impersonator" because its clinical manifestations are legion.

        (3) CT scan is the diagnostic method of choice.

            (a) **Acute SDH** appears as a hyperdense lesion that shifts and compresses adjacent brain. It is often associated with an underlying contusion. Typically, it is not lenticular shaped; usually, the collection hugs the contour of the adjacent cerebral hemisphere.

            (b) **Chronic SDH** is present bilaterally 50% of the time. It is usually a hypodense or isodense collection associated with shift and compression. Isodense hematomas can be detected with contrast-enhanced CT scan.

    c. Treatment

        (1) **Acute SDH** with decreased mentation or focal neurologic symptoms usually requires craniotomy and surgical evacuation of the dense clot.

        (2) **Chronic SDH** can often be treated initially with burr hole drainage of the lysed, liquefied clot; reaccumulation can require craniotomy for definitive drainage or subdural peritoneal shunt.

3. **SAH** may be spontaneous (e.g., aneurysm or arteriovenous malformation). The most common cause of SAH is trauma. Usually, there is a diffuse collection of blood in the subarachnoid space, which is normally filled with CSF and bathes the cerebral vessels.

    a. Spontaneous SAH due to aneurysm rupture is usually associated with sudden onset of severe headache, often associated with nausea, vomiting, stiff neck, photophobia, decreased mentation, and a history of earlier severe so-called herald headaches (i.e., heralding a catastrophic SAH; "sentinel bleed"). Certain types of **aneurysms** are associated with specific neurologic findings.

        (1) Posterior communicating artery aneurysm is associated with third nerve palsy.

        (2) Internal carotid–ophthalmic aneurysm is associated with monocular visual field cut.

    b. Diagnosis. CT scan demonstrates nearly 90% of all SAH.

        (1) If the CT scan is **negative** and shows no mass effect, then it is safe to proceed with lumbar puncture to establish diagnosis of SAH.

        (2) If CT or lumbar puncture is **positive,** an angiogram will be needed to determine the following (Fig. 27-5):

            (a) Is there one aneurysm or more than one? Fifteen percent of patients have multiple aneurysms.

            (b) If there are multiple aneurysms, which aneurysm is the one that most likely ruptured? There appears to be a correlation between aneurysm size and risk of rupture.

            (c) What is the exact orientation of the aneurysm? How can it be approached surgically? Does it possess a "clippable" neck?

            (d) Is there an abnormality? Fifteen percent of patients do not exhibit an angiographically identifiable source of SAH.

4. **Common aneurysms. Berry aneurysms** can occur at almost any junction point of any artery or any point along a vessel that receives an unusually strong stream of arterial blood. However, there are some very common aneurysms.

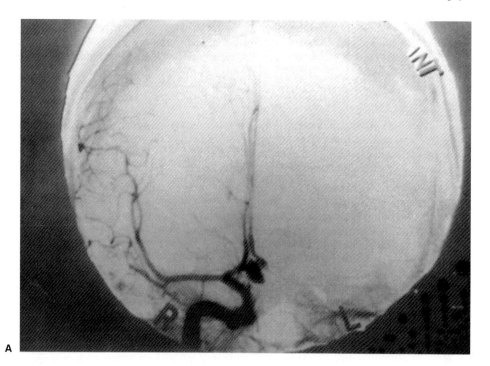

A

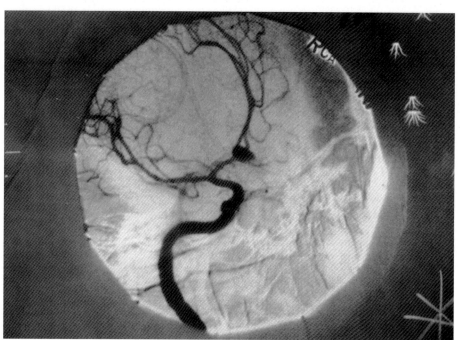

B

FIGURE 27-5 **A:** Anterior–posterior cerebral angiogram, right-sided internal carotid artery injection, demonstrating anterior communicating artery aneurysm. **B:** Oblique image, cerebral angiogram, delineating anterior communicating artery aneurysm.

    a. Internal carotid–posterior communicating artery aneurysm typically presents with third nerve palsy with a dilated ipsilateral pupil.

    b. Anterior communicating aneurysm is occasionally associated with chiasmal compression. Usually, CT scan shows a thick SAH in the frontal interhemispheric fissure.

    c. Internal carotid–ophthalmic artery aneurysm is often bilateral and is more common in female than male patients.

    d. Basilar artery aneurysms are the most frequent posterior circulation aneurysm. They are often associated with multiple cranial nerve deficits and brain stem dysfunction.

5. **Uncommon aneurysms.** There are a variety of other aneurysms besides the berry type. These aneurysms include:
   a. **Inflammatory aneurysms,** which arise secondary to infection of a cerebral artery ("mycotic aneurysm" technically refers only to fungal infection)
   b. **Atherosclerotic aneurysms,** which form ectatic or fusiform aneurysms (these seldom hemorrhage but are more likely to make their presence known by pressing on eloquent structures or by leading to thromboembolic infarcts)

C **Treatment** Surgical clipping with a small metallic clip placed around the aneurysm neck denies flow to the weakened, dilated dome of the aneurysm and is the standard treatment.

1. Interventional radiology, the obliteration of the aneurysmal sac by placement of thin metal coils by using angiographic technique, is rapidly gaining ground as the treatment of choice for aneurysms with well-defined necks. The obvious risk of the technique is vessel perforation with catastrophic consequences. However, in experienced hands, the procedure is safe and greatly simplifies patient care.

2. Some types of aneurysms in the internal carotid artery can be treated with gradual occlusion of the carotid artery in the neck to diminish the flow and induce thrombosis in the aneurysm.

3. SAH patients require extensive and often complex care in the intensive care unit to address a host of problems, such as hypertension, hyponatremia, cardiac arrhythmias, vasospasm, stroke, and hydrocephalus.

4. Inflammatory aneurysms frequently resolve with antibiotic or antifungal therapy.

D **Prognosis** The rate of bleeding from unruptured aneurysms is 2%–3% per year. Approximately one third of patients die from an SAH before they reach hospital care; another one third die during their acute hospitalization, either from rebleed before definitive clipping or from complications; and one third survive. Of the surviving one third, approximately 50% are able to return to their former lifestyle or line of work. The rest survive with impairment.

VIII TUMORS OF THE CENTRAL NERVOUS SYSTEM

A **Overview**

1. The overall incidence of brain tumors in the United States is approximately 10,000–13,000 new cases per year; 4,000 cases are spinal cord tumors.

2. CNS tumors are the most common solid tumor encountered among young patients, and they account for approximately 20% of all pediatric neoplasms.

3. **Bimodal distribution** for the frequency of brain tumors
   a. **First frequency age peak** occurs in childhood (3–10 years of age).
      (1) Among children, 50% of brain tumors occur in the posterior fossa, and 50% occur in the supratentorial compartment.
      (2) Common brain tumors occurring among children are cerebellar astrocytoma, medulloblastoma, craniopharyngioma, and brain stem glioma.
   b. **Second frequency peak** occurs in the sixth decade.
   c. Most common brain tumors occurring among **adults** are metastatic carcinoma, malignant glioma, meningioma, and pituitary adenoma.

4. **Incidence** of brain tumor according to gender
   a. There are significant genetic issues with respect to brain tumors and sex ratio. Neurofibromatosis types I and II have also been associated with chromosomal abnormalities.
   b. Most brain tumors show a preponderance among males.
      (1) **Medulloblastomas** exhibit a 5:2 male:female ratio.
      (2) **Meningiomas** reveal a 4:1 ratio favoring females over males; meningiomas also have been found to be associated with abnormalities of monosomy of chromosome 22.

B **Classification of brain tumors** The nomenclature for brain tumors is often confusing. In general, there has been an increasing trend to classify tumors based on their histologic characteristics. This is **broadly based on the cell origin.**

1. Cells derived from **astrocyte cell lines**
   a. Glial tumors (gliomas) constitute nearly 50% of brain tumors.
   b. The histology of the tumor is graded by increasing malignancy from low-grade astrocytoma to anaplastic astrocytoma to glioblastoma multiforme.
   c. Glial tumors can include oligodendrogliomas and ependymomas.
   d. Adults tend to get malignant tumors, whereas children are more prone to low-grade, midline astrocytomas in the posterior fossa.
2. **Nonglial cell tumors.** Tumors in this group include **meningiomas** (which arise from arachnoidal cells), **schwannomas** (which arise from Schwann's cells), **medulloblastomas** (which arise from primitive neuroectodermal remnants during embryologic development), **pituitary tumors** (which arise from hormonal cells in the pituitary gland), **pineal tumors** (which often arise from germ cells), and tumors arising from the blood vessels (e.g., **hemangioblastomas** and **metastatic tumors**).

C Diagnosis

1. Tumors make themselves apparent by **symptoms** that are related to several mechanisms.
   a. **Mass effect**
      (1) The brain and spinal cord are relatively intolerant of space-occupying lesions, which compete with normal tissue for space within the rigid skull or vertebral canal.
      (2) As a general principle, CNS tissues are much more tolerant of slow-growing lesions than of rapid volume change.
   b. **Eloquence**
      (1) Tumors in eloquent areas of the brain become symptomatic while relatively small as opposed to lesions in relatively "silent" areas of the brain, where the tumor becomes symptomatic first when the mass effect is great enough to affect eloquent structures at some distance.
      (2) As a general rule, the more eloquent the region in which the lesion arises, the more dramatic the patient's symptoms.
2. **CNS dysfunction** can occur because of **blood flow impairment.** Tumors can impede blood flow by several methods.
   a. Compression of normal blood vessels, depriving normal brain tissue of sufficient blood flow
   b. Tumors can produce brain dysfunction by a "steal phenomenon." As tumor metabolism increases, blood flow is diverted from normal areas of the brain, causing dysfunction.
   c. Tumors can produce metabolic impairment by growth factors and chemical messengers and interfere with normal "host" brain function.
   d. Tumors can cause seizures, either by direct mechanical irritation or by affecting normal brain metabolism through parts a, b or c above.
   e. Tumors can **obstruct CSF outflow,** which can lead to gradual enlargement of the ventricles and hydrocephalus.

D Neurologic evaluation

1. A history of either acute onset or progressive neurologic deficits should be elicited.
2. The presence of asymmetry upon examination may indicate upper motor neuron dysfunction.
3. An examination that indicates specific lobar dysfunction is highly suspicious for a focal lesion, such as a brain tumor.
4. **Additional studies** are required to pinpoint the lesion. It is important that CT and MRI scans be obtained with contrast to demonstrate disruption of the blood–brain barrier (a frequent manifestation in the vicinity of a tumor). Studies include:
   a. CT scan
   b. MRI scan
   c. Skull films
   d. Angiography
   e. PET scan

E **Specific tumors (supratentorial)**

1. **Astrocytomas** of the cerebrum are generally slow-growing, infiltrating tumors with poorly defined borders.
   a. Peak incidence is during the fourth decade of life.
   b. **Clinical presentation.** Astrocytomas often present with seizures, headaches, increased ICP, and focal neurologic deficits. CT and MRI scans show irregular nonhomogenous enhancement with a zone of edema around the tumor.
   c. **Treatment** includes:
      (1) Aggressive surgical resection with an attempt to completely resect the tumor
      (2) Radiation therapy
      (3) An additional focal radiation boost to the bed of the tumor (with brachytherapy or stereotactic radiosurgery)
      (4) Chemotherapy
   d. **Prognosis** is often related to several factors, including age of the patient, neurologic condition, and histology of the tumor.
      (1) Patients with low-grade astrocytomas have a median survival of approximately 5 years.
      (2) Patients with anaplastic astrocytomas have a median survival rate of 2 years.
      (3) Patients with glioblastomas have a median survival rate of 1 year.

2. **Ependymomas** are generally well-circumscribed tumors that occur in the vicinity of ventricles; they often metastasize through CSF pathways.
   a. **Clinical presentation** often includes increased ICP and symptoms secondary to increased ICP. MRI or CT scan shows an irregularly enhancing lesion with a well-defined border in the vicinity of the ventricle.
   b. **Treatment** includes:
      (1) Aggressive surgical resection
      (2) Radiation therapy
   c. **Prognosis.** The median survival for patients with ependymomas is 5 years.

3. **Oligodendrogliomas** are slow-growing gliomas that often have calcification in them.
   a. **Clinical presentation.** The most common presentation is seizures, and there is often a focal neurologic deficit. CT and MRI scans reveal calcified areas in nearly 40%–50% of tumors.
   b. **Treatment** includes surgical resection, with or without radiation therapy.
   c. **Prognosis.** The median survival rate is 10 years for a patient with oligodendrogliomas.

4. **Meningiomas** account for 15% of intracranial neoplasms, with a clear predilection for females. Lesions are usually adjacent to the dura with a well-defined border. Meningiomas often have variable amounts of calcium within them and are often associated with extensive edema in the adjacent brain, which is often badly compressed.
   a. **Clinical presentation** includes headache, focal neurologic deficits, and seizures. CT and MRI scans often reveal homogenous, intensely enhancing mass and well-demarcated border with normal brain.
   b. **Treatment** includes surgical excision; it can include radiation therapy. New modalities include chemotherapy for malignant meningiomas.
   c. **Prognosis** is variable, depending on factors such as location and extent of resection.

5. **Metastatic tumors.** Approximately one fifth of cancer patients will develop intracranial metastases. Metastases from lung, breast, prostate, kidney, and malignant melanomas represent the most frequent source of intracranial metastases.
   a. **Clinical presentation** includes increased ICP, obstructive hydrocephalus, focal neurologic deficit, and spontaneous intracerebral hemorrhage. CT and MRI scans often reveal well-circumscribed, enhancing masses surrounded by a ring of cerebral edema. Often, there are multiple lesions typically distributed at the junction of the gray and white matter.
   b. **Treatment** includes surgical resection if the lesion is solitary or the histology is in question. Treatment also includes steroid and whole-brain radiation therapy followed by focal radiosurgical boost.
   c. **Prognosis.** Approximately 50% of patients with a single intracranial metastasis will live for 1 year after diagnosis. Survival is increasing with more aggressive therapy, including stereotactic radiosurgery and chemotherapy.

6. **Meningiocarcinomatosis** is a special case of metastatic tumor in which the tumor spreads diffusely throughout the subarachnoid space. Typically, these patients present with evidence of meningismus and ventricular obstruction and may require shunting. Cranial nerves II, VII, and VIII are most commonly involved. Meningiocarcinomatosis is most commonly associated with leukemia, lymphoma, or breast cancer. Often, this type of tumor requires radiation therapy and intrathecal chemotherapy.

F **Specific tumors (infratentorial)**

1. **Posterior fossa tumors.** Approximately 50% of brain tumors in children are located in the posterior fossa. By contrast, only 25% of tumors in adults are in the posterior fossa.
   a. **Types.** These tumors include midline cystic cerebellar astrocytomas of the cerebellum and brain stem, medulloblastomas, ependymomas, choroid-plexus papillomas, and epidermoid tumors. **Most common** are acoustic neuromas, epidermoid cysts, meningiomas, and hemangioblastomas.
   b. **Clinical presentation.** Tumors of the posterior fossa can present with a headache secondary to ventricular obstruction. They can also present with ipsilateral ataxia and lack of coordination from lesions in the cerebellum as well as unsteady gait and truncal ataxia. In addition, loss of equilibrium and nystagmus may be present.
   c. **Treatment and prognosis** depend on tumor type and location.

2. **Medulloblastomas** are malignant tumors of the vermis and the fourth ventricle from arrest of neuroectodermal cells during embryologic development. These tumors are most frequently encountered during the first and second decades of life, with a male predominance.
   a. **Clinical presentation.** These tumors most commonly occur in the midline or lateral cerebellar hemisphere. Patients with a medulloblastoma present with cerebellar and brain stem dysfunction and increased ICP. CT and MRI scans demonstrate a nonhomogenous, enhancing mass usually adjacent to or in the fourth ventricle.
   b. **Treatment** is extensive surgical resection and radiation therapy to the site as well as the rest of the entire neuraxis to prevent CSF seeding. Radiation therapy cannot always be used in young children, and chemotherapy remains the treatment of choice after surgery.
   c. **Prognosis.** Thirty-three percent of patients survive 10 years. Survival is increased by total resection and radiation therapy.

3. **Ependymomas** arise from the floor of the fourth ventricle and are most common during childhood.
   a. **Clinical presentation.** Ependymomas usually present with obstruction of CSF pathways. There is increased ICP and disequilibrium. CT and MRI scans show a modular, multilobulated, enhancing tumor in the fourth ventricle.
   b. **Treatment.** Ependymomas are surgically resected, but often the floor of the fourth ventricle cannot be invaded to remove the tumor. Radiation therapy is usually required after removal.
   c. **Prognosis.** Median survival for patients with an ependymoma is 2.5 years.

4. **Brain stem gliomas.** These tumors occur most frequently in the first decade of life.
   a. **Clinical presentation**
      (1) Typically, this tumor presents with cranial palsies of the brain stem with gait unsteadiness and evolving myelopathy.
      (2) Hydrocephalus can occur secondary to fourth ventricular obstruction.
      (3) CT and MRI scans often demonstrate diffuse and poor enhancement of an intra-axial lesion within the brain stem.
      (4) Classic MRI appearance is sufficient for diagnosis, obviating the need for biopsy.
   b. **Treatment.** Tumors are often largely unresectable. Radiation therapy remains the mainstay of treatment.
   c. **Prognosis.** Median survival for a child with a brain stem glioma is 2 years.

5. **Cerebellar astrocytomas** have a much more benign history than astrocytomas occurring elsewhere. Like brain stem gliomas, their peak incidence is in the first decade of life, but they are generally restricted to the cerebellum. Cerebellar astrocytomas are often cystic.
   a. **Clinical presentation.** Patients typically present with cerebellar dysfunction and ipsilateral dysmetria. With progressive growth, obstructive hydrocephalus can develop. CT and MRI

scans usually reveal a multicystic or cyst-associated enhancing nodule. The nodule may be low density and is often located in the lateral cerebellar hemisphere.

  b. **Treatment and prognosis.** Tumors can be completely resected in up to 80%–90% of patients, which usually results in cure. Even patients who undergo partial resections have a median survival of 8 years.

6. **Hemangioblastomas** are the most common primary intra-axial tumor in the posterior fossa in adults.

  a. **Clinical presentation.** Patients present with cerebellar dysfunction.

    (1) **Hemangioblastomas** can be a part of von Hippel–Lindau disease with hemangioblastomas of the cerebellum and retina, in association with congenital cysts of the kidneys, pancreas, liver, and renal cell carcinoma. Approximately 10% of these patients have erythrocytosis secondary to tumor secretion of erythropoietin.

    (2) **CT and MRI scans** usually reveal a mural nodule within a cyst; the nodule is intensely enhancing.

    (3) **Angiography** reveals an intense vascular blush on this lesion.

  b. **Treatment.** Surgical resection is the treatment of choice but may be extremely difficult due to the vascularity of the tumor.

7. **Tumors of the cerebellopontile angle.** Typically, these tumors involve the cerebellopontile angle with differential involvement of cranial nerves V, VII, and VIII as well as the adjacent cerebellum. Several tumors may be involved in this location, including acoustic neuromas, meningiomas, and epidermoid cysts.

8. **Acoustic neuromas** arise from the vestibular portion of cranial nerve VIII.

  a. **Clinical presentation.** These are benign tumors that usually present with tinnitus, hearing loss, and evolving unsteadiness. Commonly, the patient first notices problems with speech discrimination followed by a gradual loss of hearing. With large tumors, there is often loss of the corneal reflex as well as facial weakness. If the tumor is quite large, it compresses the cerebellum and leads to nystagmus and gait ataxia.

  b. Enhanced CT and MRI scans often demonstrate acoustic neuroma in the internal auditory meatus. Often, the internal auditory meatus is expanded or trumpet-shaped from the lesion.

  c. **MRI** has now become the method of choice for evaluating the posterior fossa and cerebellopontile angle because these structures are better seen on MRI. With CT, bony artifacts from the petrous ridge often hide important radiographic features.

  d. **Brain stem auditory evoked potentials** and **audiometric testing** are very useful for lesions affecting the VIII nerve or a brain stem.

  e. **Treatment** involves resection or stereotactic radiosurgery.

  f. **Prognosis** is related to tumor size and extent of resection.

9. **Meningiomas** may also present in the cerebellopontile angle with precisely the same signs and symptoms as acoustic neuroma.

10. **Epidermoid cysts** also commonly occur in the cerebellopontile angle and again can present with cerebellopontile angle syndrome. Progressive dysfunction of cranial nerves V, VII, VIII, and the lower cranial nerves, along with progressive cerebellar compression, are typical.

G **Pituitary tumors**

1. **Clinical presentation.** Pituitary tumors tend to present in one of three ways.

  a. The first way is with headache and compression of the optic chiasm. Frequently, the patient presents with bitemporal hemianopsia.

  b. The second presentation is with endocrinopathy. Often, endocrinopathies consist of Cushing's syndrome (secondary to excess adrenocorticotropic hormone secretion), acromegaly (secondary to excessive growth hormone secretion), hyperprolactinema, or hypopituitarism.

  c. The third presentation is the occasional presentation of a tumor with pituitary apoplexy. This is an acute massive hemorrhage into a pituitary tumor, which may mimic the onset of a ruptured berry aneurysm. Frequently, these patients will have headache, impaired vision, extraocular muscle dysfunction, stiff neck, and endocrinopathy.

  d. In approximately 30% of the cases, the patients do not have endocrinopathy (so-called nonsecreting pituitary adenomas).

2. **Diagnostic tests**
   a. **Radioimmunoassays** are used to document the level of specific hormones in situations of endocrinopathy.
   b. **CT and MRI scans** are useful for demonstrating the erosion of the sella as well as sellar and suprasellar tumors.
   c. **Angiography** is still occasionally used in the event that there is some question about whether an intrasellar or suprasellar aneurysm may be present.
   d. **MRI** with and without contrast has now become the method of choice for diagnosis. With modern MRI techniques, flow voids associated with aneurysms are usually detectable.

3. **Treatment**
   a. Medical therapy in the form of **bromocriptine** (a dopaminergic agonist) can often be used successfully for prolactin-secreting adenomas. Bromocriptine has also proved useful for other kinds of endocrinopathies, such as in some selected patients with acromegaly.
   b. **Surgical resection** is the treatment of choice for most nonprolactin-secreting tumors and prolactinomas that are progressively symptomatic despite medical therapy. This is especially true for tumors that are impinging on the optic chiasm.
      (1) A trans-sphenoidal route can be used for small tumors with little suprasellar extension.
      (2) For tumors with extensive suprasellar mass, a frontal or pterional craniotomy may be required.
   c. **Radiation therapy** (usually in the range of 4,000–5,000 Cgy) is frequently used as an adjunct after partial surgical resection and is effective in controlling approximately 90% of pituitary adenomas that remain after surgery.

IX CONGENITAL LESIONS OF THE NERVOUS SYSTEM

A **Dysraphism** Usually, defective fusion of a raphe is associated with some findings on general physical examination. For example, examination of the back may reveal a tuft of hair, a nevus, a lipoma, abnormal blood vessels, a dimple, or a sinus tract. All of these are highly suggestive of an underlying dysraphic state.

1. **Spina bifida** results from failure of fusion of the vertebral arches.
   a. It may be totally asymptomatic and be found incidentally on spinal radiograph (spina bifida occulta), or it may be symptomatic.
   b. Spina bifida can be associated with other congenital anomalies, such as dermal sinus, diastematomyelia (splitting of the cord into halves), or neuroenteric cysts.

2. **Meningocele.** This rare lesion is a saclike posterior midline herniation of the dura mater and is usually not associated with any neurologic deficits. Repair is indicated primarily for cosmetic reasons.

3. **Myelomeningocele** is herniation of the dura mater and neural elements posteriorly as a result of incomplete closure of the spine. This lesion may be associated with hydrocephalus secondary to a Chiari malformation (i.e., an abnormally low position of the cerebellar tonsils).
   a. Surgical treatment is aimed at closure of the defect.
   b. Neurologic defects are common, and their severity is related to the location of the lesion. Patients with high lesions have a worse prognosis.

B **Hydrocephalus** literally means "water head," and the abnormality may be congenital or acquired. It is caused by an obstruction to the flow (obstructive hydrocephalus) or reabsorption (communicating hydrocephalus) of CSF.

1. **Etiology.** The most common causes are:
   a. **Sequelae of intraventricular hemorrhage** in the premature baby
   b. **Aqueductal stenosis**
   c. **Chiari malformation**
      (1) **Type I.** The fourth ventricle is above the foramen magnum, but the upper part of the cervical cord is displaced caudally.
      (2) **Type II** (most commonly seen). There is a downward herniation of the fourth ventricle and the cerebellar tonsils.
      (3) **Types III and IV.** There is progressive caudal displacement of the cerebellar vermis, pons, and medulla below the foramen magnum.

    d. Dandy-Walker syndrome, in which there is probable agenesis of the foramina of Magendie and Luschka, resulting in the filling of the posterior fossa with a large cyst and enlargement of the lateral and third ventricles

  2. Clinical findings. Patients may present with bulging fontanelles, scalp vein dilatation, a rapidly increasing head circumference, decreased upward gaze (Parinaud's syndrome), papilledema, lethargy, irritability, nausea, ataxia, and vomiting.

  3. Treatment. A CT or MRI scan is done to confirm the diagnosis, and then a shunt is placed to divert the ventricular fluid.

    a. A **ventriculoperitoneal shunt** is most commonly used.

    b. In very small infants, the absorptive surface of the peritoneum may be inadequate, warranting the placement of a **ventriculoatrial shunt.**

    c. CSF may need to be shunted to the pleural space.

X   HERNIATED DISC SYNDROME

A   **Overview**   Intervertebral discs contain a soft fibrous center, known as the nucleus pulposus.

  1. The tough fibrous covering is called the anulus fibrosis or disc capsule.

  2. Herniated or "slipped" discs occur when the nucleus pulposus herniates through a rupture or rent in the capsule.

  3. A fragment may extrude completely, in which case it is referred to as a free fragment.

  4. A herniated disc fragment may maintain its continuity with remnants of the nucleus pulposus.

  5. Typically, the disc herniates either underneath or through the posterior longitudinal ligament. It can then come to rest either on the thecal sac, spinal cord, or, more commonly, the nerve roots.

  6. Typically, if the fragment is resting against the nerve root, it produces a recognizable radiculopathic syndrome.

B   **Cervical disc syndromes**

  1. Clinical presentation. Typically, cervical disc herniation presents initially as neck pain, which is presumably secondary to inflammation of the disc capsule and the adjacent posterior longitudinal ligament.

    a. Pain may be located between the scapula, then radiate up into the neck and head.

    b. Radicular signs and symptoms often accompany cervical disc herniation, or they develop during the subacute period.

      (1) Symptoms include pain that radiates into the arm, often in a typical distribution.

      (2) Cervical disc herniation may be associated with numbness or a dysesthetic pain and weakness as well as loss of reflexes.

    c. The **most common disc herniations** are the C-6/C-7 disc herniation and the C-5/C-6 disc herniation.

      (1) The patient may have cervical muscle spasm.

      (2) The pain may be exacerbated by flexion/extension of the neck or lateral rotation as well as by pressing on the vertex of the head.

      (3) The **disc findings** are reviewed in Table 27-1.

  2. Treatment. Patients are often treated with a conservative regimen of analgesics, nonsteroidal anti-inflammatory drugs, mild muscle relaxants, bed rest, cervical collar, and cervical traction. If conservative therapy is unsuccessful, surgical removal and decompression may be required.

    a. Central and lateral herniation. An anterior approach is used for removal of the disc and decompression of the spinal cord and nerve root.

    b. Far lateral herniation. A posterior approach is used with laminectomy and foraminotomy and a posterior surgical resection of the disc.

C   **Cervical spondylosis**

  1. Clinical presentation. With progressive degenerative arthritic changes in the spine, the neural foramen can gradually impinge on the nerve root or narrow the canal.

TABLE 27-1 Cervical Disc Syndromes

	Disc Space: C4-5 Nerve Root: C5	Disc Space: C5-6 Nerve Root: C6	Disc Space: C6-7 Nerve Root: C7	Disc Space C7-T1 Nerve Root: C8
Sensory loss	Lateral arm	Radial aspect forearm; thumb; index finger web space	Posterior arm; index finger; long finger	Ulnar two fingers; medial forearm
Motor weakness	Shoulder abductors; shoulder external/ internal rotators	Biceps; brachial radialis; supinator/pronator	C6–7 wrist extensors; elbow extensors	Finger flexors; ulnar deviator of the hand
Changes in DTRs	Biceps reflex diminished	Biceps and radial reflexes diminished	Triceps reflex diminished	Finger flexor reflex diminished

DTR, deep tendon reflex.
Adapted from Freedman AH, Wilkins RH. *Neurosurgical Management for the House Officer*, Baltimore: Williams & Wilkins; 1984.

    a. This impingement can produce a radicular symptom identical to that seen with disc herniation.

    b. Gradual narrowing of the canal can produce compression of the spinal cord with a myelopathy.

    c. Spondylitic changes in the spine are best appreciated on plain radiographs or CT scan (MRI is not as useful as it is with disc herniation because it does not show bony changes as well).

  2. Treatment. Typically, these patients are treated with an osteophytectomy and discectomy if the changes are primarily at one or two levels. If multiple-level disease is present, then cervical laminectomy is the best treatment.

D | Lumbar disc herniation

  1. Overview. As in the cervical spine, disc herniation represents extrusion of nucleus pulposus through anulus fibrosis. Typically, nerve roots exit through a neural foramen one segment below the herniated disc (e.g., L-5/S-1 disc herniation irritates the S-1 nerve root).

  2. Clinical presentation. Typically, patients have a history of back pain often brought on by trauma, such as lifting or Valsalva's maneuver. Patients often report pain exacerbated by sitting or procedures involving Valsalva's maneuver (e.g., straining or bowel movements).

  3. Physical examination often shows intense lumbosacral spasm. Frequently, a positive "straight leg raising" sign, as well as radicular signs and symptoms, are present. An overview of the physical signs is reviewed in Table 27-2.

  4. Treatment. As with cervical spine problems, patients are first treated with bed rest, analgesics, antispasmodic agents, and nonsteroidal anti-inflammatory drugs.

    a. If pain does not subside, then patients undergo further study, which can include a CT scan, an MRI scan, or a myelogram (increasingly, MRI is becoming the screening study of choice for disc herniations).

    b. Typically, if the pain is unresponsive to conservative management and bed rest, then the patient will need a discectomy through a posterior approach.

E | Lumbar spondylosis   As in the neck, osteoarthritis can produce arthropathy and narrowing of the canal.

  1. Clinical presentation. The patient describes pain that is aching in nature, exacerbated by prolonged standing or walking, and ameliorated by sitting. Most often, the patient reports pain that radiates into the buttocks and down into one or both legs.

  2. Diagnosis. This condition is usually best assessed with plain films and CT scan because it is critical to see the structures of the bones in this particular syndrome. Myelogram may be necessary in some situations to get a better assessment of exactly which nerve roots are being compressed.

  3. Treatment. Conservative therapy, including heat, analgesics, and antispasmodics, may be helpful in some cases. As the disease progresses, surgical decompression by laminectomy may be required.

TABLE 27-2 Lumbar Disc Herniation Syndrome

	Disc Space: L1-2 Nerve Root: L2	Disc Space: L2-3 Nerve Root: L3	Disc Space: L3-4 Nerve Root: L4	Disc Space: L4-5 Nerve Root: L5	Disc Space: L5-S1 Nerve Root: S1	Disc space: S1-2 Nerve Root: S2-3
Distribution of sensory loss	Anterior thigh; inguinal ligament	Anterior thigh	Anterior thigh; medial leg to the medial malleolus	Lateral leg; dorsum of foot to big toe	Lateral leg; foot to small toe; sole of foot	Buttocks; perineal region; genitalia
Motor weakness	Hip flexion; hip abduction	Hip abduction; knee extension	Knee extension; foot inversion	Foot and toe extension	Foot and toe flexion	Intrinsic muscles of the foot
Reflex changes	. . .	. . .	Decreased knee jerk	Decreased or absent knee jerk	Decreased or absent ankle jerk	Sphincteric dysfunction

Adapted from Freedman AH, Wilkins RH. *Neurosurgical Management for the House Officer*. Baltimore: Williams & Wilkins; 1984.

XI   TUMORS OF THE SPINAL CORD

A **Classification**   Tumors of the spinal cord are generally classified as being intramedullary, extramedullary, intradural, or extradural. This is based on characteristic myelographic appearances. This classification is still used for both CT- and MR-based studies.

B **Types**   Common tumors of the spinal cord include astrocytomas, ependymomas, schwannomas, neurofibromas, meningiomas, metastases, chordomas, and lipomas.

1. **Astrocytomas.** As in the brain, astrocytomas of all grades can occur in the spinal cord. Most frequently, they occur in the cervical and thoracic regions. These tumors may or may not be associated with an intramedullary cyst.

2. **Ependymomas** often occur in the cervical spine and are often associated with the syrinx. A second group of ependymomas involves the filum terminale of the lumbosacral region. In general, ependymomas tend to have their peak incidence in the first and second decades of life.

3. **Schwannomas** arise from the Schwann's cells, which are associated with the spinal nerve roots. Typically, these present as dumbbell-shaped tumors protruding throughout the neural foramen. They tend to present in the third to sixth decades of life, with radiculopathy that evolves to spinal cord compression. Often, schwannomas may be multiple as part of neurofibromatosis.

4. **Neurofibromas** have their peak frequency in the third to fifth decades of life. Their clinical presentation is nearly identical to that of schwannomas and can also be associated with neurofibromatosis.

5. **Meningiomas** most typically occur in the thoracic or, less frequently, in the cervical region. They arise in the intradural extramedullary space. As with meningiomas of the brain, they occur predominantly in females.

6. **Metastatic tumors** typically occur in the vertebral body, secondary to blood supply to this region. The most frequent primary tumors occur in the lung, breast, or prostate. These tumors tend to occur extradurally and produce extramedullary compression. In contrast, some CNS tumors produce drop metastases, where the primary lesion then spreads to the subarachnoid space in the lumbosacral region. Tumors that have a propensity to do this are medulloblastomas, ependymomas, and pineal tumors that have metastasized throughout the spinal subarachnoid space.

7. **Chordomas** originate from remnants of the notochord during embryologic development. Spinal chordomas tend to be in the sacral coccygeal region or in the clival region. These lesions are destructive to bone, and it often is very difficult to get complete resections. Intense radiation treatment is often required after resection.

8. **Lipomas** can occur in intradural or extradural locations. Intradural lipomas are usually dorsal to the lumbosacral spine and often are associated with lipomeningocele and tethering of the spinal cord with a lipoma in the filum terminale.

9. **Intramedullary lesions** typically present with a gradual evolving myelopathy and often with a partial Brown-Séquard syndrome. In contrast, extradural lesions often are associated first with a radiculopathy and then with gradual spinal cord compression and myelopathy.

C **Diagnosis** is usually established by localizing the level of lesion by neurologic examination and then proceeding with radiographic studies. These studies can include CT or MRI scans with and without gadolinium. MRI is now becoming the study of choice as a relatively quick and noninvasive way to assess the spinal canal as well as the spinal cord nerve roots. In the event that MRI is nondiagnostic, the decision can be made to proceed with standard myelography with or without a postcontrast CT scan.

D **Treatment** involves the administration of high-dose steroids to help with spinal cord compression and edema. Surgical intervention is aimed at obtaining tissue diagnosis as well as decompression and stabilization. Often, with incomplete resections of metastatic tumor, radiation therapy is helpful not only in controlling the tumor but also in palliation for pain.

XII   BRACHIAL PLEXUS INJURIES

A Brachial plexopathy

1. **Anatomy.** The brachial plexus (Fig. 27-6) is an exceedingly complex anatomical structure that involves a transition from the cervical roots (C-5/T-1) to the axilla and four main nerves:
   a. Musculocutaneous
   b. Axillary
   c. Median
   d. Ulnar

2. **Clinical presentation.** Brachial plexus injuries can occur as a result of blunt, penetrating, or neoplastic injury. Most typically, brachial plexopathy is seen in the setting of trauma where the neck is severely stretched and there is a stretch avulsion injury to the brachial plexus.

3. **Physical examination.** Examination of the brachial plexus is complex because it involves not only an evaluation of the cervical cord but also an appreciation of the different motor groups and sensory areas subserved by the different nerves. In general, weakening of the scapula and weakness of the rhomboids are looked for, as is evidence of paralysis or elevation of the ipsilateral diaphragm (injury to the C-4 nerve root or phrenic nerve) or presence of Horner's syndrome.

4. **Evaluation** includes extensive electromyography as well as nerve conduction studies. Evaluation of the brachial plexus can involve a myelogram followed by a CT scan with metrizamide or, alternatively, an MRI to evaluate the nerve roots and brachial plexus.

5. **Treatment and prognosis.** Nerve root avulsions generally have a very poor prognosis. If there is residual motor and sensory function, then the patient has an excellent chance of regaining function of the nerve root. However, if the nerve root is severed, then the patient may need a cable graft to restore function in these areas.

B **Thoracic outlet syndrome** results from occlusion of the subclavian artery or vein. Thoracic outlet syndrome usually results as an aching pain in the axilla or along the forearm that is positionally dependent. If the syndrome is allowed to progress or goes undiagnosed, then weakness can occur, primarily in the intrinsic muscles of the hand. Frequently, a supraclavicular bruit is heard on physical examination. **Treatment** involves resection of an anomalous cervical rib.

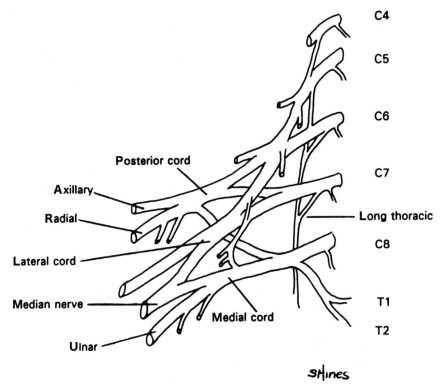

FIGURE 27-6 Simplified diagram of the brachial plexus.

chapter 28

Orthopedics

VINCENT D. PELLEGRINI, Jr. • JOHN T. RUTH • ANDREW H. BOROM

I ORTHOPEDIC PATIENT EVALUATION

A History

1. **Pain.** A thorough description of the patient's pain should be obtained, including the onset, location, duration, exacerbating factors, and character (e.g., aching, sharp, burning). What causes and alleviates the pain? Is it constant, present at rest, or only associated with activity?

2. **Mechanism of injury.** Many orthopedic complaints are related to an injury. A thorough description of the event that produced the patient's symptoms may often lead to the diagnosis. Specifically, the direction of force that acted upon a knee often gives insight into which ligaments might be injured (i.e., a patient who feels a "pop" during a twisting injury to the knee, which is followed by a large intra-articular knee effusion, often represents an acute anterior ligament rupture).

B Examination

1. **Trauma patients.** All trauma patients require a thorough palpation of all joints and bones. Specifically, the hands and feet should be inspected because fractures in these locations are often missed. The patient should always be log rolled to inspect and palpate the spine.

2. **Regional or problem-oriented complaints.** Patients with complaints about specific joints (e.g., the knee) deserve a thorough examination of that part, in addition to the joints both proximal and distal to it. The low back should also be examined because pain originating in the low back may produce symptoms more distally; this is called "referred pain."

3. **Patients with musculoskeletal tumors.** These patients deserve a complete and thorough examination to rule out the possibility of metastases.

4. **Neurovascular examination.** All orthopedic examinations should include a thorough neurovascular examination, particularly for patients who have fractures or extensive lacerations of the extremities.

C Imaging studies

1. **Plain radiographs** should include views in at least two planes and always include the joints immediately above and below the presumed area of interest. Occasionally, oblique views are necessary. These views are most useful for fracture evaluation and should afford the examiner the ability to give a thorough description of the fracture to consultants.

2. **Computed tomography (CT) scans** are useful in orthopedics to evaluate complex articular fractures as well as fractures of the spine and pelvis.

3. **Magnetic resonance imaging (MRI)** is helpful for the evaluation of meniscal tears around the knee and rotator cuff tears at the shoulder, for diagnosing and defining the extent of osteomyelitis, for evaluating avascular necrosis of the femoral head, and for determining the intraosseous and extraosseous extent of primary bone tumors or metastases. Occult fractures, not apparent on plain x-rays, such as of the scaphoid or femoral neck, are most expediently diagnosed by MRI.

4. **Bone scans** are helpful for identifying occult fractures and for localizing sites of osteomyelitis. It is important to remember that although bone scans are very sensitive, they are often not very specific.

5. Ultrasound has become popular in the evaluation of the hip in infants and children. It is also used to define and diagnose rotator cuff tears.

II TRAUMA

A Overview

1. **Orthopedic injuries** with few exceptions are **rarely acutely life threatening but can be limb threatening.** In the management of trauma patients, it is important to remember the guidelines of advanced trauma life support (**ATLS**) with strict adherence to the **ABCs** (airway, breathing, circulation; see Chapter 21).

2. The **extent of injury** to the musculoskeletal system varies according to the patient's age, the direction of the energy causing the trauma, and the magnitude of the trauma.

   a. The **patient's age** suggests the weak link in the musculoskeletal system.

   (1) **In skeletally immature patients,** the weak link is the growth plate at the ends of the long bones.

   (2) **Young but skeletally mature patients** (16–50 years of age) may be more likely to sustain ligamentous injuries because the relative strength of the mature bone exceeds the strength of the soft tissues supporting the joints.

   (3) **In late middle-aged or elderly patients** with significant osteopenia, injuries to the ligaments are uncommon. Instead, in this age group, fractures of the metaphyseal portions of long bones are prevalent (i.e., distal radius, hip). The metaphyseal area is at risk because the likelihood of osteopenia is much greater in this metabolically active area.

   b. The **direction of the trauma** may determine which structures are injured. An example is the typical knee-dash injury that occurs in motor vehicle accidents. These injuries frequently cause fractures of the patella and femur as well as posterior hip fractures or dislocations.

   c. The **magnitude of the trauma** is related to the energy imparted ($E = \frac{1}{2} mv^2$), where m = mass and v = velocity.

   (1) **High-energy injuries** (e.g., in motor vehicle accidents) tend to cause shattered or "comminuted," complex skeletal injuries, which may be open fractures.

   (2) **Low-energy injuries,** which frequently occur in sports, are more likely to cause simple, isolated injuries of ligaments, muscles, or bones.

3. **Fracture**

   a. The **radiographic appearance** of a particular fracture may give insight into the type of trauma that produced it.

   b. **Description**

   (1) **Location** may be the diaphysis (shaft), the metaphysis (juxta-articular), or through the joint surface (articular).

   (2) **Orientation** may be transverse, oblique, spiral, segmental, comminuted, or incomplete (greenstick; in the growing skeleton) (Figs. 28-1 and 28-2).

   (3) **Displacement** may be expressed in terms of bone diameters (e.g., one bone diameter of displacement = 100% displacement) in shaft fractures and in millimeters of step-off in articular fractures (e.g., tibial plateau fractures).

   (4) **Impaction** frequently occurs in the proximal humerus and may indicate stability.

   (5) **Angulation** should use the apex of the fracture as a point of reference (i.e., apex dorsal).

   (6) **Open or closed.** Open, or compound (old terminology), indicates a soft tissue injury in the region of the fracture with exposure to the external environment.

   (a) **All wounds** in the proximity of fractures should be assumed to communicate with the fracture and therefore represent open injuries until proven otherwise.

   (b) **Open fractures** are classified using the Gustilo classification (Table 28-1).

   c. **Stress fracture** implies a fracture resulting from abnormal stresses on normal bone (fatigue fracture) or normal stresses on abnormal or osteopenic bone (insufficiency fracture). Osteoporosis is a common cause of an insufficiency fracture.

   (1) **Common sites in patients with normal bone** include the tarsal bones (calcaneus), metatarsals, and tibial shaft.

   (2) **Common sites in patients with osteopenic bone** include the femoral neck, foot, pelvis, and vertebrae.

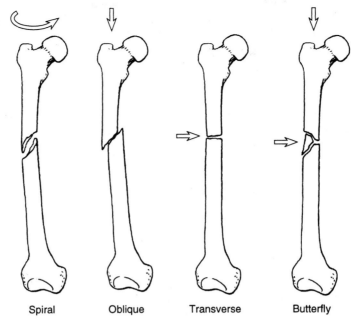

FIGURE 28-1 Fracture patterns. (Redrawn with permission from Rang M. *Children's Fractures,* 2nd ed. Philadelphia: JB Lippincott; 1983:5.)

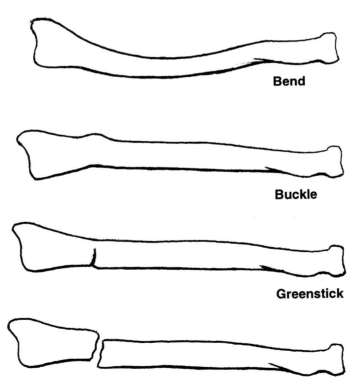

FIGURE 28-2 Fracture patterns in children. (Redrawn with permission from Rang M. *Children's Fractures,* 2nd ed. Philadelphia: JB Lippincott; 1983:2.)

TABLE 28-1   Classification of Open Fractures (Gustillo)

Grade 1: -Skin opening of 1 cm or less, quite clean; most likely from inside to outside; minimal muscle contusion; simple transverse or short oblique fractures

Grade 2: -Laceration more than 1 cm long, with extensive soft tissue damage, flaps, or avulsion; minimal to moderate crushing components; simple transverse or short oblique fractures with minimal comminution

Grade 3: -Extensive soft tissue damage including muscles, skin, and neurovascular structures; often a high-velocity injury with a severe crushing component

    3A: -Extensive soft tissue laceration, adequate bone coverage; segmental fractures, gunshot injuries

    3B: -Extensive soft tissue injury with periosteal stripping and bone exposure; usually associated with massive contamination

    3C: -Vascular injury requiring repair

Reprinted with permission from Behrens F. Fractures with soft tissue injuries. In: Browrer BD, Jupiter JB, Levine AM, Trafton PG, eds. *Skeletal Trauma* Philadelphia: WB Saunders; 1992:313.

    (3) Diagnosis
      (a) Plain radiographs are helpful if reactive healing has occurred.
      (b) Bone scans are quite sensitive but not specific.
      (c) MRI is very sensitive and has increased specificity if a linear signal change is present. The T2 image will most commonly demonstrate edema in the area of fracture.

  d. Pathologic fractures sometimes overlap with insufficiency fractures, specifically those fractures that occur in osteopenic bone. More frequently, pathologic fractures refer to a fracture occurring in a bone weakened by a tumorous condition (i.e., a primary bone malignancy, myeloma, or metastatic disease).

  e. Impending pathologic fractures refers to a lytic defect in bone, usually secondary to a metastasis, which is precariously large and weakens the bone to a worrisome degree requiring prophylactic stabilization to prevent a fracture.
    (1) This can occur with a lytic lesion greater than 2.5 cm in diameter.
    (2) Criteria include a lytic lesion that occupies 50% or more of the cortex on any radiographic view.
    (3) Also includes a lytic lesion that continues to produce pain despite radiation therapy.

B **Orthopedic urgencies** require the initiation of definitive care within 6 hours of the injury.

  1. Hip dislocations. A **reduction delayed more than 12 hours** may increase the likelihood of development of avascular necrosis of the femoral head.

  2. Open fractures
    a. Early debridement of contaminating material and devitalized tissue with stabilization has been shown to reduce the infection rate.
    b. Management
      (1) Splinting is done in the field or emergency department with removal of gross contamination and placement of sterile dressings. (Once this is done, the dressings should remain intact until the patient reaches the operating room.)
      (2) Administration of a first-generation cephalosporin (vancomycin in patients who are allergic to penicillin) should be performed in the emergency department. Use of an aminoglycoside and penicillin should be considered for patients with large wounds or for those with soil or farm contamination.
      (3) Tetanus prophylaxis is administered.
      (4) Definitive irrigation and debridement are performed in the operating room with stabilization.

  3. Penetrating injuries to joints
    a. Because of the excellent bacterial growth media provided by joint fluid, all **open-joint penetrations** require formal irrigation and debridement either via arthrotomy or arthroscopy.
    b. Common, unsuspected penetrations can occur in patients with knee-dash strikes from motor vehicle accidents.

TABLE 28-2	Common Sites and Etiologies of Compartment Syndrome
Site	**Etiology**
Calf	Tibia fractures
Forearm	Supracondylar humerus fractures
Foot	Calcaneus fracture
Thigh	Crush
Hand	Crush

    c. Intra-articular injection of 40–60 mL of sterile saline at a point distant to the laceration aids in the diagnosis because the saline will leak out through the laceration, thus confirming the intra-articular penetration.

4. Compartment syndromes

    a. Definition. A compartment syndrome involves an increase in the interstitial fluid pressure within an osseofascial compartment of sufficient magnitude to compromise the microcirculation, leading to necrosis of the muscle within the compartment and dysfunction of the nerves traversing the compartment.

    b. Sites where compartment syndromes occur are listed in Table 28-2.

    c. Diagnosis

      (1) Pain out of proportion to what would normally be expected for the injury is a diagnostic key, as is **pain with passive stretch** of the myotendinous units within the compartment.

      (2) Pain and tenseness on palpation of the compartment is also a significant diagnostic feature.

      (3) The diagnosis is **confirmed by intracompartmental pressure measurements.** A measurement of **30 mm Hg or greater** is distinctly abnormal. Inadequate tissue perfusion occurs when the intracompartmental pressure approaches 10–20 mm Hg of the diastolic blood pressure.

    d. Treatment involves surgical fascial release of all involved compartments.

5. Necrotizing fasciitis caused by group A *Streptococcus* can present as a compartment syndrome but typically is accompanied by gas production in the soft tissues. This is a rapidly ascending infection that can lead to limb loss and death if early surgical debridement is not performed.

C Orthopedic emergencies require the initiation of definitive care within 2 hours of the injury to prevent loss of life or limb.

1. Fractures and dislocations associated with vascular injury constitute **limb-threatening** injuries.

    a. Common sites include:

      (1) Distal femur

      (2) Proximal tibia

      (3) Supracondylar humerus (primarily in children)

      (4) Knee dislocations

    b. Mechanisms that can cause fractures with vascular injuries include:

      (1) Gunshot wounds

      (2) High-energy accidents (e.g., motorcycle accidents)

    c. The **diagnosis** is confirmed by:

      (1) Suspicion is based on proximity with clinical signs of vascular injury (Table 28-3).

      (2) Ankle-brachial indices less than 0.9 are indicative of a vascular injury.

      (3) Duplex Doppler ultrasonography can be used to diagnose the injury.

      (4) Formal angiography can also help to confirm the diagnosis.

      (5) A one-shot intraoperative angiogram can prove useful if the extremity is clinically ischemic with absent pulses and time does not permit a formal angiogram.

TABLE 28-3 Physical Signs of a Major Arterial Injury
Absent or comparably weak pulses
Distal cyanosis
Expanding hematoma
Pulsatile bleeding
Comparably cold extremity
Distal paralysis and paresthesias
Bleeding not controlled with direct pressure

    d. Treatment. Ideally, temporary placement of a vascular shunt followed by orthopedic stabilization of the fracture and subsequent formal vascular repair prevents disruption of formal repair by orthopedic manipulation during fracture reduction and fixation.

    e. Outcome. The amputation rate approaches 100% if warm ischemia time exceeds 6 hours.

2. Some types of pelvic ring injuries can be life threatening because of exsanguinating hemorrhage.

  a. Types

    (1) Injuries that disrupt the **sacroiliac joint** are secondary to anteroposterior compression, vertical shearing, or combined forces.

    (2) Occasionally, fractures that enter the **greater sciatic notch** can lacerate the superior gluteal artery.

  b. Diagnosis is confirmed by the following:

    (1) An initial trauma anteroposterior radiograph can show a suspicious pattern.

    (2) Pelvic instability can occur with gentle pressure over the anterior iliac crests.

  c. Management

    (1) Field and early emergency department management

      (a) Aggressive fluid resuscitation is undertaken.

      (b) A pneumatic antishock garment is applied with use of an abdominal binder.

      (c) An intra-abdominal source of hemorrhage is ruled out.

    (2) Emergent stabilization of a hemodynamically unstable patient includes:

      (a) External pelvic fixation to decrease:

        (i) Bleeding can start again from bony surfaces, and the patient can be in pain.

        (ii) Pelvic volume is decreased and, therefore, space into which bleeding can occur is decreased, thus allowing tamponade.

      (b) A pelvic angiogram is taken with embolization of bleeding vessels if external fixation and aggressive fluid replacement fail to achieve hemodynamic stabilization.

    (3) Definitive stabilization

      (a) Closed or open reduction of the sacroiliac joint, sacrum, or posterior ilium is undertaken with internal fixation.

      (b) Open reduction and internal fixation of the anterior ring or continued external fixation is achieved.

D Fractures in children

1. Overview

  a. Growth plate fractures. The growth plate is cartilaginous and, therefore, represents a weak point at the ends of the bone.

    (1) Classification. These fractures should be described using the Salter-Harris classification (Fig. 28-3).

    (2) Types. All types of growth plate fractures may be associated with growth arrest, and the parents should be advised of this.

      (a) Types 3 and 4 frequently require open reduction and fixation because they are, by definition, intra-articular fractures. These injuries cross the growth cartilage with communication of bone on both sides of the growth plate and are therefore at greatest risk of causing growth arrest.

      (b) Types 1 and 2 frequently do well with closed reduction and cast immobilization; however, some types that are very unstable may require a pin or screw fixation. Growth arrest is an unlikely sequel to these injuries.

1   **2**   **3**   **4**   **5**

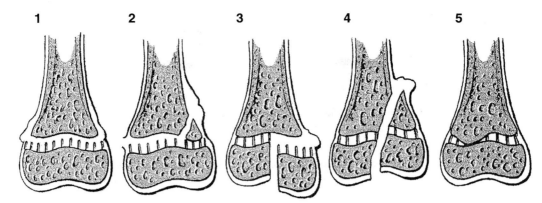

FIGURE 28-3 Salter-Harris classifications of epiphyseal fractures. (Redrawn with permission from Salter RB, Harris WR. Injuries involving the epiphyseal plate. *J Bone Joint Surg.* 1963;45A:587.)

    b. Buckle (or torus) fractures (Fig. 28-2) are incomplete fractures that occur in the metaphysis of bones adjacent to (but not involving) the growth plate.

        (1) A **common site** is the distal radius.

        (2) Treatment. Frequently, these fractures require only cast immobilization to prevent further angulation. Occasionally, a gentle closed reduction and a well-molded cast are required for more severely angulated fractures.

    c. Greenstick fractures (Fig. 28-2)

        (1) Site. Because of the flexibility and plasticity of a child's bones, some shaft fractures extend through only one side or one aspect of the cortex.

        (2) Treatment. Because of the potential for recurrent angulation despite an initial excellent closed reduction, the remaining cortex of the fractured bone should be disrupted so that the alignment of the bone can be easily obtained and maintained.

    d. Spiral fractures are unusual in children; the occurrence of a spiral fracture should always raise the question of child abuse.

        (1) A careful history obtained from the child's parents, caregiver, and siblings, as well as a complete physical examination, is important when differentiating fractures caused by accidents from those caused by child abuse.

        (2) A radiograph skeletal survey should be performed when child abuse is suspected. This usually includes anteroposterior projection of the trunk and extremities, plus anterior, posterior, and lateral views of the skull. Radiographs of the hands and feet can be requested if indicated.

        (3) Multiple fractures of varying age and stage of healing is diagnostic of child abuse. If any suspicion of abuse is present, social service/child protective consultation is mandatory.

2. Supracondylar fractures of the humerus

    a. Displaced fractures require urgent attention.

        (1) The potential for compression or entrapment of the brachial artery can lead to limb ischemia and compartment syndrome.

        (2) The potential exists for entrapment of the radial and median nerves.

    b. A **careful neurovascular examination** should be done before and after any attempts at reduction are made.

    c. Treatment. For displaced fractures, a closed (occasionally open) reduction with pin stabilization and long-arm casting is frequently the treatment of choice. If swelling is thought to be too severe, then a brief period of lateral traction followed by pinning may be indicated.

3. Fractures of both forearm bones

    a. In children, these fractures are usually managed with closed reduction and plaster immobilization. The casts must be carefully molded, and the patient must be closely observed acutely for possible compartment syndrome and to ensure that the interosseous space is preserved so that forearm rotation is maintained after healing.

b. In adolescents, an open reduction with internal fixation may be necessary if reduction is not satisfactory. Remodeling of the diaphysis is minimal after 10 years of age.

4. **Distal radius fractures**
   a. The **distal radial metaphysis** is a frequent site for buckle fractures.
   b. The **distal radial epiphyseal plate** is a frequent site for growth plate fractures. The growth plate fracture, if displaced, should have a closed reduction under anesthesia with cast immobilization.

5. **Femur fractures**
   a. **In children** between the ages of 2 and 10 years, femur fractures can most often be managed with closed reduction and plaster spica cast immobilization.
      (1) It is desirable to have 1–1.5 cm of overlap to allow for the postfracture overgrowth that frequently occurs.
      (2) If overlap exceeds this amount, then a period of traction is indicated to restore length and allow early callus formation. This is followed by spica casting.
   b. **In children 11 years and older** with an isolated femur fracture, treatment with an intramedullary rod, open plating, or external fixation is typically preferable to prolonged traction and spica casting. The physician should discuss with the parents the risks and potential benefits of all treatment options.
   c. **Regardless of the age, children who have multiple trauma or head injuries,** in which prolonged traction would interfere with nursing care or could be potentially harmful because of the child flailing in bed, should be considered as candidates for operative fracture stabilization.
      (1) **Plate or external fixation** is preferable in children between the ages of 2 and 10 years.
      (2) **Flexible intramedullary rods** may be considered in children 11 years of age and older.

6. **Supracondylar femur fractures** and fractures of the proximal tibia can be easily confused with a ligamentous knee injury during the physical examination.
   a. It is important to remember that skeletally immature individuals uncommonly have injuries to the ligaments. Rather, they frequently fracture the growth areas of the distal femur or proximal tibia, owing to the relative weakness of the junction of the growth plate with the adjacent ossifying cartilage.
   b. When a child's knee is unstable on physical examination, one should assume a periarticular growth plate injury until proven otherwise. In the setting of normal plain x-rays, stress radiographs of the knee may be helpful to ascertain the exact cause and location of the motion.

7. **Fractures of the tibia** may be open because of the subcutaneous position of the bones.
   a. These fractures can also be associated with a relatively high incidence of **compartment syndromes.**
   b. **Examination.** All patients with tibia fractures should be examined for any skin disruption, and the neurovascular status of the leg should be evaluated and documented.
   c. **Treatment.** These fractures in children are well managed with plaster immobilization. If larger open wounds are present, external fixation should be employed to allow access for wound care.

E Fractures in adults

1. **Fractures of the spine, hip, the proximal humerus, and the distal radius** at the wrist are all quite common in elderly persons with osteoporosis.
   a. In general, **distal radius fractures** can be managed with closed reduction and cast immobilization. If unstable and maintenance of satisfactory reduction is unsuccessful, internal or external fixation of the fracture may be necessary.
   b. **Proximal humerus fractures** may simply require collar and cuff immobilization. More severe fractures may require open reduction and internal fixation or prosthetic replacement. Early motion after callus development is essential to decrease shoulder stiffness.
   c. Because of the associated morbidity of bedrest and recumbency and the weight-bearing function of the **hip,** operative repair of the fracture or hemiarthroplasty is actually the conservative management and is associated with better long-term function and survival of the patient.

d. Simple osteopenic compression fractures can frequently be managed with bracing for 3–4 months. Metastatic disease should be ruled out as a cause.

2. **Humeral shaft fractures** may have an associated **radial nerve palsy.**
   a. **Generally, the palsy recovers spontaneously with immobilization.** Careful attention must be paid to the hand to prevent stiffness and contractures until the radial nerve recovers.
   b. **If the palsy develops after closed reduction,** then exploration is typically indicated to ensure that the nerve is not entrapped within the fracture site. Frequently, plate stabilization is performed at the same time.
   c. **The fracture, when isolated,** may be treated with a sling and humeral fracture brace. Early range-of-motion exercises of the shoulder and elbow and isometric exercises for the biceps and triceps are indicated as well.
   d. **The fracture in conjunction with multiple trauma,** other lower extremity fractures, or ipsilateral forearm and hand injuries frequently require intramedullary rod or plate fixation to allow use of a crutch or hand and upper extremity rehabilitation.

3. **Fractures of both forearm bones**
   a. Because of the conjoined two bone system and precise functional requirements of the forearm, these fractures require open reduction and internal fixation for optimal functional results.
   b. The consideration of compartment syndrome is important, especially in crushing injuries.

4. **Distal radius fractures**
   a. If the distal radius fracture is extra-articular and results from a relatively low-energy injury, then it can frequently be treated by closed reduction and immobilization in a well-molded, long-arm cast.
   b. If the fracture is intra-articular and results from a relatively high-energy injury (e.g., motor vehicle accident, fall from a height), then it frequently requires more aggressive treatment. Closed reduction with percutaneous pinning, external fixation, or open reduction and internal fixation may be used to obtain and maintain a satisfactory reduction.
   c. If a **distal radioulnar joint injury** is suspected, then the forearm should be immobilized in full supination.

5. **Scaphoid fractures**
   a. Wrist pain, especially in the anatomic snuff-box after a fall on an outstretched wrist, should arouse suspicion of this carpal bone injury. Healing is often delayed owing to a precarious blood supply to the bone, which is largely covered with articular cartilage.
   b. Nondisplaced fractures are treated with thumb-spica casting, whereas displaced fractures require surgical open reduction and internal fixation.

6. **Phalangeal fractures**
   a. Because of the precise, fine function of the extensor mechanism in the fingers and the problem of stiffness resulting from adherence of the tendons to the adjacent skeleton, early range-of-motion exercise of the fingers has a high priority.
   b. Percutaneous pin or plate fixation to maintain the anatomical length of the skeleton, or closed treatment by splinting with "buddy" taping of stable fractures, are acceptable methods, assuming the goal of early motion can be obtained to avoid finger contracture and dysfunction.

7. **Spinal fractures** are associated with high-energy mechanisms of injury. Automobile accidents, motorcycle accidents, and falls from heights are frequent mechanisms in spinal fractures. Associated neurologic injury must always be considered and ruled out.
   a. **General initial treatment**
      (1) **All unconscious patients** involved in motor vehicle or motorcycle accidents should be assumed to have a spinal injury until proved otherwise. Complete spinal radiographs are indicated to rule out these fractures.
      (2) All patients suspected of having a spinal injury should be immobilized on a long spine board with a cervical collar and head blocks.
      (3) A careful **neurologic examination** should be performed (including rectal examination, bulbocavernous reflex, and perirectal sensation) to distinguish between an

incomplete (i.e., some neurologic function present below the level of injury) and a complete (i.e., no function below the level of injury) neurologic injury to the spinal cord.

b. Cervical spine fractures are frequently associated with quadriplegia.

(1) If one level of injury is found, there is an increased incidence of another level of injury in the cervical spine.

(2) Cervical radiographs must include the C7-T1 junction, because as a transition zone from a mobile (cervical) to a relatively immobile (thoracic) region, it is frequently a site of injury.

c. Thoracic spine fractures

(1) When thoracic spine fractures are associated with **paraplegia,** a high-energy injury is usually implicated because of the relative stability provided in this region by the rib cage.

(2) **Simple compression fractures** may occur in elderly osteopenic patients secondary to minimal trauma (e.g., coughing).

(3) Metastatic disease can be present in patients with **thoracic spine compression fractures.**

(4) **Injuries between T1 and T10** with neurologic deficit frequently indicate a cord-level injury. **Injuries from T11-T12** may include a mixed neurologic injury consisting of conus medullaris (central) and spinal nerve roots (peripheral).

d. Lumbar spine fractures can present with a mixed neurologic injury from L1-L2 with involvement of the conus medullaris (upper motor neuron) as well as the cauda equina (lower motor neuron or root lesion). Below L2, the injury typically involves only nerve roots.

e. Treatment

(1) All patients with suspected neurologic injuries related to spinal cord injury should be started on a **steroid protocol.**

(a) **Methylprednisolone** is given as a bolus dose of 30 mg/kg body weight, followed by an infusion of 5.4 mg/kg/hour.

(b) In patients with acute spinal cord injury, this treatment protocol has been associated with improved neurologic recovery. Steroid therapy begun within the first 3 hours after an injury should continue for 23 hours. If steroids are started from 3–8 hours postinjury, they should be continued for 48 hours. If steroid therapy is not instituted in the first 8 hours, no neurologic benefit will occur.

(2) **Urgent decompression** of neural elements in patients with incomplete or progressive neural deficits or injuries at the level of the cauda equina is the optimal approach.

(3) **Spinal stabilization** with instrumentation to prevent the development or worsening of a neural deficit, and to facilitate early rehabilitation, should be performed.

(4) Patients with complete quadriplegia or paraplegia should also be considered as candidates for spinal stabilization with instrumentation on a less urgent basis to allow early rehabilitation.

8. Pelvic fractures (see II C 2)

9. Femoral shaft fractures. Early stabilization of femoral fractures has been shown to decrease pulmonary complications and to shorten intensive care unit stays in the multiply injured patient.

a. The most universally accepted method of stabilization is placement of a statically interlocked **intramedullary rod.**

b. Traction is indicated on a short-term basis if the patient is considered to be too critically ill for surgery (e.g., severe coagulopathy, marked elevation of intracranial pressure). Formal stabilization should be performed as soon as the patient's condition is stable.

c. Intramedullary stabilization is the treatment of choice for isolated femoral shaft fractures. This is due to a relatively low complication rate and superior functional outcome when compared with traction followed by cast bracing.

10. Tibial fractures frequently may be **open** and can be associated with **compartment syndromes.** These two associated problems must be anticipated and managed appropriately.

a. Isolated fractures of the tibia are generally best managed with plaster immobilization and early weight bearing. Early return to function may be facilitated by intramedullary nailing of the tibial shaft fracture.

b. Patients with multiple injuries, **open tibial fractures,** and some fracture patterns known to be associated with the development of unacceptable shortening or malalignment should be considered candidates for intramedullary rods or external fixation. Plate fixation with an open tibial fracture has limited indication because of the further stripping of crucial blood supply typically necessary to place the plate.

11. **Ankle fractures** may involve the distal fibula, lateral malleolus, or medial malleolus.
    a. **Distal fibula or lateral malleolus.** When significant displacement of the distal fibula with widening of the mortise is found on the initial radiographs, open reduction and internal fixation is most commonly indicated to provide stability to the ankle mortise.
    b. **Fractures of the medial malleolus in association with fractures of the distal fibula** may indicate ankle instability resulting from a more violent mechanism of injury. Large, displaced fragments of the medial malleolus are an indication for open reduction and internal fixation to prevent the development of nonunion and to restore the articular surface.
    c. **Spiral fractures of the proximal fibula** require a clinical and radiographic evaluation of the ankle joint. A **Maisonneuve fracture** implies disruption of the medial ankle (fracture or deltoid ligament tear), the intervening syndesmotic ligaments between the distal tibia and fibula, and proximal fibula fracture.

F **Dislocations**

1. **Shoulder**
   a. **Presentation.** Dislocations of the **glenohumeral joint** are especially common in young adults. These dislocations frequently recur in patients under the age of 40. In first-time dislocations that occur after 40 years of age, a tear of the rotator cuff should be suspected.
   b. **Management.** Shoulder dislocations are also **associated with axillary nerve palsy.** The neurologic examination should test for:
      (1) Sensation over the deltoid muscle
      (2) Active firing of the deltoid muscle

2. **Hip**
   a. **Presentation.** Dislocations of the hip occur in high-velocity injuries, especially automobile accidents. They are associated with fractures of the ipsilateral femur and patella and with contralateral hip fractures or dislocations.
   b. **Management.** Hip dislocations require prompt reduction to reduce the risk of **avascular necrosis** resulting from concomitant injury to the blood supply to the femoral head.

3. **Knee**
   a. **Presentation.** A dislocation of the knee implies severe ligamentous injury around the knee.
      (1) Ligamentous knee injuries occur most commonly in sports-related activities.
      (2) Total ligamentous disruptions and dislocations are usually the result of violent injuries and may be associated with limb-threatening neurovascular injury.
   b. **Management.** The most important consideration is the common occurrence of injuries to the **popliteal artery and vein** as well as to the **peroneal nerve.** The first step in management of a patient with a dislocated knee is to evaluate the neurovascular status of the lower extremity. Then, the ligaments and capsule around the knee are evaluated.
      (1) After a formal evaluation, a gentle closed reduction should be attempted.
      (2) **All patients with knee dislocations** deserve a formal angiographic evaluation of the femoral artery with runoff (one third will have vascular injury).

G **Musculotendinous injuries** The musculotendinous unit is most commonly disrupted by overuse but may also be disrupted by forced lengthening of the muscle.

1. **Tear of the rotator cuff**
   a. **Presentation.** Middle-aged and older patients with intermittent shoulder pain may have an episode of acute pain when the weakened tendon tears.
   b. **Management.** Most tears are small and may be treated symptomatically. However, after acute symptoms resolve, if the shoulder demonstrates poor muscular function or continued pain despite nonoperative therapy (e.g., anti-inflammatory medication, physical therapy), operative repair should be considered.

2. **Quadriceps disruptions**
   a. **Presentation.** Middle-aged and older patients, especially those with diabetes mellitus or renal disease, may acutely disrupt the quadriceps mechanism proximal to the patella.
   b. **Physical examination** shows minimal swelling and tenderness. The patient has weakness in the leg after hearing a "pop" and may be able to raise the leg if the knee is passively placed in a straight position. However, the patient is unable to initiate extension against gravity with the knee at 90 degrees of flexion.
   c. **Surgical repair** is indicated.

3. **Patellar tendon disruptions**
   a. **Presentation.** These injuries often occur in young to middle-aged athletic patients. Often, the "weekend warrior" type of athlete sustains this type of injury.
   b. A **physical examination** similar to that for a quadriceps disruption shows an inability to fully extend the knee against gravity.
   c. **Surgical repair** is indicated.

4. **Achilles tendon disruptions**
   a. **Presentation.** The patient is usually young to middle aged. Again, these injuries typically occur in the "weekend warrior" as opposed to professional athletes.
      (1) Typically, the patient feels a sharp pain or hears an audible "pop" in the posterior lower aspect of the leg. Frequently, the patient feels as if he or she has been kicked.
      (2) The patient is usually able to walk. The initial symptoms are minimal, although the patient does notice a significant decrease in plantar flexion strength.
   b. **Physical examination.** A valuable test in the diagnosis of Achilles tendon ruptures is the **Thompson test,** which is performed by squeezing the calf and observing for plantar flexion of the foot while the patient lies prone on the examination table.
      (1) This test is usually performed in comparison with the uninjured lower extremity.
      (2) If plantar flexion of the foot is greatly decreased or absent with the squeezing maneuver of the calf, then this is a positive sign of an Achilles tendon rupture.
   c. The treatment is **surgical repair** or **cast immobilization** with the ankle in plantar flexion.

5. **Acute muscle ruptures.** Any musculotendinous unit may be disrupted by forceful lengthening of the muscle. The disruption usually occurs at the musculotendinous junction but may be within the muscle belly. A typical example of a muscle belly tear is the medial head of the gastrocnemius complex in the calf. True muscular tears are best treated conservatively with immobilization or limited activity.

6. **Ankle sprains** are typically inversion injuries that involve the anterior talofibular ligament (ATFL) and less frequently the calcaneofibular ligament (CFL).
   a. **Treatment** involves rest, ice, compression, and elevation (RICE).
   b. Functional mobilization with a stirrup brace follows with weight bearing as tolerated.

III INFECTIONS

A Acute infections

1. **Osteomyelitis**
   a. **Clinical presentation.** Hematogenous osteomyelitis is common in childhood.
      (1) In the metaphysis of children's bones, there is a unique capillary venous sinusoid underneath the growth plate. Minor trauma predisposes this sinusoid to sludging and allows organisms from minor bacteremic conditions to initiate an infection.
      (2) Infection can then erupt out of the medullary space and track beneath the periosteum and cause periosteal elevation. Loss of blood supply devitalizes the bone, and the resulting necrotic bone is called a **sequestrum.** The sequestrum becomes a nidus for recurrence of infection if it is not adequately debrided. The elevated periosteum lays down extensive new bone, which is termed an **involucrum.**
      (3) If the metaphysis is intra-articular, such as in the case of the hip or shoulder, then eruption of the infection out of the medullary space can enter into the synovial cavity and result in a septic arthritis.

   b. Etiology
- **(1) Pediatric**
  - **(a)** *Staphylococcus aureus* and gram-negative rods predominate as causative organisms in **neonates.**
  - **(b)** Osteomyelitis in **young children** (i.e., 2–5 years of age) is frequently caused by *Haemophilus* species as well as by *Staphylococcus* and *Streptococcus* species.
  - **(c)** *S. aureus* is the predominant causal organism in **older children** (i.e., 5 years or older) and **adolescents.**
  - **(d)** A child with a history of minor trauma who does not improve as would normally be expected must be considered to have possibly developed osteomyelitis.
  - **(e)** A child's refusal to bear weight on an extremity demands a workup for osteomyelitis or septic arthritis.
- **(2) Adults** whose immune system is suppressed (e.g., intravenous drug users) and patients with sickle cell disease are predisposed to osteomyelitis from hematogenous spread of unusual organisms.
  - **(a)** Patients with **immunosuppression** and **intravenous drug users** are susceptible to gram-negative infections, particularly *Pseudomonas aeruginosa*
  - **(b)** In patients with **sickle cell anemia,** a particularly high incidence of *Salmonella* osteomyelitis has been observed.
  - **(c)** *Gonococcal* septic arthritis is the most common organism in adolescent, sexually active patients.

   c. Diagnosis. A careful physical examination, complete blood count, sedimentation rate, and bone scan help to confirm the diagnosis. Needle aspiration of the affected bone or joint is the definitive diagnostic test.

   d. Treatment includes appropriate intravenous antibiotics and surgical drainage. Initial antibiotic treatment should be selected to cover the most likely causes of organisms and should always include coverage for *Staphylococcus.*

2. Septic arthritis
- **a. Etiology**
  - **(1) Spontaneous joint infections** can occur in **children or adults** by the hematogenous spread of similar organisms that cause osteomyelitis.
  - **(2) Joint disease,** as well as immunosuppression such as occurs in rheumatoid arthritis, can predispose the patient to these joint infections.
- **b. Physical examination** demonstrates exquisite tenderness, effusion, and severe pain with minimal motion of the joint.
- **c. Diagnosis** is confirmed by needle aspiration of the joint with synovial fluid analysis demonstrating a markedly elevated white blood cell count with predominance of polymorphonuclear leukocytes. Synovial fluid white blood cells are greater than 50,000 with more than 90% polymorphonuclear leukocytes. The differential diagnosis includes rheumatoid arthritis and gout. A comparison of the synovial fluid analysis of septic arthritis with other types of arthritides is shown in Table 28-4.
- **d. Treatment** includes surgical decompression of the joint (either open or arthroscopic) and appropriate intravenous antibiotic therapy.
- **e. Antibiotic therapy** should not be instituted before obtaining adequate specimens for a Gram stain, culture, and sensitivity. **Penetrating wounds** that reach a bone or joint can lead to infection. A common example of this is nail puncture wounds to the **sole of the foot.** *Pseudomonas* osteomyelitis has been reported frequently when the nail puncture wound has occurred through an athletic-type shoe.

B **Chronic osteomyelitis**

1. Etiology. Chronic osteomyelitis is uncommon; however, it is seen in patients who have had severe open fractures, in immunosuppressed patients, and in patients with pressure ulcerations secondary to paraplegia.

2. Clinical presentation. Osteomyelitis involving the bony cortex is a particularly difficult problem. Cortical bone has minimal vascularity and is even less well vascularized in the face of

TABLE 28-4   Examination of the Synovial Fluid

	Normal	Group I Noninflammatory	Group II Inflammatory	Group III Septic
Gross appearance	Transparent, clear	Transparent, yellow	Opaque or translucent, yellow	Opaque, yellow to green
Viscosity	High	High	Low	Variable
White cells/mm³	<200	<2,000	5,000–75,000	>50,000, often >100,000
Polymorphonuclear leukocytes	<25%	<50%	>50%, <90%	>95%
Culture	Negative	Negative	Negative	Often positive
Glucose (mg/dL)	Almost equal to blood	Almost equal to blood	>25, lower than blood	>50, lower than blood
Associated conditions	—	Degenerative joint disease	Rheumatoid arthritis	Bacterial infections
		Trauma[a]	Connective tissue diseases (SLE, PSS, DM/PM)	Compromised immunity (disease or medication related)
		Neuropathic arthropathy[a]	Ankylosing spondylitis	Other joint disease
		Hypertrophic osteoarthropathy[b]	Other seronegative spodylo-arthropathies (psoriatic arthritis, Reiter's syndrome, arthritis of chronic inflammatory bowel disease)	
		Pigmented villonodular synovitis[a]		
		SLE[b]	Crystal-induced synovitis (gout or pseudogout)	
		Acute rheumatic fever[b]	Acute rheumatic fever	
		Erythema nodosum		

[a]May be hemorrhagic
[b]Group I or II

SLE, systemic lupus erythematosus; PSS, progressive systemic sclerosis; DM/PM, dermatomyositis/polymyositis.

Reprinted with permission from Rodnan GP, Schumacher HR. Examination of synovial fluid. In: *Primer on Rheumatic Diseases*, 8th ed. Atlanta: Atlanta Arthritis Foundation; 1983:187.

osteomyelitis. Therefore, white blood cells, as well as antibiotics, have only limited access to the site of infection.

3. **Early treatment.** Attempts to cure chronic osteomyelitis involve the removal of foreign material, including a thorough debridement of infected nonviable bone (sequestrum), open wound care, and a prolonged course of intravenous antibiotics.

4. **Late treatment.** After all devascularized bone and soft tissue have been removed, and once a stable wound base has been established, the overlying soft tissue and bone defect need to be addressed.
   a. **The bone defect can be packed with antibiotic-impregnated beads** (frequently, tobramycin or commercially available gentamicin beads) followed by rotational or free vascularized tissue coverage. Later, the flap can be elevated; the beads can be removed; and massive cancellous autografting can be performed.
   b. Use of a **ring external fixator,** such as the **Ilizarov device,** may be used to transport bone to fill defects. Occasionally, the wounds can be left open during transport, and they will close spontaneously once the defect is closed.
   c. Use of **vascularized bone grafts,** such as the free vascularized fibula or fibular transposition graft, is an option for large bone defects.

IV TUMORS

A **Primary bone tumors**

1. **Overview**
   a. **Clinical presentation.** The patient with a neoplastic bone lesion presents with pain, swelling, or occasionally, a pathologic fracture induced by minimal trauma. This is true for bony metastases as well as for benign and malignant *primary* tumors of bone.
   b. **Diagnosis.** In addition to differentiating a primary tumor from a metastatic lesion of bone, some metabolic processes, such as hyperparathyroidism and infection, must be carefully considered.
      (1) **Physical examination** demonstrates the tumor mass, allowing the selection of appropriate radiographs.
      (2) **Plain radiographs** alone often suggest the etiology and nature of the bone lesion based on its location, appearance, and the response of the surrounding normal bone (Fig. 28-4).
         (a) **Malignancy** can be expected if the films show:
            (i) A large tumor
            (ii) Aggressive destruction of bone
            (iii) Ineffective reaction of the bone to the tumor
            (iv) Extension of the tumor into soft tissue
         (b) **Benign** lesions can be expected if the films show:
            (i) A small, well-circumscribed lytic lesion
            (ii) A thick, sclerotic rim of reactive adjacent bone
            (iii) No extension into soft tissue
      (3) **Workup.** If there is any question whatsoever that the tumor is malignant, a careful workup must be performed before the biopsy. An incomplete workup or a poorly planned biopsy may prove fatal for the patient or result in loss of limb.
         (a) An **appropriate workup** includes a **CT scan and MRI** of the involved extremity to stage the tumor and delineate its extent and anatomic relationships. A **technetium-99m (^{99m}Tc) scan** is helpful in determining metastatic involvement of distant parts of the skeleton.
         (b) If **malignancy** is suspected, then a **CT scan of the chest** is important to rule out pulmonary metastases.
         (c) A **biopsy** should be performed only after staging has been completed. The biopsy should be carefully planned so that the biopsy incision can be excised with a definitive surgical resection. The biopsy is best planned and performed by the surgeon who will ultimately carry out the definitive surgical procedure.

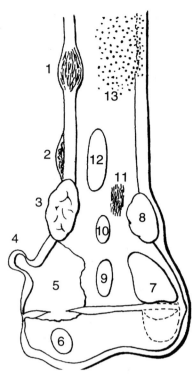

FIGURE 28-4 Schematic of the distal femur. Numbered sites represent tumor locations: **(1)** cortical fibrous dysplasia and adamantinoma; **(2)** osteoid osteoma; **(3)** chondromyxoid fibroma; **(4)** osteochondroma; **(5)** osteosarcoma; **(6)** chondroblastoma; **(7)** giant cell tumor; **(8)** nonossifying fibroma; **(9)** enchondroma or chondrosarcoma; **(10)** bone cyst or osteoblastoma; **(11)** fibrosarcoma or malignant fibrous histiocytoma; **(12)** fibrous dysplasia; and **(13)** Ewing's sarcoma or other small round tumors. (Redrawn with permission from Moser RP, Madewell JE. An approach to primary bone tumors. *Radiol Clin North Am.* 1987;25[6]:1079–1080.)

    (i) All biopsy incisions should be longitudinal on the limbs.
    (ii) Biopsy incisions should be made through a muscle belly to avoid contaminating intermuscular planes.
    (iii) Biopsy incisions should be directed away from neurovascular structures.
    (iv) Incisions should be directed through structures that can be safely and successfully resected to leave a functional limb if radical excision is later indicated.

  c. Treatment
   (1) Surgical treatment continues to be the mainstay of management for both benign and malignant tumors of the extremities. The **surgical margin** varies significantly with the aggressiveness of the lesion.
    (a) Benign tumors can be adequately treated by intralesional or intracapsular excision of the tumor with or without chemical cautery, electrocautery, or cryotherapy and with or without bone grafting of the defect.
    (b) Malignant tumors require at least a 2-cm margin.
    (c) Metastases. One or two isolated pulmonary metastases of sarcoma (especially osteosarcoma or chondrosarcoma) should be considered for surgical resection, because the literature shows that this occasionally results in a cure and certainly a prolonged life span in these patients.
   (2) Adjuvant therapy for malignant tumors
    (a) Radiation therapy
     (i) Some tumors (e.g., Ewing's tumors) are very sensitive to radiotherapy.
     (ii) Some protocols include radiation therapy initially, but in general, radiation therapy is not an important part of the protocol.
    (b) Chemotherapy, like radiation therapy, may have an important role as adjunctive therapy in anticipation of limb-sparing procedures.

      (i) Ewing's tumors are well known to be very sensitive to various chemotherapeutic regimens.

      (ii) Osteosarcoma appears to be sensitive to some chemotherapeutic agents, and work is under way to delineate the benefits, because chemotherapy may facilitate limb salvage.

2. Types of primary bone tumors

a. Tumors of bone cell origin

(1) Benign osteoid osteoma is a painful lesion that commonly involves the femur or the tibia.

    (a) Epidemiology. The tumor occurs in adolescents, and more than 50% of the tumors present in patients aged 10–20 years.

    (b) Histology. The lesions are benign and are not prone to malignant degeneration. Pathologic examination demonstrates a nidus of disorganized, dense, calcified osteoid tissue, which is histologically benign.

    (c) Treatment

      (i) Typically, aspirin offers excellent relief.

      (ii) Surgical resection or stereotactical ablation is indicated for lesions that are persistently painful. A bone graft may be necessary.

(2) Osteoblastoma is a benign, rare, painful lesion.

    (a) Epidemiology. This lesion occurs most often in the second decade of life and has a predilection for the posterior elements of the spine.

    (b) Histology. Osteoblastoma appears very similar to osteoid osteoma; one distinguishing feature is its size. An osteoblastoma is defined as a benign bone-forming lesion greater than 2 cm.

    (c) Treatment. Osteoblastomas are cured by surgical excision, if symptoms warrant. Bone grafting may be necessary.

(3) Osteosarcoma

    (a) Epidemiology. More than 60% of patients with these tumors are 10–20 years of age.

    (b) Clinical presentation

      (i) At least 60% of osteosarcomas occur about the knee at either the distal femur or the proximal tibia.

      (ii) Typically, the patient presents with pain and tumefaction.

      (iii) Radiographically, the lesion is commonly lytic, but it may be a characteristically blastic lesion of the bone and produce a classic **sunburst** appearance. An MRI scan and a CT scan show that the lesion is ill-defined with soft tissue extension.

    (c) Histology. Histologically, the tumor may be predominantly fibrogenic, chondrogenic, or osteogenic; each of the three cell types predominates in approximately equal numbers of patients. The sine qua non of osteosarcoma is production of **malignant osteoid** by the tumor stroma.

    (d) Treatment

      (i) Surgical resection is the cornerstone of management; amputation or limb salvage surgery may be required.

      (ii) Neoadjuvant chemotherapy (given before surgery) can narrow surgical margins and facilitate limb salvage. A high tumor kill rate observed in the resected specimen correlates favorably with long-term survival.

      (iii) Adjuvant chemotherapy has a beneficial effect and has increased 5-year survival rates from 10%–20% with surgery alone only to almost 60% with combined therapy.

b. Tumors originating in cartilage

(1) Enchondromas are frequently incidental findings on radiographs, although some present as pathologic fractures.

    (a) Epidemiology. The tumor occurs in patients aged 10–50 and is commonly found in the hand.

    (b) Clinical presentation

      (i) It is typically an intraosseous lytic lesion marked by characteristic "popcorn" calcifications and surrounded by reactive sclerosis.

        (ii) A tumor that appears radiographically to be an enchondroma must be suspected of being a sarcoma if the patient presents clinically with pain but no pathologic fracture.

    (c) Treatment. When an enchondroma causes a pathologic fracture, curettage and bone grafting are required, but such definitive treatment may be facilitated by first allowing the fracture to heal, especially in the small bones of the hand.

(2) Osteochondromas are benign, easily palpable tumors of bone. They are quite common.

    (a) Clinical presentation

        (i) They grow during adolescence, as does any cartilage portion of bone. If pain or growth occurs after skeletal maturity, malignant degeneration must be suspected and excisional biopsy is warranted.

        (ii) Osteochondromas may be symptomatic because of their prominence due to overlying tendon irritation or neurovascular compression.

    (b) Treatment. If symptoms warrant, osteochondromas can be excised, including the soft tissue covering and cartilage. Bone grafting is generally not necessary.

(3) Chondroblastomas are less common cartilage tumors that almost always occur within the epiphysis of long bones.

    (a) Epidemiology. More than 70% of these tumors occur during the second decade of life. They are rare if the growth plates have closed.

    (b) Clinical presentation. They are benign lesions, but a few undergo malignant degeneration.

    (c) Treatment. They frequently require excision and bone grafting.

(4) Chondromyxoid fibromas are relatively rare tumors.

    (a) Epidemiology. They usually occur in the first and second decades of life.

    (b) Clinical presentation. The tumor is a relatively large, well-defined lytic lesion with a sclerotic rim and is found in the metaphysis juxtaposed to the growth plate. It may present with pathologic fracture.

    (c) Treatment. Curettage and bone grafting may be required for treatment.

(5) Chondrosarcoma is a primary malignant tumor that occurs in adulthood and sometimes develops in pre-existing benign cartilage lesions.

    (a) Epidemiology. It occurs with an essentially constant incidence in patients from 10–70 years of age.

    (b) Clinical presentation

        (i) Typically, the tumor presents with pain and tumefaction.

        (ii) Radiographs may show a lytic lesion with or without stippled calcification. Cortical thickening and scalloping of the adjacent endosteal bone are frequently seen.

        (iii) The tumor is locally recurrent.

    (c) Treatment is surgical, and the goal is to obtain a 2-cm margin of tumorfree tissue.

c. Other primary tumors

(1) Giant cell tumors occur in the epiphyseal–metaphyseal region of long bones, especially about the knee in the femur and tibia and in the distal radius. The lesions are benign but are problematic because of their propensity to recur locally.

    (a) Epidemiology. Giant cell tumors occur in young adults and particularly in patients between the ages of 20 and 30. The patient is almost always skeletally mature.

    (b) Clinical presentation. The lesion usually extends to the subchondral plate of the joint. It is a lytic lesion and is fairly well circumscribed with some ballooning of the cortex.

    (c) Histology. The lesion is characterized histologically by the giant cells found in a benign stroma. The giant cell nuclei and the stroma nuclei are identical in appearance.

    (d) Treatment. Curettage is often accompanied by cryotherapy, phenol chemocautery, or electrocautery of the residual cavity. The lesion may be packed with methylmethacrylate bone cement, or bone grafting may be done. A recurrence usually requires wide resection of the involved bone.

(2) Unicameral bone cysts are lytic expansile lesions of bone that occur in older children in the metaphyseal region that extends to the growth plate. The proximal end of the humerus is the most common site.

(a) Clinical presentation. Typically, the patient presents with a pathologic fracture, and ultimately, the cyst may resolve in response to this trauma.

(b) Treatment. Unicameral bone cysts may be managed with intralesional steroid injections administered under radiographic control. Multiple injections may be required, which present a problem in growing children.

(3) Ewing's sarcoma is a disease of childhood and adolescence. It occurs evenly among individuals younger than 20 years of age.

(a) Clinical presentation

(i) Typically, the patient presents with significant tumefaction and pain in the involved area.

(ii) The history, physical examination, and radiographic findings mimic those of osteomyelitis.

(iii) Radiologically, the lesion is seen to be a lytic bone lesion characteristically involving the diaphysis with some periosteal reaction.

(b) Histology. Histologically, this is a tumor of small round cells, which may form pseudorosettes reminiscent of neuroblastoma. **Chromosomal translocation** t11:22 is associated with Ewing's sarcoma.

(c) Treatment. The relative roles of chemotherapy, radiation therapy, and surgical therapy are being evaluated.

(i) These tumors are sensitive to both chemotherapy and radiotherapy, and together these modalities have a significant cure rate.

(ii) However, new information suggests that patients are at risk of forming osteosarcoma in the radiated bone during early adulthood.

(4) Fibrosarcoma is a tumor that occurs in adulthood, between 20 and 70 years of age.

(a) Clinical presentation

(i) It is predominantly a lytic lesion that occurs in the femur and tibia about the knee.

(ii) It presents with pain and a radiographic appearance of a purely lytic lesion of bone.

(b) Histology. Histologic examination shows sheets of spindle cells in a herringbone pattern and with various amounts of atypism.

(c) Treatment involves wide surgical excision.

(5) Multiple myeloma

(a) Epidemiology. Whether this lesion is a primary tumor of bone or bone marrow is a matter of debate. Regardless of its classification, it is a common tumor that occurs in patients who are 30 years and older with a peak incidence at 50–60 years of age.

(b) Clinical presentation

(i) Multiple myeloma is characterized by overproduction of monoclonal immunoglobulins or immunoglobulin subchains (**Bence Jones protein**).

(ii) The initial presentation is often a pathologic fracture, frequently of the spine or long bones.

(iii) The diagnosis should be suspected when lytic lesions are found in a patient with anemia, an elevated sedimentation rate, and elevated serum calcium levels.

(c) Diagnosis

(i) The diagnosis can be made by serum or urine electrophoresis or immunophoresis in 95% of cases, but 5% of patients with myeloma are nonsecretors of M protein (immunoglobulins or Bence Jones protein).

(ii) Biopsy of the bone marrow to identify secreting and nonsecreting tumors shows plasma cells replacing the marrow. The percentage of bone marrow replacement offers some prognostic information.

(iii) Plain radiography reveals punched-out lytic lesions, with little adjacent reactive bone, that occur frequently in the spine, pelvis, proximal femur, and skull.

(iv) Bone scans are typically "cold" in the absence of pathologic fracture.

(d) Treatment is by a combination of chemotherapy and radiation therapy with palliative surgical fixation of pathologic fractures to improve the patient's quality of life.

B **Metastatic disease** Tumors metastatic to the skeleton are more common than primary musculoskeletal tumors. Primary tumors that metastasize to bone include carcinomas of the breast, lung, prostate, thyroid, and kidney, or indeed, almost any type of tumor.

1. **Diagnosis**
    a. Most bony metastatic disease presents with pain in the involved bone. Metastatic bone disease may be the initial presentation of a malignancy.
    b. **Radiographs** show most bone lesions to be lytic. With some breast tumors and most prostatic tumors, the bone lesion has a blastic appearance.
    c. **Bone scans** are helpful when a single symptomatic lytic lesion is found on initial radiographs.
        (1) If the bone scan shows multiple lesions, the likelihood of metastatic disease is high.
        (2) Bone scanning may also demonstrate a lesion that is likely to cause a fracture.
    d. **Skeletal metastases** of unknown origin are best worked up with a history and physical examination; whole-body bone scan; plain radiographs of the chest and the involved bone; and a CT scan of the chest, abdomen, and pelvis.

2. **Treatment**
    a. The treatment for most **metastatic lesions in bone** is radiation therapy. If the pain does not respond to irradiation, a pathologic fracture has probably occurred (or is about to occur) and should be surgically fixed. Pathologic fractures generally should be fixed internally, using a combination of metal implants plus methylmethacrylate bone cement to manage bone loss.
    b. **Impending pathologic fractures** (see II A 3 e)

V   ARTHRITIS

A **Classification**

1. **Degenerative joint disease**
    a. **Primary osteoarthritis** is typically seen with Heberden's nodes and asymmetric hip, knee, and spine involvement. The site of primary pathology is the articular cartilage.
    b. **Post-traumatic arthritis** of an isolated joint can occur following trauma to that joint.

2. **Rheumatoid arthritis and its variants** include the autoimmune group of inflammatory diseases in which the hyaline articular cartilage is secondarily attacked by a local invasive pannus that primarily involves the synovium.

3. **Crystal deposition diseases** include **gout** and **calcium pyrophosphate deposition disease.** These diseases usually present as an isolated hot, inflamed joint.

4. **Infectious arthritis** (see III A 2) also presents as an isolated hot, inflamed joint.
    a. This is the one form of arthritis that requires immediate emergency care.
    b. The diagnosis can be made by aspirating the joint fluid and examining it microscopically for cells, organisms, and crystals as well as by cell count and culture.

B **Nonoperative management**

1. **Pharmacologic management** is maximized by consultation with a rheumatologist.
    a. **Nonsteroidal anti-inflammatory drugs (NSAID)**
        (1) NSAIDs are especially important in rheumatoid arthritis, which requires a long-term maintenance regimen.
        (2) The crystalline and degenerative joint diseases require NSAIDs during acute flare-ups, but the natural history of these diseases is not altered by long-term management with these drugs.
    b. **Corticosteroids**
        (1) These can be used in rheumatoid arthritis when NSAIDs fail to quiet the inflammation.
            (a) They can be used systemically if multiple joint involvement or generalized disease is the problem.

(b) They can be used locally by instillation into a single joint in patients with degenerative or post-traumatic rheumatoid arthritis.

  c. **Immunosuppressants or cytotoxic agents** such as methotrexate are being used more frequently to avoid detrimental side effects of chronic steroid use and as a disease-modifying agent.

  d. **Gold and remittive agents** are indicated when the patient has not been successful with NSAIDs but are often poorly tolerated.

  e. **Anti-TNF (tumor necrosis factor) alpha** agents are a recent addition to the armamentarium in treating rheumatoid disease and have shown great promise as disease-modifying agents.

2. **Exercise and splinting** have an important place in the treatment of all forms of arthritis after the acute joint inflammation has been controlled. The exercise is designed to maintain a full range of joint motion as well as to maintain muscle strength by exercising the joint through a limited, painless arc of motion. Splinting in a functional position prevents establishment of contractures.

C **Operative management**

1. **Types of surgical procedures**
  a. **Osteotomy**
    (1) If the bone is cut and the joint is realigned, this may alter the mechanics enough to give significant, although incomplete, relief from pain.
    (2) In order for the osteotomy procedure to be successful, the disease process must not have completely destroyed the joint but must leave some remaining articular surface.
    (3) Osteotomy is designed to transfer weight bearing onto this relatively normal articular surface in the setting of noninflammatory arthritis.
    (4) Osteotomy about the hip and knee can be performed as a temporizing measure in patients too young to consider arthroplasty but who wish to preserve motion.
  b. **Arthrodesis**
    (1) In this procedure, the joint surfaces are excised and the extremity is immobilized so that the joint heals in a fixed position.
    (2) Arthrodesis is indicated for the relief of pain, especially in young individuals.
      (a) The results of arthrodesis are very durable and long lasting.
      (b) Any patient who is young or has a high functional demand should be considered for arthrodesis rather than for arthroplasty.
      (c) Arthrodesis is commonly used in the small joints of the wrist, hand, foot, and ankle in all age groups.
  c. **Arthroplasty,** or **total joint replacement,** relieves pain, preserves motion and is the most common surgical treatment for arthritis.
    (1) It can be used for joints destroyed by any of the arthritides; however, postinfectious arthritis is a relative contraindication to arthroplasty because of the increased risk of infection around the implant.
    (2) Arthroplasty is indicated for the relief of pain predominantly in patients who are usually older and less active.
    (3) At the present state of the art, the typical "life expectancy" for a hip or knee arthroplasty implant is about 15 years, depending on the functional requirements and weight of the patient. Failure is at a rate of roughly 1% per year.
    (4) Major joints such as the hip, knee, shoulder, and elbow are common sites for arthroplasty.

VI PEDIATRIC ORTHOPEDICS

A **Developmental dislocation of the hip (DDH)** is most common in female neonates, especially if the child is firstborn and was in the breech presentation. The condition is bilateral in 10% of patients.

1. **Diagnosis** can be made within the first 2 weeks after birth, once relaxin is gone from the child's circulation.

a. **Physical examination**

(1) The examiner can feel a click on reduction of the dislocated hip (**Ortolani's sign**).

(2) The examiner is able to dislocate the hip with the thigh flexed to 90 degrees (**Barlow's test**).

(3) Other physical findings (especially if the dislocation is unilateral) include asymmetry of the gluteal fold and asymmetric leg lengths, which are demonstrated by the height of the thigh when the hips are flexed to 90 degrees.

b. **Radiographs** confirm the diagnosis.

2. **Treatment.** A hip that can still be dislocated after 2 weeks of age should be treated.

a. The initial management is with a Pavlik harness.

b. Double and triple diapering probably has no significant effect on the dislocation.

c. Persistent dislocation of the hip after the commencement of ambulation typically requires surgical treatment.

B Legg-Calvé-Perthes disease

1. **Etiology**

a. Idiopathic osteonecrosis of the proximal femoral epiphysis can cause this disease.

b. This disease typically occurs in children 4–10 years old who are small for their age.

c. Males are affected more than females (5:1).

d. Clotting abnormalities and endocrinopathy (hypothyroidism) have been associated with Perthes disease.

2. **Diagnosis**

a. Patients often complain of **knee pain,** which is "referred" from the hip. In a child, this complaint should prompt an evaluation of the hip.

b. Hip irritation and limitation of internal rotation and abduction are common.

c. Radiographs of the hip demonstrate variable degrees of collapse of the femoral epiphysis.

3. **Treatment**

a. Restoration of **range of motion** and **containment** of the femoral head within the acetabulum are the cornerstones of treatment.

b. Traction followed by splinting in the abducted and internally rotated position may be tried.

c. Surgery may be necessary to redirect the femoral head into the acetabulum to allow it to reossify in a shape that matches the acetabulum and is as spherical as possible.

d. The single factor that is most predictive of a good outcome is the age at presentation (**infants <6 years old tend to do well regardless of treatment**).

C Slipped capital femoral epiphysis (SCFE)

1. **Etiology**

a. SCFE was thought initially to be idiopathic; however, new evidence may point to a subtle endocrinopathy.

b. Hypothyroidism should be suspected in children who develop SCFE before the age of 10–12 years.

c. There is a high incidence in children with renal failure and also in **African-American males** and **obese** children.

2. **Diagnosis**

a. A patient who is 10–13 years of age with hip or **knee pain** should be suspected of having SCFE.

b. Anteroposterior and **frog lateral** radiographs of the hip should be obtained in all patients who are suspected of having SCFE.

c. SCFE is bilateral in 20%–40% of patients without endocrinopathy and in 50% with endocrinopathy.

3. **Treatment.** Stabilization in situ with a single screw placed into the center of the femoral capital epiphysis is the preferred treatment.

D Scoliosis

1. **Etiology**

a. The most common form of scoliosis in the United States is the **idiopathic scoliosis** that occurs most commonly in adolescent females, beginning approximately at 11 or 12 years of age and progressing until growth is completed.

    b. Scoliosis can also be the result of neuromuscular paralysis, painful lesions, radiation, thoracic surgery, and congenital anomalies.

2. Clinical presentation

    a. Idiopathic scoliosis occurs most commonly as a right thoracic curve, but thoracolumbar, lumbar, and double major curves can occur.

    b. Thoracic curves are most noticeable because of the associated chest rotation and deformity, which create a rib hump.

    c. If the scoliosis is severe, exceeding about 90 degrees, significant cardiopulmonary complications can occur as a result of compromise of the chest cavity.

3. Treatment

    a. Braces. The **Milwaukee** and **Boston braces** are traditionally the initial form of treatment for scoliosis. They may eliminate the need for surgery in many patients.

        (1) The brace is not expected to correct a curve that is already established when the diagnosis is made but is meant to prevent *progression* of the scoliosis.

        (2) A brace is used if the curve measures about 20 degrees in a patient with significant **growth still remaining.**

        (3) The patient is placed in a brace if the scoliosis, even with a smaller angle, is clearly **progressing** during a period of observation.

    b. Surgery

        (1) Various surgical techniques are available, but the one that is most commonly performed is bone graft fusion of the spine over the area of the curve, facilitated by **rod fixation** using a segmental system with screws into the pedicles of the vertebrae.

        (2) Significant (although never complete) correction is obtained, and the long-term results are maintained by fusion of the spine in the corrected position.

E **Foot deformities** constitute a large part of pediatric orthopedic practice.

1. Etiology

    a. Idiopathic foot deformities are quite common and include **metatarsus adductus, talipes equinovalgus (clubfoot),** and **planovalgus.**

    b. A careful neurologic evaluation must be done to make sure that the foot deformity is not due to a **neuromuscular disorder.** Poliomyelitis, cerebral palsy, myelomeningocele, diastematomyelia, and Charcot-Marie-Tooth muscular atrophy can all present with foot deformities.

    c. Developmental dislocation of the hips must be ruled out whenever a child presents with a foot deformity.

2. Flatfoot seldom presents a significant problem and does not need treatment unless it causes symptoms or unless the neurologic examination is abnormal.

3. Clubfoot requires early treatment.

    a. Repeated manipulation and casting will correct the deformity in many cases.

    b. However, if the foot is relatively resistant to manipulation and casting, surgery may be indicated.

        (1) In recent years, surgical soft tissue releases before 1 year of age have shown a better prognosis than manipulation and casting.

        (2) Recurrence of the clubfoot despite correction remains a problem until the cartilaginous anlage of the child's foot has become the fixed osseous bone of the adolescent.

4. Neuromuscular foot disorders

    a. Treatment of the "neuromuscular foot" includes initial correction to a plantigrade neutral foot, either by manipulation of the very immature foot or by osteotomy and fusion of the more mature adolescent foot.

    b. Once the foot alignment is corrected, muscle transfers are carried out to prevent recurrent deformity. Tendons are transferred to replace the function of a paralyzed foot or to weaken the function of a spastic foot.

chapter 29

Pediatric Surgery

ERIC STRAUCH • CHARLES W. WAGNER

I INTRODUCTION

Pediatric surgery has evolved as a subspecialty for several reasons. First, infants and children differ from adults physiologically as well as anatomically. For example, the nutritional needs and fluid and electrolyte management for infants and children are not the same as those required for adults. Therefore, specialized knowledge is required for the care of pediatric surgical patients. Second, infants and children also differ to some extent with regard to the types of disorders that require surgical management. In infants, congenital malformations require prompt correction, and specialized knowledge is needed. The full discussion of specialized pediatric considerations is much too extensive to be covered in this chapter; therefore, only certain topics are discussed. For more complete information, the reader can consult standard textbooks on pediatric surgery.

II CONGENITAL HERNIAS (SEE CHAPTER 2, III)

A **Inguinal hernia**   Repair of an inguinal hernia remains the most common general surgical procedure in the case of the child. The defect is caused by nonfusion of the processus vaginalis and not by a breakdown of the floor of the inguinal canal.

1. **Incidence**
   a. Inguinal hernia occurs in 1%–3% of all children.
      (1) The hernia is on the right approximately 60% of the time, on the left approximately 30% of the time, and bilateral between 10% and 15% of the time.
      (2) The male:female ratio is 6:1.
   b. In premature infants, the incidence is 1½ to 2 times greater.
   c. The incidence of hernias is increased in patients with hydrocephalus who are treated with ventriculoperitoneal (VP) shunts, in patients with connective tissue disorders, and in infants and children on peritoneal dialysis.

2. **Clinical presentation**
   a. An inguinal hernia is diagnosed in infancy, and approximately 35% of patients present before 6 months of age.
   b. The classic history and clinical presentation are those of a mass or bulge in the groin, scrotum, or labia, which usually occurs during times of abdominal pain. The mass usually disappears after the straining or crying has been resolved, but it is for the most part easily reducible.
   c. If no mass is present, the physician can feel the thickened spermatic cord, which represents the nondistended hernia sac. This cord has been described as the **"silk glove" sign.**
   d. If no hernia is identified but the patient's history is both classic and reliable, most surgeons believe that surgery is indicated.

3. **Incarceration**
   a. **In boys,** the risk associated with a hernia is the chance of incarceration of the intestine.
      (1) Intestinal ischemia and obstruction can occur.
      (2) With time, the entrapped bowel becomes edematous enough to compress the spermatic vessels and cause testicular ischemia with resultant damage or necrosis.

(3) The risk of incarceration in a premature infant is 2–5 times higher than in the older child.

b. **In girls,** incarceration of the ovary is more common than incarceration of the intestine. Although ischemia of the ovary may result, it does not usually occur.

c. **Treatment** includes reduction of the incarcerated hernia, hydration of the patient, and herniorrhaphy.

   (1) These steps should all be taken within 48–72 hours.

   (2) Reduction is performed with or without sedation by gentle, continuous pressure on the incarcerated intestine.

   (3) Most hernias in children will reduce, but if the hernia cannot be reduced, emergent repair, evaluation of the intestine, and resection of necrotic intestine needs to be performed. The chance of reducing necrotic intestine is very low.

4. **Herniorrhaphy.** A hernia should be repaired soon after it is diagnosed, unless a major medical reason prohibits the use of anesthesia. In most children, the hernia can be repaired with outpatient surgery. Premature infants may have apnea and bradycardia after surgery and require overnight admission for monitoring for these conditions. Small infants with lung disease can have their hernias repaired under spinal anesthesia.

   a. **Procedure.** Herniorrhaphy in the child consists of identifying the sac, dissecting the spermatic structures free, and ligating the sac high at the internal ring of the inguinal canal. Floor repair is rarely needed.

   b. **Complications** of the procedure include damage to the vas deferens, vascular injury to the testes, recurrence of the hernia, and iatrogenic cryptorchidism.

      (1) The **recurrence rate** is reported to be approximately 1%, and the highest frequency occurs in patients with incarcerated hernias, connective tissue disorders (e.g., Ehler-Danlos or Hunter's syndrome), or increased intra-abdominal pressure (VP shunts or peritoneal dialysis [PD] catheters).

      (2) Iatrogenic cryptorchidism occurs when the testicle has been mobilized from the scrotum but has not been properly replaced. Unlike regular cryptorchidism, in which the testes may later descend, the testes remain in the abnormally high position with iatrogenic cryptorchidism.

B **Diaphragmatic hernias** are communications through the diaphragm that allow abdominal contents to migrate into the thoracic cavity.

1. **Incidence.** The incidence of this defect is 1 in 4,000 live births.

2. **Etiology.** Two underlying anatomic defects are common; both result from the failure of the surrounding tissues to fuse in utero.

   a. The **foramen of Bochdalek** is a posterolateral diaphragmatic defect.

      (1) This hernia is the most common congenital hernia (Fig. 29-1).

      (2) It occurs most often in the left hemidiaphragm and is bilateral in fewer than 10% of infants.

   b. The **foramen of Morgagni** is an anterior diaphragmatic defect. It is much less common and generally results in less severe problems.

3. **Diagnosis** of herniation of abdominal contents into the thorax is based primarily on impaired ventilatory capacity. The earlier that respiratory distress is noted in the infant (especially if it occurs during the first 24 hours), the more severe will be the impairment and the worse the prognosis.

   a. The **physical examination** reveals the following:

      (1) Tachypnea, dyspnea, use of accessory muscles for ventilation, cyanosis, and nasal flaring are evident.

      (2) Breath sounds are decreased or absent on the affected side.

      (3) Heart sounds are shifted away from the affected side.

      (4) Bowel sounds are heard in the affected hemithorax.

      (5) A scaphoid abdomen is caused by the migration of abdominal contents into the chest.

   b. A **chest radiograph** shows signs typical of herniation.

      (1) A loculated gas pattern is found in the affected hemithorax.

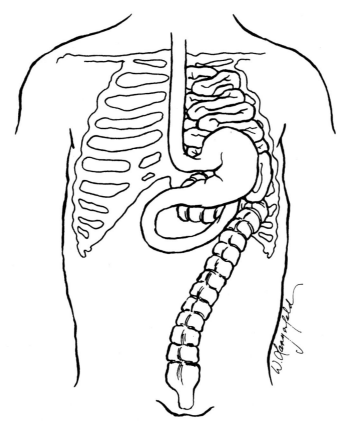

FIGURE 29-1 Bochdalek's hernia.

    (2) A mediastinal shift occurs away from the hernia.

    (3) Atelectasis occurs in the unaffected lung.

    (4) The nasogastric tube is found in the affected hemithorax after passage of the tube through the nose or mouth.

  4. Preoperative management

    a. Gastrointestinal decompression should be performed via a nasogastric or orogastric tube.

    b. A pneumothorax in the unaffected hemithorax should be sought and, if present, treated with a chest tube.

    c. Preoperative management is aimed at both respiratory insufficiency and pulmonary vascular hypertension.

      (1) Hypoxemia due to hypoplastic lung(s) causes acidosis.

      (2) Acidosis causes pulmonary vasculature to constrict, which decreases blood flow to the lung and increases the right-to-left shunt.

    d. If hypoxemia and hypercarbia can be improved with routine ventilator methods, surgical repair should then proceed.

    e. If acidosis with hypoxemia persists, preoperative use of extracorporeal membrane oxygenation (ECMO) should be considered.

    f. The hernia can be repaired while using ECMO.

    g. The use of nitric oxide (NO) is increasing as a step to improve hypoxemia. This agent is a potent pulmonary vasodilator and is mixed with the gases used in the ventilator. By dilating the pulmonary vasculature, the right-to-left shunt decreases.

  5. Operative management is based on the following principles:

    a. The herniated contents are reduced surgically back into the abdomen (through an abdominal incision), which can immediately relieve the distress.

    b. The hernia defect is repaired.

    c. An exploratory laparotomy is carried out to diagnose associated congenital anomalies (intestinal malrotation is often associated with this hernia).

    d. A chest tube can be inserted into the affected hemithorax but should not be placed on suction.

    e. The infant's acid-base balance and respiratory function are monitored carefully.

    f. A nasogastric tube is left to decompress the gastrointestinal tract.

6. **Postoperative management** is aimed primarily at maintaining adequate ventilation and perfusion and includes the following:

    a. Respiratory support on a ventilator is given as needed, and arterial blood gases are monitored.

    b. Atelectasis of either lung is treated, and the retained secretions are prevented.

    c. Chest tube suction is used on the affected side to stabilize the mediastinum in the midline.

    d. The patient is observed for contralateral pneumothorax and is treated rapidly if it occurs.

    e. Adequate gastrointestinal compression is provided.

        (1) The abdomen is small and may not be able to hold all of the contents after reduction.

        (2) The loss of the "right of domain" of the abdominal contents greatly distends the abdomen and raises intra-abdominal pressures.

        (3) Abdominal distention significantly impairs both thoracic excursion and venous return from the lower body.

    f. ECMO can also be initiated during postoperative care.

        (1) The oxygenator allows correction of hypoxemia and acidosis, thus decreasing the pulmonary vascular hypertension.

        (2) The patient is slowly weaned from ECMO so that normal pulmonary physiology can occur.

    g. If NO is used, levels of methemoglobulin are monitored. If greater than 5, one must decrease the concentration of NO in the ventilator gas mix.

    h. The use of diuretics to aid in fluid management is now being recognized as an important part of care in congenital diaphragmatic hernias.

7. The **prognosis** for the infant with a diaphragmatic hernia is a function of the preoperative severity and time of presentation of this hernia.

    a. The immediate mortality rate is approximately 35%–40%.

    b. The resolution of respiratory insufficiency in the postoperative period depends on the maturity of the contralateral lung and the control of pulmonary hypertension.

        (1) The ipsilateral lung is almost always hypoplastic when a diaphragmatic hernia is present and, therefore, does not aid in respiratory function during the immediate postoperative period.

        (2) If the infant survives, the lung eventually develops.

    c. No permanent respiratory difficulties have been noted in later life once the acute pulmonary insufficiency has resolved.

8. Patients who have been treated with ECMO have a **survival rate** of 65%. Associated risks (e.g., bleeding, cerebral infarction, recurrent hernias) keep this modality from being used routinely.

9. **Other therapeutic interventions** being investigated are high-frequency ventilation (which prevents barotrauma to the already hypoplastic lung). NO acts as a potent pulmonary vasodilator.

III   ABDOMINAL WALL DEFECTS

A **Types**   The two types of abdominal wall defects are **gastroschisis** and **omphalocele.** Although the abdominal contents are located outside of the peritoneal cavity in each type, the similarities (both developmental and therapeutic) end at that point.

1. **Gastroschisis** is an opening in the abdominal wall, immediately adjacent to the right of the umbilicus, which is located in the normal position.

    a. During fetal development, the abdominal wall is completely formed, but the peritoneal cavity does not enlarge enough to hold the abdominal contents.

  b. The protruding viscera, which consist of the midportion of the small intestine, the spleen, the stomach, the colon, and occasionally the liver, has no protective covering.

  c. The intestine is edematous, semirigid, leathery, and matted together as a result of chemical peritonitis.

  d. Associated anomalies and syndromes are rare, and intestinal atresia is the most frequent (10% of cases) anomaly.

  2. Omphalocele is an opening in the abdominal wall at the umbilicus.

  a. It is caused by incomplete closure of the somatic folds of the anterior abdominal wall in the fetus.

  b. Unless ruptured, a sac covers the extruded visceral contents, and no signs of chemical peritonitis appear.

  c. The liver and small bowel are the organs that most commonly protrude through the defect.

  d. The omphalocele may be a part of the **pentalogy of Cantrell,** which also includes:

  (1) Diaphragmatic hernia

  (2) Cleft sternum

  (3) Absent pericardium

  (4) Intracardiac defects

  e. If the caudal folds are involved, exstrophy of the bladder or cloacal exstrophy is present.

  f. Associated anomalies. Approximately 50% of these infants have one or more associated anomalies, including trisomies 13 and 18; Beckwith's syndrome; and cardiac, neurologic, and genitourinary malformations.

B **Prenatal diagnosis** may be made by the use of ultrasonography. This visualization of deep structures aids in the diagnosis of associated anomalies and in prenatal counseling as well as in early post delivery management.

C **Preoperative management** is similar in both disorders.

  1. Gastrointestinal decompression, intravenous fluids, and antibiotics are instituted.

  2. Protection of the abdominal contents is imperative, especially because the escape of moisture and heat is considerable in these patients.

  a. The **unruptured omphalocele** is left intact and protected with a sterile dressing to prevent it from drying out.

  b. Gastroschisis or a **ruptured omphalocele** is protected under a plastic covering (intestinal bag).

  3. When the patient with gastroschisis has a small defect and a swollen intestine, kinking of the vascular supply may occur at the edge of the defect. This vascular compromise may be prevented by placing the infant on his or her side. Occasionally, emergent enlargement of the defect may be necessary to protect the blood supply to the intestine.

  4. The outcome of gastroschisis is related to the condition of the intestines at the time of surgery.

D **Operative management** differs slightly for the two disorders. However, the goal in both conditions is to cover the abdominal viscera either with prosthetic material or with the abdominal wall itself.

  1. Gastroschisis. Closure is emergent, as there is no covering over the gastrointestinal tract to prevent heat and fluid losses. Primary closure involves decompressing the gastrointestinal tract and stretching the abdominal wall over the defect.

  a. If the closure is too tight, the blood supply to the intestine, abdominal wall, or lower extremities is compromised. To avoid this complication, it is better to cover the exposed organs temporarily with prosthetic materials.

  (1) Preconstructed silicon ventral wall defect silo bags are now available for staged closure. They eliminate suture lines that leak, and they also have a spring anchoring device for ease of application.

  (2) Reduction can now usually be completed by days 5–7, thus minimizing the risk of infection.

  b. A nasogastric tube is placed for decompression with either method of treatment.

2. **Omphalocele.** A ruptured omphalocele, like a gastroschisis must be covered emergently. If the sac is intact, workup for associated defects such as a cardiac anomaly can be performed. The choice of procedures includes primary closure; staged repair; or, for an unruptured omphalocele, nonoperative management. The important factor is the size of the defect.
   a. The greater the size of the defect, the less the peritoneal cavity has enlarged with adequate musculature of the abdominal wall; with a large defect, primary closure may involve too much tension.
      (1) An alternative method of treatment is to cover the defect with skin flaps, leaving the resultant ventral hernia to be repaired later on.
      (2) Silastic sheeting or preconstructed silo bags can be used to stage the repair; by keeping tension on the prosthetic sac, the Silastic sheet stretches the abdominal wall enough to accommodate the herniated viscera.
      (3) As with a staged repair of gastroschisis, closure is usually accomplished within 10 days.
      (4) **A prosthetic material such as Alloderm can be used to close the defect.**
   b. **Nonoperative management** is an alternative in patients with associated anomalies.
      (1) The sac is coated with silver sulfadiazine (Silvadene).
      (2) An eschar forms with subsequent coverage by granulation tissue.
      (3) The resultant ventral hernia can be repaired later on.
      (4) The risks associated with this method are rupture of the sac, requiring subsequent repair in an infected area; sepsis; undiagnosed intestinal atresia; and prolonged hospitalization.
   c. As with gastroschisis, a nasogastric tube is placed for decompression.

E **Postoperative management**
   1. With primary closure, respiration may be inhibited if the reduced abdominal contents compress the diaphragm. Patients may require muscular paralysis and mechanical ventilation until the abdomen stretches enough to accommodate the viscera.
   2. Venous return may be compromised owing to compression of the inferior vena cava.
      a. For vascular access, upper extremity veins should be used.
      b. The legs may show signs of venous obstruction and resultant edema.
   3. With staged repair, the patient needs to be observed after each daily reduction for both respiratory compromise and decreased venous return due to increased abdominal pressure.
   4. Patients require hyperalimentation with both primary and staged repairs, because intestinal motility and absorption are slow to return.
   5. After an unruptured omphalocele has been repaired, intestinal function is not as delayed as gastroschisis; however, hyperalimentation may still be needed.

F **Prognosis**
   1. **Gastroschisis,** although more difficult to manage initially, has very few long-term problems.
      a. Intestinal strictures may occur at the site of evisceration and will require resection later on.
      b. The **mortality rate,** approximately 30% in the past, has improved greatly with the use of hyperalimentation and is now approximately 5%. Mortality is related to sepsis and the viability of the gastrointestinal tract at the time of surgery.
      c. With resection for intestinal gangrene, short-bowel syndrome may develop.
   2. **Omphalocele.** The outcome for an omphalocele is related to the size and location of the defect and to the presence of associated anomalies. The overall mortality rate ranges from 20%–60%.

IV ESOPHAGEAL ATRESIA AND TRACHEOESOPHAGEAL MALFORMATIONS

Esophageal atresia and tracheoesophageal malformations occur once in every 3,000 live births. They encompass a spectrum of lesions that can vary greatly in their time of presentation and in their treatment. A high incidence of associated maldevelopments in other organ systems may complicate the treatment of these patients.

A **Types of lesions** (Fig. 29-2)
   1. **Esophageal atresia** (proximal pouch) **with a distal tracheoesophageal fistula** is the most common type; it occurs in 86% of patients.

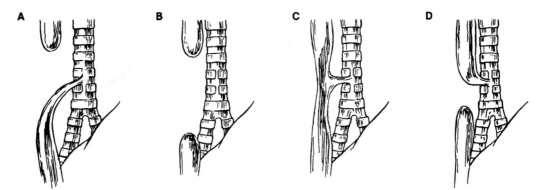

FIGURE 29-2   Esophageal atresia. **A:** Esophageal atresia with distal tracheoesophageal fistula. **B:** Proximal and distal blind pouches without fistula. **C:** H fistula. **D:** Esophageal atresia with proximal tracheoesophageal fistula. (Adapted from Altman RP, et al. Pediatric surgery. In Guzetta PC, Anderson KD, Altman RP et al. eds. *Principles of Surgery,* 7th ed. New York: McGraw-Hill; 1989:1724.)

   2. Pure esophageal atresia (proximal and distal blind pouches) without a fistula occurs in 7% of patients.

   3. Tracheoesophageal fistula without atresia (the H fistula) occurs in 5% of patients.

   4. A proximal and a distal tracheoesophageal fistula are combined with a proximal atresia (the least common type) in 2% of patients.

B **Associated anomalies**   In approximately 40% of these patients, other malformations are present in one or more organ systems.

   1. An **endocardial cushion defect** affects the heart, which is the most common single involved organ.

   2. The **VACTERL complex,** a well-recognized anomaly complex, involves **v**ertebral, **a**nal defects, **c**ardiac anomalies, **t**rache**o**esophageal fistula, **r**enal and **l**imb dysplasia.
   a. The complex may be fully or partially demonstrated; that is, one or any combination of lesions may occur.
   b. If it seems to be partial, the complete complex must be ruled out.

C The **diagnosis** of esophageal atresia and tracheoesophageal fistula is usually made soon after birth, when the affected infant exhibits some form of respiratory distress.

   1. Physical examination
   a. Aspiration of material from the upper pouch causes some symptoms.
      (1) The infant may appear to be salivating excessively and may drool continuously.
      (2) The aspiration may also cause coughing spasms, intermittent choking, or cyanosis that develops when the infant is feeding.
   b. Continuous aspiration of gastric secretions occurs if a fistula is present. This aspiration is more severe and more harmful than that from the upper pouch.
   c. Tachypnea and signs of pneumonia may develop.
   d. A scaphoid abdomen due to the unused gastrointestinal tract accompanies pure atresia.
   e. Attempts to pass a tube through the nose into the stomach will fail, because the tube will stop in the blind pouch of the esophagus, thus confirming the suspicion of esophageal atresia.

   2. Radiographs of both the chest and the abdomen are important in order to make a diagnosis and to prepare for treatment.
   a. The chest film will show the blind upper pouch and also the failure of passage by the gastric tube.
   b. A gasfree abdomen is characteristic of pure atresia.
   c. Hyperventilation, atelectasis, or pneumonia must be evaluated so that the proper surgical approach (i.e., immediate vs. delayed repair) can be chosen.

d. Identification of the aortic arch is also necessary for proper surgical management. The use of echocardiography may also assist in determining not only the aortic anatomy but also any associated congenital heart anomalies (see IV B).

e. The length of the esophageal defect can be measured on a lateral film.

D **Preoperative management**   Several steps should be taken once the diagnosis is made.

1. **Decompression** of the proximal pouch by means of a sump tube with constant suction (Replogle tube) is required.

2. An **upright position** is maintained, using a chalasia chair.

3. **Gastrostomy** is performed if delayed repair is chosen.
   a. This procedure prevents further gastric aspiration.
   b. It also provides a route for preoperative feedings if surgery is delayed for an extended period.

4. Stretching the proximal pouch daily in a pure atresia shortens the distance between the esophageal ends in preparation for eventual repair.

E **Operative management**   **Primary repair** at the time of presentation can be undertaken if the defect measures less than 2 cm and no signs of pneumonitis are present. **Delayed repair** may be needed if the defect is greater than 2 cm or extends the length of 2½ vertebral bodies. At the time of surgery, the approach is the same for either immediate or delayed repair.

1. Broad-spectrum antibiotic therapy is begun.

2. If not previously undertaken, a gastrostomy may be performed, although this measure is controversial.

3. An extrapleural dissection through the hemithorax opposite the aortic arch is currently favored to prevent empyema from occurring as the result of an anastomotic leak.

4. The tracheoesophageal fistula is repaired.

5. A primary esophagostomy is performed.
   a. The distal esophagus must be carefully dissected because the blood supply is tenuous.
   b. An adequate length of esophagus is necessary to create a tensionfree anastomosis and is obtained by dissecting the proximal pouch. The use of myotomies may aid in gaining length for closure.

6. A drain is placed in the extrapleural space.

F **Postoperative management** is directed at potential pulmonary and esophageal problems.

1. The infant is extubated as soon as possible to protect the tracheal repair.

2. Vigorous pulmonary toilet is necessary to clear up any previous pneumonia and to prevent the need for reintubation.
   a. Reintubation may disrupt the esophageal repair, the tracheal repair, or both.
   b. A degree of tracheal malacia compromises pulmonary function.
   c. Chest percussion is mandatory to prevent early postoperative problems.

3. The infant is kept upright, because esophageal function will not yet be adequate for swallowing oral secretions.

4. Esophagotracheal suction is done carefully and with a specifically defined length of tubing. Disruptions of the esophagus can occur during placement of a suction catheter through the anastomotic line.

5. The esophagus is evaluated after 7 days by means of a swallow study.
   a. If no leak is present, oral feedings are started; if feedings are tolerated, the extrapleural drain is removed.
   b. Before evaluation after 7 days, the gastrostomy (if present) may be used for continuous feedings.

6. **Surgical follow-up** is very important. Certain well-recognized problems sometimes develop, and they can have a drastic effect on the outcome in these patients.

   a. Esophageal dysmotility and its concomitant problems are major concerns.
      (1) The patient may develop a **dilated proximal pouch** with resultant aspiration or tracheal compression.
      (2) The patient may also have severe **gastroesophageal reflux** and aspiration.
         (a) Anastomotic stricture, once thought to be solely related to ischemia at the suture line, is now considered to be a consequence of esophagitis from gastroesophageal reflux.
         (b) If gastroesophageal reflux is implicated in postoperative problems, an **"antireflux" procedure** (usually a Nissen fundoplication) is recommended.
   b. Recurrent fistulas were formerly considered to be a relatively common potential problem, but in recent studies, they have occurred in fewer than 10% of patients.

7. The **prognosis** is related to the size of the patient, the condition of the lungs, and the presence or absence of associated anomalies. Patients have been grouped into three categories:
   a. Group A—100% survival: Patients weigh more than 2,500 g, have no associated anomalies, and have no signs of pneumonitis.
   b. Group B—80% survival: Patients have one of the following conditions:
      (1) Patients weigh 1,800–2,500 g.
      (2) Patients weigh more than 2,500 g but have mild pneumonitis.
      (3) One or more associated anomalies is present but is not life threatening.
   c. Group C—43% survival: Patients have one of the following conditions:
      (1) Patients weigh less than 1,800 g.
      (2) Patients have severe pneumonitis.
      (3) Patients have a life-threatening anomaly.

V   **MALROTATION OF THE INTESTINE**

Malrotation of the intestine is the abnormal placement and fixation of the midgut into the peritoneal cavity (Fig. 29-3). The involved portion of the gut includes all of the small intestine from the ampulla of Vater to the proximal two thirds of the transverse colon. Malrotation can occur independently or can be associated with other malformations, such as diaphragmatic hernia, omphalocele, and gastroschisis.

A **Overview**

1. Normal in utero development. The midgut develops extra-abdominally. It then migrates intraperitoneally, where it undergoes a 270-degree rotation. The results are as follows:
   a. The cecum ends up in the right lower quadrant.

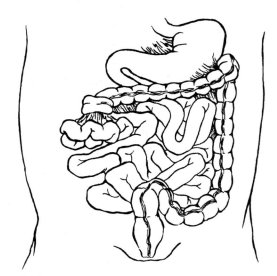

FIGURE 29-3 Malrotation and volvulus of the midgut.

    b. The right colon becomes fixed in the right paracolic gutter.

    c. The duodenum becomes fixed in the retroperitoneal location, with the superior mesenteric artery passing over the duodenum.

  2. Displacements caused by malrotation

    a. The cecum is not in the right lower quadrant, and the duodenum does not pass posteriorly to the superior mesenteric artery.

    b. Instead of the base of the small bowel being fixed from the ligament of Treitz to the cecum in the right lower quadrant, the whole midgut is anchored on the superior mesenteric artery.

    c. Various stages of fixation of the cecum can be seen, but it is usually fixed to the right upper quadrant with the fibrinous bands (Ladd's bands) that extend across the second portion of the duodenum.

  3. Sequelae to malrotation. Two serious problems may accompany this lesion, which must, therefore, be handled expeditiously.

    a. Intestinal obstruction can result from adhesive bands across the second portion of the duodenum fixing to the right upper quadrant.

    b. A **midgut volvulus,** which is more serious than intestinal obstruction, can also occur.

      (1) This volvulus develops when the intestine twists on its vascular pedicle (the superior mesenteric artery) and causes ischemia as well as obstruction of the entire midgut.

      (2) The result can be catastrophic, and gangrene of the entire small bowel can occur.

  4. Symptomatic malrotation is now being recognized in the older child. This is manifested by an atypical type of abdominal pain or vomiting caused by a partial or intermittent duodenal obstruction. Volvulus is rare in this group, but cases have been reported.

B **Clinical presentation**

  1. Bilious vomiting is the usual presenting symptom.

  2. Passage of a bloody stool is a late occurrence and implies ischemia, with necrosis of the bowel mucosa, bowel wall, or both.

  3. The infant may appear normal, with hemodynamic stability, or may be dehydrated and in shock.

C **Early diagnosis** of malrotation is crucial to prevent the development of a volvulus with resultant intestinal gangrene. Therefore, when malrotation in an infant is suspected and cannot be ruled out, all efforts are made to confirm the diagnosis rapidly.

  1. Radiographs are very useful when making the diagnosis.

    a. The **plain film** may demonstrate the "double-bubble" sign, which is produced by intestinal gas confined to the stomach and duodenum, with small amounts of gas in the residual, unused gastrointestinal tract. In a newborn with bilious vomiting, this sign is an indication for surgery.

    b. The **upper gastrointestinal series** may demonstrate an abnormally located ligament of Treitz, the presence of the duodenum to the left of midline, a duodenal obstruction, or a "beaked" end in the barium column at the point of the intestinal twist.

  2. Prompt **surgical exploration** is imperative if the diagnosis of malrotation is suspected but cannot be ruled out, because most infants with obstructive malrotation have a volvulus.

D **Operative management** Surgical procedures for malrotation vary with the presence or absence of volvulus and the status of the intestine.

  1. Simple malrotation is treated by the **Ladd procedure.**

    a. This procedure consists of releasing the adhesive bands and mobilizing the duodenum. The goal is to broaden the mesentery of the intestine as much as possible and to separate the duodenum and ascending colon.

    b. The cecum is placed in the left upper quadrant and the duodenum in the right lateral abdomen so that both organs will be in positions that should prevent intestinal obstruction or ischemia.

    c. An appendectomy is performed, and the remaining abdominal contents are examined for other anomalies, such as a duodenal web.

2. **Malrotation with volvulus** requires several **preliminary steps.**
   a. The first step is a counterclockwise detorsion of the midgut volvulus.
   b. The bowel is then examined for viability and for areas of necrosis.
      (1) If small areas of gangrene are present, resection is performed, followed by the Ladd procedure.
      (2) If large amounts of the midgut appear necrotic, long lengths of bowel are not resected. Instead, the bowel is untwisted, and the abdomen is closed and then re-explored 24 hours later. This second look allows marginally viable tissue to recover, with the hope of minimizing the amount of bowel to be resected.

E Prognosis

1. The recurrence of a **midgut volvulus** after surgical exploration and a Ladd procedure occurs in as many as 10% of cases, usually in the immediate postoperative period.
2. The long-term sequelae are minimal after repair of **simple malrotation.** However, when **extensive intestinal resection** is required, the result depends strongly on the amount of intestine remaining. Extreme resections result in severe malabsorption and even in death.

VI INTESTINAL ATRESIA

A Duodenal atresia and stenosis occur because the second portion of the duodenum fails to recanalize in the early embryonic stages. The lesion may be complex, partial, or in the form of a web (which is identified by an upper gastrointestinal study).

1. **Associated anomalies**
   a. **Trisomy 21** occurs in 30% of infants with duodenal malformations.
   b. **Cardiac lesions** and various elements of the **VACTERL** complex are present in many infants.
   c. An **annular pancreas** may be present, with the pancreas forming a ring around the duodenum. This anomaly is now thought to result from the malformation, rather than being a cause of duodenal stenosis.

2. The **diagnosis** is usually made from two simple findings.
   a. Bilious vomiting that occurs soon after birth in a nondistended infant suggests a high obstruction.
   b. Abdominal radiographs show the classic **double-bubble sign,** which involves air in the stomach and a proximally dilated duodenum.
      (1) This sign suggests duodenal obstruction but can also be seen with malrotation.
      (2) Although duodenal atresia or stenosis in itself is not life threatening, malrotation is life threatening (see V).
         (a) If delay in treatment is being considered in the patient with a double-bubble radiograph, a barium contrast study is necessary to rule out malrotation.
         (b) This study may be a barium enema to localize the cecum or an upper gastrointestinal study to see the duodenal sweep.

3. **Preoperative management**
   a. Gastric decompression and fluid resuscitation are performed as needed.
   b. Broad-spectrum antibiotic therapy is begun.
   c. Because these lesions have a high association with other more critical anomalies, stabilization and evaluation of these lesions can be done before surgery. However, this combination can be done only if malrotation is ruled out as the cause of duodenal obstruction.

4. **Operative management** has as its goal the re-establishment of a patent gastrointestinal tract.
   a. The site of obstruction is identified.
   b. Usually a duodenoduodenostomy can be performed. If this cannot be done, a duodenojejunostomy is a good alternative. Gastrojejunostomy is contraindicated.
   c. If a **web** is present, the duodenum is opened at the site of obstruction, the web is excised, and the duodenum is closed. Care must be taken to identify the ampulla of Vater, because it is also located on the mesenteric side of the web.

  d. If an **annular pancreas** is present, care is taken not to damage this structure.
    (1) In no circumstance is the pancreas divided.
    (2) The annular pancreas is not the obstructing lesion (as is the duodenal stenosis), and the mortality rate is extremely high among patients whose annular pancreas is divided.
    (3) The annular pancreas can usually be bypassed by a duodenoduodenostomy.
  e. Because 15% of the patients have other gastrointestinal atresias, a thorough search is undertaken to ensure the patency of the entire gastrointestinal tract.
  f. A nasogastric tube is used for gastrointestinal decompression.
5. **Postoperative management** is simple but requires patience.
  a. Gastrointestinal decompression is important to protect the suture line and to prevent possible aspiration.
  b. The return of gastrointestinal function is slow, not only because of gastric and duodenal dysfunction but also because the distal intestine is small owing to disuse.
  c. Nutritional support by hyperalimentation is usually needed.
6. **Prognosis.** Long-term results of surgery are good. Mortality in these patients is related to prematurity of the infant and to associated anomalies.

B **Jejunal, ileal, and colonic atresias** are caused by in utero vascular accidents that result in ischemia of a segment of bowel, with consequent stenosis or atresia. The **ileum** is most commonly affected; the **jejunum** and **colon** are affected less often. The severity of the lesion is related to the size of the vascular arcade that was affected in utero.
1. **Associated anomalies.** Because they are not embryonic maldevelopments, associated anomalies are much less common than with duodenal atresia. However, approximately 10% of patients have **cystic fibrosis.** DNA studies to identify the cystic fibrosis gene are now available and can be used if a sweat test is inadequate or unavailable. Patients with these atresias should have a sweat chloride test by 2 months of age to rule out cystic fibrosis.
2. **Clinical presentation.** The diagnosis is suspected when an infant develops bilious vomiting after 24 hours of life.
  a. The degree of abdominal distention varies with the level of the obstruction.
  b. The passage of meconium does not rule out an atresia, because the gastrointestinal tract was intact before the vascular accident.
  c. All patients with small bowel or colonic atresia should have an early evaluation for cystic fibrosis.
3. **Diagnosis**
  a. **Abdominal radiographs** show various degrees of obstruction, depending on the level of the atresia or stenosis.
    (1) The picture can be confused with meconium ileus.
    (2) In atresia, air–fluid levels are present; whereas a meconium ileus shows only distended bowel, without fluid levels, and a soap-bubble appearance.
  b. **Contrast studies** are helpful in both diagnosis and management.
    (1) A contrast enema will reveal colonic lesions and perhaps low ileal lesions.
    (2) Hirschsprung's disease, meconium ileus, and other congenital disorders may also be ruled out, making diagnosis of the atresia more certain.
4. **Preoperative management** includes gastrointestinal decompression and fluid replacement. Begin broad-spectrum antibiotic therapy.
5. **Operative management.** Surgery is performed to re-establish intestinal continuity.
  a. The current **procedure of choice** is an end-to-end intestinal anastomosis.
    (1) This procedure may be difficult to accomplish because of the marked size disparity of the bowel—the proximal bowel is dilated, and the distal, unused bowel is small.
    (2) Because of the variations in size, tapering of the proximal bowel may aid in the repair.
  b. The distended bowel has been found to have varying degrees of impaired motility. Therefore, gastrointestinal function may be extremely slow to return.
  c. A nasogastric tube is placed to allow decompression, prevent aspiration, and protect the suture line.

  d. A thorough abdominal examination for **multiple atresias** is performed. Their overall occurrence rate is 6%, but the frequency is high with ileal atresia and very low with colonic atresia.

  e. In a patient with **both an atresia and meconium ileus,** the distal intestine may contain inspissated small bowel secretions. In this situation, the site of inspissation should be irrigated with a 4% acetylcysteine (Mucomyst) solution to relieve any potential obstruction before the atresia is repaired.

6. Postoperative management involves decompression and patience.
  a. Hyperalimentation may be needed until the gastrointestinal tract begins to function.
  b. Malabsorption, if present, may prolong the recovery time.

7. Prognosis. Because associated anomalies are few, survival is a function of the prematurity of the infant. Current results show a survival rate of almost 100%.

C "Apple-peel" atresia, a severe form of small bowel atresia, is known by this name because of its appearance.

  1. This atresia occurs during a large vascular accident to one or more of the mesenteric arcades in utero.

  2. Stenting procedures have been developed to preserve gastrointestinal length in patients with both apple-peel and multiple atresias.

  3. In these patients, return of gastrointestinal function is very prolonged, and malabsorption is common.

VII ■ IMPERFORATE ANUS (FIG. 29-4)

Abnormal termination of the anorectum has a clinical spectrum that ranges from a fistulous opening in the perineal area or a colourethral fistula to a completely blind ending of the rectum. The incidence of these malformations ranges from 1 in 1,500 to 1 in 5,000 births. The male:female ratio is 2:1.

A Types   Although many classifications have been proposed for an imperforate anus, the simplest division is on the basis of sex and the relationship to the levator ani.

  1. Infralevator (low) type. The rectum passes through the puborectalis sling. This type is more common in girls.

  2. Supralevator (high) type. The rectum does not pass through the puborectalis sling. This type is more common in boys.

B Associated anomalies are common in patients with an imperforate anus, and this congenital defect is associated with the VACTERL syndrome.

  1. The **genitourinary tract** is the most commonly involved organ system.
    a. Malformations include renal agenesis, renal dysplasia, hypospadias, epispadias, bladder exstrophy, vaginal atresia, and cloacal exstrophy.
    b. These findings have been reported in up to 40% of patients with imperforate anus.

  2. Other organ systems involved are:
    a. Gastrointestinal tract (in 15%), most often as a tracheoesophageal fistula
    b. Heart (in 7%)
    c. Skeletal system (in 6%)
      (1) Defects include hemivertebrae, sacral agenesis, and spina bifida.
      (2) Although sacral agenesis may not physically affect the patient, it may have implications for the successful functioning of the surgically created anus for continence, constipation, and toilet training at a later age.

C Diagnosis of an imperforate anus appears easy; however, determination of the extent of the **lesion** is critical for management.

  1. Physical examination. The first step is a thorough examination of the perineum and, in girls, the vaginal vault.

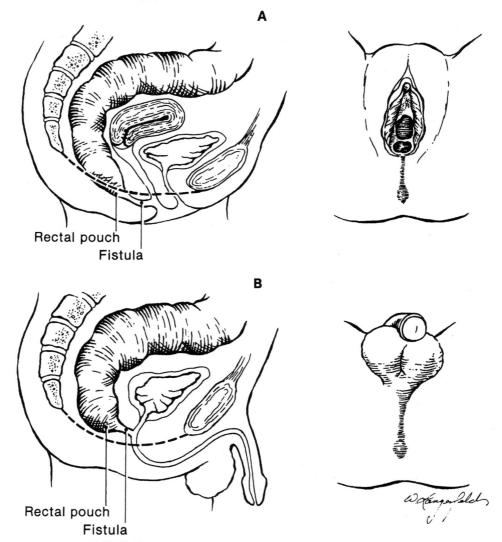

A

Rectal pouch

Fistula

B

Rectal pouch

Fistula

FIGURE 29-4 Imperforate anus in the female **(A)** and in the male **(B)**.

a. A fistula may be found in the perineal area.
b. The patient may have a fistulous tract, which opens:
   (1) In girls, posterior to the vagina within the vestibule
   (2) In boys, to the posterior urethra
c. In boys, meconium in the urine should be sought. This condition occurs only when a fistula is present between the rectal pouch and the urinary tract.
d. Problems in patients with fistulas
   (1) They may develop symptomatic **urinary tract infections.**
   (2) They may also develop a **hyperchloremic acidosis** caused by reabsorption of chloride by the colonic mucosa.
      (a) This acidosis is characterized by lethargy, tachypnea, and elevation of the serum chloride and the blood urea nitrogen (BUN).
      (b) Although the condition may resolve in time, treatment with bicarbonate may be required; and, if the condition is severe or cannot be corrected, the rectal pouch–urinary tract fistula may need to be divided before the definitive procedure is undertaken.

2. **Radiographs.** If no external fistula is identified, the surgeon must determine whether the rectum has traversed the puborectalis sling. Using a cross-table lateral radiograph of the pelvis, the surgeon can identify the extent of the rectum by visualizing the end of the infracolonic air.
   a. A line drawn from the posterior portion of the symphysis pubis to the tip of the coccyx (the **pubococcygeal line**) aids when differentiating the infralevator type from the supralevator type.
   b. Air visible in the bladder suggests a posterior urethral fistula, which implies a supralevator type.
   c. If the distance from the tip of the colonic air column to the anal dimple is greater than 2 cm, the lesion is the supralevator type. An ultrasound examination may prove more accurate in defining the distance.

D **Operative management**

1. **Infralevator type.** If an **external fistula** is identified, several alternatives are available for the initial management.
   a. If the fistula can be dilated, it may function satisfactorily until the patient is older, at which time the opening can be relocated to the correct site (the **Pott's anal transfer**).
   b. If the mucosa is close to the opening, the fistula may be enlarged by a procedure known as a **Denis Browne cutback.**
   c. These procedures are performed more commonly in girls, because the infralevator type of imperforate anus occurs more often in girls.
2. **Supralevator type.** The treatment for the supralevator type of imperforate anus is, first, the formation of a colostomy, followed by the formation of a neorectum and anus.
3. The sagittal posterior anoplasty (Peña procedure) has been used for reconstruction of all levels of imperforate anus. The goal is to bring the rectum down to the perineum within the sphincter complex to try and maximize continence.

E **Postoperative management** depends on the type of imperforate anus. Basically, the **goal of treatment** in these patients is to have a socially accepted, continent child. These children require patience during toilet training; they are usually trained between 3 and 5 years of age.

1. **Infralevator types** of anus require constant dilatations until the stool obtains bulk.
2. **Supralevator types** of anus require colostomy care until the definitive procedure can be performed. With the formation of a new anus, the patient may require dilatations to prevent strictures.

F **Prognosis**

1. The mortality rate among patients with an imperforate anus is directly related to the associated anomalies.
2. Functional morbidity is directly related to:
   a. Inappropriate management
   b. Associated neurologic dysfunction due either to spina bifida or to sacral agenesis with poorly developed neuromuscular control in the lower pelvis
3. The development and use of either irrigating stomas or cecostomy buttons for prograde enemas have shown a simple solution for a poor outcome (constipation or soilage).

VIII **HIRSCHSPRUNG'S DISEASE**

A **Overview**

1. Hirschsprung's disease is caused by the congenital absence of parasympathetic ganglia cells in the wall of the gastrointestinal tract.
   a. As a result, the affected portions of the bowel are unable to relax and allow effective peristalsis to occur.
   b. Hirschsprung's disease always involves the rectum and extends proximally with no skip areas. Any other part of the gastrointestinal tract, or even the entire tract, may also be involved.

2. Male predominance is 4:1, except when the entire colon is involved. In that situation, the frequency ratio is reversed, with females predominating.

3. Approximately 30% of patients with Hirschsprung's disease have a relative afflicted with the disease.

B **Clinical presentation**   Hirschsprung's disease may go **undiagnosed** for years after birth. It should be **suspected** in any patient with a chronic unexplained illness and an abnormal bowel pattern dating back to early infancy.

1. Newborns with Hirschsprung's disease present with a history of nonpassage of meconium.
  a. Meconium is usually passed within 24 hours after birth in term infants and within 48 hours in premature infants.
  b. Distention and bilious vomiting are common.
  c. Physical examination in the newborn reveals a distended abdomen.
    (1) Occasionally, loops of stool-filled bowel may be palpated.
    (2) A rectal examination shows the ampulla or rectal vault to be empty and the sphincter tone to be increased. Classically, when the examining finger is removed, an explosion of watery stool occurs.

2. Infants and older children have a history of obstipation and constipation as well as failure to thrive.
  a. Bouts of diarrhea, vomiting, and abdominal distention may herald the development of enterocolitis.
  b. Enterocolitis is sometimes associated with Hirschsprung's disease. If left untreated, it has a high mortality rate (up to 50%).

C **The diagnosis** is confirmed by radiographic and tissue studies.

1. Abdominal radiographs reveal air–fluid levels and a distended bowel. Often, no air is seen in the rectum.

2. Barium enema shows spasm and a narrowed lumen in the affected bowel.
  a. A **transition zone** is often present, showing a dilated proximal gut and a narrowed distal gut.
    (1) This zone represents the most distal area in which ganglia cells are present.
    (2) In most patients, this zone is in the rectosigmoid segment of the colon.
    (3) The ratio of the diameter of the sigmoid colon to the diameter of the rectum on contrast enema is greater than 1 in patients with Hirschsprung's disease.
  b. In patients with total colonic Hirschsprung's disease or with a longer segment involving the small bowel, the findings may not be as clear, and the transition zone may not be identified. The sigmoid–rectum ratio is not helpful.

3. A **follow-up radiograph** is obtained in 24 hours when the barium enema is inconclusive in a newborn with suspected Hirschsprung's disease. The appearance of residual barium in the bowel is very suggestive of Hirschsprung's disease.

4. Tissue confirmation
  a. Biopsy specimens are examined for the presence of Auerbach's plexus in the muscular layer. The specimen can be obtained by either of two procedures.
    (1) Seromuscular biopsy of the bowel wall at laparotomy
    (2) Full-thickness transrectal biopsy, which requires general anesthesia
  b. Suction biopsy technique is currently used as the first step.
    (1) With this procedure, the biopsy specimen is examined for Meissner's plexus in the submucosal layer.
    (2) The procedure can be performed at the bedside, with little risk to the patient.
    (3) Although the procedure is simple, it produces small specimens and requires an experienced pathologist for a correct interpretation.
    (4) Staining for acetylcholinesterase (which is increased in Hirschsprung's disease) may aid in the histologic diagnosis.

D **Preoperative management**   Once the diagnosis has been made, the patient is prepared for surgery.

1. If enterocolitis is present preoperatively, the patient requires parenteral antibiotics and gastric decompression. In addition, rectal decompression and irrigations with saline or an antibiotic solution are performed.

2. The classic surgical approach is to perform a colostomy in an area of intestine that has ganglia cells.

3. Once the gastrointestinal tract is patent, the child can be fed orally.

E Operative management There are a variety of different operative approaches for Hirshsprung's disease. Many surgeons will do a primary pullthrough at the time of diagnosis if the patient is stable. If not, a colostomy will need to be performed to relieve the obstruction and allow enteral feedings.

1. **Goals of surgery.** Although different operative procedures are available for the definitive repair, all have two goals in common:
   a. Removal of most or all of the involved intestine
   b. Re-establishment of a functional, continent gastrointestinal tract by bringing well-inervated intestine to the anus.

2. **Procedures.** The four most commonly performed are the Swenson, Duhamel, and Soave procedures, and the recently described transanal approach. These procedures can be performed in a tradional open fashion or laparoscopically assisted.
   a. **Swenson's procedure** is the standard operation, but it is difficult to perform and is not used today by most pediatric surgeons.
      (1) The involved colon is excised to within 1 cm of the anal mucocutaneous margin.
      (2) The bowel is then sutured to the cuff of distal anorectal segment, thus establishing gastrointestinal continuity.
   b. **Duhamel procedure**
      (1) The involved colon is excised to the level of the peritoneal reflection within the abdomen.
      (2) The proximal normal bowel is tunneled between the sacrum and the rectum and is then anastomosed end-to-side to the low anorectum.
   c. **Soave procedure**
      (1) In this operation, the involved colon is also excised to the level of the peritoneal reflection.
      (2) The mucosa is removed in the remaining rectum.
      (3) The proximal normal bowel is pulled through the stripped anorectal segment and is sutured to the anorectal junction.
   d. **Transanal approach**
      (1) In this operation, the rectal mucosa is dissected from the rectal wall transanally up to the peritoneal reflection.
      (2) The abdomen is entered transanally through the rectal wall.
      (3) The proximal normal bowel is pulled through the stripped anorectal segment is and sutured to the anorectal junction.

3. **Sequelae.** Enterocolitis may occur after these operations because the internal sphcinter is still abonormally innervated. Because the mortality rate is high if untreated, early diagnosis and treatment are critical.

F The **prognosis** for infants properly treated for Hirschsprung's disease is good.

1. Anal dilatation may be necessary intermittently if constipation occurs secondary to the retained aganglionic internal anal sphincter.

2. Problems of incontinence and fecal soiling occur occasionally.

3. **Postoperative constipation** may reflect a group of patients with poor gastrointestinal motility as a spectrum of the disease. These patients have responded to prokinetic agents. Recent studies have raised the question of poor neurotransmission as a problem with Hirschsprung's disease. However, if constipation persists, biopsy at the surgical anastomosis should be considered to document ganglion cells at this site.

IX **DISORDERS OF INFANCY**

A **Pyloric stenosis** In this condition, hypertrophy of the muscular layer of the pylorus causes gastric outlet obstruction. The classic symptom is nonbilious projectile vomiting.

1. The **etiology** of the condition is unknown. However, certain consistent elements imply a hereditary, genetic basis.
   a. It is a male-predominant disease; the male:female ratio is 4:1.
   b. The offspring of a female with pyloric stenosis have a 10-fold greater chance of developing pyloric stenosis, whereas offspring of a male with pyloric stenosis have a four-fold greater chance of developing pyloric stenosis.
   c. The condition is more common in whites than in blacks.

2. **Clinical presentation.** Pyloric stenosis occurs early in life, usually between the age of 2 weeks and 2 months.
   a. The history is one of nonvomiting at birth, a gradual onset of vomiting, and final progression to nonbilious projectile vomiting.
   b. Vomiting may lead to dehydration.
   c. A hypochloremic, hypokalemic metabolic alkalosis may be present; this condition varies with the degree of dehydration.
   d. Jaundice is present in 10% of the infants. It is thought to be caused by a deficiency of glucuronyl transferase and resolves after surgical treatment of the pyloric stenosis.
   e. With the improvement of survival of premature infants with various other anomalies, a group of older (2–4 months of age) infants is developing pyloric stenosis. It is unclear whether this situation represents a delay in diagnosis because of parenteral feeding or a true older presentation. However, the diagnosis should be considered in this subgroup if feeding problems develop or persist.

3. **Diagnosis**
   a. The **physical examination** can often provide the diagnosis.
      (1) Palpation of a midepigastric mass in the right upper quadrant of an infant with projectile vomiting is the sine qua non of pyloric stenosis. However, finding the mass may require experience, persistence, and patience.
      (2) Complete evacuation of the stomach by a nasogastric tube may aid in finding the mass.
   b. Ultrasonography, however, has become the most common method of diagnosis due to the case of the study and "the lost art of physical exam." Although the examination does not require a cooperative patient, it does rely on the experience of the person performing the study. The criteria for diagnosis are documented.
      (1) The length of the pylorus is measured; if greater than 15 mm, pyloric stenosis is suspected.
      (2) The width of the muscular wall is measured; if greater than 4 mm, pyloric stenosis is suspected.
   c. **Upper gastrointestinal series** may be helpful in the diagnosis. The findings include:
      (1) Gastric retention of 3–4 hours
      (2) Elongation and narrowing of the antrum
      (3) A "string" sign or "railroad track" sign (one or two thin barium tracts, respectively, through the pylorus)
      (4) A mass effect on the antrum
      (5) Nonprogression of a peristaltic wave through the pylorus to the duodenum

4. **Preoperative management**
   a. Correction of the alkalosis and volume deficits is necessary.
      (1) The conditions are corrected by fluid replacement and potassium supplementation.
      (2) Adequate hydration is determined by voiding patterns (the normal infant voids 4 to 5 times a day).
      (3) Alkalosis correction is measured by the serum bicarbonate, which should be less than 28 mEq/dL, or serum chloride, which should be greater than 92 mEq/dL before surgery is considered.
   b. **Nasogastric decompression** may also be instituted to protect against aspiration and to aid in the quicker return of gastric motility in the postoperative period.

5. **Operative management.** The surgical procedure is pyloromyotomy. This procedure involves an incision of the serosa over the pylorus and division of the hypertrophic muscle of the antrum but not the duodenum. The stomach is not entered.

6. **Postoperative management**
   a. The patient may be started on feedings of glucose and water or an electrolyte infant formula (e.g., Pedialyte) 4–6 hours after surgery.
   b. Vomiting occurs in 50%–80% of patients because of gastric atony or acute gastritis.
      (1) This vomiting is usually self-limited and has been decreased with preoperative gastric decompression.
      (2) Occasionally, the patient will benefit from gastric lavage with half-strength bicarbonate solution.
   c. Feedings are advanced on a prescribed schedule, and full feedings are usually reached by 24 hours after surgery. The patient may be discharged at this point.
   d. **Complications**
      (1) **Duodenal perforation** is the major complication.
         (a) Its danger is not so much its occurrence as the problem of its being overlooked at the time of surgery.
         (b) The perforation is handled by a simple repair, nasogastric decompression for 24–48 hours, and antibiotics.
         (c) If it is recognized and handled appropriately, the major difficulty is an extended hospital stay.
         (d) If the perforation is missed, the morbidity is severe, and the incidence of mortality is significant.
      (2) **Apnea** may also occur in the early postoperative period.
         (a) The patient should, therefore, have an apnea monitor in place for the first 24 hours postoperatively.
         (b) Postoperative apnea is associated with a serum carbon dioxide level greater than 28 mL/dL.
      (3) An **incomplete pyloromyotomy** may cause recurrent symptoms. This operation can be evaluated best with ultrasonography. Pyloric measurements decrease to normal 2–4 weeks after a complete pyloromyotomy.

7. **Prognosis.** Once adequately treated, pyloric stenosis does recur, and long-term studies indicate no sequelae such as ulcer disease, food intolerance, or hiatal hernia. In addition, no problems with growth and development occur.

B **Biliary atresia** is a disease that affects the development of the biliary duct system both intra- and extrahepatically. It occurs once in every 25,000 births.

1. The **etiology** of the disease is unknown. Many possible causes have been implicated but not confirmed, including viral infections, hereditary factors, neonatal hepatitis, and malformation of the extrahepatic ductal system. Biliary atresia appears to develop after birth. Although isolated fetal cases have been described in Japan, no cases have been reported in the United States.

2. **Types.** Classically, biliary atresia is divided into correctable and uncorrectable types. However, the current belief is that biliary atresia represents a progressive spectrum of disease and that these divisions have little bearing on the eventual outcome.
   a. **Correctable biliary atresia** occurs in 20% of the cases.
      (1) A **normal common bile duct** becomes atretic at some distal point.
      (2) It is called "correctable" because the duct can be anastomosed to a jejunal conduit.
   b. **Uncorrectable biliary atresia. No macroscopic biliary system** is present in the portal triad. Until the Kasai operation, no procedure had been successful in establishing bile drainage of the liver.

3. **Clinical presentation.** Clinically, the child presents from 4 weeks to 4 months of age as a healthy but jaundiced infant with few other complaints. Some patients have associated light stools.
   a. Laboratory studies show conjugated hyperbilirubinemia.
   b. Liver function studies may or may not be abnormal, depending on the degree of liver damage from cholestasis.

4. **Diagnosis.** The most important rule of thumb is that **persistent jaundice** beyond the first month of life must be evaluated. This condition may not affect the outcome in patients with medical causes of conjugated hyperbilirubinemia (for whom no effective therapy may exist). However, the prognosis of surgery for biliary atresia is related to the age at diagnosis.

a. The workup is designed to differentiate true anatomic obstruction of the biliary tree from other causes of hyperbilirubinemia.

(1) **TORCH** (**t**oxoplasmosis, **o**thers, **r**ubella, **c**ytomegalovirus, and **h**erpes simplex virus) titers are checked for possible infection.

(2) Serum electrophoretic patterns are examined for α_1-antitrypsin deficiency.

(3) **Ultrasonography** is performed to identify the gallbladder and the fibrotic bile duct at the portohepatis. If the gallbladder is not seen or the fibrotic ducts are not located, an exploratory laparotomy should be strongly considered instead of further tests.

(4) **Nuclear scans** using technetium 99m (^{99m}Tc)-labeled iminodiacetic acid derivatives look for biliary excretion into the gastrointestinal tract. The accuracy of these tests may be enhanced with the administration of phenobarbital sodium (PBS). PBS stimulates liver enzymes and improves the excretion of bile in patients without biliary atresia.

(5) **Percutaneous liver biopsy** is very helpful in experienced hands. If it shows bile duct proliferation in the face of hepatocellular necrosis, biliary atresia should be suspected.

b. If biliary atresia cannot be ruled out by these methods, the child should undergo a **diagnostic laparotomy.**

(1) If an **intraoperative cholangiography** demonstrates a normal patent biliary system, a **wedge biopsy** of the liver is taken and the surgical procedure is ended.

(2) If patency cannot be demonstrated, the porta hepatis is explored in an effort to find the atretic duct.

(3) If an extrahepatic duct can be found, a Roux-en-Y loop of jejunum is anastomosed to it. This is the so-called **correctable biliary atresia.**

(4) If the common duct cannot be found, the dissection is then carried to the hilus of the porta hepatis and a **Kasai procedure** (hepatoportal enterostomy) is performed. This involves anastomosing a loop of jejunum to the liver hilus, incorporating the area where the common bile duct should be.

5. **Prognosis**

a. Two factors influence the outcome of the Kasai operation:

(1) At surgery, the patient is **less than 10 weeks old.**

(a) The best results are obtained in patients 8–12 weeks old.

(b) To date, there have been no long-term survivors among patients who had repairs done when they were more than 20 weeks old. This is caused by the irreversible liver damage that results from cholestasis.

(2) The **microscopic stage** of the biliary tree is examined from the hilar dissection specimen.

(a) Patients with ductules greater than 120 μm in diameter have a good prognosis.

(b) Patients with ductules smaller than 70 μm have a very poor prognosis.

(c) A "gray zone" occurs when the ductules are between 70 and 120 μm. Although bile drainage may occur, resolution of the jaundice and reversibility of the liver disease may or may not occur.

b. Currently, approximately 60% of the patients with biliary atresia undergo a **surgical repair.**

(1) However, only a little more than one half of these patients have a resolution of jaundice and a return to normal liver function.

(2) One third of all patients with biliary atresia who undergo surgery will be treated successfully by current surgical techniques. (These results were obtained in the United States.)

c. Biliary atresia remains the primary indication for liver transplantation in the pediatric population.

(1) More than 50% of the patients with failed hepaticoportenterostomies can be treated successfully with transplants. The limiting factor is the availability of donor organs.

(2) Recently, the use of split liver grafts has shown promise. This allows a donor liver to be anatomically divided and used in two recipients.

(3) Living related liver transplants (using segments of the left lobe) have also been successful.

(4) Because of these advancements, some transplant centers advocate transplant as the primary procedure.

C **Necrotizing enterocolitis** (NEC) is an ischemic disorder of the intestine in the newborn.

1. **Etiology.** Although the etiology and underlying mechanism of NEC is not completely understood, it is probably multifactorial. Ischemic injury to an immature intestine in a host with an immature immune system in the presence of bacteria can result in NEC.

2. **Clinical presentation**
   a. The **basic defect** is an ischemic or hypoxic insult, which causes intestinal mucosal sloughing. This may lead to bacterial invasion and subsequent intestinal gangrene and perforation.
   b. The patients are usually born prematurely or have a low birth weight (75% weigh <2,000 g at birth). The disease usually occurs within the first 2 weeks of life.
   c. The **first signs** are usually intolerance to formula and abdominal distention. These signs may be associated with the passage of either heme-positive or grossly bloody stools.
   d. **Associated perinatal problems** include premature rupture of the membranes, prolonged labor, amnionitis, umbilical artery catheterization, respiratory distress, apneic episodes, cyanosis, or delivery-room resuscitation.

3. **Diagnosis**
   a. **Laboratory findings** include leukopenia, thrombocytopenia, a low hematocrit, low serum sodium levels, metabolic acidosis, and coagulation defects.
   b. **Abdominal radiographs** are used to aid in the diagnosis and to follow the patient's clinical course. The initial findings include distended, edematous intestines; intramural air (pneumatosis); portal vein gas; an isolated persistent distended loop of bowel; or free intraperitoneal air, suggesting intestinal perforation.

4. **Medical management.** The primary management remains medical. This includes gastrointestinal decompression with a large oral or nasogastric tube, parenteral antibiotic therapy, treatment with fluids, and nutritional support.

5. **Operative management.** Although the disease is primarily a medical disorder, approximately 40% of all infants who develop necrotizing enterocolitis require surgery for its complications (e.g., perforation, gangrene, or intestinal stricture).
   a. An **absolute indication** for surgery in the acute stage is **intestinal perforation.**
      (1) This perforation can usually be documented by the abdominal radiograph.
         (a) A cross-table lateral or left lateral decubitus position is used.
         (b) Films are obtained every 4–6 hours or as clinically indicated.
      (2) If perforation occurs, it is **treated** by resection of the involved intestine.
         (a) The gastrointestinal tract is diverted with either a jejunostomy or an ileostomy and colostomy.
      (3) Primary reanastomosis of the normal bowel is performed only in patients with limited disease or an isolated perforation.
      (4) In the severely ill patient with perforation or in the micropremature infant (<1,000 g), a major resective procedure may not be tolerated. In this situation, placement of peritoneal drains (using local anesthesia) at the bedside has proved successful. This can be either a stabilizing step or definitive therapy, depending on the clinical response of the patient.
   b. **Relative indications** for surgery
      (1) Signs of peritonitis (erythema or edema of the abdominal wall) increase.
      (2) The patient fails to stabilize after 12 hours of optimal medical treatment (the patient shows persistent acidosis, apnea, or hypothermia).
      (3) A persistent distended loop of bowel is seen on serial radiographs.
      (4) An abdominal mass is palpated.

      (5) A stricture with subsequent intestinal obstruction occurs in approximately 30% of cases.

         (a) This problem occurs usually 3–6 weeks after the acute episode.

         (b) Strictures are treated by resection and primary anastomosis once the patient is prepared nutritionally for surgery.

  6. Postoperative management includes continued medical management of the primary disease as well as routine postsurgical care.

    a. The infant is treated with antibiotics, gastrointestinal decompression, and hyperalimentation.

    b. The disease may progress, requiring further surgery for additional perforations. Recurrent necrotizing enterocolitis occurs in approximately 4% of patients.

    c. Oral feedings are not started until 10–14 days after the acute disease resolves. Dietary adjustments may be necessary until the mucosa has regenerated and undergone functional maturation.

    d. The enterostomy can be closed during the initial hospitalization or later on.

    e. Management of the stoma can be difficult.

      (1) Local problems include prolapse, degeneration of the surrounding skin, or mucosal irritation.

      (2) Physiologic problems include fluid losses, electrolyte abnormalities, and intolerance of the diet.

      (3) Early recognition and treatment of these difficulties are necessary to prevent further complications.

  7. Prognosis

    a. The mortality rate is 20% among patients who require only medical management for NEC.

    b. The mortality rate among patients requiring surgery is up to 50%, reflecting the greater severity of the disease in this group.

    c. Birth weight also affects outcome, and the overall mortality is 40% in patients weighing less than 1,500 g and 0%–20% in patients weighing more than 2,500 g.

    d. Long-term morbidity is related to the quantity and function of the remaining intestine and other comorbidities related to prematurity after recovery from NEC.

      (1) A patient who has had an extensive bowel resection may develop a short-bowel syndrome (see Chapter 12, II E) requiring a change of diet or nutritional support. This syndrome has been reported to occur in approximately 8% of all patients with NEC. However, NEC is the major cause of short-bowel syndrome in children (20%–50% of all patients).

      (2) Comorbidities include intraventricular cerebral hemorrhage, chronic pulmonary insufficiency, or associated cardiac problems.

X   SOLID TUMORS

The two most common solid tumors of childhood are Wilms' tumor and neuroblastoma. Although **other tumors** occur (e.g., rhabdomyosarcoma, Ewing's tumor, osteogenic sarcoma, various brain tumors), neuroblastoma and Wilms' tumor illustrate the multidisciplinary approach that is currently used in the management of tumors that occur in childhood. They are also outstanding examples of successful management (Wilms' tumor) and the need for continued research to improve current poor results (neuroblastoma).

A Wilms' tumor can involve either the entire kidney or a part of it. Bilateral involvement occurs in 3%–10% of the cases.

  1. Etiology. Mesodermal, mesonephric, and metanephric origins have been proposed for this tumor.

  2. Incidence. It has been estimated that 500 new cases of Wilms' tumor occur each year in the United States.

  3. Clinical presentation

    a. An asymptomatic flank mass is usually discovered by the parents or during a routine physical examination. The mass is smooth, lobulated, and commonly mobile.

b. Other complaints or findings include abdominal pain, hematuria, and anorexia.

c. Hypertension occurs in approximately 10% of patients.

d. The patient is between 1 and 4 years of age at presentation; most patients are between 1 and 3 years of age.

e. The tumor rarely crosses the midline but may appear to cross because of its size.

4. Associated anomalies

a. Wilms' tumor has been associated with congenital anomalies, such as aniridia, hemihypertrophy, Beckwith's syndrome, sexual ambiguity, cryptorchidism, urinary tract anomalies, and abnormal karyotypes.

b. Congenital mesoblastic nephroma is a distinct renal tumor of infancy related to Wilms' tumor.

    (1) To date, approximately 70 cases have been reported.

    (2) The tumor usually presents soon after birth as an abdominal mass.

    (3) Nephrectomy alone is the current therapy and provides a cure.

5. Diagnosis. Imaging studies to aid in the diagnosis of Wilms' tumor should define the nature of the abdominal mass, the organ of origin, the status of the contralateral kidney, the presence of tumor in the renal vein or vena cava, and the presence or absence of distal metastases.

a. A **chest radiograph** will reveal metastasis to the lung, which is the most common site.

b. Ultrasonography with a Doppler examination can identify the organ of origin, the opposite kidney, and the presence of renal vein or vena cava involvement.

c. Venograms are useful if the ultrasound cannot define tumor involvement of the vena cava.

d. A **computed tomography (CT) scan** can identify both the tumor and lung metastasis, but the sensitivity for the metastasis is high and is not used currently in the staging of Wilms' tumor.

6. Staging of Wilms' tumor is as follows:

a. Stage I: The tumor is limited to the kidney and is completely excised. The surface of the renal capsule is intact. The tumor was not ruptured before or during removal. There is no residual tumor apparent beyond the margins of resection.

b. Stage II: The tumor extends beyond the kidney but is completely removed. There is regional extension of the tumor (i.e., penetration through the outer surface of the renal capsule into the perirenal soft tissues). Vessels outside the kidney substance are infiltrated or contain tumor thrombus. The tumor may have been biopsied, or there has been local spillage of tumor confined to the flank. There is no residual tumor apparent at or beyond the margins of excision.

c. Stage III: A residual nonhematogenous tumor is confined to the abdomen.

    (1) Lymph nodes on biopsy are found to be involved in the hulus, the periaortic chains, or beyond.

    (2) There has been diffuse peritoneal contamination by tumor, such as spillage or tumor beyond the flank before or during surgery or tumor growth that has penetrated through the peritoneal surface.

    (3) Implants are found on the peritoneal surface.

    (4) The tumor extends beyond the surgical margins either microscopically or grossly.

    (5) The tumor is not completely resectable because of local infiltration into vital structures.

d. Stage IV: Hematogenous metastases can occur with deposits beyond stage III (e.g., lung, liver, bone, or brain).

e. Stage V: Bilateral renal involvement is evident at diagnosis. An attempt should be made to stage each side according to the aforementioned criteria on the basis of the extent of disease before a biopsy.

7. Management of Wilms' tumor involves a **multidisciplinary approach.**

a. Surgery is the mainstay of treatment.

    (1) The timing of surgery depends on the stage of the tumor (i.e., stage IV or V).

    (2) The operation includes:

        (a) An exploratory laparotomy

        (b) Examination of the opposite kidney

        (c) Resection of the tumor

        (d) Periaortic node dissection or sampling

(3) Because of the relatively good prognosis, even with extensive disease, resection of other organs in an effort to remove the tumor is acceptable.

(4) Venacaval extension requires the removal of the tumor thrombus. This operation may require a cardiopulmonary bypass to assist in the resection.

b. Chemotherapy currently involves the use of dactinomycin (actinomycin D) and vincristine.

(1) Currently, chemotherapy is used in all stages (I–V) for varying cycles, depending on the histology (see X A 8).

(2) Dactinomycin and vincristine are given preoperatively in stages IV and V disease.

(3) Adriamycin is added to the chemotherapy regimen for patients with advanced disease.

c. Radiotherapy is used to treat extensive disease (stages III–V). The numerous **complications** after high-dose radiotherapy include secondary cancers in children; interference with growth and development of bones, joints, and muscles; radiation pneumonitis; radiation enteritis; and cardiotoxicity.

8. **Prognosis.** Survival appears to be related to the histology of the tumor, which is reported as favorable (FH) and unfavorable (UH) and dictates treatment protocols. Current 2-year survival rates by stage and histology are as follows:

a. Stage I (FH)—97%

b. Stage II (FH)—95%

c. Stage III (FH)—88%

d. Stage IV (FH)—85%

e. Stages I–III (UH)—80%

f. Stage IV (UH)—55%

g. Stage V—50%

B **Neuroblastoma** is a neoplasm of adrenal and neural crest origin.

1. **Incidence.** It occurs in 1 of every 10,000 live births and is the most common extracranial solid tumor of childhood. It occurs in the early age group, with 50%–60% presenting by 2 years of age.

2. **Types.** The following are several **major variants** of neuroblastoma.

a. Classic neuroblastoma is a highly undifferentiated, immature malignant tumor that is unencapsulated and diffusely infiltrates the surrounding tissue.

b. Ganglioneuroma is a benign, well-encapsulated tumor containing fully differentiated mature ganglia cells.

c. Ganglioneuroblastoma is an intermediate or transitional form consisting of both primitive undifferentiated neuroblasts and mature differentiated ganglia cells. It can occur with or without encapsulation.

3. **Etiology.** Although they may occur anywhere along the sympathetic chain, the majority (65%) of these tumors arise from adrenal or nonadrenal retroperitoneal sites.

4. **Clinical presentation**

a. Most patients **present** with a complaint of an abdominal mass.

b. Neurologic symptoms may occur, resulting from compression of nerve trunks or from extension of the tumor into the extradural space (**"dumbbell" tumor**).

c. Horner's syndrome has been reported.

d. Other symptoms include acute cerebellar ataxia and **opsoclonus** (i.e., sustained, irregular multidirectional, spontaneous conjugate eye movements).

e. Metastatic spread can involve the liver, lungs, skin, bone marrow, and bone.

(1) Skin lesions are firm, nontender, and bluish; a biopsy will provide the diagnosis.

(2) The orbit is a common site of bony metastasis with consequent periorbital ecchymosis and proptosis.

(3) More than 50% of patients have metastatic disease at presentation.

5. The **diagnosis** of the tumor may be obtained by various laboratory methods.

a. Bone marrow aspiration may reveal typical neuroblastoma cells.

b. Urinalysis. The tumor may synthesize various catecholamines.

(1) The excretion products include vanillylmandelic acid (VMA) and homovanillic acid.

(2) These acids can be checked in both spot urine samples and in 24-hour urine collections.

c. Radiologic studies

(1) Skeletal surveys or bone scans may show metastatic lesions.

(2) Chest radiographs will confirm or rule out pulmonary metastasis.

(3) Ultrasonography acts as a screening tool to define the organ of origin and to rule out Wilms' tumor.

(4) Calcifications are seen much more often on abdominal radiographs in neuroblastoma than in Wilms' tumor.

(5) A CT scan gives complete details of the tumor as well as being sensitive to identifying metastatic disease.

(6) If spinal cord extension of a paraspinal neuroblastoma, the presence of a "dumbbell" tumor, or neurologic symptoms are suspected, magnetic resonance imaging (MRI) is very helpful in defining the exact extent of cord involvement.

d. Liver function is documented, and routine blood studies are done. Anemia will be present in approximately 40%–60% of the patients at the time of diagnosis.

6. Staging for neuroblastoma is as follows using the International Neuroblastoma Staging System (INSS) classification:

a. Stage 1: A localized tumor is present with complete gross excision, with or without microscopic residual disease; representative ipsilateral lymph nodes are negative for tumor microscopically (nodes attached to and removed with the primary tumor may be positive).

b. Stage 2A: A localized tumor is treated with incomplete gross excision; representative ipsilateral nonadherent lymph nodes are negative for tumor microscopically.

c. Stage 2B: A localized tumor is present with or without a complete gross excision, with ipsilateral nonadherent lymph nodes that are positive for tumor. Enlarged contralateral lymph nodes must be negative microscopically.

d. Stage 3: An unresectable unilateral tumor infiltrates across the midline, with or without regional lymph node involvement; or a localized unilateral tumor is present with contralateral regional lymph node involvement; or a midline tumor is present with bilateral extension by infiltration (unresectable) or by lymph node involvement. The midline is defined as the vertebral column. Tumors originating on one side and crossing the midline must infiltrate to or beyond the opposite side of the vertebral column.

e. Stage 4: This stage involves any primary tumor with dissemination to distant lymph nodes, bone, bone marrow, liver, skin, or other organs (except as defined for stage 4S).

f. Stage 4S: A localized primary tumor (as defined for stage 1, 2A, or 2B) is present, and dissemination is limited to the skin, liver, or bone marrow (limited to infants younger than 1 year of age). Marrow involvement should be minimal (i.e., <10% of total nucleated cells identified as malignant by bone biopsy or bone marrow aspirate). More extensive bone marrow involvement would be considered to involve stage IV disease. The results of the metaiodobenzylguanidine (MIBG) scan (if performed) should be negative for disease in the bone marrow.

7. Medical/surgical management. A rational approach to the treatment of neuroblastoma requires a combined approach using the surgeon, radiation oncologist, chemotherapist, and pediatrician.

a. Surgery. Although complete surgical removal is desirable, most patients (60%) present with metastatic disease. Neuroblastoma differs from Wilms' tumor, in which aggressive surgery in the face of advanced disease is associated with good results.

b. Radiation is used as an adjuvant for resected or partially resected primary tumors and as palliative therapy for symptomatic metastases.

c. Chemotherapy includes the use of cyclophosphamide, vincristine, adriamycin, and dacarbazine (DTIC). The exact therapeutic protocol has not been developed, and other agents are under investigation.

d. An **autologous bone marrow transplant with a tumor cell purge** is being used for advanced stages or recurrent disease, and survival rates are much better than those achieved with standard therapy.

8. Prognosis. Neuroblastoma remains as one of the few childhood tumors that has not responded dramatically to modern antitumor therapy. A child diagnosed today has the same dismal prognosis as a child diagnosed more than 20 years ago.

a. **Factors that influence survival**
   (1) **Age.** The younger the child at diagnosis, the better will be the outlook; this variable is independent of staging.
   (2) **Stage.** The more advanced the disease, the worse will be the prognosis; however, stage D (S) has a relatively good prognosis (70% survival).
   (3) **Location.** An abdominal neuroblastoma has a worse outlook than has an extra-abdominal neuroblastoma.
   (4) **Site of metastasis.** Patients presenting with bony lesions have a mortality rate of almost 100%.
   (5) **Presentation.** Patients presenting with opsoclonus have a higher survival rate than do those who present without it.
   (6) **Biologic markers** are currently being used to define a study group as low risk in an effort to limit transplantation in order to reduce morbidity.
b. **Overall survival rates** are as follows:
   (1) **Stage A**—90%
   (2) **Stage B**—80%
   (3) **Stage C**—60%
   (4) **Stage D**—10%
   (5) **Stage D (S)**—70%

9. The two major pediatric cancer study groups (Pediatric Oncology Group and Children's Cancer Group) are currently merging into one unit. This merger will standardize study data and will result in an effort to improve therapy and general outcome.

10. Other studies now being undertaken in the long-term outcome for survivors relate to possible second malignancies and fertility as well as mental and physical development. These studies are confined not just to solid tumors but also to hematologic cancer.

chapter 30

Laparoscopic Surgery

JOHN L. FLOWERS • W. BRADFORD CARTER
DAVID D. NEAL • JAMES A. WARNEKE

I HISTORY

A **Technical advances**

1. The idea of visual inspection of the abdomen without open celiotomy was demonstrated by Kelling in 1901. He performed peritoneal "celioscopy" of a canine abdomen by using a cystoscope after air insufflation. In 1910, H. C. Jacobaeus used this technique on humans.

2. In the 1940s, Goetz, and later Veress, developed a spring-loaded obturator needle for safe insufflation. On penetration of the peritoneum, the obturator springs over the needle to prevent inadvertent perforation or laceration of the abdominal organs. Coupled with the gas-flow insufflator with continuous pressure monitoring designed by Semm in 1964, this advance allowed for the establishment and maintenance of a controlled pneumoperitoneum.

3. When **fiberoptic light sources** replaced incandescent lights in the 1960s, a new generation of laparoscopic exploration and procedures became possible. The addition of **computer chip cameras** greatly facilitated resolution of the video image, and fine detail and precise surgery became a reality.

B **Operative milestones**

1. **In the 1960s, Semm replaced 75% of open gynecologic operations with laparoscopy,** with an overall complication rate of 0.28%. This demonstrated the safety and cost effectiveness of laparoscopy.

2. Laparoscopic appendectomy was pioneered by DeKok (1977) and Semm (1982). Use of laparoscopy decreased removal of normal appendices by 50% in young female patients who presented with equivocal signs of appendicitis.

3. Laparoscopy in general surgery was first used for liver biopsy under direct vision.

4. Warshaw used laparoscopy to stage pancreatic cancer in 1986, with an accuracy of 93%.

5. **Laparoscopic cholecystectomy** was first performed in Europe; initially by Erich Muhe (1985) in Germany, then by Dubois, Mouret, and Perrisat (1987) in France. The procedure was introduced and popularized in the United States by McKernan and Saye (1988), and Reddick.

6. By the early 1990s, the technical feasibility of a laparoscopic approach was demonstrated for virtually all major open abdominal surgical procedures. Since that time, research has focused on the appropriate indications for laparoscopic procedures and documentation of complication rates and cost-effectiveness of the laparoscopic approach. Significant progress has been made in the areas of video technology, laparoscopic surgical instrumentation, and the physiology of laparoscopy as well.

II GENERAL PRINCIPLES

A **Differences between laparoscopy and laparotomy**   A critical concept in understanding laparoscopy is that it is merely **a different method of surgical access to the abdominal cavity.** It is **not a fundamentally superior technology and does not replace laparotomy.** Like all other procedures, it has advantages and disadvantages when compared with standard laparotomy. The fundamental technical differences between laparoscopy and laparotomy are:

1. **Pneumoperitoneum.** Laparoscopy requires creation of a pneumoperitoneum in order to visualize intra-abdominal organs. Gas (usually carbon dioxide) is insufflated into the peritoneal cavity at a pressure of 12–15 mm Hg, elevating the abdominal wall and allowing visualization of the peritoneal cavity.

2. Small airtight cylindrical **"operating ports"** or "trocars" are required for insertion of surgical instruments into the abdomen. Common sizes include 2-, 3-, 5-, 10-, 11-, and 12-mm diameters. Larger operating ports (15 mm, 18 mm, 30 mm) are sometimes used for insertion of large instruments and removal of specimens. Larger airtight plastic sleeves are also available for introduction of the surgeon's entire hand during a variant of laparoscopy known as "hand-assisted laparoscopic surgery".

3. A laparoscope with an attached video camera is inserted through an operating port into the abdomen in order to view the intra-abdominal contents. The image is transmitted to television monitors, permitting the entire operating room staff to see a high-quality magnified image of the operative field.

4. Laparoscopic instruments are dramatically different in appearance compared with traditional surgical instruments due to the mechanical constraints of the operating parts. Most instruments are 27–32 cm in length, making them ergonomically less efficient. Though steady improvement has occurred, they remain relatively clumsy when compared with traditional surgical instruments.

B **Advantages of laparoscopy**

1. **Potential advantages of laparoscopy (when compared with laparotomy)** are:
   a. Improved visualization of anatomy
   b. Less tissue trauma and physiologic stress
   c. Less postoperative pain
   d. Shorter hospital stay
   e. Earlier return to normal activity after discharge
   f. Improved cosmetic result
   g. Decreased perioperative complication rates (especially superficial wound infection, incisional hernia, and pulmonary dysfunction such as hypoxia and atelectasis)

2. Proving these potential advantages is easier said than done. It must be emphasized that **except for laparoscopic cholecystectomy and a few other procedures, laparoscopy has proved to be superior to open surgery in very few instances.** Quantifying patient outcome variables such as postoperative pain and return to normal activity is difficult and highly subjective. Length of hospital stay varies widely with geography, indication for surgery, and economic variables. Complication rates are dependent on multiple factors that are incompletely understood. Clinical outcomes after specific laparoscopic procedures are currently the subject of intense investigation.

3. Most surgeons adept at advanced laparoscopy, however, agree that all of the potential advantages listed in item 1 are possible in certain circumstances. A well-planned and executed laparoscopic procedure, performed expeditiously by a properly trained surgeon in an appropriate patient, can lead to a truly impressive result.

C **Disadvantages**

1. Most of the disadvantages of laparoscopy are the result of the technical and mechanical factors that, ironically, are also responsible for the advantages of laparoscopy. Cumbersome instruments that are small in diameter must be inserted at a fixed angle through the abdominal wall. The use of suction is limited by the need for a constant pneumoperitoneum in order to see the operative field. Other disadvantages are:
   a. **Tactile sensation is lost.** This is the single biggest disadvantage of laparoscopy. The inability to place a hand in the abdomen and feel tissue makes it very difficult to locate masses and find correct tissue planes. It also decreases the safety of blunt dissection and increases operative time.
   b. **Depth perception is diminished.** The use of a television monitor makes laparoscopy two-dimensional. Tasks requiring fine motor skills, such as sewing and dissection around major blood vessels, are more difficult than during laparotomy.

    c. **Hemostasis is difficult.** Intraoperative bleeding during laparoscopy is harder to manage for two reasons. Sudden severe hemorrhage is nearly impossible to control, as a hand cannot be used to tamponade bleeding and the ability to suction is limited. Second, limited means are available to manage the constant low-level bleeding that may occur in a patient taking aspirin or in a patient with an acute inflammatory process such as acute cholecystitis.

    d. **Suturing is difficult.** Several factors make laparoscopic suturing substantially more difficult and time consuming than suturing during open surgery. These include fixed angles of instrument insertion; long, cumbersome needle holders; loss of depth perception; and the need for a cooperative camera holder.

    e. **Laparoscopy is resource intensive.** Compared with laparotomy, laparoscopy requires relatively delicate and expensive equipment that requires more knowledge and sophistication on the part of the operating room staff to operate and maintain.

    f. **Cost-effectiveness of laparoscopy is uncertain.** In general, laparoscopic procedures use more expensive equipment and supplies and more disposable instrumentation than laparotomy, increasing the in-hospital costs associated with laparoscopy. This cost increase is amplified by longer operating times seen during the surgeon's learning curve. Theoretically, this cost increase will be offset by more rapid return to normal activity and lower complication rates, though this is difficult to objectively measure. The true cost-effectiveness of laparoscopy will only be determined by numerous outcome studies on a procedure-by-procedure basis.

2. Many of the disadvantages of laparoscopy can be offset to some degree by the use of additional technologies, such as intraoperative endoscopy and laparoscopic ultrasound during laparoscopy. As newer technologies are developed, their usefulness in overcoming current disadvantages of laparoscopy will be evaluated.

D **Patient preparation**

1. **Preoperative preparation** for laparoscopic surgery is essentially the same as for laparotomy. Before surgery, the **patient's overall physical condition is assessed,** and special attention is paid to:
    a. Optimal stabilization of underlying medical problems
    b. Assessment of fluid and electrolyte balance
    c. Assessment of coagulation status

2. **General anesthesia** is employed in nearly all advanced laparoscopic procedures. **Pneumoperitoneum is poorly tolerated in awake patients** because of the discomfort of abdominal distention and the resulting sensation of dyspnea as well as shoulder pain caused by diaphragmatic irritation. Local anesthesia may be used with success in properly selected patients:
    a. Diagnostic laparoscopy, especially short procedures limited to the pelvis
    b. Conscious pain mapping for chronic abdominal pain
    c. Some types of extraperitoneal inguinal hernia repair

3. **Intraoperative conduct**
    a. **The abdomen is prepped and draped widely** in all cases so that an urgent laparotomy can be performed if necessary.

    b. An **orogastric or nasogastric tube and urinary catheter are inserted to decompress the stomach and bladder** in order to avoid injury to these structures during creation of the pneumoperitoneum.

    c. **Antithromboembolic pumps are applied** to the lower extremities to minimize the possibility of deep venous thrombosis (DVT). Physiologic changes occur during laparoscopy that create the potential for increased risk of postoperative DVT, but the true incidence of DVT and pulmonary embolism following most laparoscopic operations is unknown. All patients undergoing laparoscopic surgery should be considered at "moderate risk" for postoperative DVT. At the present time, the same general recommendations that are widely used for DVT prophylaxis during open surgery should be used during laparoscopic procedures.

    d. **Appropriate anesthetic monitoring is necessary,** especially end-tidal CO_2 monitoring. Patients with underlying cardiopulmonary diseases are at risk for acidosis, and a lower threshold for use of more invasive devices such as arterial lines and pulmonary artery catheters is necessary in this group.

E **General operative technique**   Though every surgical procedure is different, all laparoscopic procedures share several common steps:

1. **Room setup.** Attention to detail is critical. Patient position, placement of television monitors, location of the operating team, and preoperative testing of the video system to ensure proper function can all make the difference between a failed or successful procedure.

2. **Establishment of intra-abdominal access.** Though laparoscopy may be performed by using one of several specialized mechanical abdominal wall lifting devices, **virtually all laparoscopic procedures performed today use a pressurized carbon dioxide (CO_2) pneumoperitoneum** to elevate the abdominal wall and allow visualization of the peritoneal cavity.

   a. CO_2 is used because it is readily available, inexpensive, and does not support combustion. It also is absorbed readily by the peritoneal cavity, has a high diffusion coefficient, and is rapidly excreted by respiration. Nitrous oxide and inert gases such as argon have also been used but are not widely popular today. Filtered CO_2 is insufflated into the peritoneal cavity at a **pressure of 12–15 mm Hg in adults.** Higher pressures may impede venous return and cardiac output.

   b. Safe, airtight entry into the peritoneal cavity is necessary to create a pneumoperitoneum. Any of three common methods may be used:

      (1) **Closed pneumoperitoneum method.** An umbilical incision is made, and a spring-loaded obturator needle (Verres needle) is inserted through the abdominal wall into the peritoneal cavity. CO_2 is insufflated through the needle until the desired pressure is achieved. The Verres needle is removed, and an appropriate-sized operating port is placed through the incision into the abdomen.

      (2) **Laparoscopic-assisted method.** A specialized disposable operating port with a transparent plastic cutting tip is necessary. A laparoscope is placed in the operating port while the port is advanced under laparoscopic guidance directly through the abdominal wall. Gas is then insufflated directly through the operating port into the peritoneal cavity.

      (3) **Open pneumoperitoneum method.** A 10- to 20-mm incision is made at the umbilicus, and standard surgical instruments are used to dissect directly through the abdominal wall under direct vision into the peritoneal cavity. A specialized operating port with a blunt obturator and cork-shaped attachment (Hasson cannula) is used to prevent bowel injury and gas leakage around the site, which tends to be less airtight.

   c. **Exploratory laparoscopy.** After establishment of pneumoperitoneum, a few minutes are taken to perform diagnostic laparoscopy. The posterior aspect of the anterior abdominal wall and the surfaces of organs are carefully inspected for abnormalities. Special attention is paid to the area of the initial puncture into the abdomen to check for entry trauma. Visualization of these structures is often superior to that allowed with standard abdominal incisions.

   d. **Insertion of accessory operating ports.** Anywhere from three to six total ports are necessary to accomplish most advanced laparoscopic procedures. Their position varies according to procedure and the patient's body habitus. In general, placement of ports on the arc of a circle with the target organ at its center will allow a successful result.

   e. **Hand-assisted laparoscopic surgery (HALS),** also known as "handoscopy," is a hybrid alternative to conventional laparoscopy. After starting a typical laparoscopic procedure, a small laparotomy incision (6–8 cm) is made that allows the surgeon to introduce his hand into the abdomen. This allows exposure and dissection maneuvers with the surgeon's hand while under videoendoscopic control. HALS requires the use of a specialized baglike device that provides an airtight seal around the incision and the surgeon's wrist and forearm while maximizing freedom of movement.

      (1) **Advantages of HALS.** Restores tactile sensation; improves traction, dissection, and tissue exposure; improves control of bleeding; aids handling and extraction of large or bulky specimens.

      (2) **Disadvantages of HALS.** Requires additional incision that increases surgical trauma; alters port placement and operative strategy; presence of surgeon's hand minimizes free space in abdomen; induces hand and back fatigue in surgeon; increased costs due to pneumatic sleeve

At the present time, HALS has not been widely adopted as an alternative to traditional laparoscopy. It is used mainly to prevent conversion of difficult laparoscopic cases to laparotomy and may have a role in training laparoscopic surgeons in new procedures.

F **Relative contraindications** are factors that increase the risk of complications or exacerbate comorbid conditions. They apply generally to most laparoscopic surgical procedures.

1. **Severe cardiopulmonary disease.** The increased abdominal pressure associated with pneumoperitoneum will decrease venous return and worsen pulmonary compliance, causing complications such as acidosis, hypotension, and arrhythmia in these patients.

2. **Generalized peritonitis** is usually best treated with laparotomy, although diagnostic laparoscopy is useful in equivocal cases.

3. **Prior abdominal operations** and adhesion formation increase the technical difficulty and potential danger of laparoscopy. Severe adhesions may make it difficult to place operating ports in proper position and limit the potential working space in the abdomen. They can also increase operating time and increase the likelihood of injury to abdominal organs. Unfortunately, it is not possible to predict the number or severity of intra-abdominal adhesions prior to surgery. Ultimately, the surgeon's judgment is needed to decide whether persisting with a laparoscopic approach or converting to laparotomy is the best choice when faced with significant adhesions.

4. The **risk of hemorrhage in severe coagulopathic states** is a contraindication for laparoscopy. These patients should be treated with open techniques that allow direct intervention at potential bleeding sites.

5. **Morbidly obese patients** have a very thick abdominal wall, which can hinder operating port placement and free movement of laparoscopic instruments. Excessive intra-abdominal pressure (>20 mm Hg) may be necessary in some patients to elevate the abdominal wall and achieve adequate visualization of the peritoneal contents. The emergence of laparoscopic bariatric surgery over the past several years has led to increased use of laparoscopy in this patient population.

6. The enlarging uterus of **advanced pregnancy** may preclude sufficient intraperitoneal space to perform laparoscopic procedures. Most surgeons do not recommend the use of laparoscopy past the 20th week of gestation.
    a. However, laparoscopic appendectomies and cholecystectomies have been performed successfully during the second trimester and even in the early third trimester.
    b. Laparoscopy does not appear to add additional risk to the fetus greater than that experienced during open abdominal procedures.

7. **Portal hypertension,** especially when associated with varices, significantly increases the risk of hemorrhage and is best approached with traditional open surgical techniques.

G Physiologic changes associated with pneumoperitoneum

1. Carbon dioxide insufflation and absorption through the peritoneum produces **hypercarbia** and **acidosis,** although this quickly resolves postinsufflation.

2. The pneumoperitoneum produced by pressure insufflation will **decrease venous return** by compression of major retroperitoneal veins, thus decreasing cardiac output. Decreased flow rates and velocities are also seen in major veins of the legs and pelvis. This is one of the factors that may predispose patients to postoperative DVT.

3. The pneumoperitoneum also **increases systemic vascular resistance** and increases mean arterial pressure.

4. **Respiratory function is compromised** by decreased pulmonary compliance, due to the elevation of the diaphragm that occurs during pneumoperitoneum.

H Immunologic and metabolic effects of laparoscopic surgery Numerous studies in both animals and humans have shown that a laparoscopic surgical procedure results in significantly less surgical trauma and physiologic stress than an equivalent open surgical procedure. One area where these differences can be objectively measured is in the metabolic and immune response of the host. Potential advantages of laparoscopy include:

1. **Lesser catabolic response.** Lower levels of insulinlike growth factor and more modest increases in counter-regulatory hormones (cortisol, catecholamines) are seen after laparoscopic cholecystectomy than in open cholecystectomy.

2. **Attenuation of the inflammatory response.** Compared with open surgery, laparoscopy results in smaller increases in interleukin-6 (IL-6) and C-reactive protein (CRP) levels and less elevation of the erythrocyte sedimentation rate (ESR).

3. **Less cell-mediated immunosuppression** (as measured by lymphocyte proliferation) occurs after laparoscopy than after laparotomy. Total lymphocyte counts are higher and better preservation of delayed-type hypersenstivity is seen after laparoscopic procedures.

   It is hypothesized that the lesser degree of immunosuppression seen during some laparoscopic procedures may result in fewer postoperative complications and improved outcomes after cancer surgery, such as a lower incidence of local recurrence or systemic metastases. However, the effect of laparoscopy on tumor biology in humans is complex and poorly understood. In fact, some research suggests that a carbon dioxide pneumoperitoneum is potentially harmful due to local immunosuppression from impaired macrophage function in the peritoneal cavity. It is not possible to draw any definitive conclusions about the effects of laparoscopy on tumor biology in humans at the present time.

I Complications

1. **General morbidity and mortality. The overall mortality rate and incidence of major complications after laparoscopic procedures is similar to that seen with open procedures.** The types of complications are similar as well.

   a. A **wound infection rate of 0.1%–2%** is acceptable in "clean" surgical wounds and should be comparable to wound infection rate of the open technique for any specific procedure. Wound infection rates during laparoscopic intestinal surgery are higher, especially in the larger extraction incision used to remove the specimen (10%–15%).

2. **Complications specific to laparoscopy.** A few complications seen after laparoscopic procedures are due specifically to laparoscopic techniques or instrumentation and are therefore not seen during open procedures. These include:

   a. **Complications due to needle or operating port insertion:**

      (1) **Abdominal wall vessels or nerves may be injured** due to direct trocar laceration in about **1%–4%** of cases. Abdominal wall hematomas may occur as well. Avoiding placement of trocars through the rectus abdominus muscle limits these complications.

      (2) **Abdominal wall herniae** may occur through 10-mm or larger trocar sites. They usually occur at the umbilicus.

      (3) **Abdominal organ injury** may occur, especially with adhesions from previous surgery. Placement of an orogastric tube and urinary catheter prior to insufflation may decrease the risk of bladder or bowel perforation but does not eliminate the risk of this complication.

   b. **Complications due to pneumoperitoneum:**

      (1) **Pneumomediastinum, pneumothorax, or subcutaneous emphysema.** These are usually the result of excessive insufflation pressures (>20 mm Hg), though subcutaneous emphysema is common after many routine, uncomplicated laparoscopic procedures.

      (2) **Decreased cardiac output and cardiac arrhythmia** can occur due to compression of intra-abdominal venous return or acidosis from hypercarbia. In rare cases, sudden cardiovascular collapse may occur, usually in patients with prior existing cardiopulmonary disease. These complications are prevented by proper anesthetic monitoring and careful attention to end-tidal CO_2 levels.

      (3) **Postoperative shoulder pain** occurs in 10%–20% of patients. It is referred pain from the diaphragm believed to be due to either stretching of the diaphragm by the pneumoperitoneum or direct irritation of the diaphragm by CO_2. The pain resolves spontaneously and causes no long-term morbidity.

      (4) **Gas embolism** may occur due to direct placement of an insufflation needle into a vessel or carbon dioxide flow directly into an open vessel exposed in dissection. This extremely rare complication may be fatal if not recognized and promptly treated.

   c. Complications due to laparoscopic instrumentation. Examples include **thermal or mechanical injury** to underlying bowel, blood vessels, or diaphragm from the electrocautery or other thermal energy sources. Fortunately, major bowel or vascular injuries occur in <1% of cases. Mortality is 5% following inadvertent bowel injury during laparoscopy. Visceral injuries may also be caused by **excessive traction** on organs due to the loss of tactile feedback. These complications almost always require reoperation and may be life threatening if missed. Constant vigilance and a high index of suspicion are necessary to prevent and recognize them.

III LAPAROSCOPIC PROCEDURES

  A **Laparoscopic cholecystectomy**

    1. Indications include:

      a. Patients with **biliary colic** or symptomatic cholelithiasis

      b. Patients presenting with **acute cholecystitis**

      c. Patients with evidence of **biliary dyskinesia** or chronic cholecystitis with gallstones

      d. Other conditions: Very large gallstones (>3 cm), gallbladder polyps
      Note: **Asymptomatic cholelithiasis** in diabetic patients is no longer felt to be an indication for cholecystectomy. Cholecystectomy for asymptomatic gallstones in other high-risk groups (organ transplant patients, other immunosuppressed patients) is controversial.

    2. Contraindications

      a. Absolute contraindications: Suspicion of malignancy, uncontrolled coagulopathy

      b. Relative contraindications: Severe gallbladder inflammation (acute or chronic), hepatic cirrhosis, portal hypertension, biliary fistula

    3. Complications

      a. Common bile duct injuries occur four to five times more often during laparoscopic cholecystectomy than with the open technique. The incidence varies from **0.2%–1%,** with most estimates around 0.5%. Common bile duct injury is one of the most devastating consequences of laparoscopic cholecystectomy, producing duct obstruction and jaundice, cholangitis, or peritonitis. This complication requires laparotomy and major biliary reconstruction.

      b. A **bile leak** may develop from the gallbladder bed or cystic duct stump. Cystic duct stump leaks are most commonly due to a metal clip or tie coming off the duct. Leaks can be difficult to diagnose because they usually occur after discharge and have nonspecific symptoms such as fever, failure to thrive, nausea, vomiting, and abdominal pain. If suspected, the patient should undergo either an **abdominal ultrasound or computed tomography (CT) scan** to diagnose any fluid collections. If one is present, it usually can be drained percutaneously. This is typically followed by a **hydroxy iminodiacetic acid (HIDA) biliary scan and endoscopic retrograde cholangiopancreatography (ERCP)** to diagnose the level of leak or obstruction. A biliary drain (internal stent) is also placed in the bile duct to the duodenum to allow free drainage of bile. Most leaks can be controlled by a combination of percutaneous drainage and ERCP drainage. Obstructions are usually surgically repaired, though some partial obstructions can be managed by endoscopic or percutaneous balloon dilation.

      c. A **retained common bile duct stone** occurs in about 10% of patients with common bile duct stones found during cholecystectomy. Management is the same as for primary common bile duct stones.

      d. The conversion rate to open cholecystectomy ranges from 2%–10%. Factors prompting a laparotomy include any situation that hinders the accurate identification of biliary anatomy such as uncontrolled bleeding, dense adhesions, severe acute cholecystitis, or suspected common bile duct injury.

    4. Management of common bile duct stones. Several generally accepted options are used at present, depending on surgeon preference and available resources:

      a. Preoperative ERCP to clear the common bile duct of stones prior to laparoscopic cholecystectomy

      b. Laparoscopic cholecystectomy, **intraoperative cholangiography, and common bile duct exploration during the same procedure**

    c. Laparoscopic cholecystectomy followed by **postoperative ERCP** to clear the common bile duct

    d. Laparoscopic cholecystectomy followed by ERCP is most commonly performed option today. However, it is preferable to perform **laparoscopic cholecystectomy and intraoperative cholangiography with stone extraction if the surgeon is skilled in this technique.**

    e. **Cholangitis** is best treated **with endoscopic drainage with ERCP and antibiotics.** A laparoscopic cholecystectomy can be performed during the same hospitalization, after resolution of the cholangitis.

5. Controversies and conclusions

    a. Many studies have compared laparoscopic cholecystectomy with open cholecystectomy. **Laparoscopic cholecystectomy has been demonstrated to be safe and cost-effective when compared with open cholecystectomy and is the procedure of choice in most biliary tract diseases requiring cholecystectomy.**

    b. Controversies

       (1) The use of intraoperative cholangiography (IOC). IOC is indicated for two reasons: the detection of common bile duct stones and the identification of biliary anatomy. Though some surgeons practice "routine" IOC, most surgeons use IOC "selectively." Advantages of IOC include rapid recognition (and thus repair) of biliary injuries and skill development for more advanced biliary tract procedures. Disadvantages include increased operating time and expense. At the present time, there is no compelling evidence that routine IOC decreases the likelihood of common bile duct injury during laparoscopic cholecystectomy.

B Laparoscopic appendectomy

1. Indications. Laparoscopic appendectomy is technically possible in nearly all patients with suspected acute or chronic appendicitis, including many with perforation and/or abscess. However, it is most useful in the following situations:

    a. Obese patients. Avoids a large open incision and improves visualization

    b. Patients in whom the diagnosis is uncertain. Visualization of the peritoneal cavity and diagnostic accuracy is much better with laparoscopy.

    c. Females of child-bearing age. This group of patients has a 30% likelihood of having some other diagnosis when operated on for suspected acute appendicitis.

2. Relative contraindications

    a. An **appendiceal abscess** is best treated by one of two methods: either percutaneous drainage and interval appendectomy several weeks later or open appendectomy and drainage

    b. Known or suspected **appendiceal tumors**

3. Complications

    a. In general, the types of complications are no different than those seen with open appendectomy (bleeding, wound infection, intra-abdominal abscess, incisional hernia, cecal fistula or perforation)

    b. The conversion rate to the open technique ranges from 3%–10% and is usually caused by bleeding; abscess or extensive abdominal contamination; or difficulty localizing, exposing, or dissecting the appendix.

4. Controversies and conclusions

    a. At least 20 prospective, randomized trials have compared open and laparoscopic appendectomy, with several meta-analyses of these data. **Laparoscopic appendectomy is as safe and effective as open appendectomy.** However, there appear to be specific advantages and disadvantages associated with the procedure when compared with open appendectomy.

    b. Advantages. Most data show slightly shorter hospital stay, lower incidence of wound infection, more rapid resumption of diet, and less postoperative pain.

    c. Disadvantages. Nearly all data show that laparoscopic appendectomy is more expensive and takes longer to perform than open appendectomy. The risk of postoperative intra-abdominal abscess also appears to be greater after laparoscopic appendectomy.

    d. Summary. Laparoscopic appendectomy is considered the preferred approach by most surgeons in obese patients and in those in whom the diagnosis is uncertain. Laparoscopic appendectomy probably offers no benefit in males with an obvious diagnosis of acute appendicitis. It is unclear whether the recovery benefits of laparoscopic appendectomy outweigh

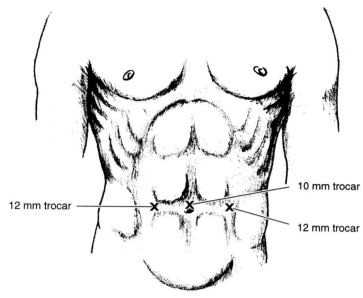

FIGURE 30-1 Trocar replacement for the laparoscopic hernia repair, rectosigmoid colectomy, and the pelvic lymphadenectomy. (Redrawn with permission from United States Surgical Corporation. Copyright 1992, United States Surgical Corporation. All rights reserved.)

the higher incidence of abscess formation associated with laparoscopy. Further randomized studies are needed to clarify the cost-effectiveness, diagnostic accuracy, and incidence of postoperative complications of the two procedures.

C **Laparoscopic inguinal-femoral hernia repair**

1. **Indications.** Patient selection for laparoscopic inguinal hernia remains controversial. Widely accepted indications for the laparoscopic approach include a **recurrent hernia** and **simultaneous repair of bilateral herniae.**

2. **Contraindications**
   a. **Absolute.** Inability to tolerate general anesthesia (open repair can be performed under local anesthesia in most cases), infarcted bowel in the hernia sac (not safe to place mesh in this circumstance)
   b. **Relative.** Prior bladder or prostate surgery, hernia repair in children

3. **Technique.** Laparoscopic hernia repair can be performed from an intraperitoneal or preperitoneal approach.
   a. The **intraperitoneal procedure** requires general anesthesia and changes an open regional operation into a major abdominal procedure. Dissection in the peritoneal cavity increases the risk of bowel injury, adhesion formation, and postoperative small bowel obstruction. **Most surgeons performing laparoscopic hernia repair use some variation of the preperitoneal procedure.**
   b. The **preperitoneal procedure** remains extraperitoneal and avoids these possible complications as well as those of insufflation and pneumoperitoneum. This procedure can be performed with spinal or epidural anesthesia in some patients, thereby avoiding the consequences of a general anesthetic. Because of its advantages, the preperitoneal approach is recommended. A 1-cm infraumbilical incision is created in the midline. The anterior rectus fascia on the side of the hernia is opened, and the rectus muscle is mobilized laterally. A balloon-dissecting trocar is introduced anterior to the posterior rectus fascia, gently advanced to the pubis in the preperitoneal space, and expanded with 700 cc of saline, opening up the preperitoneal space. A working space is maintained by insufflating carbon dioxide to 8 mm Hg pressure in the extraperitoneal space. Two additional operating ports are placed into the preperitoneal space (Fig. 30-1). The hernia sac is reduced, and the pubis, inguinal ligament, spermatic cord structures, Cooper ligament, and epigastric vessels are exposed. Polypropylene mesh is then secured with a laparoscopic hernia stapler to

the pubis, Cooper and inguinal ligaments, and the lateral abdominal wall, completing the repair.

   4. **Complications**
      a. The risk of **recurrent hernia** after laparoscopic hernia repair is **1%–5%** within the first 5 years of surgery. This is comparable to the recurrence rate after open inguinal hernia repair. Reliable long-term recurrence rates for laparoscopy are not yet known.
      b. **Genitofemoral and lateral femoral cutaneous nerve injuries** can result in significant postoperative groin and thigh pain. They are usually caused by inadvertent staple placement too close to the nerves. Knowledge of the anatomic courses of these nerves prevents staple applications in these areas.
      c. **Adhesion formation** from an intraperitoneal repair can lead to small bowel obstruction. The surgeon must be careful when placing the balloon-dissecting trocar. It can easily penetrate the peritoneum, forcing conversion to an intraperitoneal approach and thus the problems associated with that approach.
      d. **Injury to bowel, bladder, or major blood vessels.** Though rare, these injuries occur more commonly after laparoscopic than open repair.

   5. **Controversies and conclusions.** Recent large meta-analyses and randomized trials have begun to clarify the role of laparoscopic inguinal hernia repair.
      a. **Advantages.** Earlier return to normal activity, less postoperative pain and numbness
      b. **Disadvantages.** Longer operative times, higher risk of rare serious injuries (viscera and vessels)
      c. **Summary.** Laparoscopic hernia repair can be performed safely and with similar short-term recurrence rates to open hernia repair. The potential advantages of a laparoscopic approach have been offset to some extent by improvements in the open technique, including routine use of prosthetic mesh. More data is needed to determine long-term recurrence rates and cost-effectiveness of the laparoscopic approach.

D **Laparoscopic incisional hernia repair**

   1. **Indications.** Any **symptomatic** abdominal wall fascial defect, **asymptomatic defects >4 cm² in area, "Swiss-cheese" abdomen** (multiple small fascial defects)

   2. **Contraindications**
      a. **Absolute.** Loss of abdominal domain
      b. **Relative.** Incarcerated incisional hernias, patients with cirrhosis or portal hypertension, patients with a history of long-term peritoneal dialysis (they may develop a thick inflammatory peel in the abdomen). Also, hernias of the lateral abdominal wall and lumbar region are much more technically difficult than anterior abdominal wall hernias near the umbilicus.

   3. **Technique.** The abdomen is usually entered laterally, away from the umbilicus, as most incisional hernias involve the midline. Three or four operating ports are placed laterally on one or both sides of the hernia. Lysis of adhesions is usually necessary to visualize the hernia defect. **Great care must be taken during this step to avoid injury to underlying organs.** There are often additional hernia defects seen during laparoscopy that were not appreciated on physical exam. The size of the hernia defect(s) is measured, and an appropriate-sized piece of prosthetic mesh is chosen. Polytetrafluorethylene (Gore-Tex) is used most commonly. The mesh should be sufficiently large to overlap the edges of the hernia defect by 2–3 cm in all directions. The mesh is rolled and placed into the abdomen, where it is then deployed over the hernia defect and is secured using sutures, metal tacks, or both.

   4. **Complications**
      a. **Recurrent hernia.** Initial data show 5%–10% recurrence rates at 1–2 years after surgery.
      b. **Seroma.** Ten to 20% of patients develop a fluid collection between the nonporous polytetrafluorethylene and the skin. They resolve spontaneously in most cases, but aspiration is occasionally necessary.
      c. **Bowel or bladder injury** occurs in about 2% of cases. Bowel injuries that go undetected during the original surgery are often fatal.
      d. **Infection.** Wound infection occurs in about 1.5%–2% of patients. A few cases require removal of mesh.

5. **Controversies and conclusions.** Laparoscopic ventral hernia repair has been demonstrated to be a safe and effective method of repairing abdominal wall hernias. It can be performed in complex surgical patients with moderate morbidity and low short-term recurrence rates. However, data from existing studies are difficult to compare due to heterogeneous patient populations, different surgical techniques, and variable surgeon experience. More data is necessary to determine morbidity, cost-effectiveness, and long-term recurrence rates when compared with open ventral hernia repair.

E **Laparoscopic surgery of the esophagus and stomach**

1. **Laparoscopic esophageal myotomy.** Also known as laparoscopic **"Heller myotomy"**
   a. **Indications.** The primary indication is for **achalasia** of the esophagus, a motor disorder characterized by a hypertensive lower esophageal sphincter and aperistalsis of the body of the esophagus. The procedure may also be performed using a thoracoscopic approach.
   b. **Contraindications**
      (1) Other esophageal motility disorders such as **diffuse esophageal spasm** or **"vigorous" achalasia** that require a longer myotomy that must be performed through the chest.
      (2) Severe advanced achalasia with "megaesophagus" or **"sigmoid esophagus"** (this condition usually requires esophagectomy)
   c. **Technique.** A vertical cut is made through the outer longitudinal and inner circular smooth muscle layers, taking great care to avoid perforation of the esophageal mucosa. **The length of the myotomy should be at least 7 cm,** and it is important to carry the incision down **onto the stomach wall for 1–2 cm** to completely destroy the lower esophageal sphincter. A fundoplication is often performed with the myotomy because destruction of the lower esophageal sphincter results in symptomatic gastroesophageal reflux in about 20% of patients.
   d. **Complications**
      (1) **Inadequate myotomy,** resulting in persistent dysphagia after surgery
      (2) **Esophageal perforation,** which may be life threatening if not immediately recognized.
   e. **Controversies and conclusions**
      (1) **Most surgeons consider laparoscopic esophageal myotomy the procedure of choice in patients with achalasia.** Data shows that the laparoscopic approach has similar efficacy and safety to open esophageal myotomy with advantages in postoperative recovery. Other therapies such as balloon dilatation, botulinum toxin injection, and medical therapy are not effective long-term treatments in most patients. Further studies are needed to define cost-effectiveness and long-term efficacy of the procedure.
      (2) **Controversies.** The main controversy is technical—whether or not to add a fundoplication to esophageal myotomy to prevent gastroesophageal reflux after destruction of the lower esophageal sphincter. Most experienced laparoscopic surgeons add some type of fundoplication to the myotomy, as it adds no significant morbidity to the procedure. However, there is some disagreement and no true consensus regarding this step.

2. **Fundoplication for gastroesophageal reflux disease (GERD)**
   a. **Indications.** Severe gastroesophageal reflux disease, characterized by:
      (1) **Failure of medical therapy** with proton pump inhibitors
      (2) **Severe nonhealing esophagitis** despite aggressive medical therapy
      (3) **Complications of GERD.** Esophageal stricture, recurrent pneumonia or aspiration, severe asthma
         Note: Barrett's esophagus is a controversial indication for fundoplication (III E 2e 2b)
   b. **Contraindications**
      (1) **Shortened esophagus.** Severe long-standing GERD causes fibrosis and shortening of the length of the esophagus. This results in severe dysphagia or inadequate symptom relief after surgery if an esophageal-lengthing procedure is not performed. A laparoscopic approach should be undertaken with caution in patients with a hiatal hernia larger than 5 cm.
      (2) **Prior laparoscopic fundoplication** is considered a relative contraindication, though experienced laparoscopic esophageal surgeons have reported success in this group of patients.

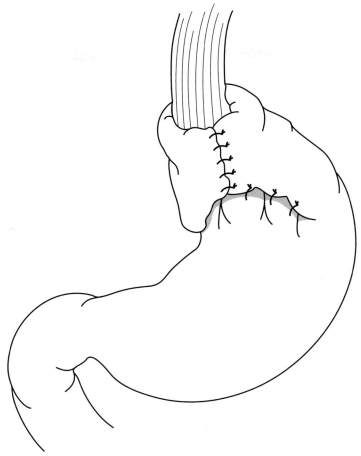

FIGURE 30-2   Completed laparoscopic Nissen fundoplication for gastroesophageal reflux disease.

   c. Technique. Numerous variations in technique exist, but two main procedures are performed in the United States. **All antireflux procedures have two common features: repair of a hiatal hernia,** when present, and **augmentation of lower esophageal sphincter pressure.**

     (1) Full (360°) fundoplication (Nissen fundoplication). The esophagus is mobilized for a distance of at least 5 cm, avoiding injury to the vagus nerve. The crura of the diaphragm are reapproximated with sutures, which repairs any present hiatal hernia. The fundus of the stomach is mobilized, with division of the short gastric vessels in most cases. The fundus of the stomach is wrapped around the esophagus and is sutured to itself. Several technical points must be adhered to so that the fundoplication is "short" and "floppy" to minimize postoperative symptoms (Fig. 30-2).

     (2) Partial 270° fundoplication (Toupet fundoplication). The procedure is similar to the 360° fundoplication with two differences: The crura are not sutured together (the posterior aspect of the fundoplication is sutured to the crura to prevent recurrent hiatal hernia), and the wrap encompasses only the posterior 270° of the esophagus, resulting in a lower pressure gradient across the gastroesophageal junction. This procedure is **used primarily in patients with poor esophageal motility** and is also frequently added to esophageal myotomy for control of postoperative gastroesophageal reflux (Fig. 30-3).

   d. Complications

     (1) Esophageal perforation ($<$1%) may occur. If unrecognized and unrepaired, this may be life threatening.

     (2) Pneumothorax or pneumomediastinum from violation of the pleura during mediastinal dissection may occur.

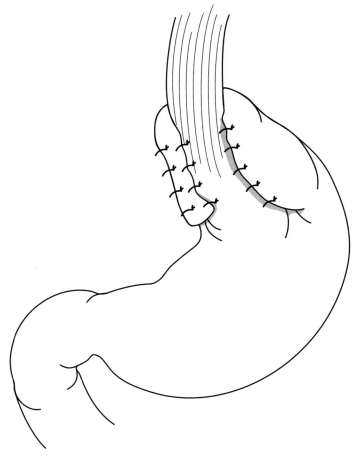

FIGURE 30-3 Completed laparoscopic Toupet fundoplication (part Nissen fundoplication).

    (3) Splenic injury may occur during mobilization of the fundus and division of the short gastric vessels.

    (4) Complications of the fundoplication fall into two general categories:

        (a) Mechanical failure. This results from either dehiscence of the suture line or, more commonly, herniation of an intact fundoplication through the diaphragm into the chest (recurrent hiatal hernia). Mechanical disruption occurs in up to 10%–20% of patients at 5 years after surgery. When it occurs, it may be totally asymptomatic, or it can result in significant dysphagia or recurrent GERD symptoms.

        (b) Fundoplication dysfunction due to improper construction. If the wrap is too long or too tight, the result is significant **dysphagia** or **inability to belch** or vomit. Vagal nerve injury may also result in poor gastric emptying. This symptom complex is known as "gas bloat syndrome" or "post-Nissen syndrome."

  e. Controversies and conclusions

    (1) Laparoscopic fundoplication is considered the procedure of choice in patients requiring surgical therapy for GERD. It provides good to excellent relief of "typical" symptoms in 85%–90% of patients. Careful patient selection and preoperative evaluation is necessary to achieve these results.

    (2) Controversies. Numerous aspects of GERD treatment and surgical therapy continue to be debated. Some of the more important controversies are:

        (a) Medical versus surgical therapy. This topic is too detailed to discuss within the parameters of this text. However, increasing clinical data suggest that surgical therapy may be preferable to long-term medication in some patient populations. More data is needed to clarify this issue, especially the long-term efficacy and cost-effectiveness of laparoscopic fundoplication.

(b) Use of **laparoscopic fundoplication in patients with Barrett's esophagus.** Until recently, the mere presence of Barrett's esophagus was not felt to be an indication for fundoplication, as earlier data showed no reliable regression of Barrett's esophagus after surgical treatment. However, newer studies clearly show arrest of progression, relief of symptoms, and regression of metaplasia in some patients with Barrett's esophagus. The treatment of this complication of GERD is complex and in evolution; the choice of surgical therapy in patients with Barrett's esophagus should be considered on a case-by-case basis.

(c) **Preoperative evaluation** of surgical candidates with GERD. "Standard" preoperative evaluation usually consists of upper endoscopy, evaluation of esophageal motility, and 24-hour pH monitoring. Some surgeons believe that 24-hour pH monitoring and esophageal motility studies are unnecessary in some or most patients. The development of newer and less invasive studies such as impedance monitoring and wireless pH probes is likely to have some impact in this area.

3. **Laparoscopic surgery for peptic ulcer disease.** All traditional surgical procedures for peptic ulcer disease are possible by using a laparoscopic approach, including parietal cell vagotomy (highly selective vagotomy), truncal vagotomy and pyloroplasty, and truncal vagotomy and antrectomy. Due to the effectiveness of medical therapy, **elective ulcer procedures are performed infrequently.** Little data exists comparing the effectiveness of laparoscopic and open ulcer surgery.

   a. **Indications**

      (1) **Intractability.** Parietal cell vagotomy is usually indicated.

      (2) **Bleeding.** Usually, the bleeding point is oversewn, and a vagotomy and pyloroplasty are performed. Combined endoscopic and laparoscopic techniques are helpful if equipment and expertise is available.

      (3) **Obstruction.** Either vagotomy or pyloroplasty or vagotomy and gastric resection have been used in the few reported laparoscopic procedures for this indication.

      (4) **Perforation.** This is the most frequent indication for laparoscopic intervention in patients with peptic ulcer disease. Irrigation of the abdomen and use of an omental patch (Graham patch) in patients with small anterior duodenal ulcer perforations and minimal contamination of the peritoneal cavity is readily performed.

   b. **Contraindications**

      (1) **Suspicion of malignancy in a gastric ulcer**

      (2) **Severe bleeding or sepsis with hemodynamic instability** should be treated with laparotomy.

      (3) **Long-standing perforation** with severe generalized peritonitis or extensive abdominal contamination

   c. **Technique.** The critical steps of all procedures are essentially identical to their open counterparts.

      (1) **Parietal cell vagotomy.** The parietal cell mass is denervated, thus selectively eliminating vagal stimulus for gastric acid secretion. The anterior vagal trunk is identified and preserved. The small branches innervating the lesser curve of the stomach are divided by using an ultrasonic scalpel or surgical clips. The distal 5 cm of the esophagus are also skeletonized. The terminal branches innervating the antrum (the "crow's foot") are preserved so that gastric emptying is normal.

      (2) **Vagotomy and pyloroplasty.** The vagotomy is performed by mobilizing the esophagus and locating the anterior and posterior trunks. Visualization is usually superior to that seen during laparotomy. The trunks are divided between surgical clips and a 1-cm segment is excised. The pyloroplasty is performed by mobilizing the duodenum (Kocher maneuver) and making a 3-cm horizontal incision centered over the pylorus but perpendicular to the muscle fibers. The incision is then closed vertically in one or two layers (Heineke-Mikulicz pyloroplasty).

      (3) **Vagotomy and antrectomy.** The vagotomy is performed as for vagotomy and pyloroplasty. The antrectomy is performed by dividing the stomach and duodenum at the appropriate landmarks by using a laparoscopic stapling device. The anastomosis (usually a Billroth II reconstruction) may be either handsewn or stapled.

    d. **Complications** are generally the same as those seen after open ulcer surgery:

       (1) **Incomplete vagotomy.** Inadequate dissection and division of vagal fibers during either parietal cell or truncal vagotomy may result in persistent hyperacidity and persistence or recurrence of peptic ulcers.

       (2) **Parietal cell vagotomy. Delayed gastric emptying** due to excessive denervation at the crow's foot or perforation of the lesser curvature of the stomach from ischemia are two unique complications of this procedure.

       (3) **Postgastrectomy syndromes.** Just as after traditional gastric surgery, laparoscopic vagotomy or ablation of the pylorus may result in postgastrectomy syndromes such as diarrhea, dumping syndrome, afferent loop syndrome, and nutritional deficiencies.

  4. **Other gastric procedures.** Essentially all traditional gastric surgical procedures have been performed by using a laparoscopic approach. Most are used infrequently, with the exception of Roux-en-Y gastric bypass for morbid obesity.

    a. **Gastrojejunostomy** may be performed for benign or malignant obstruction of the duodenum, such as for palliation of unresectable pancreatic cancer.

    b. **Insertion of gastrostomy or jejunostomy tubes** for feeding or decompression

    c. **Wedge-resection of gastric masses.** Combined endoscopic and laparoscopic approaches are being used with increasing frequency for treatment of ulcers and gastric polyps.

    d. **Major gastric resection, including esophagogastrectomy,** is performed in small numbers at some centers. Though the technical feasibility of these operations is clearly established, their utility as routine procedures is uncertain. Specifically, laparoscopic resection for potentially curable cancer of the esophagus or stomach is NOT considered the approach of choice at the present time.

F **Laparoscopic surgery for morbid obesity** The introduction of laparoscopic techniques and increasing awareness of the obesity epidemic has dramatically increased the number of surgical procedures performed for morbid obesity. Several different laparoscopic surgical procedures are currently performed, including Roux-en-Y gastric bypass, vertical banded gastroplasty, biliopancreatic diversion, and adjustable gastric banding. The majority of surgeons in the United States perform **laparoscopic Roux-en-Y gastric bypass,** though adjustable gastric banding is gaining popularity.

  1. **Indications.** It is assumed that candidates for surgery have failed vigorous attempts at nonsurgical methods of weight loss. Most surgeons follow the recommendations of a 1991 National Institutes of Health (NIH) consensus conference, which are based on both the patient's degree of obesity and comorbid conditions. Degree of obesity is measured by body mass index (**BMI**), defined as the patient's weight in kilograms divided by the square of their height in meters:

    a. **BMI >40 kg/m^2** without the presence of significant comorbidity

    b. **BMI between 35–40 kg/m^2 with the presence of certain comorbidities,** including severe cardiopulmonary problems (sleep apnea, pickwickian syndrome, obesity-related cardiomyopathy), severe diabetes mellitus, or physical problems interfering with lifestyle (severe joint disease, interference with employment)

  2. **Contraindications.** Prior to the operation, patients must clearly understand the long-term lifestyle and physiologic changes that will occur after surgery. All patients in whom open obesity surgery is appropriate are potential candidates for a laparoscopic approach, though several relative contraindications exist. They include **BMI >50** ("superobesity"), **age >60 years, severe psychiatric illness,** and **lack of motivation or understanding** to follow postoperative care programs.

  3. **Technique.** Numerous variations in technical details exist, though the basic elements of the procedures are fairly constant.

    a. **Roux-en-Y gastric bypass.** The stomach is divided by using a stapler into two portions: a very small 15- to 30-mL proximal gastric pouch that serves as the new food reservoir, and the remainder of the stomach, which is left in situ and drains into the duodenum. The proximal pouch is then connected to a Roux limb about 50–60 cm in length to re-establish gastrointestinal continuity.

    b. **Gastric banding.** A tunnel is created behind the proximal stomach. A 15-mL balloon is placed into the stomach by the anesthesiologist at the gastroesophageal junction to determine where to place the gastric band. A device consisting of a Silastic band and attached balloon (the gastric band) is placed around the outside of the stomach and is sutured in place to prevent slippage. The gastric band functionally divides the stomach into a small proximal pouch and the remainder of the stomach. The balloon is attached to a subcutaneous inflation port, which allows the size of the gastric pouch to be adjusted postoperatively.

4. **Complications.** Gastric bypass and gastric banding are very different procedures in terms of surgical trauma and physiologic changes. Gastric bypass requires division of the stomach; two surgical anastomoses; and bypass of the stomach, duodenum, and proximal small intestine. Gastric banding places a small, inert cuff around the proximal stomach without entering or bypassing any of the gastrointestinal tract. Their morbidity differs accordingly.
   a. **Roux-en-Y gastric bypass.** Anastomotic complications include **anastomotic leak** (3%–5%), **anastomotic stricture** (5%–12%), **marginal ulcer** (2%–8%), **internal hernia** causing small bowel obstruction (1%–2%). Metabolic complications include **dumping syndrome** (2%–5%), **gallstone formation,** and **vitamin and mineral deficiency** (especially iron, Vitamin B_{12}, folate, and calcium).
   b. **Gastric banding.** Most complications are **band related,** such as **erosion, stenosis,** and **slippage** of the band. They occur in about **3%–8%** of patients.

5. **Controversies and conclusions**
   a. **Surgical outcomes after gastric bypass.** There are two ways to measure the success of a surgical procedure for morbid obesity: the degree of weight loss and the resolution of comorbidities such as diabetes and sleep apnea. Typical weight loss after gastric bypass (laparoscopic or open) is 50%–70% of excess weight at 1 year and 70%–80% at 3–5 years. Sleep apnea, diabetes, hypertension, and cholesterol and lipid disorders improve or completely resolve in many patients with successful weight loss.
   b. **Conclusions. Both laparoscopic gastric bypass and gastric banding are safe and effective methods of short-term weight loss,** though long-term efficacy for both procedures cannot yet be determined.
      (1) **Laparoscopic gastric bypass appears to be a more effective weight loss procedure than laparoscopic gastric banding,** though it is associated with a higher rate of serious complications.
      (2) **Weight loss and resolution of comorbidities appears similar after open and laparoscopic gastric bypass,** though definitive conclusions cannot yet be drawn. Limited evidence suggests the following: Fewer serious complications occur after laparoscopy; operating time is longer after laparoscopy; laparoscopy results in less blood loss, fewer ICU visits, reduced length of hospital stay, and earlier return to normal activity.
      (3) The appropriate role and indications for various laparoscopic procedures remains uncertain. Most surgeons in the United States favor gastric bypass. Gastric banding has the advantage of being easily reversible and may play a role in young, elderly, and highly motivated patients and in those with lower BMIs (30–40 kg/m^2).

G **Laparoscopic colectomy**

1. **Indications.** Laparoscopic colectomy is commonly performed for most elective conditions requiring colon resection. It is not frequently used in emergency cases. The utility of laparoscopy depends on the anatomic location of the lesion, the body habitus of the patient, and the acuity of the problem.
   a. Colon polyps, including incompletely resected polyps at colonoscopy and familial polyposis
   b. Arteriovenous malformations (elective resection for bleeding)
   c. Diverticular disease (elective resection for bleeding or recurrent episodes of diverticulitis)
   d. Formation and takedown of intestinal stomas
   e. Sigmoid or cecal volvulus
   f. Repair of rectal prolapse, particularly sigmoid resection and rectopexy
   g. Crohn's disease or ulcerative colitis (particularly ileocecal and left colon resection)
   h. Elective resection of potentially curable colon cancer
   i. Palliative resection of incurable colon cancer (obstruction or bleeding in a patient with unresectable liver metastases)

2. **Contraindications**
    a. **Acute inflammatory processes.** Patients with acute diverticulitis or severe active inflammatory bowel disease are very difficult from a technical standpoint and may be more prone to complications such as ureteral injury.
    b. **Large or bulky inflammatory masses or tumors**
    c. **Rectal cancer** is considered a relative contraindication. There is insufficient data available regarding the efficacy of the laparoscopic approach for routine use in cancers below approximately 15 cm from the anal verge.
3. **Technique.** The difficulty of laparoscopic colectomy is highly dependent on the disease process, the location of the lesion, and the degree of obesity. The right colon and sigmoid colon are easiest to resect, the descending colon and rectum are intermediate in difficulty, and both flexures and the transverse colon are hardest to resect. Polyps and arteriovenous malformations are relatively easy to resect, and acute and chronic inflammatory conditions are much more difficult.
    a. **Intraoperative colonoscopy should be used liberally** to localize lesions such as polyps and to determine margins of resection.
    b. Two types of laparoscopic colectomy are currently used:
        (1) **Laparoscopic-assisted colectomy.** This is the most popular procedure. The colon is mobilized completely by using laparoscopy. Division of the colon and colon mesentery may be performed either inside the abdomen or extracorporeal, whichever is easiest. A suitable incision is then made for extraction of the specimen and performance of the anastomosis. The two ends of the colon are then anastomosed outside the body just as for open colectomy.
        (2) **Intracorporeal colectomy.** The entire procedure including mobilization, division of the colon and its mesentery, and anastomosis of the colon are performed under laparoscopic guidance. However, an incision is still necessary for specimen extraction. A good example of this procedure is sigmoid resection with transanal end-to-end anastomosis (EEA) stapled anastomosis.
        (3) **Hand-assisted laparoscopic surgery.** Colon resection is one of the more frequent indications for the use of HALS. It facilitates blunt dissection of peritoneal attachments and tactile localization of masses and inflammation. Some surgeons use HALS as an intermediate step between true laparoscopic colectomy and conversion to open colectomy.
4. **Complications**
    a. **Hemorrhage.** This complication may occur from either the mesentery or the suture or staple line. Laparotomy may be necessary for control.
    b. **Infection**
        (1) Superficial wound infection
        (2) Intra-abdominal abscess
    c. **Anastomotic leak.** Occurs in approximately 5% of cases
    d. **Postoperative small bowel obstruction.** Recent data suggest that laparoscopic colectomy results in significantly fewer episodes than open colectomy (2%–4% vs. 10%–12%)
5. **Controversies and conclusions**
    a. **Laparosopic colectomy is technically challenging** when compared with other laparoscopic procedures for a variety of reasons.
    b. **Outcomes after laparoscopic colectomy are difficult to generalize;** studies often compare several different surgical procedures performed for a variety of different indications performed in heterogeneous patient populations by surgeons with varying experience.
    c. **Advantages of laparoscopic colectomy** include **decreased hospital stay and recovery time, decreased incidence of wound complications,** and **decreased need for pain medication** and subsequent respiratory embarrassment. **Disadvantages of laparoscopic colectomy** when compared with open colectomy are **longer operative times** and relatively **high technical difficulty.**
    d. The use of laparoscopic colectomy in patients with **potentially curable colon cancer.** Recent data show that **laparoscopic colectomy and open colectomy are equivalent oncologic procedures** with similar overall survival, diseasefree survival, wound recurrence, and surgical complications. **Appropriate patient selection and surgeon experience are critical factors in**

achieving this equivalence. Oncologic equivalence between open and laparoscopic colectomy **has NOT been demonstrated for rectal cancer.**

H Diagnostic laparoscopy

1. **Indications**
   a. **Acute pelvic or lower abdominal pain.** The differentiation of acute appendicitis from other problems (e.g., pelvic inflammatory disease, ovarian torsion, or hemorrhagic cyst of ovary) is greatly facilitated by laparoscopy.
   b. **Tubal ectopic pregnancy.** Fallopian tube excision or incision with evacuation of the tubal pregnancy can be accomplished laparoscopically.
   c. **Ovarian torsion or infarction.** Laparoscopic treatment options include detorsion or resection of the ovary.
   d. **Infertility.** Laparoscopy is invaluable in establishing some causes of infertility, including adhesions, endometriosis, and tubal stricture. Adhesiolysis and endometriosis ablation are possible laparoscopic procedures. Additionally, egg harvest for in vitro fertilization is accomplished with the laparoscope.
   e. **Staging of uterine or cervical malignancy.** Intra-abdominal disease can be staged with aortic and iliac lymph node sampling.
   f. **Ovarian masses.** Laparoscopy can be used to differentiate benign from malignant ovarian lesions. Additionally, staging of ovarian malignancy with intra-abdominal washings and biopsies can be accomplished with laparotomy.
   g. **Abdominal trauma** to diagnose injuries
   h. A **suspected abdominal catastrophe** or abscess in a **critically ill ICU patient**

I Laparoscopic hysterectomy

1. **Indications**
   a. **Menorrhagia, chronic cervicitis, dysmenorrhea,** and **leiomyoma** may all be indications for a hysterectomy. In these routine cases, there is minimal advantage in a laparoscopic approach (except in cases of a large uterus or significant myomata).
   b. The presence of an **adnexal mass** associated with an indication for hysterectomy would indicate a laparoscopic evaluation and treatment.
   c. Patients **postcesarean section** or patients **with chronic pelvic inflammatory disease** are poor candidates for vaginal hysterectomy but have been successfully treated with laparoscopic hysterectomy.

2. **Contraindications.** A potentially curable malignancy is best treated with en bloc resection through a laparotomy.

J Laparoscopic staging of malignancy is being used with increasing frequency in a variety of different roles. The exact role of many of these procedures is uncertain and depends on treatment algorithms for different diseases at different institutions.

1. **"Formal" staging procedures.** These usually include exploratory laparoscopy, formal lymph node sampling or dissection, liver biopsy, and other interventions as needed for the particular disease process. Examples include gastrointestinal cancers (esophagus, lung, stomach), genitourinary cancers (testicular, bladder, prostate), lymphoma, and gynecological cancers (uterus, cervix). Results may be used to select neoadjuvant treatment prior to definitive surgery.

2. **Directed staging procedures** to assess resectability for cure, such as for pancreatic cancer. The abdomen is inspected for evidence of occult distant metastases, the presence or absence of local invasion into surrounding organs is determined, and specific lymph nodes may be sampled.

3. **Biopsy of specific abnormalities detected on imaging studies** or screening exams. Examples include evaluation of suspicious masses or areas on CT or positron emission tomography (PET) scans during follow-up for colon cancer, directed liver biopsy for any reason, and excisional biopsy of suspicious retroperitoneal lymph nodes in patients with lymphoma.

K Other laparoscopic procedures Many additional procedures are routinely performed depending on surgeon expertise and clinical volume at different institutions. Though they may be the

"procedure of choice" among some surgeons, it is difficult to make broad statements about long-term efficacy and morbidity, as many of the procedures are performed infrequently by the average general surgeon. A few notable examples follow, but the list is by no means all inclusive.

1. **Laparoscopic adrenalectomy** is regarded as the procedure of choice for most patients with benign adrenal tumors. It is contraindicated in patients with adrenocortical carcinoma and malignant pheochromocytoma.

2. **Laparoscopic splenectomy** is ideal in patients without severe splenomegaly or uncorrectable coagulopathy, such as those with well-controlled idiopathic thrombocytopenic purpura (ITP). It is more difficult in patients with splenic abscess and is relatively contraindicated in patients with malignancy, excluding staging procedures. In appropriate patients, laparoscopic splenectomy confers clear recovery advantages over open splenectomy.

3. **Laparoscopic liver resection.** All types of resection, from wedge resection to true anatomic resection, have been reported. The procedure is more popular in France and Japan than in the United States. Though technical feasibility has been established, the procedure is not widely performed at present.

4. **Laparoscopic adhesiolysis** for chronic partial bowel obstruction or chronic abdominal pain can be effective in carefully selected patients. A few relatively small series have reported 50%–75% improvement in quality of life. Long-term follow-up is not available.

5. **Laparoscopic donor nephrectomy** is considered the procedure of choice for harvest of renal allografts in appropriate patients. Allograft function from laparoscopic donors is equivalent to that of kidneys from open donors, with significant improvements in recovery time and morbidity to the kidney donor.

Study Questions for Part VII

Directions: *Each of the numbered items in this section is followed by several possible answers. Select the ONE lettered answer that is BEST in each case.*

1. In which of the following situations would the best results be obtained for an emergency department thoracotomy?

- A Cardiac arrest in a construction worker after falling from a scaffold eight stories high
- B Cardiac arrest following a motor vehicle accident with expulsion of the individual from the car
- C Cardiac arrest following a gunshot wound to the abdomen
- D External cardiac massage that has failed after more than 10 minutes in a trauma patient
- E Cardiac arrest following a stab wound to the chest

2. A trauma patient undergoes exploratory laparotomy for severe blunt injury with a positive diagnostic peritoneal lavage. After splenorrhaphy is performed for a splenic laceration, a retroperitoneal hematoma overlying the pancreas is explored. The pancreas is found to be transected overlying the vertebral bodies. What is the optimal management of this injury?

- A Sump drainage
- B Resection of the distal pancreas
- C End-to-end repair of the pancreatic duct
- D Whipple resection
- E Anastomosis of the jejunum to the severed pancreatic duct

3. A 21-year-old male is brought to the emergency room after an assualt with a baseball bat. He has suffered obvious head trauma. He opens his eyes spontaneously, does not speak but makes incomprehensible sounds, and localizes to pain. What is his Glasgow Coma Scale (GCS) score?

- A 8
- B 9
- C 10
- D 11
- E 12

QUESTIONS 4–5

A 50-year-old man is brought to the emergency department immediately after suffering full-thickness burns over the entire surface of both upper extremities and the anterior chest and abdomen. His weight is approximately 155 pounds. Initial fluid resuscitation has been started with lactated Ringer's solution.

4. The initial resuscitation rate should be approximately which of the following?

- A 300 mL/hour
- B 600 mL/hour
- C 900 mL/hour
- D 1,200 mL/hour
- E 1,500 mL/hour

The patient responds to treatment.

5. After 8 hours, the fluid rate should be changed to which of the following?

- A 300 mL/hour
- B 600 mL/hour
- C 900 mL/hour
- D 1,200 mL/hour
- E 1,500 mL/hour

6. A 22-year-old previously healthy male presents with a 2-month history of fevers, night sweats, and a 20-pound weight loss. On physical examination, he is found to have palpable cervical and inguinal lymphadenopathy. A computed tomography (CT) scan of the chest and abdomen reveals mediastinal and abdominal para-aortic enlarged lymph nodes. Excisional biopsies are performed on a cervical and inguinal lymph node. Both of these biopsies reveal lymphocyte-depleted Hodgkin's disease. What should be the next step in the management of this patient?

- [A] Radiation therapy
- [B] Surgical debulking of the enlarged lymph nodes followed by chemotherapy
- [C] Staging laparotomy to include splenectomy, liver biopsy, and biopsies of intra-abdominal lymph nodes
- [D] Systemic chemotherapy
- [E] Mediastinoscopy

7. A 55-year-old patient with alcoholism who is still actively drinking presents to the emergency department with hematemesis. The bleeding stops, and he undergoes upper endoscopy. This reveals large varices in the gastric fundus. Physical examination is notable for splenomegaly and the absence of ascites. His prothrombin time is 14 seconds, but his bilirubin and albumin are normal. An ultrasound and Doppler examination of the abdomen reveal a small nodular liver, a large spleen, calcifications throughout the pancreas, a thrombosed splenic vein, and patent superior mesenteric and portal veins with hepatopetal flow. What is the recommended treatment for this patient?

- [A] Orthotopic liver transplant
- [B] Peritoneovenous shunt
- [C] Mesocaval shunt
- [D] Distal splenorenal shunt
- [E] Splenectomy

QUESTIONS 8–9

A 65-year-old woman with no other significant past medical history presents with a large mass in the right breast. The mass measures approximately 6 cm in diameter and appears to be fixed to the chest wall. In addition, bulky adenopathy is present in the right axillary region. The patient states that the mass has been enlarging for the last several years.

8. Following mammography, what should be the next step in this patient's evaluation?

- [A] Fine-needle aspiration
- [B] Incisional or core biopsy
- [C] Excisional biopsy
- [D] Modified radical mastectomy
- [E] Radical mastectomy

The diagnosis for this patient is invasive ductal carcinoma. A mammogram reveals no other lesions in the right breast and no abnormalities in the left breast. A chest radiograph, bone scan, and liver function tests are normal.

9. What should the next step in the management of this patient involve?

- [A] Neoadjuvant chemotherapy
- [B] Radiation therapy to the breast and axilla
- [C] Radical mastectomy
- [D] Modified radical mastectomy
- [E] Simple mastectomy

10. A 47-year-old patient with a history of left-sided nephrectomy for trauma 20 years ago presents with right flank pain and hematuria. Laboratory studies reveal a creatinine of 2.5 mg/dL. Which of the following is the appropriate management plan?

 A Hydration overnight, followed by repeat evaluation of serum creatinine
 B Intravenous pyelography (IVP)
 C CT scan of abdomen and pelvis with oral and intravenous contrast
 D Ultrasonography followed by urgent cystoscopy
 E Percutaneous nephrostomy tube placement

11. Which of the following are potential sequelae of benign prostatic hyperplasia?

 A Bladder stone formation
 B Recurrent urinary tract infections secondary to prostatitis
 C Prostate cancer
 D Bladder cancer
 E Organic impotence

12. A 68-year-old man undergoes a CT scan of the abdomen as part of the evaluation for some mild abdominal tenderness after a motor vehicle collision. The scan reveals no evidence of trauma, but a 4-cm solid left renal mass is noted. There is evidence of thrombus in the inferior vena cava. Which of the following treatments is not indicated?

 A Preoperative chemotherapy and radiation to downstage tumor
 B Resection of the left adrenal gland
 C Resection of the para-aortic lymph nodes
 D Resection of the left kidney
 E Incision of vena cave and removal of thrombus

13. A 23-year-old man has a solid mass in his left testis. When it is removed, the pathology reveals an embryonal carcinoma with a teratoma. A CT scan of the chest and abdomen reveals 8 cm of lymphadenopathy in the periaortic nodes. What is the recommended treatment?

 A Modified nerve-sparing retroperitoneal lymph node dissection
 B Full bilateral retroperitoneal lymph node dissection
 C Chemotherapy with paclitaxel (Taxol), gemcitabine, and cisplatin
 D Chemotherapy with cisplatin, etoposide, and bleomycin
 E Chemotherapy plus retroperitoneal radiation

14. Which testicular cancer cell type is extremely radiosensitive?

 A Embryonal carcinoma
 B Yolk sac tumor
 C Seminoma
 D Choriocarcinoma
 E Teratocarcinoma

15. A 21-year-old male patient is brought to the emergency department for evaluation after a motor vehicle accident. As part of this secondary survey, the patient is found to have blood at the urethral meatus. What is the next maneuver?

 A Foley catheter insertion followed by cystogram
 B Urethrogram
 C IVP
 D CT scan
 E Diagnostic peritoneal lavage

16. A 24-year-old woman was admitted to the hospital complaining of dysuria and urinary frequency. She had a temperature of 101°F, pyuria, and bacteriuria. Her chest was clear and her abdomen normal on physical examination. Tenderness was noted at the costovertebral angle. With which of the following should this patient be treated?

 A Antibiotics for 1 day
 B Antibiotics for 1 week

C Antispasmodics
D Fluids and observation
E Bethanechol

17. A 47-year-old woman is undergoing a left mastectomy for a large breast cancer. Postoperative chemotherapy is planned. Which of the following is not true?

A A tissue expander can be placed at the time of the initial operation to provide reconstruction.
B A latissimus dorsi flap can provide adequate tissue for reconstruction.
C Reconstruction must be delayed until after treatment for the primary tumor is complete.
D A contralateral reduction mammoplasty can provide symmetry.
E Nipple reconstruction is typically performed as a separate procedure.

18. A 68-year-old woman has a Mohs' excision on the tip of her nose. A full-thickness skin graft with a tie-over dressing is used. On the fifth postoperative day, the dressing is removed, and the graft is pink. What is the most likely reason for this?

A Imbibition
B Inosculation
C Infection
D Fibrination
E Collagenesis

19. A 5-year-old boy sustains a laceration to the cheek. It is bleeding profusely. What is the best way to initially control the bleeding?

A Direct pressure
B Clamps
C Cautery
D Suture ligature
E Dissolving clips

20. Which of the following is the best treatment for melanoma?

A Surgical excision
B Chemotherapy
C Radiation therapy
D Immunotherapy
E Regional hyperthermic perfusion

21. A 21-year-old male suffers a severe comminuted fracture of the right lower extremity with considerable soft tissue loss after a motorcycle accident. He has exposed bone and tendon in his wound after external fixation. Which is the appropriate management?

A Split-thickness skin graft
B Full-thickness skin graft
C Allograft followed by full-thickness skin graft
D Z plasty
E Muscle flap

22. The son of a 74-year-old woman calls her primary care physician for advice. He says that his mother has been complaining of headache and vertigo for several hours and is vomiting. Apart from a deep venous thrombosis in her left leg 2 months ago, she has been healthy. They shared dinner the night before, and she had been fine. She now is asking for a prescription for the same motion sickness pills that she used to help her son when she drove him to camp. What should the physician do?

A Call in a prescription for droperidol
B Make arrangements to see the patient in clinic tomorrow
C Make arrangements to see the patient in clinic today
D Recommend that the patient be taken to the emergency department in an ambulance
E Order a ventilation/perfusion ($\dot{V}/\dot{Q}$) scan to rule out pulmonary embolism

23. Which of these statements is true?

- A Brain metastases occur more frequently than primary brain tumors.
- B The Cushing's response is the tachycardia and hypertension seen with mass lesions of the pituitary.
- C The Cushing's response is bradycardia and hypotension seen with terminal brain herniation.
- D The Cushing's response is the maintenance of cerebral perfusion pressure against variations in systemic blood pressure.
- E Primary brain tumors are more common than metastatic brain tumors.

QUESTIONS 24–25

A 38-year-old previously healthy female presents with a single partial seizure. Physical examination is unremarkable. A CT head scan shows a lesion that enhances with contrast measuring 1.5×1 cm in the tip of the right temporal lobe surrounded by a rim of local edema.

24. What is the best way to proceed?

- A Stereotactic needle biopsy
- B Open biopsy
- C Tumor resection
- D Electroencephalography (EEG)
- E Brain magnetic resonance imaging (MRI), chest radiograph

25. If this patient's lesion is resected and it turns out to be a glioblastoma, which of the following is true?

- A The patient's median expected survival is 2 years.
- B Additional surgery is not meaningful.
- C The patient's prognosis is unchanged by radiation therapy.
- D Age is an important prognostic factor for this tumor.
- E The clinical presentation of the tumor was uncommon for this patient.

26. Which of the following major joint dislocations constitutes the most dire surgical emergency?

- A Hip dislocation
- B Knee dislocation
- C Shoulder dislocation
- D Elbow dislocation
- E Subtalar dislocation

27. A 37-year-old intoxicated man is struck by the bumper of a car while he is crossing the street. He sustains a comminuted closed proximal one-third tibia and fibula fractures. The fractures are stabilized with an external fixator 1 hour after the man arrives at the trauma bay. Approximately 2 hours after surgery, he has a severe pain that is not controlled by intravenous morphine. The physical examination demonstrates 2+ dorsalis pedis and posterior tibial pulses, increased swelling of the leg, decreased sensation and paresthesias of the first web space, and exquisite pain with active and passive motion of the toes. What should be the next step in treatment?

- A Four compartment fasciotomies of the leg
- B Femoral angiography with runoff
- C Elevation of the leg above the heart
- D Continued observation
- E Repeat plain radiographs of the leg

28. Which of the following describes the most appropriate treatment regimen for a newly diagnosed primary osteogenic sarcoma of the distal femur?

- A Above-knee amputation and chemotherapy
- B Radiation therapy

> C Limb-salvage surgery with marginal excision
>
> D Neoadjuvant and adjuvant chemotherapy with surgical excision
>
> E A combination of chemotherapy and radiation therapy

29. A 2,600-g newborn without any obvious anomalies turns blue during her first feeding. An attempt at passing an oral gastric tube to decompress the stomach is unsuccessful. Which of the following statements is correct?

> A The most likely form of tracheal esophageal malformation is a blind pouch without a tracheal fistula.
>
> B No further workup for other anomalies is indicated owing to the normal appearance of the patient.
>
> C Because the orogastric tube does not pass, it should be removed to prevent gagging.
>
> D Primary repair can be undertaken if the defect is less than 2 cm in length
>
> E If the lung fields are clear to auscultation after the cyanotic episode, an immediate chest radiograph would not aid in the newborn's management.

30. Which of the following statements about laparoscopic surgery is true?

> A Due to the minimally invasive nature of laparoscopy, preoperative evaluation of patients is less critical than for laparotomy.
>
> B Routine use of orogastric tubes and urinary catheters is unnecessary during advanced laparoscopic procedures.
>
> C The abdomen is always prepared and draped for potential laparotomy.
>
> D Antithromboembolic pumps are not needed during laparoscopic procedures, as the risk of deep venous thrombosis is less than for laparotomy.
>
> E Spinal anesthesia is sufficient for most advanced laparoscopic procedures.

31. Which of the following physiologic changes occurs as a result of carbon dioxide pneumoperitoneum?

> A Decreased pulmonary compliance due to diaphragm elevation and increased abdominal pressure
>
> B Metabolic alkalosis from systemic absorption of carbon dioxide
>
> C Increased cardiac output as a result of increased venous return
>
> D Decreased systemic vascular resistance
>
> E Decreased mean arterial pressure

32. A 32-year-old woman undergoes a laparoscopic cholecystectomy for biliary colic. Forty-eight hours after the operation, she complains of fever and right upper quadrant pain. Laboratory studies reveal an elevated white blood cell count as well as an elevated total bilirubin. Which of the following is not part of the initial management?

> A CT scan of the abdomen
>
> B Hydroxy iminodiacetic acid (HIDA) biliary scan
>
> C Surgical exploration
>
> D Endoscopic retrograde cholangiopancreatography (ERCP)
>
> E Broad spectrum antibiotics

33. Which of the following is true about pediatric hernias?

> A The incidence is roughly equal in males and females, with males becoming more common as age increases.
>
> B Congenital pediatric hernias are bilateral 50% of the time.
>
> C Inguinal hernias often close spontaneously in children, and repair should be delayed until 2 years of age.
>
> D Incarcerated hernias in children should never be reduced. Emergency repair is mandatory.
>
> E Right-sided inguinal hernias are twice as common as left-sided inguinal hernias.

34. A victim of a motor vehicle accident who was thrown from the vehicle is brought to the emergency department. The patient is unconscious and hypotensive. He is found to have a dilated left pupil, decreased breath sounds over the right chest, a moderately distended abdomen, an unstable pelvis, and severe bruises over the thighs. After resuscitation with 2 L of crystalloid and 2 units of type-specific packed red blood cells, the patient remains hypotensive with a systolic blood pressure in the low 80s. What is the least likely explanation for this patient's hypotension?

- A External blood loss
- B Bleeding into the chest
- C Retroperitoneal bleeding
- D Severe closed head injury
- E Femoral fractures

35. An adult male is brought to the emergency department for evaluation and treatment following injury in a house fire. The patient was found in a closed room. He has singed facial hair and full-thickness burns over approximately 30% of his body surface area. All of the following are important in his initial stabilization and treatment *except* which?

- A Endotracheal intubation
- B Intravenous fluid resuscitation
- C Insertion of a ureteral catheter
- D Tetanus toxoid administration
- E Systemic antibiotics

36. Which of the following is not associated with an increased incidence of invasive ductal carcinoma of the breast?

- A Sclerosing adenosis
- B Lobular carcinoma in situ
- C Atypical ductal hyperplasia
- D Epithelial hyperplasia
- E Papillomatosis

37. With the increasing use of ultrasound, prenatal diagnosis of abdominal wall defects is becoming more common. You are asked to consult a family with this prenatal diagnosis. Which of the following points and discussion is not true?

- A Closure may require more than a single operation.
- B If gastroschisis is strongly suspected, amniocentesis is essential to rule out chromosomal abnormalities.
- C Total parenteral nutrition is frequently used.
- D The outcome of this category of patient is related both to the integrity of the gastrointestinal tract or to associated anomalies.
- E One of the primary goals of treatment with abdominal wall defects is to protect the exposed contents of the abdomen.

38. A patient is involved in a high-speed motor vehicle collision. The patient has a GCS score of 7 on arrival. Which of the following is not indicated?

- A Emergent intubation
- B Placement of an intraventricular catheter
- C Nasogastric tube to prevent aspiration
- D Spinal cord immobilization
- E Urgent CT scan of the brain

39. Disadvantages of laparoscopy when compared with laparotomy include all of the following *except* which?

- A Difficulty controlling severe bleeding
- B Poorer visualization of the operative field
- C Greater difficulty placing sutures
- D Loss of tactile sensation
- E Higher operating room costs

40. Laparoscopic cholecystectomy is indicated for all of the following conditions *except* which?

- [A] Biliary dyskinesia
- [B] Initial treatment in patients with severe cholangitis
- [C] Acute cholecystitis
- [D] Symptomatic cholelithiasis
- [E] Biliary pancreatitis

Directions: *The group of items in this section consists of lettered options followed by a set of numbered items. For each item, select the lettered option(s) that is(are) most closely associated with it. Each lettered option may be selected once, more than once, or not at all.*

QUESTIONS 41–44

Match the correct treatment with each inflammatory or infectious process of the breast.

- [A] Surgical drainage
- [B] Excision of sinus tract
- [C] Antibiotics
- [D] Nonsteroidal anti-inflammatory drugs (NSAIDs)

41. Mastitis

42. Abscess

43. Chronic subareolar abscess

44. Mondor's disease

QUESTIONS 45–49

For each clinical situation, match the appropriate diagnosis.

- [A] Acute tubular necrosis
- [B] Hyperacute rejection
- [C] Graft versus host disease
- [D] Acute rejection
- [E] Chronic rejection

45. Occurs when there is cross-match incompatibility

46. Usually a temporary condition or poor renal function that lasts from 1–14 days related to preservation, ischemia, and reperfusion of the transplanted kidney

47. Can usually be successfully treated with high doses of immunosuppression, such as methylprednisolone

48. More prevalent in small bowel transplantation than in other organ transplants related to the large amount of lymphoid tissue associated with the graft

49. Slow decline in renal function over months or years resulting from humoral and cellular events that are generally not treatable or reversible

QUESTIONS 50–51

For each question, match the appropriate immunosuppressive agent.

[A] Corticosteroids
[B] Tacrolimus
[C] Cyclosporine
[D] Antithymocyte globulin
[E] Mycophenolate

50. A calcineurin inhibitor that became the mainstay of immunosuppressive regimens in the 1980s and continues as the basis of many immunosuppressive regimens with toxicities that include hypertension, gingival hyperplasia, and nephrotoxicity

51. An antimetabolite used as part of triple immunosuppression therapy

QUESTIONS 52–55

Match the gastrointestinal anomaly with the listed statement.

[A] Malrotation
[B] Duodenal atresia
[C] Small bowel (jejunal and ileal) atresia
[D] Imperforate anus

52. While considering a vascular accident, there is an associated finding of cystic fibrosis in a patient with this gastrointestinal problem.

53. Although part of the VATER complex (vertebral defects, imperforate anus, tracheoesophageal fistula, and radial and renal dysplasia, it is associated more commonly with renal malformations.

54. Complete intestinal necrosis is the most feared complication.

55. There is a high association with trisomy 21.

Answers and Explanations

1. The answer is E (Chapter 21, I D 3 a [2] [a]–[c]). Emergency department thoracotomies should only be performed by trained personnel and for specific indications. The best results and the highest salvage rates have been obtained with emergency thoracotomy following cardiac arrest from penetrating injury to the chest (patient E). In general, major blunt trauma (patients A and B) and failed external cardiac massage lasting for 10 minutes (patient D) are relative contraindications. A patient whose heart stops after a gunshot wound to the abdomen (patient C) has likely exsanguinated and will not benefit from an emergency thoracotomy.

2. The answer is B (Chapter 21, I D 5 b [4] [c] [iii]). Retroperitoneal hematomas overlying the duodenum and pancreas should be explored. In this case, the pancreas has been transected overlying the vertebral bodies. The optimal treatment for this condition is distal pancreatic resection. The remaining pancreas will provide adequate exocrine and endocrine function. Direct repair of the pancreatic duct and pancreatic tissue would be extremely difficult and likely associated with a high incidence of fistula and infection. Whipple procedure involves resection of the head of the pancreas and the duodenum and is not indicated for this injury. Pancreaticojejunostomy is used for refractory pancreatic fistulas but would not be optimal treatment in this situation. Most pancreatic injuries can be handled by simple sump drainage, provided that they do not involve transection or major pancreatic ductal injury.

3. The answer is D (Chapter 21, I C). He receives 4 points for eye opening, 2 for best verbal response, and 5 for best motor response.

4–5. The answers are 4-B and 5-A (Chapter 21, II C 2 a, b; Chapter 21, II C 2 a, b). The burn involves approximately 36% of the body surface area (BSA). According to the Parkland formula, 4 mL/kg of body weight/percent BSA burned of lactated Ringer's solution should be administered during the first 24 hours. Half of this amount should be given during the first 8 hours after injury and the remainder over the next 16 hours.

6. The answer is D (Chapter 22, III G 3 a–c). This patient has Hodgkin's disease. Involvement of lymph nodes on both sides of the diaphragm with the presence of "B" symptoms (fever, night sweats, and weight loss) makes this stage IIIB. Hodgkin's disease is not a surgical disease. The surgeon's involvement is to establish a diagnosis by biopsy or, in some cases, to assist with staging of the disease. Stage IIIB Hodgkin's disease is treated by systemic chemotherapy. Radiation therapy would be used in some lower-stage lesions. Surgical debulking would not add anything to the treatment. Since the diagnosis has been established, mediastinoscopy would add nothing further in this particular patient.

7. The answer is E (Chapter 22, III B 2 a–c). The patient described has left-sided or sinistral portal hypertension secondary to splenic vein thrombosis. Pancreatitis is the most common etiology of splenic vein thrombosis. This patient is an alcoholic, and the calcifications of the pancreas are suggestive of chronic pancreatitis. The small, nodular liver seen on ultrasound is suggestive of cirrhosis, but this diagnosis would be established histologically. In any event, even if the patient has cirrhosis, he would be Child-Turcotte-Pugh (CTP) class A based on his laboratory values and the absence of encephalopathy and ascites. Orthotopic liver transplantation would not be indicated because of the patient's CTP class and his active drinking. A peritoneovenous shunt is sometimes used for the treatment of refractory ascites, which this patient does not have. The occluded splenic vein rules out a distal splenorenal shunt. A mesocaval shunt would decrease portal pressure in the right or portomesenteric aspect of the abdomen, but not on the left side because of the splenic vein thrombosis. Bleeding gastric varices secondary to splenic vein thrombosis is the one instance of portal hypertension that is cured by splenectomy.

8–9. The answers are 8-B and 9-A (Chapter 23, II F 2, 3; Chapter 23, IV F 5 a). Although fine-needle aspiration can be performed, it may not be conclusive to warrant further treatment. A core needle biopsy can easily be performed on a mass of this size. Excision is inappropriate in masses larger than 5 cm. Definitive surgical therapy should not be performed until after neoadjuvant chemotherapy is given.

10. The answer is D (Chapter 25, II D, E). An obstruction calculus in a patient with a single kidney represents an indication for emergency surgery. Hydration alone is insufficient and may lead to permanent renal impairment. Radiographic studies with intravenous contrast may cause nephrotoxicity with impaired renal function. Percutaneous nephrostomy tube placement should be reserved for cases in which cystoscopy and retrograde pyelography and stent placement fail.

11. The answer is A (Chapter 25, III B 1). Bladder stone formation due to urinary stasis is a known sequelae of benign prostatic hyperplasia (BPH), and with severe obstructive symptoms, patients can have bilateral hydroureteral nephrosis and renal failure, commonly known as obstructive azotemia. Recurrent prostatitis is caused by bacterial or nonbacterial infection of the prostate and has no correlation with BPH. Bladder and prostate cancer or organic impotence are not directly associated with BPH.

12. The answer is A (Chapter 25, IV D). Renal cell carcinoma is very chemotherapy resistant. A left radical nephrectomy includes the left kidney, adrenal gland, and investing and fascia as well as a regional lymphadenectomy. Removal of tumor thrombus from the inferior vena cava is indicated.

13. The answer is D (Chapter 25, IV E 6 a [3], b [3]). Men with metastatic nonseminomatous testicular carcinoma, and in this case with bulky retroperitoneal disease, are best treated initially with systemic chemotherapy. The agents of choice are cisplatin, etoposide, and bleomycin.

14. The answer is C (Chapter 25, IV E 5 a). Seminomas are uniquely radiosensitive among testicular tumors. Other nonseminomatous tumors, on the other hand, respond to chemotherapy and are generally radioresistant.

15. The answer is B (Chapter 25, VII D 2). The finding of blood at the urethral meatus or an elevated prostate gland suggests a urethral tear. Passage of a Foley catheter may exacerbate a urethral tear. Intravenous pyelogram (IVP) and computed tomography (CT) can detect injuries to the kidney, ureters, and bladder, but not injuries to the urethra. The patient must have a carefully performed urethrogram before any other urologic manipulation.

16. The answer is B (Chapter 25, I C; II B 4). The signs and symptoms of the patient suggest a renal infection. Simple pyelonephritis responds well to antibiotic therapy but requires more than 1 day of therapy to prevent recurrences. However, single-day therapy is adequate for bladder infections. Antispasmodics may minimize some of the symptoms of frequency, but bethanechol can be expected to increase such symptoms.

17. The answer is C (Chapter 26, I D). Breast reconstruction can be performed either at the time of mastectomy or as a delayed procedure. Timing is not dependent on adjuvant treatment.

18. The answer is B (Chapter 26, I B 3 a [2]). Skin grafts are initially held in place by fibrin bonds. Imbibition is from passive movement of nutrient to the graft from the donor tissue. When inosculation, or vascular budding, occurs, the graft turns pink from return of circulation to the graft.

19. The answer is A (Chapter 26, I F 1 a). Direct pressure is the best initial way to control bleeding. Blind clamping or ligatures should never be placed, because this may injure underlying nerves. Clamps, cautery, sutures, ligatures, and clips may be necessary, but this should only be performed under a very controlled situation, preferably in the operating room.

20. The answer is A (Chapter 26, II E 6 a). Surgical excision remains the definitive treatment for melanoma. All of the other options are adjuvant treatments.

21. The answer is E (Chapter 26, I B). Bone denuded of periosteum and tendons does not support skin grafts. These areas require muscle flaps for coverage.

22. The answer is D (Chapter 27, VII A 1 b). The patient has symptoms referable to the central nervous system. Her age makes stroke likely. Having had a recent venous thrombosis, she will likely be on anticoagulant therapy. Thus, a hemorrhage should be suspected. There is no information about motor weakness; therefore, the cerebellum is a more likely location than the cerebrum. The vertigo also implicates the cerebellum. The posterior fossa is a very tight compartment, intolerant of mass effects. Uncontrolled hypertension leads to progression of clot size and is the mechanism for rapid symptom progression and death. Even without clot growth, there is a risk for development of hydrocephalus. The patient needs to be evaluated emergently, her blood pressure normalized if elevated, and a CT scan performed to look for the suspected cerebellar hemorrhage. She will then need either surgery or observation in the intensive care unit. Pulmonary embolism is far less likely than stroke and usually presents with dyspnea. Thus, the ventilation/perfusion ($\dot{V}/\dot{Q}$) scan is not indicated. The son is not vomiting, so the food they had shared is unlikely to be causing her symptoms. Droperidol is given intravenously and would be of little use to the patient at home even if all she really needed was an antiemetic.

23. The answer is A (Chapter 27, VIII E; IV B 2). The Cushing's response is the combination of bradycardia and hypertension. Metastatic cancers greatly outnumber primary brain neoplasms. Even if only one fifth of cancers cause brain metastases, these still outnumber primary tumors.

24. The answer is E (Chapter 27, VIII E 1, 5). Late onset seizure should be considered to be caused by a brain tumor until proved otherwise. CT head scan appearance is only suggestive of etiology; it cannot be fully depended on to distinguish between primary tumors and metastases. Magnetic resonance imaging (MRI) can reveal additional small lesions often not visible on CT. Multiple lesions would suggest metastases rather than primary tumor, as primary parenchymal tumors are usually but not always solitary. A lesion found on chest radiograph suggests a brain metastases since primary brain tumors do not spread to the lungs. If MRI shows multiple lesions, the surgeon can target the safest one for biopsy. If there is only one lesion, suggesting a primary brain neoplasm, its location in the tip of the nondominant hemisphere allows for radical resection.

25. The answer is D (Chapter 27, VIII F 4). Younger patients with glioblastomas tend to survive longer than the elderly, and supratentorial location is more common than infratentorial location in adults. The median expected survival for a patient with a glioblastoma is 1 year. Aggressive cytoreductive surgery improves survival. The difficult issue is the postoperative quality of life. Survival is improved by radiation, although the time gained is weeks or months, not years. The tumor was located in the anterior temporal lobe where seizures are a common presentation.

26. The answer is B (Chapter 28, II F 3 b). Dislocation of the knee is accompanied by a 30%–33% incidence of injury to the popliteal vasculature (and nerve). A pre- and postreduction neurovascular examination is mandatory, and any suggestion of altered perfusion (ankle-brachial index (ABI) <0.9, decreased pulses, signs of ischemia) requires an evaluation of the vascular supply distal to the knee. Frank tears or intimal injuries can occur. Dislocation of the hip can lead to avascular necrosis of the femoral head, especially if reduction is delayed for longer than 12 hours; however, this injury is not limb threatening. Shoulder dislocation is associated with axillary nerve trauma and rotator cuff tears in older people. Simple (no fracture) elbow or subtalar dislocations tend to be stable following reduction.

27. The answer is A (Chapter 28, II B 4 d). Compartment syndrome is common after high-energy trauma, particularly that which has a component of crushing injury. The diagnosis is made clinically by pain out of proportion to that expected from the injury and pain with passive stretch of muscles in the involved compartment. Intracompartmental pressure monitoring can be used to confirm the diagnosis or to make it in an obtunded patient. Femoral angiography would be indicated if vascular injury were suspected. Elevation of the leg can actually exacerbate compartment syndrome by decreasing the arterial inflow pressure if elevation is excessive. Plain radiographs and continued observation are not indicated, because excessive delay in treatment can result in irreversible ischemia. Fasciotomies must be performed to relieve the compartment syndrome.

28. The answer is D (Chapter 28, IV A 2 a [3] [d] [i]–[iii]). Primary osteogenic sarcoma occurs most frequently in adolescence and young adulthood and appears most commonly about the knee (distal femur and proximal tibia). The combination of neoadjuvant (before surgery) and adjuvant chemotherapy, with surgical resection to achieve at least a wide (2-cm cuff of normal tissue) surgical margin, has increased the 5-year diseasefree survival rate to more than 60%. Radiation is not indicated when clean surgical margins are obtained.

29. The answer is D (Chapter 29, IV A, B, C, F 7). A primary repair at time of presentation can be undertaken if the defect is less than 2 cm in length. A blind proximal pouch with a distant tracheo-esophageal fistula is the most common type of malformation. There is a 40% incidence of associated anomalies in one or more other organ systems. Decompression of the proximal pouch is important to reduce aspiration. A radiograph can help to demonstrate the anatomy.

30. The answer is C (Chapter 30, II D 3 a). Since all laparoscopic procedures have the potential to be converted to laparotomy, preoperative preparation must be as thorough as for open abdominal surgery. The bladder and stomach are decompressed with a urinary catheter and an orogastric tube, respectively, to avoid injury during creation of the pneumoperitoneum. Prophylaxis against deep venous thrombosis is necessary, as risk factors for that condition are inherent in laparoscopy. General anesthesia is needed for the vast majority of advanced laparoscopic procedures; spinal anesthesia cannot achieve a high enough level without respiratory embarrassment.

31. The answer is A (Chapter 30, II G 1–4). Physiologic changes associated with carbon dioxide pneumoperitoneum are complex and interdependent, but several generalizations can be made. Pulmonary compliance is decreased from diaphragmatic elevation and increased intra-abdominal pressure. Hypercarbia causes acidosis, not alkalosis. Cardiac output is usually decreased due to decreased venous return, and blood pressure and systemic vascular resistance are increased.

32. The answer is C (Chapter 30, III A). Bile duct injuries or bile leaks after laparoscopic cholecystectomy should not initially be managed by surgical exploration. Resuscitation, antibiotics, and appropriate imaging to define the anatomy of the problem are the first steps.

33. The answer is E (Chapter 29, II A). Sixty percent of pediatric inguinal hernias are right sided, 30% are left sided, and 10%–15% are bilateral. The male:female ratio is 6:1. Inguinal hernias do not close spontaneously like umbilical hernias and should be repaired when diagnosed. Incarcerated hernias are managed with reduction followed by hydration and repair.

34. The answer is D (Chapter 21, I D 5 b [5] [a], [b], [d], [e]; I D 4 a [1] [c]). Multiple trauma patients with hypotension and hypovolemic shock are rarely, if ever, hypotensive secondary to head injury. The treating physician must look for another cause of hypotension, which is almost always blood loss. The blood loss can be from five different areas: (1) external blood loss from lacerations or an open wound (details should be obtained from the rescue workers at the scene of the accident; (2) intrathoracic blood loss; (3) intra-abdominal blood loss; (4) retroperitoneal bleeding almost always associated with pelvic fractures; and (5) bleeding into the thighs secondary to femur fractures, which can cause shock. In the patient described, the closed head injury would be the least likely mechanism for this continued hypotension.

35. The answer is E (Chapter 21, II B 1; C 1, 2 c (1), (2); E 3, 4). The patient described is at a high risk for suffering an inhalation injury. Delayed airway obstruction can develop rapidly during the first 24–48 hours after injury. It is best to perform endotracheal intubation early before respiratory problems develop, as later intubation can be difficult. Vigorous intravenous fluid resuscitation is indicated for all patients who have full-thickness burns involving more than 20% BSA. Since urine output must be followed very closely, an indwelling ureteral catheter is mandatory in the management of these patients. Tetanus toxoid with or without hyperimmune immunoglobulin should be given if the patient's tetanus immunization status is not current. Systemic antibiotics are usually not indicated in the initial management of burn patients.

36. The answer is A (Chapter 23, III B). Epithelial hyperplasia, atypical ductal hyperplasia, and papillomatosis are proliferative lesions of the breast that carry an increased risk of invasive ductal carcinoma of the breast. Papillomatosis is simply a description of the pattern the cells assume (papillary). Lobular carcinoma in situ of the breast carries an increased risk bilaterally for an invasive breast cancer, which can be ductal or lobular. Sclerosing adenosis is a proliferation of the acini that appear to invade, but it is not a malignant or premalignant lesion.

37. The answer is B (Chapter 29, III). The general category of abdominal wall defects consists of gastroschisis and omphaloceles. The primary goal of treatment is to protect the exposed or potentially exposed gastrointestinal tract. This is done either by abdominal wall closure, scarification of the omphalocele sac, or covering with Silastic or silicon material with staged reduction and closure. Although coverage is complete and the gastrointestinal tract is functional, nutrition is usually accomplished by total parenteral nutrition. The outcome for the patient is dictated by the integrity and viability of the gastrointestinal tract (gastroschisis) or associated anomalies (omphalocele). Chromosomal abnormalities may be present in patients with omphaloceles but not with gastroschisis.

38. The answer is C (Chapter 27, V C, D). An orogastric tube should be placed until a fracture of the skull base can be excluded. Nasogastric have been demonstrated to enter the skull through basilar fractures. A GCS less than 8 requires intubation and intracranial pressure monitoring. Pinal cord immobilization should be practiced for all trauma patients. A CT scan will greatly aid diagnosis.

39. The answer is B (Chapter 30, II C). It is generally agreed that improved visualization of the operative field due to magnification and improved light delivery to remote areas of the abdomen are an advantage of laparoscopy over laparotomy. Difficulty controlling severe bleeding, greater difficulty placing sutures, loss of tactile sensation, and higher operating costs are clear disadvantages of laparoscopy as compared with laparotomy.

40. The answer is B (Chapter 30, III A 1, 2). Laparoscopic cholecystectomy is indicated for most symptomatic biliary conditions, including biliary colic, acute cholecystitis, biliary dyskinesia, and biliary pancreatitis, after resolution of pancreatitis. However, initial therapy for cholangitis is hydration, broad spectrum antibiotics, and drainage of the common bile duct. Cholecystectomy is performed at a later time, after resolution of sepsis.

41–44. The answers are 41-C, 42-A, 43-B, and 44-D (Chapter 23, III A). Cellulitis of the breast (mastitis) requires treatment with antibiotics to cover staphylococcus and streptococcus infection. An acute abscess requires surgical drainage. A chronic recurrent abscess requires excision of the sinus tract to avoid recurrence. Mondor's disease is a phlebitis of the superficial veins, and although self-limited, treatment with nonsteroidal anti-inflammatory drugs can alleviate the discomfort.

45–49. The answers are 45-B, 46-A, 47-D, 48-C, and 49-E (Chapter 24, I G 1; Chapter 24, V E 1; Chapter 24, I G 2; Chapter 24, VII E 1; Chapter 24, I G 3). Hyperacute rejection occurs when the serum of the recipient has preformed antidonor antibodies. Before transplantation, the recipient's blood is examined for the presence of cytotoxic antibodies specifically directed against antigens on the donor's T lymphocytes (cross-match test). Hyperacute rejection cannot be treated but can be avoided. Kidney transplants are occasionally associated with a period of acute tubular necrosis, which is a temporary condition thought to be related to conditions that occur during obtaining and preserving the kidney. It occurs rarely in living donor transplants. High doses of immunosuppression—either methylprednisolone or antithymocyte globulin or OKT3—are used to treat acute rejection. This diagnosis is usually made via the detection and workup of graft dysfunction and may include a biopsy. Acute rejection can be treated and is reversible. Chronic rejection usually has an insidious onset and is multifactorial, involving both cell-mediated and humoral arms of the immune system. In lung transplantation, it is known histologically as bronchiolitis obliterans. Generally, there is no known effective therapy. Because the small bowel is rich in lymphoid tissue, graft versus host disease has become more prevalent in this group of recipients than in other organ transplants. This is caused by the proliferation of donor-derived immunocompetent cells with a number of clinical presentations, including skin rash.

50–51. The answers are 50-C and 51-E (Chapter 24, I H 4 a; Chapter 24, I H 6). Calcineurin inhibitors block the calcineurin-dependent pathway of helper T-cell activation and include cyclosporine and tacrolimus, which are both used in maintenance immunosuppressive regimens. Cyclosporine became the mainstay of immunosuppressive regimens in the early 1980s and is now in a new formulation known as Neoral. Associated side effects include nephrotoxicity, hypertension, tremor, and hirsutism. Tacrolimus, which was introduced more recently, is also a profound inhibitor of T-cell function, with many similar side effects as cyclosporine. Corticosteroids inhibit all leukocytes and have numerous side effects, including excessive weight gain, diabetes, and cushingoid facies. Mycophenolate is an antimetabolite that impairs lymphocyte function by blocking purine biosynthesis via inhibition of the enzyme inosine monophosphate dehydrogenase.

52–55. The answers are 52-C, 53-D, 54-A, 55-B (Chapter 29, V A 3; VI A, B 1; VII B1, 2). Gastrointestinal anomalies vary greatly. The difference between duodenal atresia and the other small bowel atresias is a developmental (duodenal) accident versus a vascular accident (jejunum and ileum). Therefore, chromosomal abnormalities (most commonly, trisomy 21) appear with duodenal problems. The exception to this general rule is the associated incidence of cystic fibrosis with small bowel atresias. Malrotation, although it causes an obstruction, may also pose a vascular problem. This is related to the midgut volvulus, which can cause total ischemia to the intestine. Renal malformations occur in 40% of the imperforate anus, either as a VACTERL (Chapter 29 IV B 2) complex or related to the disease itself (urethral fistula).

Index

NOTE: Page numbers followed by *t* indicate table; those followed by *f* indicate figure.